DATE DUE

JA 15 95			
JE 11 95			
95			
AP 98			
MY 98			
AG 98			
JY 30 98			
NO 13 98			
FE 16 99			
NO 27 01			
DE 12 01			
JE 11 03			

DEMCO 38-296

Fitness and Sports Medicine:
An Introduction

David C. Nieman, D.H.Sc., M.P.H.

Bull Publishing Company
Palo Alto, California

Bull Publishing Company
P.O. Box 208
Palo Alto, California 94302-0208
(415) 322-2855

ISBN 0-915950-91-X

Distributed in the U.S. to the trade by:
Publishers Group West
4065 Hollis Street
Emeryville, CA 94608

Library of Congress Cataloging-in-Publication Data
Nieman, David C., 1950-
    Fitness and sports medicine: an introduction/ David C. Nieman.
        p.   cm.
    Rev. ed. of: Sports medicine fitness course. 1986.
    Includes bibliographical references.
    ISBN 0-915950-91-X : $39.95
    1. Exercise—Physiological effect. 2. Physical fitness.
3. Sports medicine. I. Nieman, David C., 1950-   Sports medicine
fitness course. II. Title.
QP301.N53   1990   89-71187
613.7—dc20   CIP

Designed by: Detta Penna
Illustrations by: Wayne Harlow
Photos by: William Andress
Production Manager: Helen O'Donnell
Compositor: The Cowans
Printer: Banta Company
Text Face: Palatino
Display Face: Avant Garde

To my late father, Herbert A. Nieman,
who instilled within me his love of books and scholarship.

Overview of Contents

Detailed Table of Contents

Chapter 9   Nutrition and Physical Performance   221

Chapter 14 Additional Benefits of Physical Activity 409

Chapter 15 Precautions for Physical Activity 423

Appendixes   449

Index   571

List of Tables

Preface

Nearly four years have passed since the publication of the first edition of the *Sports Medicine Fitness Course*. During this time, much progress has been made in advancing our understanding of public policy issues in physical activity, testing and conditioning for physical fitness, and the benefits and precautions of physical activity. Every attempt has been made in the second edition (as in the first) to assist the reader who desires to participate in the American College of Sports Medicine Health/Fitness Instructor certification process. (See especially Chapter 3).

In this second edition, I have attempted to bring you up to date with the current information and facts in sports medicine. There are nearly 2,000 references from the literature in this book, with an average of more than 125 references per chapter. To aid you in understanding this information, there are 186 tables and 229 illustrations and photographs.

Two additional special features have been added to this edition to enhance its use as a textbook. These are the "Sports Medicine Insight," and the "Physical Fitness Activity." The Sports Medicine Insight precedes the end-of-chapter summary, and highlights interesting topics of special concern in sports medicine. The Physical Fitness Activity outlines practical and useful laboratory activities for students, and follows the listing of references in each chapter.

The chapters of this second edition have been reordered and reorganized in such a way that there is a more natural progression of information. The reader will find it most satisfactory to start with Chapter 1, and continue chapter by chapter to the end of the book. The book is organized into four parts. Part 1 deals with public policy issues in physical activity. Part 2 describes the various tests for each of the three major elements of physical fitness: cardiorespiratory endurance, body composition, and musculoskeletal fitness. Part 3 reviews the basics of exercise physiology, the process of writing exercise prescriptions, and the relationship between nutrition and performance. Part 4 summarizes current understanding regarding the association of physical activity and heart disease, obesity, aging, psychological health, diabetes, cancer, and other concerns. In addition, a complete review of the precautions of exercise is given in Chapter 15.

The appendix has been greatly improved. Appendix B contains 62 tables of physical fitness testing norms. Addresses of professional organizations and equipment suppliers are listed in Appendix C. A comprehensive glossary is found in Appendix F. This edition also is completely indexed.

Two ancillaries are available with this book from Bull Publishing. Nearly 150 transparency masters have been prepared and are contained in a separate syllabus. The physical fitness test norms and formulas used in this book have been beautifully organized into an outstanding computer software package. This software program allows you to input test data, print results that are classified in comparison to national norms, and monitor progress over time.

The software package was developed by Dr. Mark Brittingham. The software is available from ESHA Research (see next page).

Production of this book has involved the assistance of many people. I want to thank my wife, Cathy, who has graciously supported me throughout all phases of this endeavor. I also thank David Bull of Bull Publishing for his vision and prowess in editing, and my secretary, Rebecca Buchanan, whose administrative skills have multiplied my productivity.

The Fitness Pro!
A Special Software Program

designed for

Fitness and Sports Medicine:
An Introduction

The Fitness Pro! software provides ACSM Medical Status, several Risks Analyses, and fast, accurate calculations of the physical fitness test norms and formulas used in this book.

The program enables the reader to input test data, calculate fitness tests, compare to national norms, and monitor progress. Results are quickly calculated and can be printed for permanent records.

Functions include: ACSM Medical Status, Cardiac and Stroke Risk Analysis, Body Fat Percentage (5 methods), $\dot{V}O_{2max}$ (12 methods), Strength and Flexibility (YMCA and more); Blood Pressure, Body Circumference, Goals and Lifestyle section to develop calories expended; and Exercise Prescription.

The Fitness Pro! was developed by Mark Brittingham, PhD, and is available directly from ESHA Research, Salem, Oregon. Designed for IBM and compatibles—650K and 1.3 Mg hard drive needed.

To order, or for more information, call or write:

ESHA Research—Nutrition and Health Systems
P.O. Box 13028
Salem, OR 97309

Phone: 503-585-6242   FAX: 503-585-5543

Part 1

Trends/Definitions

Chapter 1

Exercise in America

"The increasing costs associated with health care will compel public policy to emphasize measures such as physical fitness to enhance health."—U.S. Public Health Service, 1980

Health Objectives for the Nation

The focus of public health has changed in recent years. From an emphasis on mainly trying to reduce sickness and death, attention has turned more and more to *health promotion*.[1]

America began to get serious about health promotion during the 1970s. Health promotion is defined as the science and art of helping people change their lifestyle to move toward a state of optimal health.[2] This modern emphasis on health promotion is inspired in part by the World Health Organization's definition of *Health*: "Health is physical, mental, and social well-being, not merely the absence of disease and infirmity."

In 1979, the Surgeon General issued a Report on Health Promotion and Disease Prevention, *Healthy People*.[3] Noting that the Nation's first public health revolution against infectious diseases had been very successful, a challenge was issued to begin encouraging a second public health revolution—this time against *chronic diseases*, or lifestyle-related diseases such as heart disease, cancer, and stroke, which together with accidents account for 75 percent of all deaths in America.

With the release of the Surgeon General's Report, the Public Health Service launched an unprecedented, decade-long initiative, calling on professionals and lay people alike to take steps to reduce preventable death and disease, and setting a target date of 1990.

Following up on the Surgeon General's report, *Promoting Health/Preventing Disease: Objectives for the Nation* was published in 1980.[4] It set out 226 health objectives for 1990, emphasizing 15 areas of particular importance. In response to the growing body of evidence that regular physical activity produces significant benefits, both physically and mentally, "Physical Fitness and Exercise" was specified as one of those 15 areas.[4]

In 1991, a new document was published, *Healthy People 2000: National Health Promotion and Disease Prevention Objectives*, outlining an agenda for action, providing a strategy for improving the health of the nation.[5]

Physical Fitness and Exercise Objectives for the Year 2000

In response to the growing body of evidence that regular physical activity produces significant benefits, both physically and mentally, the Public Health Service specified 12 objectives to increase physical activity and fit-

---

Table 1.1 Year 2000 Objectives to Increase Physical Activity and Fitness

Year 2000 Goals (selected)	Best Estimate of Current Status
Risk Reduction	
Increase to at least 30% the proportion of people aged 6 and older who engage regularly, preferably daily, in light to moderate physical activity (less than 50% $\dot{V}O_{2max}$) for at least 30 minutes per day.	22% (5 times/week) 12% (7 times/week)
Increase to at least 20% the proportion of people aged 18 and older and to at least 75% the proportion of children and adolescents aged 6 through 17 who engage in vigorous physical activity (greater than 50% $\dot{V}O_{2max}$) that promotes the development and maintenance of cardiorespiratory fitness 3 or more days per week for 20 or more minutes per occasion.	12% (age ≥18 yrs) 66% (ages 10–17)
Reduce to no more than 15% the proportion of people aged 6 and older who engage in no leisure-time physical activity.	24% (of adults)
Increase to at least 40% the proportion of people aged 6 and older who regularly perform physical activities that enhance and maintain muscular strength, muscular endurance, and flexibility.	No baseline data
Services and Protection	
Increase to at least 50% the proportion of children and adolescents in 1st through 12th grade who participate in daily school physical education.	36%
Increase to at least 50% the proportion of school physical education class time that students spend being physically active, preferably engaged in lifetime physical activities.	27%
Increase the proportion of worksites offering employer-sponsored physical activity and fitness programs as follows:	
• 50–99 employees: 20%	14%
• 100–249 employees: 35%	23%
• 250–749 employees: 50%	32%
• 750 employees: 80%	54%
Increase community availability and accessibility of physical activity and fitness facilities.	

Source: U.S. Department of Health and Human Services, Public Health Service. Healthy People 2000: National Health Promotion and Disease Prevention Objectives (1991). DHHS Publication No. (PHS) 91-50212. Government Printing Office, Washington, DC 20402-9325.

---

ness in Americans by the year 2000.[5] Table 1.1 summarizes seven of the objectives.

Components of Public Policy

Accomplishing the physical fitness and exercise objectives for the year 2000 will entail a coordinated effort by educational systems, mass media, local, state, and federal governments, health care providers, private industry, volunteer organizations, and the American public. Formation of public policy to reach these objectives involves four basic considerations:[8, 9]

1. The severity of the problem
2. The certainty with which we know the causes and solutions
3. The cost of the solutions
4. The methods of implementation

The Severity of the Problem

The country faces two related problems—(1) the problem of chronic disease; and (2) the problem of inactivity.

The Problem of Chronic Disease in the United States

The severity of the chronic disease problem is appalling. As Figure 1.1 demonstrates, since 1900 there has been a dramatic shift in cause of death away from infectious disease to chronic disease. Diseases of the heart, cancer, and stroke accounted for only 22 percent of all deaths in 1900. By 1985, they accounted for 64 percent.

The facts and figures for the major chronic diseases will be reviewed in Part 4. While progress is being made with several of these diseases, much work remains to be done. (See Sports Medicine Insight 1.1.) The important role of exercise for each of these diseases will also be discussed in Part 4.

The Problem of Inactivity in this Country

A Brief Historical Review

Early Concepts of Exercise During the late 1800s, as America experienced increasing urbanization and industrialization, the health of Americans became a growing concern to many leaders.[11] Social reformers such as Dr. Oliver Wendell Holmes, Catharine Beecher, and Dr. Dioclesian Lewis were leaders in encouraging Americans to exercise more.

In the schools, several progressive colleges hired medical doctors to teach students health, light gymnastics with dumbbells, European gymnastics, and anthropometric measurements. Most of the programs were based upon German and Swedish gymnastic programs, which consisted of marching, free exercises with rings and clubs, and apparatus work on balance board, rings, and vaulting box.[12]

The emphasis of these programs was on the health-related value of proper physical exercise. Muscle strength and size were seen as most important. Sports and play and cardiorespiratory exercise were not generally included.[13]

Around the turn of the century, however, public interest and participation in sports grew strongly.[14] This was mirrored in the schools as leadership shifted from medical doctors to "physical educators" who promoted sports and games as the best way to develop intellectual awareness and moral and social behavior, along with physical fitness.[15] The promotion of exercise for physical fitness, however, became secondary to the development of game and sport skills (motor fitness), and the attainment of psychosocial goals.[16]

This was the beginning of a furious debate that has continued to this day—should physical education emphasize health-related physical activities (exercises that develop the heart, lungs, and musculoskeletal system), or should it emphasize motor-fitness-related activities (exercises that develop coordination, balance, agility, speed, and power)?[17] (See the discussion of terms in Chapter 2.)

Several major events of the 1940s and 1950s prompted Americans to take a closer look at both school physical education programs and adult fitness.

The Fitness Awakening Statistics on draftees during World War II spurred the media to report that school sports programs were not adequately developing students' physical fitness. Out of nine million registrants examined for the armed services in early 1943, almost three million were rejected for physical or mental reasons.[12] The chief of Athletics and Recreation for the Army responded by recommending at the 1943 War Fitness Conference that "physical education through play must be discarded and a more rugged program substituted."[12]

After World War II, heart disease reached epidemic proportions.[18] Obesity became a major public health problem, and health care costs skyrocketed.[10] In the midst of these health problems, however, the public was still focusing on such men as Charles Atlas and Jack La Lanne, who emphasized muscular strength and muscle size.

The first evidence of national fitness awareness concerned the young. The shocking results of the Kraus-Weber tests of minimum muscular fitness of school children were released in 1953.[19] The tests consisted of six simple movements of key muscle groups. Of U.S. children 59% failed, while only 8.7 percent of European children failed.[20] When President Eisenhower learned of this study, he immediately called for a special White House Conference, which was finally held in June, 1956. As a result, the President's Council on Youth Fitness and a President's Citizens Advisory Committee on the Fitness of American Youth were formed.

A surge in public concern about adult fitness took place in the late 1960s. In 1967, Oregon track coach Bill Bowerman toured New Zealand and discovered "jogging." He returned to America and wrote, *Jogging*,[21] igniting the first running boom in the United States, with the book selling over 300,000 copies.

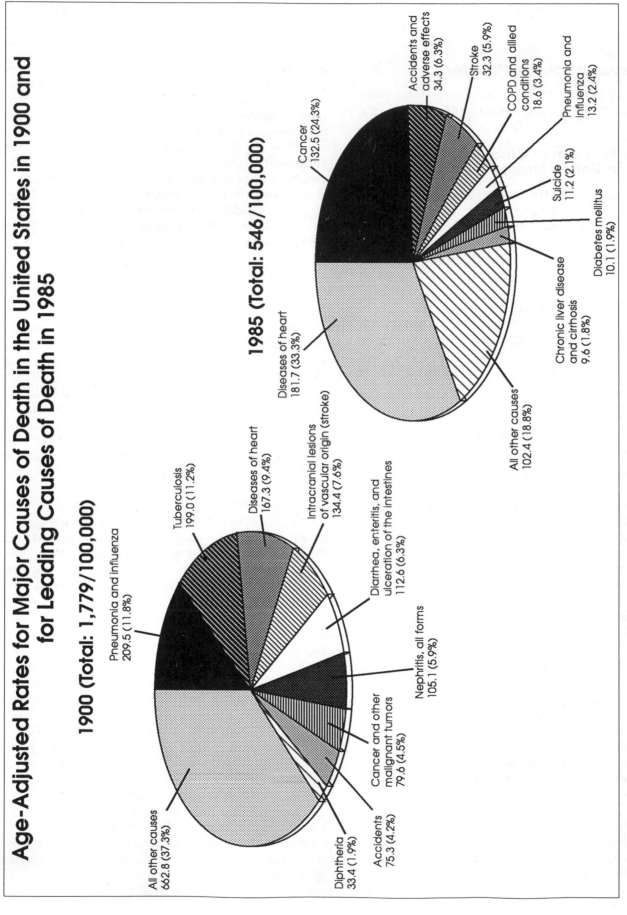

Age-Adjusted Rates for Major Causes of Death in the United States in 1900 and for Leading Causes of Death in 1985

1900 (Total: 1,779/100,000)

Pneumonia and influenza
209.5 (11.8%)

Tuberculosis
199.0 (11.2%)

Diseases of heart
167.3 (9.4%)

Intracranial lesions
of vascular origin (stroke)
134.4 (7.6%)

Diarrhea, enteritis, and
ulceration of the intestines
112.6 (6.3%)

Nephritis, all forms
105.1 (5.9%)

Cancer and other
malignant tumors
79.6 (4.5%)

Accidents
75.3 (4.2%)

Diphtheria
33.4 (1.9%)

All other causes
662.8 (37.3%)

1985 (Total: 546/100,000)

Cancer
132.5 (24.3%)

Accidents and
adverse effects
34.3 (6.3%)

Stroke
32.3 (5.9%)

COPD and allied
conditions
18.6 (3.4%)

Pneumonia and
influenza
13.2 (2.4%)

Suicide
11.2 (2.1%)

Diabetes mellitus
10.1 (1.9%)

Chronic liver disease
and cirrhosis
9.6 (1.8%)

All other causes
102.4 (18.8%)

Diseases of heart
181.7 (33.3%)

Figure 1.1 A dramatic shift in cause of death away from infectious disease to chronic disease took place between 1900 and 1985. *Source:* U.S. Department of Health and Human Services. Prevention '86/'87: Federal Programs and Progress. U.S. Government Printing Office: Washington, D.C., 1987.

In 1968, Dr. Kenneth H. Cooper, a medical doctor for the Air Force, published his book, *Aerobics*[22] followed two years later by *The New Aerobics*.[23] In these books, Cooper challenged Americans to take personal charge of their lifestyles, and to counter the epidemics of heart disease, obesity, and rising health care costs by engaging in regular exercise. Cooper emphasized, however, that the best exercise for stimulating the heart, lungs, and blood vessels is *aerobic*:

> *"I'll state my position early. The best exercises are running, swimming, cycling, walking, stationary running, handball, basketball, and squash, and in just about that order . . . Isometrics (static muscle contractions against immovable objects), weight lifting and calisthenics, though good as far as they go, don't even make the list, despite the fact that most exercise books are based on one of these three, especially calisthenics.[21]"*

These two books provided the necessary theoretical fuel for an adult fitness revolution that soon gripped the country. Millions took up the "aerobic challenge" and began jogging, cycling, walking, and swimming programs.[24] Ken Cooper's wife, Mildred Cooper, joined her husband in 1972, writing *Aerobics for Women*.[25] Within nine years, these three books on aerobics sold over 6 million copies and were translated into 15 foreign languages, and into braille.[24]

In 1972, Frank Shorter won the Olympic marathon gold medal in Munich. The extensive television coverage of both this marathon, and later of Shorter's silver medal effort in 1976 (Montreal), helped to spawn the road racing movement that has since become so popular.[26] (See Figure 1.2.)

Running, which quickly became a symbol of the American exercise movement, was promoted by a spate of successful books by Henderson,[27] Ullyot,[28] Sheehan,[29] and others, climaxed by *The Complete Book of Running* by Jim Fixx.[30] Fixx's book topped the bestseller lists for nearly two years, second in history only to *Games People Play*.[31] In the space of one year, 1977 to 1978, the magazine *Runner's World* tripled its circulation from 85,000 to 270,000.[32]

A Summary of the Surveys

Many surveys have been conducted to evaluate the magnitude of the present fitness revolution in the United States. Unfortunately, there has been little design consistency among these surveys;[33,34] nevertheless, some generalizations can be drawn from the most reliable and relevant of the sources available.[5, 6, 7, 33–38]

1. As was stated earlier, *only 11 percent of the adult population* exercises with the intensity, duration, and frequency generally recommended for cardiovascular benefit.[6] (See also Chapter 8.) If intensity is ignored, 28 percent of all American adults are considered very physically active.[38] Forty percent of American adults report that they exercise or play sports regularly, but more than a third of these exercise less frequently and intensely than is recommended for heart and lung fitness (though some health benefits are probably gained). Approximately 27 percent of the population is considered completely sedentary, and 33 percent irregularly active.[5, 38]

2. *Those in the upper socio-economic status (SES) group* (based on income, education, and occupation), are more physically active than those of lower SES. Managers and professionals are more

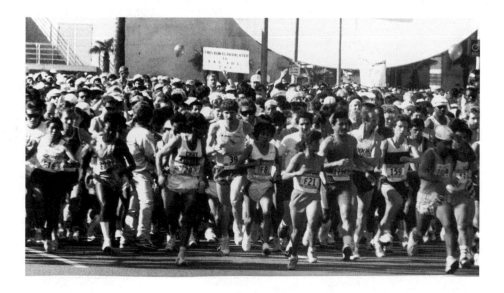

Figure 1.2 Running has become a symbol of the modern fitness revolution.

active in their leisure time than other white-collar workers, who in turn exercise more frequently than blue-collar workers.

Figures 1.3 and 1.4 show the relationship between amount of education and income and the percent of U.S. adults who exercise appropriately.

Interestingly, there appears to have been a narrowing of the education gap (for both men and women) between 1971–5 and 1983. During that period the difference between college graduates and those without a college degree diminished (when asked whether they engaged in "much exercise").[34]

Figure 1.3 Among adults, higher levels of education are associated with more exercise.[38]

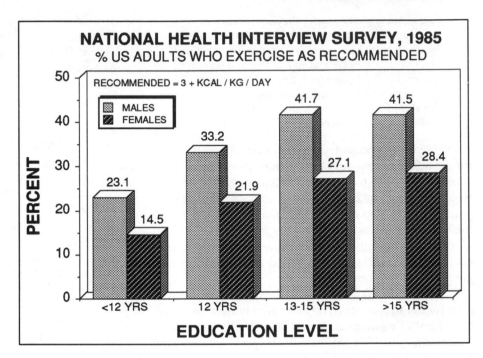

Figure 1.4 Among adults, higher levels of family income tend to be associated with more exercise.[38]

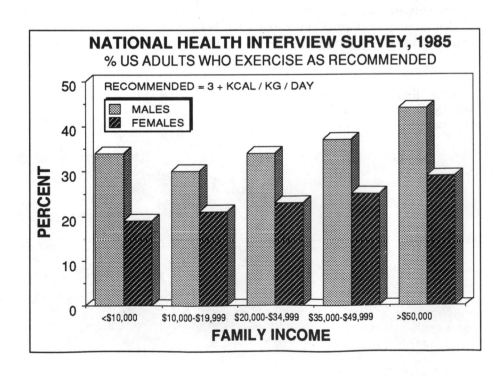

3. *With increasing age,* people become less physically active, though this is not considered an inevitable result of aging. In 1985, 49 percent of young male adults (18–29 years) and 30 percent of young female adults reported exercising appropriately, whereas only 24 percent of elderly males and 12 percent of elderly females reported appropriate levels of physical activity.[34, 38] (See Figure 1.5.)

4. *Five forms of exercise are consistently most popular:* walking for exercise, swimming, calisthenics, bicycling, and jogging-running. Jogging-running and calisthenics have grown the most in popularity since the 1970s. All of these activities have several important features in common: they are aerobic, inexpensive, do not require co-ordination with others for participation, can be done close to home, and are typically flexible in their scheduling. Presumably, popular activities in the future will have these features as well.

In the 1986 National Sporting Goods Association survey of exercise participation,[39] a participant was defined as someone seven years of age or older who took part in the activity at least six times during that year. Swimming was the most popular activity, with 72.6 million participants, exercise walking was second, with 53.5 million participants, and bicycling third, with 49.7 million. Exercising with equipment (use of any type of exercise equipment, such as weights, stationary bikes, and rowing machines) drew the most new participants for the third consecutive year—6.9 million, followed closely by exercise walking, with 6.8 million new participants.

5. *Males and females* differ in their exercising, with males exercising more than females. In 1985, 34 percent of males exercised appropriately, compared to only 22 percent of females.[38] Although both genders tend to be equally likely to participate in conditioning activities (such as walking, bicycling, and calisthenics), males are more likely to be involved in sports, intense activities, or activities performed more frequently.

6. *The proportion of the population that is physically active* during its leisure time clearly has increased substantially in recent years. However, there are no reliable statistics to gauge trends in activity—in part, at least, because no satisfactory definition of physical activity has ever been used even twice in comparable studies.[34]

Studies have variously shown that at any given age, the prevalence of activity increased from 1978 to 1982, and again from 1982 to 1985, and that between 1971 and 1985 there was a steady decline from 41 percent to 27 percent among adults classified as completely sedentary.

Five Gallup Polls (1961, 1977, 1980, 1982, 1984) have used the question "Aside from work

Figure 1.5 With increasing age, a decreasing proportion of both U.S. males and females are classified as physically active.[38]

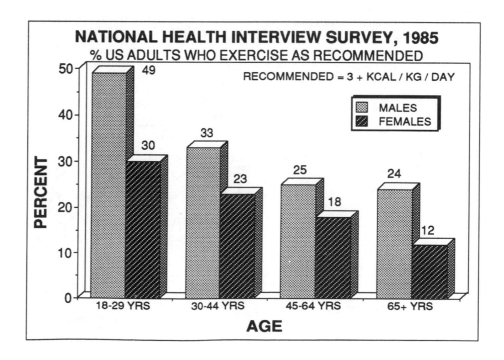

NATIONAL HEALTH INTERVIEW SURVEY, 1985
% US ADULTS WHO EXERCISE AS RECOMMENDED
RECOMMENDED = 3 + KCAL / KG / DAY

you do at home or at a job, do you do anything regularly, that is, on a daily basis, that helps keep you physically fit?" Positive responses have increased from 24 percent to 59 percent during the polling period. (Results may reflect changes in perception as much as changes in practices.) The 1981 Canada Fitness Survey revealed pronounced increases in sports participation when compared to a 1976 survey.[34] Similarly, recent years have seen considerable growth in sales of sports equipment and supplies, circulation of sports and fitness magazines, medical articles on fitness and sports, and membership in the American College of Sports Medicine.

7. *For some activities, rates of increase are slowing.* Rates of participation rose dramatically from 1975 to 1984, and then dropped slightly in 1985. The marathon appears to have been losing popularity since 1983, while interest in 10 kilometer events has risen. The rate of increase of participation in the running movement was most pronounced in the 70s, and appears to be slowing in the mid-80s.[34]

8. *Regionally, people in the northeast and the south* are less physically active, people in the west most active.[38] (See Figure 1.6.) In California, for example, a survey in 1983 showed that 59 percent of adults participated in active physical

sports at least once a week[40]—of those over 60, the percentage was an amazing 50 percent.

9. *There is little difference among races* in terms of activity during leisure time (when age and socio-economic status are held constant).

10. *Since 1976, women and older people have increased their* leisure-time physical activities to a greater extent than the population in general.[34, 41]

11. *About 40 percent of the U.S. population have jobs* that require at least a moderate amount of physical work.[38] Among men under 45 years of age, about two thirds of those with 12 years of education or less have physically demanding jobs, in contrast with about one-fifth of college graduates.

Youth Fitness Studies

Baseline data on the health-related fitness level of school-aged children were made available in 1984 with the release of the First National Children and Youth Fitness Study (NCYFS I),[41] in 1985 with The President's Council on Physical Fitness and Sports School Population Fitness Survey,[43] and in 1987 with the Second National Children and Youth Fitness Study (NCYFS II).[44-47] Results from these three surveys have caused much public concern about the fitness of American youth. (See Figure 1.7.)

Figure 1.6 Regionally, the Northeast and the South have the lowest proportion of physically active residents; the West has the highest proportion.[38]

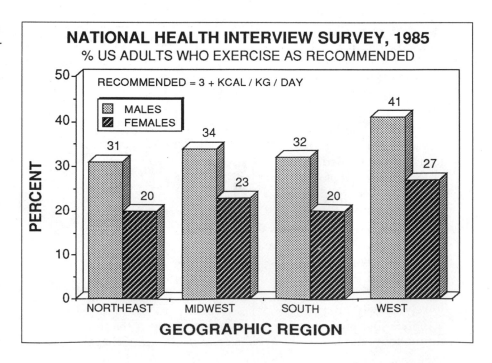

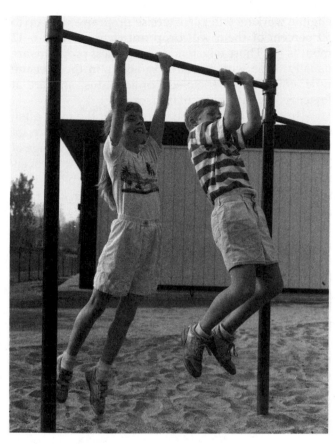

Figure 1.7 National surveys on the fitness status of American children and youth have aroused much public concern.

Important findings from these three surveys include the following:[42-47]

- **Body fat higher:** The NCYFS showed that American young people have become fatter since the 1960s.

- **Daily P.E. taken by minority of students:** Virtually all (97%) of first through fourth graders were found to be enrolled in P.E. programs. However, only 36.3 percent of students in grades 5–12 take P.E. daily. For grades 11 and 12, less than 50 percent of students have any P.E. at all.

- **Present P.E. programs have wrong emphasis:** P.E. programs do not emphasize activities which teach the physical skills needed for active lifestyles that promote health and physical fitness. For older students especially, physical educators continue to rely heavily on competitive sports and other activities that students cannot readily continue throughout adulthood.

- **Cardiovascular exercise appropriate in only 50 percent:** Half of American children and youth are not getting enough exercise to develop healthy cardiorespiratory systems.

- **Activity outside of P.E. is greater:** The typical student reports getting over 80 percent of his/her physical activity outside of P.E. class. Activity peaks in the summer. Year round, the average student spends 760 minutes per week in sports, games, and exercises. The majority of youth participate in physical activity through community organizations.

- **Students scoring higher are more active:** For students with higher fitness scores (in the one-mile run, skinfold tests, and musculoskeletal tests), greater activity was reported during non-summer months. In addition, such students were more likely to be enrolled in P.E. classes that emphasized a wide variety of activities. Greater participation in community organizations was also reported.

- **Upper body strength poor for many:** For girls ages 9 to 17, 55 percent could not perform more than one pull-up. For boys ages 6 to 12, 40 percent could not do more than one pull-up; 25 percent could not do any. Girls did not improve with age in dynamic upper arm strength. Boys steadily improved in this area, from ages 12 to 17.

- **Flexibility better among girls than boys:** Girls scored significantly better in flexibility than boys, and increased sharply from age 7 to 16. Forty percent of boys ages 6 to 15 could not reach beyond their toes.

- **Endurance low:** Approximately 50 percent of girls ages 6 to 17 and 60 percent of boys ages 6 to 12 could not run a mile in less than 10 minutes.

- **No improvement since 1965:** A comparison of the 1985 test results with those from 1958, 1965, and 1975 show little overall change.

The information from these three surveys suggests that current physical education programs may be inadequate to promote lifetime physical fitness. These results and others are causing physical educators to realize that curriculum changes are needed.[46, 49-52]

How Well Do We Know the Causes and the Solutions?

There are multiple causes of heart disease, hypertension, obesity, cancer, diabetes, osteoporosis, and other chronic diseases, but inactivity is involved in each, either directly or indirectly.[53, 54] (See Part 4 of this book, exploring the role of exercise in both the treatment and prevention of chronic disease.)

We still have much to learn about the relationship between physical activity and health. Some have questioned whether there is sufficient evidence to support a major drive to promote exercise and physical fitness as part of a comprehensive health promotion/disease prevention strategy. Obviously, the Public Health Service has concluded that there is enough evidence. While this evidence needs further documentation and analysis, and there is much more to learn, this is not reason to withhold public action.[55]

The relationships between physical activity, physical fitness, demographic and cultural status, health, and disease are complex, but this should not deter investigators (see Figure 1.8).[9] Research must continue to untangle this web so that more meaningful instruction can be given to Americans.

One of the greatest challenges for the future is to devise methods of encouraging sedentary and irregularly active Americans (60 percent of all adults) to become more active. Statistics are quite dismal. At the worksite, considered one of the most promising places for adults to obtain regular exercise, only 20 percent of

eligible workers will join exercise programs, and up to 50 percent of them will drop out over the first 6–12 months.[56-58] Those who tend to join fitness programs are usually those who are already active in their leisure time, enjoy upper socio-economic status, and are at lower risk of cardiovascular disease.[57]

In other words, those who need it the most often don't sign up for fitness programs. Furthermore, of those who do sign up, within six months an average of 30–70 percent will drop out. Dropouts tend to be overweight, low in self-motivation, and blue collar. They complain of program inconvenience and lack of time, and lack of spousal support.

Even in well-structured programs for cardiac patients, 30–70 percent of them will drop out, the majority within the first 3 months.[59] Continued deterioration in exercise participation continues, leveling off at 50–70 percent attrition at 12–24 months. This is remarkable in light of the benefits of exercise, especially for these patients who stand to benefit the most.

National goals call for regular participation in aerobic exercise by 90 percent of youth and 50 percent of adults by year 2000.[5] Much work needs to be done in creating an environment that will help build motivation for regular exercise. See Chapter 8, where factors asso-

Figure 1.8 Relationships between physical activity, physical fitness, health benefits, and sociodemographic variables. (Adapted from: Powell KE, Paffenbarger RS. Workshop on Epidemiologic and Public Health Aspects of Physical Activity and Exercise: A Summary. *Public Health Rep* 100:118–126, 1985).

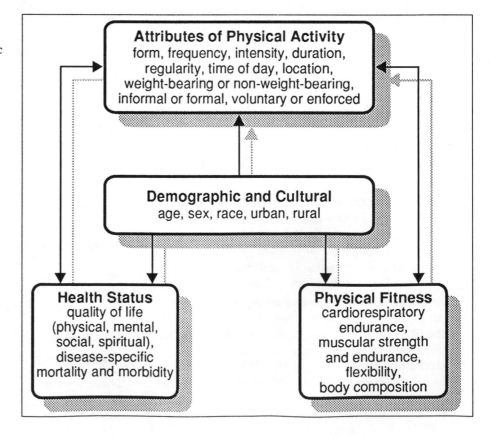

ciated with compliance and noncompliance are reviewed.

The Cost of the Solution

Measures to build participation in physical activity involve economic costs, and they involve potential risks of injury (musculoskeletal, cardiovascular, psychological, etc.).[60] The potential risks will be discussed in Chapter 15. They are numerous, but with gradual implementation and careful education, they can be greatly reduced.

The Economic Costs

Figure 1.9 portrays the mounting costs of health care. Total medical expenditures in the United States during 1929 were only $3.6 billion, or 3.5 percent of the Gross National Product (GNP).[61] By 1960, national health expenditures totaled $26.9 billion, 5.2 percent of the GNP. In 1985, $442.6 billion was spent on health care, 10.6 percent of the GNP. Annual health expenditures are expected to be considerably over $400 billion during the rest of the 1980s and on into the 1990s.[62]

One fourth of this medical bill is picked up by business through health insurance premiums.[62] Federal, state, and local governments pay most of the rest of the medical bill, which is indirectly passed on to each American. Illness and accident related costs, including health, disability, and life insurance, workers compensation, and sick leave, now constitute roughly 10 percent of payroll costs.[63]

Financial Incentives for Health Promotion

Several forces are leading hospitals, businesses, and health-fitness centers to reevaluate the balance between health care and health promotion.[64] The diagnosis-related-groups (DRG) system has now been imposed upon hospitals by Medicare administrators, leading to a stricter payment structure. The National Center for Health Statistics has reported that the average length of stay for hospital patients decreased from 7.8 days in 1965 to 6.6 days in 1984. Hospital admissions fell 2.4 percent in 1984. The public is looking more to self-care, as the fitness-health revolution continues to gain support from both the federal government and the media. These forces are creating more of an interest in health promotion on the part of both hospitals and physicians.[64, 65]

The last 10 years has brought major changes in employer attitudes toward workplace health promotion programs.[66] Interest in worksite health programs has increased as growth in health care costs have cut into profits. Changes in the organizational structures of health care facilities (in particular, the growth of the for-profit health care sector and the need to contain costs) are changing perceptions.

Figure 1.9 National health expenditures have increased dramatically since 1929. *Source:* National Center for Health Statistics: Health, United States, 1987. DHHS Pub. No. (PHS) 88-1232. Public Health Service. Washington D.C. U.S. Government Printing Office, 1988).

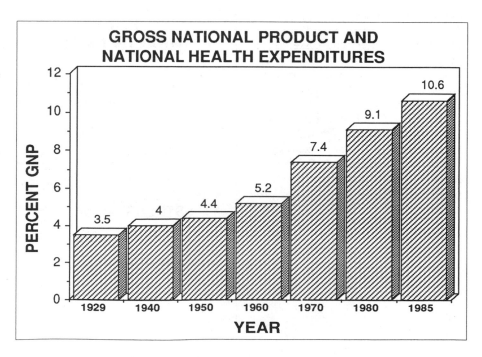

Based on a recent survey, almost 60 percent of worksites with 50 or more employees had worksite health promotion activities in 1985.[66] (See Figure 1.10.)

At most worksites with programs (85.4 percent), all employees are eligible to participate. Only 30 percent, however, offer them to employee dependents. When worksites seek outside program assistance, they turn to voluntary, not-for-profit organizations (57.1 percent), private for-profit providers-consultants (50 percent), local hospitals (44 percent), and insurance companies (43 percent).[66]

Smoking cessation and alcoholism treatment programs appear most likely to be cost-beneficial.[63] Smoking-related health problems cost U.S. businesses $26 billion per year in lost productivity and $7–8 billion in smoking-related medical costs. Workers who smoke are 50 percent more likely to be hospitalized than nonsmokers, have 2 times as many job-related accidents as nonsmokers, and have absenteeism rates approximately 50 percent higher than nonsmokers.[66]

Alcoholics have lower life expectancies, and consume medical care resources at a much higher rate than nonalcoholics.[67] Treatment of alcoholics decreases overall health care utilization following alcoholism treatment, making such treatment cost effective.

Benefits of Worksite Exercise Programs

Today, a growing number of companies, especially large ones, have worksite physical fitness programs. (See Figure 1.11.)

What benefits can be expected from worksite exercise programs specifically?[68] A summary of the major research in this area was developed through a cooperative effort by the Office of Disease Prevention and Health Promotion, U.S. Department of Health and Human Services, and a team of researchers from the Institute for Aerobics Research, Dallas.[69] (See Table 1.2.)

In general, the research results support the notion that worksite exercise programs improve fitness and help reduce health risks. The findings consistently show improvements in aerobic capacity and exercise habits, as well as in other fitness-related measures. In most cases, health risk factors such as smoking and elevated blood lipids also respond to the worksite programs. The impact of these programs on job performance, including productivity and job-related attitudes, is less well established. More research is needed in this area.

Impact of Exercise on Absenteeism

Employers are very interested in the relationship between worksite exercise programs and "bottom-line" variables, such as absenteeism and medical care costs. The results from the few programs that measured these variables show mostly favorable effects.

■ Among Canadian Life employees, there were modest differences in absenteeism between those that were and those that were not in the fitness

Figure 1.10 Smoking control leads the list of most common worksite health promotion activities. Exercise programs are offered by 22 percent of worksites nationwide with 50 or more employees. *Source:* The Office of Disease Prevention and Health Promotion. U.S. Public Health Service. U.S. Department of Health and Human Services. *Disease Prevention/ Health Promotion: The Facts.* Palo Alto: Bull Publishing Company, 1988.

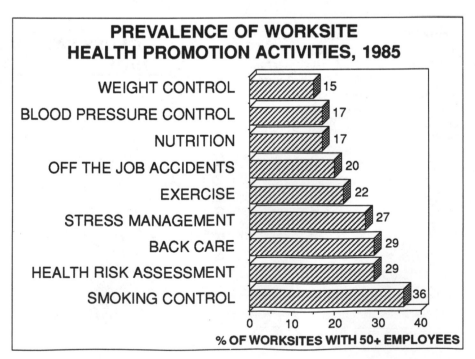

PREVALENCE OF WORKSITE HEALTH PROMOTION ACTIVITIES, 1985

Activity	%
WEIGHT CONTROL	15
BLOOD PRESSURE CONTROL	17
NUTRITION	17
OFF THE JOB ACCIDENTS	20
EXERCISE	22
STRESS MANAGEMENT	27
BACK CARE	29
HEALTH RISK ASSESSMENT	29
SMOKING CONTROL	36

% OF WORKSITES WITH 50+ EMPLOYEES

Figure 1.11 Larger companies tend to provide employees with physical fitness programs more than companies with fewer employees. *Source:* Washington Business Group on Health. Physical Fitness Programs in the Workplace, 1987. 229-1/2 Pennsylvania Ave., SE, Washington, D.C. 20003.

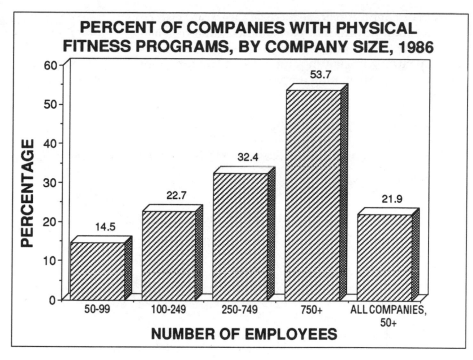

program.[72] However, the average absentee rate of "high adherent" participants dropped almost 50 percent the year they first participated in the fitness program.

- At the New York State Education Department, there was a net reduction of 4.7 hours of sick leave per employee per year for all participants.[84]
- At Prudential, there was a 20.1 percent reduction in average disability days for one group of program participants.[85]
- At Tenneco, there was a trend for exercisers to have fewer sick hours than nonexercisers, although this difference was statistically significant only for female employees.[86]
- At both the Dallas and H-E-B Independent School Districts, there were reductions in absences of 1.25 days per year and 0.43 days per year, respectively, for program participants relative to those not enrolled. These absenteeism reductions yielded actual savings of $149,578 for the Dallas district and $4,127 for the H-E-B district.[75, 77]

Impact of Exercise on Medical and Health Care Costs

Direct medical and health care cost savings also have been documented in several studies of worksite exercise programs. Most studies report the short-term (one- to two-year) effects.

- For example, in the Canadian Life program,[73] researchers showed that the total costs for medical care increased by 35 percent in a company without a program but only by one percent at Canadian Life.
- At Prudential,[85] researchers found a 45.7 percent ($262.15) reduction in average major medical costs for one group of program participants. The higher the level of fitness achieved during the program, the lower the post-entry medical care costs.
- Similarly, there was a 48.2 percent ($553) difference between exercisers and nonexercisers at Tenneco.[86]
- An average $253.42 reduction in medical care costs was reported for the comprehensive program participants at the H-E-B Independent School Districts.[77]

Two long-term medical care studies extend the findings of the short-term programs.

- The Los Angeles County Firefighters showed a 45 percent reduction in workers' compensation costs during the first 10 years of their program. Compensation costs, especially those for back injuries, were substantially lower for those firefighters who were most flexible, those strongest, and those who had the highest physical work capacity.[81]
- At Blue Cross and Blue Shield of Indiana, long-term (4.75-years) there was a difference of $519.09

in discounted average medical care costs between a group of program participants and a matched group.[71] For every $1.00 in medical care costs spent on participating employees, $1.73 was spent on nonparticipating employees.

Cost-Benefit of Worksite Exercise Programs

Worksite exercise programs are not free; so, in an attempt to factor in the costs associated with conducting

Table 1.2   Summary of Research Findings on Worksite Exercise Programs[69]

Documented Benefits

Worksite	Ref #	Fitness	Health Risks	Job Perf	Absenteeism	Health Costs	CBA
AT&T	70	0/+	+	+		+	+
Blue Cross	71					+	+
Canadian Life	72, 73	+		0	+	+	
Control Data	74	+	+				
Dallas ISD	75	+	+	+	+		
Exxon	76	+	+				
H-E-B ISD	77				+	+	+
Johnson & Johnson	78	+	0/+				
Kimberly-Clark	79	+	+		+		
LA City Fire	80	+	+		+		
LA County Fire	81	+	+		+		
Mobil Oil	82	+	+				
NASA	83	+	0/+	0/+			
NY State Ed Dept	84	+	+		+		
Prudential	85	+	0/+		+	+	+
Tenneco	86, 87			0/+	0/+	0/+	
Xerox	88	+	+				

Definition of Terms

Fitness:	aerobic capacity, physical work capacity, exercise habits and patterns, strength, flexibility, body composition
Health Risks:	smoking, blood pressure, blood lipids, psychological factors
Job Performance:	productivity, attitudes, satisfaction, commitment
Absenteeism:	disability and sick leave, turnover
Health Costs:	medical and health care costs
CBA:	cost-benefit analysis

Rating Key

+ = Beneficial effect of exercise program

0 = Neutral or minimal effect

+/0 = Mixed findings

Blank = No data reported

these programs, several researchers have published cost-benefit analyses.

∎ At Prudential, with a facility-based program that includes physical examinations, laboratory testing, exercise classes and instruction, educational seminars, and periodic rescreening, researchers estimated that for every $1.00 spent on the programs, Prudential realized a $1.91 savings in short-term disability and medical care costs.[85]

∎ At the H-E-B Independent School District, in a program that used the existing facilities and resources of the school district, the benefit-to-cost ratio for program participants during the experimental period was $1.41.[77]

∎ In the Blue Cross and Blue Shield of Indiana program, the benefit-to-cost ratio for the entire five years of the program was 1.45.[71]

Future Growth Predicted for Worksite Health Programs

Projections for the next decade indicate that worksite health programs will continue to grow in importance.[66] Most experts are predicting, however, that construction of on-site fitness facilities will decline as companies attempt to make better use of existing facilities and community resources and encourage self-help programs in the employees' homes, and as other alternative health promotion programs are offered.[66] Chapter 8 will deal with principles of successful exercise program management at the worksite and elsewhere.[89, 90]

Methods of Implementation
General Recommendations

To accomplish the year 2000 Objectives for the Nation, the Public Health Service has recommended several "Prevention/Promotion Measures":[5]

∎ Using television and radio public service announcements to provide information on appropriate physical activity and its benefits.

∎ Providing information in school and college-based programs.

∎ Providing information in health care delivery systems, including making queries about exercise habits a part of routine clinical history.

∎ Encouraging health care providers, especially HMOs, community health centers, and others in organized settings to prescribe appropriate exercise as part of weight loss regimens complementary to the management of severe chronic diseases,

and to give patients 65 years and older and the handicapped more detailed information on appropriate physical activity.

∎ Adopting an exercise component by community service agencies (such as the American Red Cross and the American Heart Association).

∎ Assuring that all programs and materials related to diet and weight loss have an active exercise component.

∎ Tailoring education programs to the needs and characteristics of specific populations.

∎ Providing physical fitness and exercise programs to school children, and ensuring that those programs emphasize activities for all children, rather than just competitive sports for relatively few.

∎ Providing physical fitness and exercise programs in colleges.

∎ Providing worksite-based fitness programs, linked to other health enhancement components encouraging an active outreach effort.

∎ Incorporating exercise and fitness protocols as regular clinical tools of health providers.

∎ Increasing the availability of existing facilities and promoting the development of new facilities by public, private, and corporate entities (e.g., fitness trails,[91, 92] bike paths, parks, pools).

∎ Upgrading existing facilities, especially in inner city neighborhoods, and involving the population to be served at all levels of planning.

In addition, the following legislative, regulatory, and economic measures were advocated:

∎ City council support of bicycle and walking paths for travel to and from work and school.

∎ Developing and operating local, state, and National park facilities appropriate for physical fitness activities in urban areas.

∎ Increasing the number of school-mandated physical education programs that focus on health-related physical fitness.

∎ Establishing state and local councils on health promotion and physical fitness.

∎ Allowing expenditure of funds for fitness-related activities under Federally funded programs guided by Federal regulations.

∎ Tax incentives for the private sector to offer physical fitness programs for employees.

∎ Encouraging employers to permit employees to exercise on company time and/or giving employees flexible time for use of facilities.

■ Offering health and life insurance policies with reduced premiums for those who participate in regular vigorous physical activity.

The Medical Care Setting

The medical care encounter provides an ideal situation for promoting physical activity.[89] Patients want and expect physicians to be concerned about their health habits. They say that their physician's advice encourages them to become more active.

Yet studies show the majority of physicians do not counsel their patients about physical activity.[89] One study showed that doctors tend to harbor doubts about their own effectiveness in counseling patients about their health risks, and also state that lack of insurance reimbursement is an obstacle to providing nutrition and exercise counseling.[93] It appears that there are important deficiencies in the medical students' knowledge of the physiology of exercise and physical training.[94]

Community Settings

The largest number and greatest variety of physical activity programs are found in community settings.[89] A number of public organizations, including health-care organizations, sponsor organized programs which enable participants to be more active through a variety of physical activity programs.

Unfortunately, there have been virtually no controlled studies of the effects of community-based physical activity programs. It does appear, however, that community-based programs that use mass media as a regular means of communicating with constituents are successful in increasing both awareness and interest in physical activity, but probably not in changing attitudes or exercise behavior in the short term.[89]

School Settings

Schools represent the ideal setting for influencing the physical activity of children and teenagers.[89] The ideal school program should:[90]

■ Have compulsory physical education throughout both primary and secondary grades.

■ Have daily instruction, with a total of 150 to 300 minutes of physical education instruction per week for elementary students. One-sixth to one-third of the total elementary school schedule should be devoted to physical activity.

■ Include a wide variety of activities to interest and provide success for all students, both boys and girls.

■ Emphasize activities that can be continued for a lifetime and have positive influences on health, such as swimming, running, and individual recreation, as opposed to team sports.

■ Include properly trained teachers with specialties in physical fitness and education.

■ Include adequate facilities and equipment, using existing resources in the community when necessary, such as community swimming pools, playing fields, and outdoor recreation areas.

■ Emphasize the joy of fitness and physical exercise. The common practice of using exercise as punishment (for example, pushups and jogging laps) should be emphatically discouraged.

In 1988, the American College of Sports Medicine (ACSM) released an opinion statement on physical fitness for children and youth.[95] ACSM urged that physical fitness programs for children and youth be developed with the primary goal of encouraging lifelong exercise to enhance cardiorespiratory fitness and health. Recommendations for action include an improved fitness focus in school, home, and community programs, emphasizing health-related rather than athletic-related physical fitness programs.

ACSM also recommends that physical fitness test scores be interpreted in relation to acceptable extrinsic standards, rather than by average population norms. It is illogical to declare that American children and youth are physically unfit as a group and then use group norms to interpret their fitness.

Sports Medicine Insight
The Wellness Revolution

As this chapter indicates, a growing number of Americans are entering the fitness movement. The fitness movement, however, is only one part of a much larger "wellness revolution" that is sweeping the United States. Let's consider some facts about this wellness revolution.[9]

The Hopeful Facts About the Wellness Revolution

1. **Increasing life expectancy:** The age-adjusted death rate in 1985 is the lowest ever recorded in the United States. Life expectancy in 1985 was 74.7 years.

2. **Death rates for heart disease are decreasing:** Between 1973 and 1985, the American death rate for stroke fell 50 percent, and for heart disease, 35 percent. Heart disease deaths, however, are still the leading cause of death in America, now closely followed by cancer deaths. For Americans aged 25–64, the positions are reversed, with cancer the leading cause of death. For cancer generally, both incidence and mortality increased during the 10-year period from 1975 to 1984.

3. **Diets are improving:** A U.S. Department of Agriculture (USDA) survey of adults in 1985 found that Americans now consume 36 percent of Calories in the form of fat, down slightly from the 1970s. Other surveys show that the percentage of people consuming poultry and fish remained fairly constant between 1977 and 1985, while the consumption of beef and pork decreased. Consumption of whole milk and eggs also declined, while intake of low-fat and skim milk products increased.

4. **Cigarette consumption is falling:** Between 1982 and 1983, the age-adjusted incidence rate for lung cancer declined for white males from 82.7 to 79.3 new cases per 100,000 population. This decline of 4.1 percent is the first significant decrease in lung cancer for any race-sex group in the United States, and is related to reduced cigarette smoking by white males.

5. **Alcohol consumption is falling:** Per capita rates of alcohol consumption rose approximately 21 percent during the 1960s, and 10.3 percent during the 1970s. Overall per capita consumption reached a plateau in 1980 and 1981 and subsequently declined, ending in 1984 at 1977 levels.

6. **Death rates for the elderly are falling:** In 1900, only about 4 percent of the population was elderly; by 1984 the number was approximately 28 million, or roughly 12 percent of the population. By the year 2030, the percentage will be 18 percent. Between 1950 and 1985, there was an 18 percent drop in the age-adjusted mortality rate for older adults—much of this because of the decline in death rates for stroke (50 percent) and heart disease (24 percent). Cancer, however, has risen steadily since 1950, in large part because of increased deaths from lung cancer among women.[10]

Health Promotion Concerns

When the U.S. Public Health Service published the set of national disease prevention objectives for 1990, it set up a system for tracking progress.[38] Some of the major findings are as follows (the results of the exercise portion of the survey were summarized earlier):

▪ Eighty-five percent of U.S. adults had had their blood pressure checked within the past year. More than 90 percent of U.S. adults were aware that high blood pressure increased the risk of heart disease.

▪ About one-half of adults had experienced at least a moderate amount of stress in the past 2 weeks. People with higher education and income were more likely to feel that they had experienced stress than people with lower education and income. Four in ten adults felt that stress had at least some effect on their health in the past year.

▪ About 30 percent of those 18 years or older smoked cigarettes in 1985. Young adults who had not completed high school were more than twice as likely as college graduates to be smokers. Ninety percent of U.S. adults recognized that smoking increases one's chances of getting heart disease.

▪ Thirteen percent of men and 3 percent of women drank an average of two drinks (1.0 ounce of ethanol) or more per day—an amount termed "heavier drinking" by the National Institute on Alcohol Abuse and Alcoholism. Among men under 45 years of age, those with less education had higher rates of heavier drinking, whereas those 45 and over reported heavier drinking among the college-educated.

▪ Over half of U.S. children 4 and under were breast fed at some time, but less than one-fourth were breast fed for 6 months or more.

▪ Fifty-five percent of U.S. adults ate breakfast almost every day. The older the age group, the more likely they were to eat breakfast daily.

▪ Twenty-nine percent of adults rarely or never ate snacks. Those 65 and over were twice as likely to avoid snacks as those age 18–29.

▪ In 1985, about one-fourth of the adult population was 20 percent or more above desirable body weight, about one-third of those ages 45–64. Thirty-six percent of black women were overweight, compared to 21 percent of white women. Among middle-aged women, 55 percent of black women were overweight, compared to 28 percent of white women. About 56 percent of overweight people were trying to lose weight in 1985.

Summary

1. The year 2000 health objectives for the nation, with emphasis on the physical activity and fitness objectives, were reviewed.

2. Public health policy is a complex function of four areas: the severity of the problem; the certainty with which we know the cause of and solution to the problem; the cost of the solution; and the methods of implementation.

3. The problem of inactivity in this country can be viewed in a historical context, showing how concepts of healthful exercise have changed. A turning point in adult fitness awareness took place in 1968 with the publication of Dr. Ken Cooper's first book, *Aerobics*.

4. Many surveys have tried to evaluate the magnitude of the present fitness revolution. Only 28 percent of the American public are exercising appropriately. The 1990 goal of having more than 60 percent of adults exercising appropriately is unrealistic.

5. Those exercising effectively tend to be of upper socio-economic status, young, male, and from the West.

6. Three major surveys of child and youth fitness have been conducted during the 1980s. They show that large numbers of American children and youth perform at less than desirable levels. Of particular concern are test results showing low upper body strength and cardiorespiratory fitness. Skinfold measurements show larger fat percentages than 20 years ago.

7. The causes and solutions to the problem are not simple. Exercise program compliance statistics are quite dismal. Even in well-structured programs, close to half of the participants will drop out within the first 6–12 months. One of the greatest challenges for the future is to devise methods to aid sedentary and irregularly active Americans (now 60 percent of all adults) in becoming more active.

8. The cost of the apparent solution (widespread public health programs to facilitate increased physical activity) involve potential risks (musculoskeletal, cardiovascular, psychological) and economic burdens. Economic considerations are leading many institutions to reevaluate the relative costs of health care and health promotion. Nearly 60 percent of worksites with 50 or more employees offered health promotion activities for their employees in 1985.

9. Exercise programs are offered by 22 percent of worksites with 50 or more employees. A review of 17 studies shows that fitness status can be improved, and absenteeism and health risks and costs lowered through worksite exercise programs.

10. Helping Americans to exercise more at school, the workplace, and during leisure time will require efforts on several fronts, including employers, schools, homes, local, state, and federal governments, and medical care providers.

References

1. Breslow L. Setting Objectives for Public Health. Ann Rev Public Health 8:289–307, 1987.

2. O'Donnell MP. Definition of Health Promotion: Part II: Levels of Programs. Am J Health Promotion 1(2):6–9, 1986.

3. Office of the Assistant Secretary for Health and Surgeon General: Healthy People: The Surgeon General's Report On Health Promotion and Disease Prevention. DHEW (PHS) Publication No. 79-55071. U.S. Government Printing Office, Washington, D.C., 1979.

4. Department of Health and Human Services: Promoting Health/Preventing Disease: Objectives for the Nation. U.S. Government Printing Office, Washington, D.C., Fall 1980.

5. Public Health Service, U.S. Department of Health and Human Services (1991). *Healthy People 2000: National Health Promotion and Disease Prevention Objectives*. DHHS Publication No. (PHS) 91-50212. Superintendent of Documents, Government Printing Office, Washington, DC 20402-9325.

6. Caspersen CJ, Christensen GM, Pollard RA. Status of the 1990 Physical Fitness and Exercise Objectives—Evidence from NHIS 1985. Public Health 101:581–592, 1986.

7. Powell KE, Spain KG, Christenson GM, Mollenkamp MP. The Status of the 1990 Objectives for Physical Fitness and Exercise. Public Health Rep 101:15–21, 1986.

8. Mason JO, Powell KE. Physical Activity, Behavioral Epidemiology, and Public Health. Public Health Rep 100:113–115, 1985.

9. Powell KE, Paffenbarger RS. Workshop on Epidemiologic and Public Health Aspects of Physical Activity: A Summary. Public Health Rep 100: 118–126, 1985.

10. U.S. Department of Health and Human Services. Public Health Service. Office of Disease Prevention and Health Promotion. Prevention '86/'87: Federal Programs and

Progress. U.S. Government Printing Office: Washington, D.C., 1987.

11. Spears B, Swanson RA. History of Sports and Physical Activity in the United States. Dubuque, Iowa: W.C. Brown Co., 1978.

12. Rice EA, Hutchinson JL, Lee M. A Brief History of Physical Education. New York: The Ronald Press Co., 1958.

13. Siedentop D. Physical Education, Introductory Analysis. Dubuque, Iowa: W.C. Brown Co., 1972.

14. Bucher CA. Foundations of Physical Education. Saint Louis: C.V. Mosby Co., 1972.

15. Corbin DH. Recreation Leadership. Englewood Cliffs, N.J.: Prentice-Hall, Inc., 1970.

16. Pate RR. A New Definition of Youth Fitness. Physician Sportsmed 11:77–83, 1983.

17. Misner JE. Are We Fit to Educate About Fitness? JOPERD, November/December, 1984, pp. 26–28.

18. Report of Inter-Society Commission for Heart Disease Resources. Circulation 70:157A–205A, 1984.

19. Kraus H., Hirschland RP. Muscular Fitness and Health. JAMA, 17–19, December, 1953. See also: Kraus H, Hirschland RP. Minimum Muscular Fitness Tests in School Children. Res Q Am Assoc Health Phys Educ 25:178–188, 1954.

20. See discussion: Is American Youth Physically Fit? U.S. News & World Report, Aug. 2, 1957, pp. 66–77.

21. Bowerman WJ, Harris WE. Jogging. New York: Grosset & Dunlap, 1977 (Copyright 1967).

22. Cooper KH. Aerobics. New York: Bantam Books, Inc., 1968.

23. Cooper KH. The New Aerobics. New York: M. Evans and Company, Inc., 1970.

24. Cooper KH. The Aerobics Way. New York: M. Evans and Company, Inc., 1977.

25. Cooper M, Cooper KH. Aerobics for Women. New York: M. Evans and Co., Inc., 1972.

26. Higdon H. Running After 40. Runner's World. August, 1978, p. 36.

27. Henderson J. Long Slow Distance: The Humane Way to Train. Mountain View, California: World Publications, 1969.

28. Ullyot J. Women's Running. Mountain View, California: World Publications, 1976.

29. Sheehan GA. Dr. Sheehan on Running. Mountain View, California: World Publications, 1976.

30. Fixx JF. The Complete Book of Running. New York: Random House, 1977.

31. Leavy J, Okie S. The Runner: Study Tells A Lot About the Man on the Run. The Atlanta Journal and Constitution. November 18, 1979, p. 13-D.

32. Higdon H. Running After 40. Runner's World. August, 1978, p. 36.

33. Stephens T, Jacobs DR, White CC. A Descriptive Epidemiology of Leisure-Time Physical Activity. Public Health Rep 100:147–158, 1985.

34. Stephens T. Secular Trends in Adult Physical Activity: Exercise Boom or Bust? Res Quart Exerc Sport 58:94–105, 1987.

35. Thomas GS, Lee PR, Franks P, Paffenbarger RS. Exercise and Health: The Evidence and the Implications. Cambridge, Massachusetts: Oelgeschlager, Gunn & Hain, Publishers, Inc., 1981.

36. Lupton CH, Ostrove NM, Bozzo RM. Participation in Leisure-Time Physical Activity. JOPERD, November/December, 1984, pp. 19–23.

37. Powell KE, Paffenbarger RS. Workshop on Epidemiologic and Public Health Aspects of Physical Activity and Exercise: A Summary. Public Health Rep 100:118–126, 1985.

38. National Center for Health Statistics, C. A. Schoenborn. 1988. Health Promotion and Disease Prevention: United States, 1985. Vital and Health Statistics. Series 10, No. 163. DHHS Pub. No. (PHD) 88–1591. Public Health Service. Washington: U.S. Government Office.

39. National Sporting Goods Association, 1699 Wall St., Mt. Prospect, IL, 60056, (312/439-4000).

40. Hypertension Control Program, Adult Health Section, Department of Health Services. 1983 California Hypertension Survey.

41. Who is the American Runner? Runner's World, August, 1984, pp. 46–51, 156–168.

42. Office of Disease Prevention and Health Promotion, Public Health Service. Summary of Findings from National Children and Youth Fitness Study, JOPERD, January 1985, pp. 2–90.

43. Youth Physical Fitness in 1985. The President's Council on Physical Fitness and Sports School Population Fitness Survey. President's Council on Physical Fitness and Sports. 450 Fifth St NW, Suite 7103, Washington, D.C., 20001.

44. Ross JG, Pate RR, Delpy LA, Gold RS, Svilar M. New Health-Related Fitness Norms. JOPERD, November/December, 1987, pp. 66–70.

45. Pate RR, Ross JG. Factors Associated With Health-Related Fitness. JOPERD, November/December 1987, pp. 93–96.

46. Ross JG, Pate RR. The National Children and Youth Fitness Study II: A Summary of Findings. JOPERD, November/December 1987, pp. 51–56.

47. Ross JG, Delpy LA, Christenson GM, Gold RS, Damberg CL. The National Children and Youth Fitness Study II: Study Procedures and Quality Control. JOPERD, November/December 1987, pp. 57–62.

48. Hovell MF. An Evaluation of Elementary Students' Voluntary Physical Activity During Recess. Res Quart Exerc Sport, 49:460–474, 1978.

49. Franks BD. Physical Fitness in Secondary Education. JOPERD, November/December, 1984, pp. 41–43.

50. Anonymous. Scanning Sports. Physician Sportsmed 15(8):33, 1987.

51. The American Alliance for Health, Physical Education, Recreation and Dance. Health Related Physical Fitness Test Manual. 1900 Association Drive, Reston, Virginia 22091: AAHPERD, 1980.

52. Safrit MJ, Wood TM. The Health-Related Physical Fitness Test: A Tri-State Survey of Users and Non-Users. Res Quart Exerc Sport 57:27–32, 1986.

53. Blair SN, Jacobs DR, Powell KE. Relationships Between Exercise or Physical Activity and Other Health Behaviors. Public Health Rep 100:172–180, 1985.

54. Siscovick DS, Laporte RE, Newman JM. The Disease-Specific Benefits and Risks of Physical Activity and Exercise. Public Health Rep 100:180–188, 1985.

55. Stamler J, Epstein F. Coronary Heart Disease: Risk Factors as Guides to Preventive Action. Prev Med 1:27–48, 1972.

56. Shephard RJ. Motivation: The Key to Fitness Compliance. Physician Sportsmed 13:88–101, 1985.

57. Dishman RK, Sallis JF, Orenstein DR. The Determinants of Physical Activity and Exercise. Public Health Rep 100:158–171, 1985.

58. Shephard RJ. The Impact of Exercise Upon Medical Costs. Sports Med 2:133–143, 1985.

59. Martin JE. Exercise and Health: The Adherence Problem. Behavioral Medicine Update 14:16–24, 1982.

60. Koplan JP, Siscovick DS, Goldbaum GM. The Risks of Exercise: A Public Health View of Injuries and Hazards. Public Health Rep 100:189–195, 1985.

61. National Center for Health Statistics: Health, United States, 1987. DHHS Pub. No. (PHS) 88–1232. Public Health Service. Washington, D.C., U.S. Government Printing Office, 1988.

62. Gray HJ. The Role of Business in Health Promotion: A Brief Overview. Prev Med 12:654–657, 1983.

63. Hollis JF. The Effectiveness of Worksite Health Promotion Efforts, 1986. Greater Portland Business Group on Health: Employee Health Education and Wellness Task Force. 221 N.W. 2nd Avenue, Portland, Oregon 97209.

64. Rogers CC. Does Sports Medicine Fit in the New Health Care Market? Physician Sportsmed 13:116–127, 1985.

65. Clubs, YMCAs and Hospitals: The New Allies. Athletic Business, May 1985, pp. 22–29.

66. The Office of Disease Prevention and Health Promotion. U.S. Public Health Service. U.S. Department of Health and Human Services. Disease Prevention/Health Promotion: The Facts. Palo Alto: Bull Publishing Company, 1988.

67. Holder HD, Blose JO. Alcoholism Treatment and Total Health Care Utilization and Costs: A Four-Year Longitudinal Analysis of Federal Employees. JAMA 256:1456–1460, 1986.

68. Anonymous. New Study Links Unhealthy Behavior to Higher Medical Costs. Employee Health & Fitness 9(6):61–64, 1987.

69. Washington Business Group on Health. Physical Fitness Programs in the Workplace, 1987. 220-1/2 Pennsylvania Ave., SE, Washington, D.C. 20003. Reported in Employee Health & Fitness (April):44–46, 1987.

70. Spilman MA, Goetz A, Schultz J, Bellingham R, Johnson D. Effects of a Corporate Health Promotion Program. J Occup Med 28:285–289, 1986.

71. Gibbs JO, Mulvaney D, Henes C. Reed RW. Work-site health promotion: Five-Year Trend in Employee Health Care Costs. J Occup Med 27:826–830, 1985.

72. Cox MC, Shephard RJ, Corey P. Influence of an Employees Fitness Programme Upon Fitness, Productivity, and Absenteeism. Ergonomics 24:795–806, 1981.

73. Shephard RJ, Corey P, Renzland P, Cox M. The Influence of an Employee Fitness and Lifestyle Modification Program Upon Medical Care Costs. Can J Public Health 73:259–263, 1982.

74. Naditch MP. The Staywell Program. In: Matarazzo JD, Weiss SM, Herd JA, Miller NE, Weiss SM (eds). Behavioral Health: A Handbook of Health Enhancement and Disease Prevention. New York: Wiley-Interscience, 1984, pp. 1071–1078.

75. Blair SN, Smith M, Collingwood TR, Reynolds R, Prentice MC, Sterline CL. Health Promotion for Educators: Impact on Absenteeism. Prev Med 15:166–175, 1986.

76. Yarvote PM, McDonagh TJ, Goldman ME, Zuckerman J. Organization and Evaluation of a Physical Fitness Program in Industry. J Occup Med 16:589–598, 1974.

77. Rogers T, Cole JA, Erwin PG. "Heart at Work": Cost-Benefit Analysis of a New Worksite Health Promotion Program. In: Proceedings of the Seventh Annual Meeting of the Society of Behavioral Medicine. San Francisco: Society of Behavioral Medicine, 1986, pp. 10–11.

78. Blair SN, Piserchia PV, Wilbur CS, Crowder JH: A Public Health Intervention Model for Work-site Health Promotion: Impact on Exercise and Physical Fitness in a Health Promotion Plan After 24 Months. JAMA 255:921–926, 1986.

79. Smoczyk CM, Dedmon RE. Health Management Program Kimberly-Clark Corporation. Am Behav Scientist 28:559–576, 1985.

80. Barnard RJ, Anthony DF. Effect of Health Maintenance Programs on Los Angeles City Firefighters. J Occup Med 22:667–669, 1980.

81. Cady LD, Thomas PC, Karwasky RJ. Program for Increasing Health and Physical Fitness of Fire Fighters. J Occup Med 27:110–114, 1985.

82. Horne WM. Effects of a Physical Activity Program on Middle-Aged Sedentary Corporation Executives. Am Indus Hygiene Assoc J 36:241–245, 1975.

83. Durbeck DC, Heinzelmann F, Schacter J, et al. The National Aeronautics and Space Administration—U.S.

Public Health Service Health Evaluation and Enhancement Program. Am J Cardiol 30:784–790, 1972.

84. Bjurstrom LA, Alexiou NG. A Program of Heart Disease Intervention for Public Employees. J Occup Med 20:521–531, 1978.

85. Bowne DW, Russell ML, Morgan JL, Optenberg SA, Clarke AE. Reduced Disability and Health Care Costs in An Industrial Fitness Program. J Occup Med 26:809–815, 1984.

86. Baun WB, Bernacki EJ, Tsai SP. A Preliminary Investigation: Effect of a Corporate Fitness Program on Absenteeism and Health Care Cost. J Occup Med 28:18–22, 1986.

87. Bernacki EJ, Baun WB. The Relationship of Job Performance to Exercise Adherence in a Corporate Fitness Program. J Occup Med 26:529–531, 1984.

88. Pauly JT, Palmer JA, Wright CC, Pfeiffer GJ. The Effect of a 14-Week Employee Fitness Program on Selected Physiological and Psychological Parameters. J Occup Med 24:457–463, 1982.

89. Iverson DC, Fielding JE, Crow RS, Christenson GM. The Promotion of Physical Activity in the United States Population: The Status of Programs in Medical, Worksite, Community, and School Settings. Pub Health Rep 100:212–224, 1985.

90. Wynder EL. The American Health Foundation. The Book of Health. New York: Franklin Watts, 1981, pp. 337–340.

91. Parcourse, Ltd. 3701 Buchanan Street, San Francisco, California 94123 (415/931-9444).

92. Fit-Trail. Southwood, P.O. Box 240457, Charlotte, North Carolina, 28224 (704/554-8000).

93. Rosen MA, Lodgsdon DN, Demak MM. Prevention and Health Promotion in Primary Care: Baseline Results on Physicians from the INSURE Project on Lifecycle Preventive Health Services. Prev Med 13:535–548, 1984.

94. Young A, Gray JA, Ennis JR. Exercise Medicine: The Knowledge and Beliefs of Final-Year Medical Students in the United Kingdom. Med Educa 17:369–373, 1983.

95. American College of Sports Medicine. Opinion Statement on Physical Fitness in Children and Youth. Med Sci Sports Exerc 20:422-423, 1988.

Physical Fitness Activity 1.1— What Is Your Personal Exercise Program?

In this chapter, the exercise habits of Americans were fully described. The 1985 National Health Interview Survey (NHIS) by the National Center for Health Statistics is presently one of the best data sources for this type of information. Data from NHIS have been collected continuously since 1957. In 1985, a special section on Health Promotion and Disease Prevention was included. A total of 33,630 interviews were completed, covering a wide range of health promotion topics including general health habits, injury control, high blood pressure, stress, exercise, smoking, alcohol use, dental care, and occupational safety and health.

In this Physical Fitness Activity, you will be answering questions on exercise taken directly from the NHIS Health Promotion and Disease Prevention. Fill in the blanks in the table on the next page, and then summarize your exercise program by answering the questions (listed below).

Physical Fitness Activity Questions

1. Summarize your answers to the NHIS questionnaire by filling in the following:

    A. What was your average *frequency per week* of exercise during the last 2 weeks?

    _____ average frequency/week

    Note: Total the number of times in past 2 weeks and divide by 2. For example, if you jogged 2 times in the past 2 weeks, biked 2 times, and played soccer once, your average frequency per day would be 5 divided by 2, or 2.5 times/week.

    B. What was your average *duration per exercise session in minutes*?

    _____ average duration per exercise session (in minutes)

    Note: Total the number of minutes spent in exercise during past 2 weeks and divide by number of exercise sessions. For example, if the jogging sessions lasted 15 minutes each, the biking sessions 30 minutes each, and soccer 40 minutes, the average duration per exercise session in minutes would be 130 min/5 = 26 minutes per session.

    C. In how many exercise sessions per week did you tend to have *at least a moderate increase in heart rate* and breathing?

    _____ average number of exercise sessions/week at moderate heart rate levels

    Note: Add the total number of sessions in which your heart rate was at least at moderate levels, and divide by 2. For example, if all exercise sessions in the previous section were at moderate levels, the answer would be 2.5 sessions per week at moderate heart rate levels.

How do you compare with American College of Sports Medicine standards?

The American College of Sports Medicine recommends that people exercise at least three times per week, for at least 20 to 30 minutes, at moderate-to-hard intensity levels (at least 50 percent maximal oxygen capacity). (See Chapter 8.)

Source: National Health Interview Survey, Health Promotion and Disease Prevention. National Center for Health Statistics, T. Stephens and Schoenborn. 1988. Adult Health Practices in the United States and Canada. Vital and Health Statistics. Series 5, No. 3. DHHS Pub. No. (PHS) 88–1479. Public Health Service. Washington, D.C.: U.S. Government Printing Office.

National Health Interview Survey
Health Promotion and Disease Prevention Supplement
Section R: Exercise (Adapted)

A			B	C	D			
In the past 2 weeks, have you done any of the following exercises, sports, or physically active hobbies?			How many times in the past 2 weeks did you [play/go/do] (*activity in A*)?	On the average, about how many minutes did you actually spend (*activity in A*) on each occasion?	What usually happened to your heart rate or breathing when you undertook (*activity in A*). Did you have a small, moderate, or large increase, or no increase at all in your heart rate or breathing?			
	Yes	No	Times	Minutes	Small	Moderate	Large	None
1. Walking for exercise	___	___	___	___	___	___	___	___
2. Jogging or running	___	___	___	___	___	___	___	___
3. Hiking	___	___	___	___	___	___	___	___
4. Gardening/yard work	___	___	___	___	___	___	___	___
5. Aerobic dancing	___	___	___	___	___	___	___	___
6. Other dancing	___	___	___	___	___	___	___	___
7. Calisthenics	___	___	___	___	___	___	___	___
8. Golf	___	___	___	___	___	___	___	___
9. Tennis	___	___	___	___	___	___	___	___
10. Bowling	___	___	___	___	___	___	___	___
11. Biking	___	___	___	___	___	___	___	___
12. Swimming	___	___	___	___	___	___	___	___
13. Yoga	___	___	___	___	___	___	___	___
14. Weight lifting	___	___	___	___	___	___	___	___
15. Basketball	___	___	___	___	___	___	___	___
16. Baseball	___	___	___	___	___	___	___	___
17. Football	___	___	___	___	___	___	___	___
18. Soccer	___	___	___	___	___	___	___	___
19. Volleyball	___	___	___	___	___	___	___	___
20. Handball/raquetball	___	___	___	___	___	___	___	___
21. Skating	___	___	___	___	___	___	___	___
22. Skiing	___	___	___	___	___	___	___	___
23. Any other type of exercise not mentioned here	___	___	___	___	___	___	___	___
List here _____	___	___	___	___	___	___	___	___

Chapter 2

Physical Activity, Exercise, and Physical Fitness: Definitions

Over the years, I have come to look upon physical fitness as the trunk of a tree that supports the many branches which represent all the activities that make life worth living: intellectual life, spiritual life, occupation, love life and social activities.—Thomas Kirk Cureton, Jr.

Introduction

During the fall of 1984, the Centers for Disease Control conducted a workshop on "Epidemiologic and Public Health Aspects of Physical Activity and Exercise."[1] Experts were invited to prepare papers and attend the workshop. Before the preparation of the review papers, the Behavioral Epidemiology and Evaluation Branch (BBEB) within the Division of Health Education, Center for Health Promotion and Education, Centers for Disease Control, prepared a manuscript discussing the definitions of physical activity, exercise, and physical fitness. This paper was circulated among the participants, and the definitions discussed here were adopted.[2]

Physical Activity

Physical activity is defined as any bodily movement produced by skeletal muscles that results in energy expenditure.[2] The energy expenditure can be measured in kilocalories (kcal) or kilojoules (kJ). One kcal is essentially equivalent to 4.184 kJ.

Everyone performs physical activity in order to sustain life. The amount, however, varies considerably from one individual to another, based on personal lifestyles and other factors.

Total 24-hour energy expenditure consists of three major categories (as will be discussed in more detail in Chapter 11):[3]

1. **Resting metabolic rate (RMR)**—*Resting metabolic rate* is generally the largest component of energy expenditure for most people except for some athletes. This is the amount of energy expended to maintain body systems while resting quietly in a comfortable environment several hours following meals or physical activity.

2. **Thermic effect of physical activity**—The second largest component of daily energy expenditure for most people is the energy expended for physical activity. The amount of this energy expenditure represented by muscular work depends on the duration and intensity of the physical activity.

   Energy is expended in physical activity during occupational duties, leisure-time activities, and even sleep. Table 2.1 outlines the average energy expenditure of American adults in various types of occupations.[4] The 24-hour kilocalorie totals represent the contribution of both resting metabolic rate and energy expended during physical activity.

Notice (from Table 2.1) that endurance athletes tend to have energy expenditure patterns quite similar to those of sedentary office workers, except for the large amount of energy expended during short but intense training sessions. When endurance athletes are compared to workers in heavy labor occupations, the total energy expenditure is nearly the same, but once again, the athletes' energy expenditure patterns are characterized by short but intense sessions whereas heavy laborers expend the majority of their kilocalories in lower intensity physical activity. The nutritional implications of

these different energy expenditure patterns will be discussed in Chapter 9.

Table 2.2 outlines the average energy intakes of Americans.[5-8] Results from the latest survey (1985),[8] show that the average American male is consuming about 2600 kcal/day, and the average American female about 1600 kcal/day. These energy intake levels approximate closely the average energy expenditures of sedentary males and females.

3. **Thermic effect of food (TEF)**—The third component of energy expenditure is the *thermic effect of food* or the energy expended above RMR over the several hours (usually four to six)

Table 2.1 Patterns of Average Daily Physical Activity and Energy Expenditure for Athletes and Nonathletes

Males	Sedentary (Office)	Light Occupation	Heavy Occupation	Endurance Training	Heavy Sports Training
Rest/Maintenance					
sleep	8 hrs/530 kcal	8 hrs/530 kcal	8 hrs/530 kcal	8 hrs/600 kcal	8 hrs/600 kcal
sit/stand	14 hrs/1700 kcal	6 hrs/750 kcal	6 hrs/750 kcal	12 hrs/1500 kcal	10 hrs/1250 kcal
Physical Activity					
45% $\dot{V}O_{2max}$	2 hrs/350 kcal	10 hrs/1500 kcal	6 hrs/1125 kcal	3 hrs/525 kcal	2 hrs/400 kcal
45–70% $\dot{V}O_{2max}$	< ... >	< ... >	4 hrs/1200 kcal	< ... >	3 hrs/1500 kcal
70+% $\dot{V}O_{2max}$	< ... >	< ... >	< ... >	1 hr/1100 kcal	1 hr/750 kcal
Total 24 hrs	2580 kcal	2780 kcal	3605 kcal	3725 kcal	4500 kcal

Females	Sedentary (Office)	Housewife	Endurance Training	Heavy Sports Training
Rest/Maintenance				
sleep	8 hrs/400 kcal	8 hrs/420 kcal	8 hrs/460 kcal	8 hrs/460 kcal
sit/stand	15 hrs/1100 kcal	12 hrs/990 kcal	12 hrs/1290 kcal	10 hrs/1170 kcal
Physical Activity				
45% $\dot{V}O_{2max}$	1 hr/130 kcal	4 hrs/550 kcal	3 hrs/400 kcal	3 hrs/430 kcal
45–70% $\dot{V}O_{2max}$	<...>	<...>	<...>	2 hrs/940 kcal
70+% $\dot{V}O_{2max}$	<...>	<...>	1 hr/790 kcal	1 hr/590 kcal
Total 24 hrs	1630 kcal	1960 kcal	2940 kcal	3590 kcal

Source: Adapted from Brotherhood JR. Nutrition and Sports Performance. Sports Med 1:350–389, 1984. With permission from ADIS Press Limited, Auckland 10, New Zealand.

Table 2.2 Energy Intake by American Adults (Kcal) and Percent Kilocalories as Fat (%Fat) from Various National Surveys

Population Studied		Name of Study	Kcal	(%Fat)
Men	35 to 59 yrs	LRCP[a]	2600	(40%)
Women	35 to 59 yrs		1750	(39%)
Men	35 to 57 yrs	MRFIT[b]	2500	(38%)
Men	18 to 75 yrs	NHANES[c]	2400	(37%)
Women	18 to 75 yrs		1600	(37%)
Men	19 to 64 yrs	NFCS[d]	2300	(42%)
Women	19 to 64 yrs		1500	(41%)
Men	19 to 50 yrs	CSFII[e]	2560	(36%)
Women	19 to 50 yrs		1588	(37%)

[a]Lipid Research Clinics Program (1972–1975)[5]
[b]Multiple Risk Factor Intervention Trial (1973–1975)[5]
[c]National Health and Nutrition Examination Survey (1976–1980)[6]
[d]Nationwide Food Consumption Survey (1977–1978)[7]
[e]Nationwide Food Consumption Survey, Continuing Survey of Food Intakes by Individuals (1985)[8]

following a meal.[3] The largest part of the energy expended immediately following meals is due to the metabolic costs of processing the meal, and include the costs of digestion ("internal exercise" by the muscular gastrointestinal tract), absorption, transport, and storage. The TEF accounts for approximately 10 percent of daily energy expenditure, but can vary depending on the amount and the composition of the diet (high-carbohydrate diets elevate the TEF more than high-fat diets). (See Chapter 11.)

Exercise

Exercise is not synonymous with physical activity.[2] It is a subcategory of physical activity. Exercise is physical activity that is planned, structured, repetitive, and purposive in the sense that improvement or maintenance of physical fitness is an objective.[2] Virtually all conditioning and many sports activities are considered as exercise because they are generally performed to improve or maintain physical fitness. Household and occupational tasks are usually accomplished with little regard to physical fitness. However, a person can structure work and home tasks in a more active form, and thus build up physical fitness at the same time the tasks are accomplished. Many people find this more motivating than "running in circles" for exercise.

Physical Fitness

Physical Fitness has been defined as:

> "The ability to carry out daily tasks with vigor and alertness, without undue fatigue and with ample energy to enjoy leisure-time pursuits and to meet unforeseen emergencies."[9]

Because modern day tasks require so little energy expenditure, and because of the human tendency to equate leisure time with inactivity, some researchers would add three other reasons (in addition to providing energy for work, leisure, and emergency) for being physically fit:

1. To help avoid hypokinetic diseases (such as heart disease, hypertension, diabetes, osteoporosis, and others). (See Part 4.)
2. To make the most of mental capacities. (See Chapter 13.)
3. To feel good, energetic, buoyant.

In other words, a good level of physical fitness may not be needed any more to work in a world dominated by technological innovations, but it is needed to make the most of mental potentialities, to avoid the many chronic diseases that plague Americans today, and to feel good, energetic, and that you are making the most of what life has to offer. The focus of fitness is not so much just to have minimal amounts of energy to barely make it through the day, but more to live an integrated, meaningful, joyous, and satisfying, "self-actuated" life.[9]

Rene Dubos spoke of health as a mirage. You can reach for it, but never fully grasp it. Physical fitness is the same way. Fitness is not so much a possession as a procession; not so much something to have as a way to be. One can never say, "I am physically fit." Instead, one is always within the process, seeking to attain a goal that in itself is unattainable.

One can subjectively measure physical fitness by determining how much energy one has for doing what is enjoyable in life, and experiencing all the natural adventure possible. From snow skiing to mountain climbing, country cycling to weekend backpacking, those who are physically fit have the energy to maximize their enjoyment of all the natural resources of their environment.

Physical fitness has also been described as:[10]

"... the ability to last, to bear up, to withstand stress, and to persevere under difficult circumstances where an unfit person would give up. Physical fitness is the opposite to being fatigued from ordinary efforts, to lacking the energy to enter zestfully into life's activities, and to becoming exhausted from unexpected, demanding physical exertion .... It is a positive quality, extending on a scale from death to 'abundant life.'"

How to obtain this energy and zest for life is the subject of Part 3 of this book. Basically, when the heart, lungs, blood vessels, and muscles are regularly stimulated through physical activity, in time, every physical movement throughout the day is somewhat easier. This means that more energy is available for active leisure-time as well as emergencies, accompanied by both physiological and psychological benefits.

In light of these thoughts, I submit the following definition for physical fitness:

Physical fitness is a dynamic state of energy and vitality that enables one to carry out daily tasks, to engage in active leisure-time pursuits, and to meet unforeseen emergencies without undue fatigue. In addition, those who are physically fit have a decreased risk of hypokinetic diseases, and are more able to function at the peak of their intellectual capacity, while enjoying a "joie de vivre."

The Measurable Elements of Physical Fitness

This definition of physical fitness is philosophical. Variables such as vigor, alertness, fatigue, and enjoyment are not easily measured. To clarify the meaning of physical fitness, it is important to identify the components that can actually be measured and defined and developed separately from each other. Although there has been misunderstanding in the past, and confusion regarding the measurable elements of physical fitness, there is now a growing consensus on this important matter.[12]

The most frequently cited components fall into two groups: one related to health and the other related to skills that pertain more to athletic ability in sports.[2, 11, 12] Figure 2.1 summarizes the components of *health-related fitness* and *skill-related fitness* with examples of the continuum of physical activities that covers the entire range of sports.

Notice that these activities demand these components in varying degrees. While some physical activities such as archery, bowling, and table tennis demand and develop mainly skill-related attributes, others such as walking, running, and stairclimbing are almost entirely health-related. Some activities such as soccer, handball, basketball, and skating require high levels of both components.

The Elements of Skill-Related Fitness Defined

While the elements of skill-related fitness are important for participation in various dual and team sports, they have little significance for the day-to-day tasks of Americans or for their general health.[2, 13] Thus, people with poor athletic skills should understand that they can still be healthy, through the development of the health-related components of physical fitness. Just as importantly, the person who excels in throwing a ball or swinging a golf club should understand that the related athletic activity may leave the core elements of health-related physical fitness underdeveloped.[13] The trend today in public policy recommendations is to emphasize the development of the health-related fitness elements, and to push for their prominence in school, worksite, and community programs.

The elements of skill-related fitness are:

Agility—Relates to the ability to rapidly change the position of the entire body in space, with speed and accuracy.

Balance—Relates to the maintenance of equilibrium while stationary or moving.

Coordination—Relates to the ability to use the senses, such as sight and hearing, together with body parts in performing motor tasks smoothly and accurately.

Speed—Relates to the ability to perform a movement within a short period of time.

Power—Relates to the rate at which one can perform work (strength over time).

Reaction time—Relates to the time elapsed between stimulation and the beginning of the reaction to it.

The Elements of Health-Related Fitness Defined

Each of the components of health-related physical fitness can be measured separately from the others, with specific exercises applied to the development of each. The levels of the health-related components of

THE MEASUREABLE ELEMENTS OF PHYSICAL FITNESS

HEALTH-RELATED FITNESS	SKILL-RELATED FITNESS

1. CARDIORESPIRATORY ENDURANCE
2. BODY COMPOSITION
3. MUSCULOSKELETAL
   a. flexibility
   b. muscular strength
   c. muscular endurance
	1. AGILITY
	2. BALANCE
	3. COORDINATION
	4. SPEED
	5. POWER
	6. REACTION TIME

THE SPORTS CONTINUUM

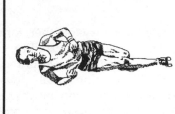

HEALTH-RELATED FITNESS	BOTH	SKILL-RELATED FITNESS
AEROBIC DANCING CALISTHENICS CROSS COUNTRY SKIING ROPE JUMPING ROWING SNOWSHOEING BACKPACKING BICYCLING RUNNING STAIRCLIMBING SWIMMING WALKING WEIGHT LIFTING	BASKETBALL HANDBALL ICE SKATING RACQUETBALL ROLLER SKATING SOCCER SQUASH	ARCHERY BOWLING FENCING GOLF TABLE TENNIS VOLLEYBALL BADMINTON BASEBALL DOWNHILL SKIING FOOTBALL TENNIS

Figure 2.1 Most physical activities exist on a continuum between health- or skill-related fitness. Adapted from Caspersen CJ, Powell KE, Christenson GM. Physical Activity, Exercise, and Physical Fitness: Definitions and Distinctions for Health-related Research. Public Health Rep 100:126–131, 1985.

physical fitness need not vary together; for example, a person may be strong but lack flexibility, or a person may have good heart and lung endurance, but lack muscular strength.[2] To develop "total" physical fitness for health, each of the five components discussed below must be included within the exercise prescription. (See Chapter 8.)

Cardiorespiratory Endurance

Cardiorespiratory endurance can be defined as the ability to continue or persist in strenuous tasks involving large muscle groups for extended periods of time.[14, 15] It is the ability of the circulatory and respiratory systems to adjust to and recover from the effects of whole-body exercise or work.[13]

For many people, being in good shape means having good cardiorespiratory endurance, exemplified by such feats as being able to run, cycle, and swim for prolonged periods of time. (See Figure 2.2). To most fitness leaders, cardiorespiratory endurance is the most

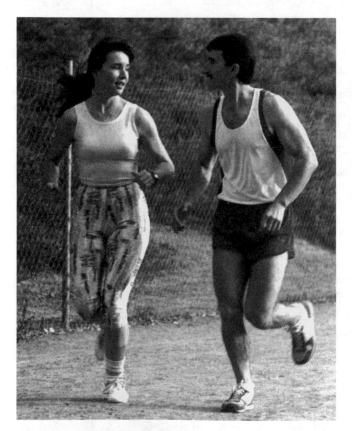

Figure 2.2 Cardiorespiratory endurance can be defined as the ability to continue or persist in strenuous tasks involving large muscle groups for extended periods of time. Jogging or running is one example.

important of the health-related physical fitness components.[13]

High levels of cardiorespiratory endurance indicate a high physical work capacity, which is the ability to release relatively high amounts of energy over an extended period of time.[16] As will be explained in Part 4, there are many benefits associated with cardiorespiratory endurance. Testing for cardiorespiratory endurance will be the subject of Chapter 4; conditioning for cardiorespiratory endurance will be covered in Part 3.

Dr. Kenneth H. Cooper, who coined the term *aerobics,* which is merely another term for cardiorespiratory endurance, gives this definition:[17]

> "Aerobics refers to a variety of exercises that stimulate heart and lung activity for a time period sufficiently long to produce beneficial changes in the body. Running, swimming, cycling, and jogging—these are typical aerobic exercises. There are many others . . . They have one thing in common: by making you work hard, they demand plenty of oxygen. That's the basic idea. That's what makes them aerobic."

Body Composition

Body composition refers to the body's relative amounts of fat and lean body tissue, or fat-free mass (muscle, bone, water).[15, 16, 18] (See Figure 2.3.) Body weight can be subdivided simply into two components: fat weight and fat-free weight. Fat-free weight comprises all the tissue of the body except for chemical fat.[15] Obesity is defined as an excessive accumulation of fat weight.

Percent body fat, the percent of total weight represented by fat weight, is the preferred index for evaluating a person's body composition.[15] The optimal body fat level for men is less than 15 percent; they are considered obese when their body fat percentage is above 25 percent. The optimal body fat level for women is less than 21 percent, and they are considered obese when their body fat percentage is above 32 percent.

Chapters 5 and 11 will describe how to measure body fat accurately, theories of obesity, the impact of obesity on health, and how to treat obesity.

Musculoskeletal Fitness

Musculoskeletal fitness is comprised of three components: flexibility, muscular strength, and muscular endurance.

1. **Flexibility** is defined as the functional capacity of the joints to move through a full range of

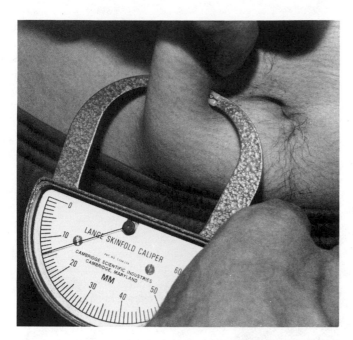

Figure 2.3 Body composition is the body's relative amounts of fat and lean body tissue, or fat-free mass (muscle, bone, water). Chapter 5 will review procedures for measuring body fat through the use of skinfold calipers.

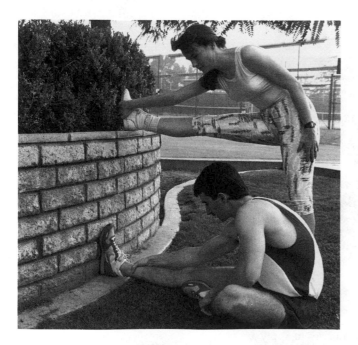

Figure 2.4 Flexibility is defined as the functional capacity of the joints to move through a full range of movement.

movement.[14] (See Figure 2.4.) Flexibility is specific to each joint of the body. Muscles, ligaments, and tendons largely determine the amount of movement possible at each joint.[18] Common flexibility exercises include touching the floor with the hands while the legs are nearly straight, or spreading the legs far out to the side.

Chapter 6 will explain how to test for flexibility; Chapter 8 will discuss the principles of flexibility exercise; Chapter 6 will explore the benefits.

2. **Muscular strength** is the maximal one-effort force that can be exerted against a resistance.[14] (See Figure 2.5.) It is the absolute maximum amount of force that one can generate in an isolated movement of a single muscle group.[19] The stronger the individual, the greater the amount of force that he or she can generate. Common muscular strength exercises include weight lifting with heavy weights.

Chapters 6 and 8 will discuss how to test and develop muscular strength.

3. **Muscular endurance** is defined as the ability of the muscles to apply a submaximal force repeatedly or to sustain a muscular contraction for a certain period of time.[14] (See Figure 2.6.) Common muscle endurance exercises are sit-ups, push-ups, chin-ups, or repetitions of lifting weights. Chapters 6 and 8 will describe how to test and develop muscular endurance.

Sports Medicine Insight
What is Health Promotion?

Three definitions of health promotion have been proposed in the literature.[20-22]

O'Donnell, who is the editor of the *American Journal of Health Promotion*, has written extensively on health promotion.[20] He defines health promotion as the science and art of helping people change their lifestyles to move toward a state of optimal health. The focus is on behaviors that result in improved lifestyle, because only when people take action, only when their behaviors change, do they improve their health.

Health promotion programs have three levels, according to O'Donnell: awareness, behavior change, and supportive environments. Awareness programs increase the participant's understanding of or interest in health related topics. Lifestyle change programs are designed to help participants change physical and emotional health related behaviors (starting to exercise, quitting smoking, learning to manage stress, and so forth).

Lifestyle change programs have a greater chance of success if they take place over time, involve a multistep process, and include a combination of educational, behavior modification and experiential components.

The third level, supportive environments, concerns the importance of the environment in determining behavior. Families, friends, organizational cultures, community laws, and other forces shape these environments. If environments can be created that encourage a healthy lifestyle, there is a greater chance of helping people sustain long-term lifestyle change.

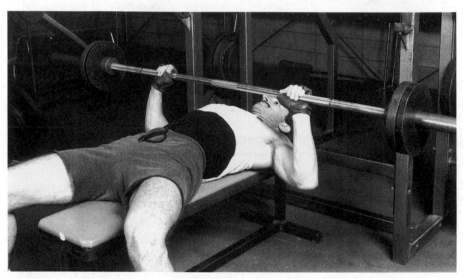

Figure 2.5 Strength is the maximal one-effort force that can be exerted against a resistance.

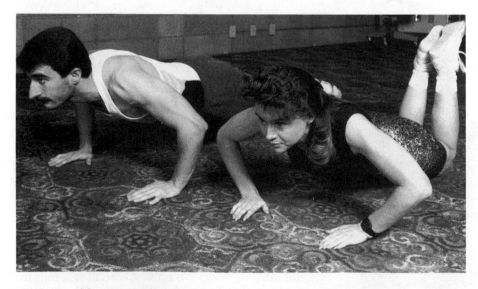

Figure 2.6 Muscular endurance is defined as the ability of the muscles to apply a submaximal force repeatedly or to sustain a muscular contraction for a certain period of time.

Self-responsibility is a central theme in health promotion. A health promotion program will be most successful when it provides the skills and environment necessary for the participant to take responsibility for making choices that are consistent with good health habits.[20]

In 1987, the American Public Health Association published a technical report on the criteria for the development of health promotion.[21] Health promotion was defined as a wide variety of individual and community efforts to encourage or support health behavior and environmental improvement goals and objectives, determined, usually on the basis of epidemiological data, to be important.

Health promotion may involve educational, organizational, economic, and environmental interventions targeted toward specific lifestyle behaviors and environmental conditions that are harmful to health— e.g., smoking, alcohol and drug misuse, inadequate/ inappropriate diet, sedentary patterns of daily living, high stress levels, environmental conditions related to worksite exposure to toxins or the risk of personal injury from accidents, etc. Health education was defined as learning experiences designed to assist individuals, groups or communities in the voluntary control of their own health, as they define it.

This document presented a set of five criteria intended to serve as guidelines for establishing the feasibility and/or the appropriateness of such programs.

1. A health promotion program should address one or more risk factors that are carefully defined, measureable, modifiable, and prevalent among the members of a chosen target group— factors that constitute a threat to the health status and the quality of life of target group members.

2. A health promotion program should reflect a consideration of the special characteristics, needs, and preferences of its target group(s).

3. Health promotion programs should include interventions that will clearly and effectively reduce a targeted risk factor.

4. A health promotion program should identify and implement interventions that make optimum use of available resources.

5. From the outset, a health promotion program should be organized, planned, and implemented in such a way that its operation and effects can be evaluated.

Dr. L. W. Green, a renowned public health educator, has written that health promotion can be defined as any combination of health education and related organizational, economic, and environmental supports for individual, group, and community behavior conducive to health.[22]

The behavior in question ultimately is that of the person whose health is at risk (or whose health enhancement is sought), but the processes of change often must include institutional decision-makers and collectives of people acting in concert as groups, neighborhoods, organizations, communities, and electorates. Behavior at all of these levels and education through all of these channels is the object of health promotion.

Settings for health promotion include most notably schools, worksites, homes, and health care settings. Channels for health promotion include the mass media, parents, teachers, counselors, physicians, nurses, self-help groups, and other individuals and media— through which information, training, and persuasion may assist in producing voluntary adaptations of behavior.

Effective programs to modify or develop health behavior must include some combination of health education and organizational, economic, and environmental supports for that behavior. Environmental supports can be political, physical, economic, social, and legal in nature.

Summary

1. "Physical activity," "exercise," and "physical fitness" are terms that describe different concepts. Physical activity is defined as any bodily movement produced by skeletal muscles that results in energy expenditure. Total energy expenditure is the sum of the energy expended in basal metabolism, the thermic effect of physical activity, and the thermic effect of food. Physical activity includes sleep, and occupational and leisure-time activities.

2. Exercise is a subcategory of physical activity which is planned, structured, repetitive, and purposive in the sense that improvement or maintenance of physical fitness is an objective.

3. A comprehensive definition of physical fitness is: Physical fitness is a dynamic state of energy and vitality that enables one to carry out daily tasks, to engage in active leisure-time pursuits, and to meet unforeseen emergencies without undue fatigue. In addition, physically fit indi-

viduals have a decreased risk of hypokinetic diseases, and are better able to function at their peak intellectual capacity while experiencing a sense of "joie de vivre."

4. The measurable elements of physical fitness fall into two groups, "skill-related fitness" and "health-related fitness." The former include agility, balance, coordination, speed, power, and reaction time. The latter include cardiorespiratory endurance, body composition, and musculoskeletal fitness, which includes flexibility, muscular strength, and muscular endurance.

References

1. Centers for Disease Control. Workshop On Epidemiologic and Public Health Aspects of Physical Activity and Exercise. Public Health Rep 100:113–224, 1985.

2. Caspersen CJ, Powell KE, Christenson GM. Physical Activity, Exercise, and Physical Fitness. Definitions and Distinctions for Health-Related Research. Public Health Rep 100:126–131, 1985.

3. Danforth E. Diet and Obesity. Am J Clin Nutr 41:1132–1145, 1985.

4. Brotherhood JR. Nutrition and Sports Performance. Sports Med 1:350–389, 1984.

5. Goor R, Hosking JD, Dennis BH, et al. Nutrient Intakes Among Selected North American Populations in the Lipid Research Clinics Prevalence Study. Composition of Fat Intake. Am J Clin Nutr 41:299–311, 1985.

6. National Center for Health Statistics, Caroll MD, Abraham S, Dresser CM. Dietary Intake Source Data. United States 1976–80, Second National Health and Nutrition Examination Survey. Vital and Health Statistics. Series II–No. 231. DHHS Pub. No. (PHS) 83–1681. Public Health Service. Washington. U.S. Government Printing Office, March 1983.

7. Nutrient Intakes. Individuals in 48 States, Year 1977–78. Consumer Nutrition Division, Human Nutrition Information Service, U.S. Department of Agriculture, Hyattsville, Maryland 20782. Nationwide Food Consumption Survey 1977–78, Report No. I–2, May 1984.

8. U.S. Department of Agriculture, Human Nutrition Information Service. 1985. Nationwide Food Consumption Survey, Continuing Survey of Food Intakes by Individuals. Women 19–50 Years and Their Children 1–5 Years, 1 Day, 1985. U.S. Dept. of Agric., Rpt. No 85–1. Men 19–50 Years, 1 Day, 1985. U.S. Dept. of Agric., Rpt. No 85–3.

9. President's Council on Physical Fitness and Sports. Physical Fitness Research Digest. Series 1, No. 1. Washington, DC, 1971.

10. Combs BJ, Hales DR, Williams BK. An Invitation to Health: Your Personal Responsibility. Menlo Park. The Benjamin/Cummings Publishing Co., Inc., 1980.

11. Clarke HH. Application of Measurement to Health and Physical Education. Englewood Cliffs. Prentice-Hall, Inc., 1967.

12. Pate RR. A New Definition of Youth Fitness. Physician Sportsmed 11:77–83, 1983.

13. Johnson BL, Nelson JK. Practical Measurements for Evaluation in Physical Education. Minneapolis: Burgess Publishing Co., 1979.

14. Hockey RV. Physical Fitness. The Pathway to Healthful Living. Saint Louis. CV Mosby Co., 1973.

15. AAHPERD. Technical Manual: Health Related Physical Fitness, 1984. 1900 Association Drive, Reston, VA 22091.

16. Blair SN, Falls HB, Pate RR. A New Physical Fitness Test. Physician Sportsmed 11:87–95, 1983.

17. Cooper KH. The New Aerobics. New York: M. Evans and Company, Inc., 1970.

18. Getchell B. Physical Fitness. A Way of Life. New York: John Wiley and Sons, 1983.

19. Pollock ML, Wilmore JH, Fox SM. Exercise in Health and Disease. Evaluation and Prescription for Prevention and Rehabilitation. Philadelphia. WB Saunders Company, 1984.

20. O'Donnell MP. Definition of Health Promotion. Part II: Levels of Programs. Am J Health Promotion 1(2):6–9, 1986.

21. APHA Technical Report. Criteria for the Development of Health Promotion and Education Programs. Am J Public Health 77:89–92, 1987.

22. Green LW. Modifying and Developing Health Behavior. Ann Rev Public Health 5:215–236, 1984.

23. Thomas Kirk Cureton, Jr., *Physical Fitness and Dynamic Health*. The Dial Press, 1965.

Physical Fitness Activity 2.1— Ranking Activities by Health-Related Value

As discussed in this chapter, there are five measurable elements of health-related fitness:

The Measurable Elements of Health-Related Physical Fitness

Cardiorespiratory Endurance

Body Composition

Flexibility

Muscular Endurance ⎫ *Musculoskeletal*

Muscular Strength ⎭ *Fitness*

Sports and other forms of physical activity vary in their capacity to develop each component. In this physi-

cal fitness activity, you will be ranking different sports and exercises in terms of their capacity to promote such development, using a five point scale for each of the five health-related fitness components. Answer the questions to the best of your ability, and then *compare your answers in a group session with your teacher or your local fitness expert.*

Rate each physical activity or sport in terms of its capacity to develop each of the five health-related components: 1 = not at all; 2 = somewhat or just a little bit; 3 = moderately; 4 = strongly; 5 = very strongly. Then answer the following question.

1. What five activities received the highest total score (add the five component scores for each activity)?

   #1 Overall activity _____

   #2 Overall activity _____

   #3 Overall activity _____

   #4 Overall activity _____

   #5 Overall activity _____

Physical Activity	Cardio-respiratory	Body Composition	Flexibility	Muscular Endurance	Muscular Strength	Total
Archery						
Backpacking						
Badminton						
Basketball						
non-game						
gameplay						
Bicycling						
pleasure						
15 mph						
Bowling						
Canoeing, Rowing, Kayaking						
Calisthenics						
Dancing						
social and square						
aerobic						

Physical Activity	Cardio-respiratory	Body Composition	Flexibility	Muscular Endurance	Muscular Strength	Total
Fencing						
Fishing						
bank, boat, or ice						
stream, wading						
Football (Touch)						
Golf						
power cart						
walking, with bag						
Handball						
Hiking, Cross Country						
Horseback Riding						
Paddleball, Racquetball						
Rope Jumping						
Running						
12 min per mile						
6 min per mile						
Sailing						
Scuba Diving						
Skating						
ice						
roller						
Skiing, Snow						
downhill						
cross country						
Skiing, Water						
Sledding, Tobogganing						
Snowshoeing						
Squash						
Soccer						
Stair Climbing						
Swimming						

Physical Activity	Cardio-respiratory	Body Composition	Flexibility	Muscular Endurance	Muscular Strength	Total
Table Tennis						
Tennis						
Volleyball						
Walking, Briskly						
Weight Training, Circuit						
Brick Laying, Plastering						
Painting, Masonry						
Shoveling Light Earth						
Splitting Wood						
Digging Ditches						

Part 2

Testing

Chapter 3

Physical Fitness Testing Concepts

"Obviously, there is no precise and completely reliable way of gauging a person's physical fitness. The real test is intuitive, and the truly fit person can know that he is truly fit only by sensing that he is deriving the most possible satisfaction from living."—Thomas K. Cureton

Before the Exercise Program Begins

This chapter will focus on some of the preliminary considerations that are considered necessary when individuals start an exercise program. Preliminary information includes the following:

1. The American College of Sports Medicine Classification Categories
2. Medical/health status questionnaire
3. Determination of cardiovascular disease risk
4. Medical evaluation and the graded exercise test
5. Informed consent
6. Physical fitness testing concepts and the purposes of testing
7. Choosing a physical fitness testing battery

The American College of Sports Medicine Classification Categories

The American College of Sports Medicine has advised that people wishing to enter an exercise program should be classified first, according to one of the categories described in Table 3.1.

Medical/Health Status Questionnaire

To classify an individual according to the ACSM categories, the *Medical/Health Status Questionnaire* should be given to each potential participant.

The medical/health status questionnaire should include the following:[1,2]

- Personal and family history of cardiovascular disease
- Personal medical history
- Cardiovascular risk factors (lifestyle habits such as smoking, diet, exercise, alcohol intake, stress, social networks, working environment)
- Present medications and treatment
- History of chest discomfort, pressure, pain, and other symptoms

Table 3.1 Classification of Individuals by Health Status Prior to Exercise Testing or Exercise Prescription

Category	Description
Apparently Healthy	Those who are asymptomatic* and apparently healthy with no more than one major coronary risk factor.**
Individuals at Higher Risk	Those who have symptoms suggestive of possible cardiopulmonary or metabolic disease (see next category) disease and/or two or more major coronary risk factors.
Individuals with Disease	Those with known cardiac, pulmonary, or metabolic disease (diabetes, thryoid disorders, renal disease, liver disease).

*Major symptoms or signs suggestive of cardiopulmonary or metabolic disease include: 1) pain or discomfort in the chest or surrounding areas that appear to be ischemic (deficiency of blood supply due to obstruction of the circulation) in nature; 2) unaccustomed shortness of breath or shortness of breath with mild exertion; 3) dizziness or fainting; 4) difficulty in breathing when standing or sudden breathing problems during the night; 5) ankle edema; 6) rapid throbbing or fluttering of the heart; 7) severe pain in leg muscles during walking; known heart murmur.

**If an individual has two or more of the following coronary risk factors, he would be classified as an individual at higher risk:
1. Diagnosed hypertension or systolic blood pressure ≥160 or diastolic blood pressure ≥90 mmHg on at least two separate occasions, or on antihypertensive medication.
2. Serum cholesterol ≥ 240 mg/dl.
3. Cigarette smoking.
4. Diabetes mellitus (if over age 30 with a long history of this disease, should be classified as "individual with disease.")
5. Family history of coronary or other atherosclerotic disease in parents or siblings prior to age 55.

Source: Adapted from the American College of Sports Medicine. *Guidelines for Exercise Testing and Prescription* (4th edition). Philadelphia: Lea & Febiger, 1991.

Examples of medical/health status questionnaires can be found in several different books.[1,2,3] (See Appendix A for an example of an employee wellness program medical/health status questionnaire used at the Loma Linda University Center for Health Promotion.)

The information obtained with the questionnaire will enable each participant to be classified according to an ACSM category. In addition, questionnaire data enhance a professional's ability to interpret exercise testing data.[2] In Chapter 8, emphasis will be placed upon using the medical/health status questionnaire to individualize the exercise prescription. The more background information obtained, the greater the ability to meet individual needs.

In some circumstances, particularly when testing large numbers of people in relatively short time periods, a shorter, simpler medical/health questionnaire is preferable. A simple, brief medical questionnaire called the *Physical Activity Readiness Questionnaire* (PAR-Q) has been used very successfully in Canada.[4] (See Figure 3.1.) The PAR-Q appears to be a valid screening instrument for both submaximal exercise step testing and for beginning moderate and gently progressive (but not heavy or violent) exercise programs.[5] Moderate and gradually progressive exercise has been found to be generally safe for those who are at low risk for heart or metabolic diseases.

Cardiovascular Disease Risk Factor Analysis

The medical/health status questionnaire can assist exercise leaders in determining participants' risk of cardiovascular disease (CVD). A full description of the major CVD risk factors will be given in Chapter 10. The six major risk factors according to ACSM were listed in Table 3.1. Table 3.2 outlines optimal, moderately high, and high risk values for the three primary CVD risk factors (high blood pressure, cigarette smoking, and high levels of serum cholesterol).

Medical Evaluation and the Graded Exercise Test

A careful evaluation of individuals prior to exercise testing or participation in an exercise program is important to assure safety, to aid in diagnosis of cardiovascular disease, to assess heart and lung fitness, to make appropriate recommendations for an exercise program, to follow the progress of the exercising individual, to identify those who need more comprehensive testing, and for developing rapport with the participant.[1] An exercise test can only be interpreted properly when

PHYSICAL ACTIVITY READINESS QUESTIONNAIRE (PAR-Q)
A Self-administered Questionnaire for Adults

PARTICIPANT IDENTIFICATION

____

____

____

____

____

PAR-Q & YOU

PAR-Q is designed to help you help yourself. Many health benefits are associated with regular exercise, and the completion of PAR-Q is a sensible first step to take if you are planning to increase the amount of physical activity in your life.

For most people physical activity should not pose any problem or hazard. PAR-Q has been designed to identify the small number of adults for whom physical activity might be inappropriate or those who should have medical advice concerning the type of activity most suitable for them.

Common sense is your best guide in answering these few questions. Please read them carefully and check the ❑ YES or NO opposite the question if it applies to you.

YES	NO	
❑	❑	1. Has your doctor ever said you have heart trouble?
❑	❑	2. Do you frequently have pains in your heart and chest?
❑	❑	3. Do you often feel faint or have spells of severe dizziness?
❑	❑	4. Has a doctor ever said your blood pressure was too high?
❑	❑	5. Has your doctor ever told you that you have a bone or joint problem such as arthritis that has been aggravated by exercise, or might be made worse with exercise?
❑	❑	6. Is there a good physical reason not mentioned here why you should not follow an activity program even if you wanted to?
❑	❑	7. Are you over age 65 and not accustomed to vigorous exercise?

IF YOU ANSWERED

YES to one or more questions

If you have not recently done so, consult with your personal physician by telephone or in person BEFORE increasing your physical activity and/or taking a fitness test. Tell him what questions you answered YES on PAR-Q, or show him your copy.

programs

After medical evaluation, seek advice from your physician as to your suitability for:
- unrestricted physical activity, probably on a gradually increasing basis.
- restricted or supervised activity to meet your specific needs, at least on an initial basis. Check in your community for special programs or services.

NO to all questions

If you answered PAR-Q accurately, you have reasonable assurance of your present suitability for:
- A GRADUATED EXERCISE PROGRAM- A gradual increase in proper exercise promotes good fitness development while minimizing or eliminating discomfort.
- AN EXERCISE TEST- Simple tests of fitness (such as the Canadian Home Fitness Test) or more complex types may be undertaken if you so desire.

postpone

If you have a temporary minor illness, such as a common cold.

Figure 3.1 The Physical Activity Readiness Questionnaire (PAR-Q) is useful in health fair or mass testing situationsfor screening out individuals at risk for cardiovascular or metabolic disease.[5]

Table 3.2 Categorization of the Primary Risk Factors and Blood Values

Risk Factor	Optimal Value	Moderately High Risk	High Risk
Blood Pressure	<120/80 mm Hg	140/90 • 160/95 mm Hg	>160/95 mm Hg
Cigarettes/Day	None	10 – 20	20+
Cholesterol (mg/dl)			
Age 20–29	<160	160 – 220	+220
Age 30–39	<180	180 – 240	+240
Age 40+	<190	190 – 260	+260
Total Chol/HDL Ratio	<3.5	4.5 – 5.0	+5.0

See Chapter 10 for an overview of these risk factors.

physicians and exercise leaders have adequate background knowledge concerning the individual being tested.

A physical examination for any individual is recommended, the depth of evaluation depending on the health status of the individual. Laboratory tests such as total cholesterol and high-density lipoprotein cholesterol are helpful in determining whether an individual fits in the higher risk category. The most important part of the pretest evaluation, however, is the medical history.[1]

In general, most individuals, except for those with known serious disease, can begin a moderate exercise program such as walking (40–60% $\dot{V}O_{2max}$) without a medical evaluation or exercise test.[1] Whenever one is in doubt about his/her own personal safety while exercising, a medical routine evaluation is recommended. Exercise testing is not recommended as a routine screening procedure in adults who have no evidence of heart disease. Risk of serious medical complications during exercise is low unless an individual is at high risk for cardiovascular disease.

Guidelines for exercise testing and physician supervision are given below.

Apparently Healthy Individuals

Apparently healthy individuals can begin moderate (intensities of 40 to 60% $\dot{V}O_{2max}$) exercise programs, such as walking or increasing usual daily activities, without the need for exercise testing or medical examination.[1] This is especially true when the moderate exercise program proceeds gradually, and the individual is alert to the development of the signs and symptoms listed in Table 3.1.

Prior to starting a vigorous exercise program (>60% $\dot{V}O_{2max}$), apparently healthy men above the age of 40 or women above the age of 50 would do well to have a medical examination and a maximal exercise test (with physician supervision). The distinction between moderate and vigorous exercise is an important one. While untrained individuals can usually exercise moderately safely and comfortably for about 60 minutes, vigorous exercise cannot be sustained for more than 15 to 20 minutes, and results in a significant increase in heart rate and breathing.

At any age, the information garnered from a maximal exercise test is useful to establish an effective and safe exercise prescription. Submaximal testing up to 75% of age-predicted maximal heart rates can be conducted without physician supervision, but provides less valuable information for exercise prescription or fitness status determination.

Exercise testing is relatively safe with only one death per 20,000 tests reported in the literature.[1] In one clinic, no deaths after more than 70,000 maximal exercise tests has been reported.

Individuals at Higher Risk

Individuals at higher risk are those with two or more major coronary risk factors and/or symptoms suggestive of heart, lung, or metabolic disease (metabolic diseases include diabetes mellitus, thyroid disorders, kidney disease, liver disease, and other less common forms) (see Table 3.1). A maximal GXT prior to beginning a vigorous exercise program is desirable for high risk individuals of any age, especially in those with symptoms.[1] For those without symptoms, an exercise test or medical examination may not be necessary if moderate exercise (such as walking) is undertaken gradually with appropriate guidance. The maximal GXT should be physician supervised. Although submaximal exercise tests are of little diagnostic value for individuals at higher risk, if such a test is given for fitness assessment purposes, it is not necessary to have a physician present if the patient has no symptoms of disease.

Patients with Disease

A complete medical evaluation with a physician-supervised maximal GXT is recommended before starting an exercise program for all individuals with known heart, blood vessel, lung, or metabolic disease. Test results can help the physician make appropriate decisions to ensure the safety of exercise for the patient, and also allow progress to be monitored.[1]

Table 3.3 summarizes the major points from this section.

These American College of Sports Medicine (ACSM) guidelines are in agreement with other published recommendations. The National Heart, Lung, and Blood Institute's 1981, 40-page consumer booklet entitled "Exercise and Your Heart" advises that people at low risk for heart disease and without symptoms do not need to see a physician before starting an exercise

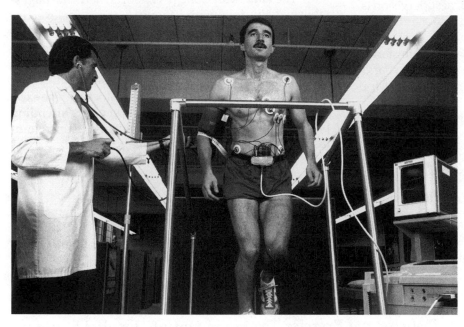

Figure 3.2 For people of all ages, information from the maximal graded exercise test is valuable in establishing an effective and safe exercise prescription.

Table 3.3 Guidelines for Exercise Testing and Participation

	Apparently Healthy Younger*	Older	Higher Risk No Symptoms	Higher Risk Symptoms	With Disease
Medical exam and diagnostic exercise test recommended prior to:					
Moderate exercise (40–60% $\dot{V}O_{2max}$)	No**	No	No	Yes	Yes
Vigorous exercise (>60% $\dot{V}O_{2max}$)	No	Yes	Yes	Yes	Yes
Physician supervision recommended during exercise test:					
Sub-maximal testing	No	No	No	Yes	Yes
Maximal testing	No	Yes	Yes	Yes	Yes

*≤40 years for men, ≤50 years for women
**The "no" responses in this table mean that an item is "not necessary."
  The "no" response does not mean that the item should not be done.
  The "yes" response means that an item is recommended.

Source: Adapted from: American College of Sports Medicine. Guidelines for Exercise Testing and Prescription (4th edition). Philadelphia: Lea & Febiger, 1991.

program.[6] The American Heart Association in 1981 simply stated that "older sedentary individuals may also wish to seek medical advice."[7]

Some argue that while it might be ideal for everyone to see a doctor and have a treadmill-EKG test before starting an exercise program, this is neither practical, economically feasible, nor desirable.[2] It is simply unrealistic to recommend comprehensive medical evaluations for the total population.

If a GXT is administered for a diagnostic purpose, or is performed on people who have or are at high risk for cardiovascular disease, direct medical supervision is necessary.[1,2] On the other hand, nondiagnostic tests of apparently healthy people for purposes of physical fitness status determination can be safely administered without direct physician supervision. The YMCA and many other fitness centers have been doing this for years.

Astrand, the European exercise physiologist who has done much to mold thought and opinion about exercise over the last two decades, summarizes this discussion as follows:[8]

"Anyone who is in doubt about the condition of his health should consult his physician. But as a general rule, moderate activity is less harmful to the health than inactivity. You could also put it this way: A medical examination is more urgent for those who plan to remain inactive than for those who intend to get into good physical shape."

Contraindications for Exercise and Exercise Testing

Although most people in the United States can be safely evaluated and started on an exercise program, there are some who should not exercise. The risks for such people outweigh the benefits.

The American College of Sports Medicine has established the following *contraindications* for exercise and exercise testing in out-of-hospital settings.[1] A contraindication means that most experts would agree that it is inadvisable for the individual to be exercise tested or to engage in active exercise. These contraindications should be diagnosed only by medical doctors. The exercise leader should draw the attention of the attending physician to this ACSM contraindication listing (summarized in Box 3.1).

Informed Consent

Like it or not, we live in an increasingly litigious society.[9] Today's exercise program director, recreation adminis-

---

Box 3.1   Contraindications for Exercise and Exercise Testing in Out-of-Hospital Settings

Absolute Contraindications

A recent significant change in the resting ECG suggesting infarction or other acute cardiac events

Recent complicated myocardial infarction

Unstable angina

Uncontrolled ventricular dysrhythmia

Uncontrolled atrial dysrhythmia that compromises cardiac function

Third degree heart block

Acute congestive heart failure

Severe aortic stenosis

Suspected or known dissecting aneurysm

Active or suspected myocarditis or pericarditis

Thrombophlebitis or intracardiac thrombi

Recent systemic or pulmonary embolus

Acute infection

Significant emotional distress (psychosis)

Relative Contraindications (Benefits of evaluation often exceed risk)

Resting diastolic blood pressure over 120 mm Hg; systolic over 200 mm Hg

Moderate valvular heart disease

Known electrolyte abnormalities (hypokalemia, hypomagnesemia)

Fixed rate artificial pacemaker (rarely used)

Frequent or complex ventricular ectopy

Ventricular aneurysm

Cardiomyopathy including hypertrophic cardiomyopathy

Uncontrolled metabolic disease (diabetes, thyrotoxicosis, myxedema, etc.)

Chronic infectious disease (mononucleosis, hepatitis, AIDS, etc.)

Neuromuscular, musculoskeletal, or rheumatoid disorders which would make exercise difficult

Advanced or complicated pregnancy

Source: Adapted from American College of Sports Medicine. Guidelines for Exercise Testing and Prescription. Philadelphia: Lea & Febiger, 1991.

trator, or exercise testing program director is much more likely to be sued than his or her predecessors.

By law, any subject, patient, or client who is exposed to possible physical, psychological, or social injury must give informed consent prior to participation in a program.[10] *Informed consent* can be defined as the knowing consent of an individual or his legally authorized representative, able to exercise free power of choice without undue inducement or any element of force, fraud, deceit, duress, or other form of constraint or coercion.

The subject should read the Informed Consent Form, and then sign in the presence of a witness, indicating that the document has been read and consent given to participation under the described conditions. The consent form should be written so as to be easily understood by each participant, in the language in which the person is fluent.

Separate forms should be used for diagnostic exercise testing and for the exercise program itself. (See Boxes 3.2 and 3.3 for sample forms.) The following items should be included in the informed consent form.[1, 2, 3, 10]

Box 3.2   Consent to Graded Exercise Testing and Other Physical Fitness Tests

Testing Objectives:

I understand that the tests that are about to be administered to me are for the purpose of determining my physical fitness status, including heart, lung, and blood vessel capacities for whole body activity, body composition (ratio of body fat to muscle, bone, and water), muscular endurance and strength, and joint flexibility.

Explanation of Procedures:

I understand that the tests which I will undergo will be performed on a treadmill, bicycle, or steps. The tests are designed to increase the demands on the heart, lung, and blood vessel system. This increase in effort will continue until exhaustion or other symptoms prohibit further exercise. During the test, heart rate, blood pressure, and electrocardiographic data will be periodically measured. Body composition will be determined through use of skinfolds or underwater weighing to determine levels of body fat versus fat-free weight. Muscular endurance and strength will be determined through use of body calisthenics and/or equipment. The sit-and-reach test will be used to determine the flexibility of the hip joint.

Description of Potential Risks:

I understand that there exists the possibility that certain abnormal changes may occur during the testing. These changes could include abnormal heart beats, abnormal blood pressure response, various muscle and joint strains or injuries, and in rare instances, heart attack. Professional care

throughout the entire testing process should provide appropriate precaution against such problems.

Benefits to be Expected:

I understand that the results of these tests will aid in determining my physical fitness status, and in determining potential health hazards. These results will facilitate a better individualized exercise prescription.

I have read the foregoing information and understand it. Questions concerning these procedures have been answered to my satisfaction. I also understand that I am free to deny answering any questions during the evaluation process or to withdraw consent and discontinue participating in any procedures. I have also been informed that the information derived from these tests is confidential and will not be disclosed to anyone other than my physician or others who are involved in my care or exercise prescription without my permission. However I am in agreement that information from these tests not identifiable to me can be used for research purposes.

Participant's Signature _____

Date _____

Witness Signature_____

Date _____

1. A general statement of the background of the program and objectives.

2. A fair explanation of the procedures to be followed.

3. A description of any and all risks attendant to the procedures.

4. A description of the benefits that can reasonably be expected.

5. An offer to answer any of the subject's queries.

6. An instruction that the subject, client, or patient is free to withdraw consent and to discontinue participation in the program at any time without prejudice to the person.

7. An instruction that, in the case of questionnaires and interviews, the participant is free to refuse to answer specific items or questions.

8. An explanation of the procedures to be taken to insure the confidentiality of the information derived from the participant.

While it should be understood that execution of an informed consent form does not protect the exercise or medical director from legal action, if the program is in accordance with established guidelines and run by

---

Box 3.3 Consent for Physical Fitness Program

General Statement of Program Objectives and Procedures:

I understand that this physical fitness program may include exercises to build the cardiorespiratory system (heart and lungs), the musculoskeletal system (muscle endurance and strength, and flexibility), and to improve body composition (decrease of body fat in individuals needing to lose fat, with an increase in weight of muscle and bone). Exercises may include aerobic activities (treadmill walking/running, bicycle riding, rowing machine exercise, group aerobic activity, swimming, and other such activities), calisthenics, and weight lifting to improve muscular strength and endurance, and flexibility exercises to improve joint range of motion.

Description of Potential Risks:

I understand that the reaction of the heart, lung, and blood vessel system to such exercise cannot always be predicted with accuracy. I know there is a risk of certain abnormal changes occurring during or following exercise which may include abnormalities of blood pressure or heart rate, ineffective functioning of the heart, and in rare instances, heart attacks. Use of the weight lifting equipment, and engaging in heavy body calisthenics, can lead to musculoskeletal strains, pain, and injury if adequate warm-up, gradual progression, and safety procedures are not followed. Safety procedures are listed on the wall of the fitness facility. In addition, trained staff members will be supervising during all times to help ensure that these risks are minimized. The staff are trained in CPR and first aid, and regularly practice emergency procedures. Equipment is inspected and maintained on a regular basis.

Description of Potential Benefits:

I understand that a program of regular exercise for the heart and lungs, muscles and joints, has many associated benefits. These may include a decrease in body fat, improvement in blood fats and blood pressure, improvement in psychological function, and a decrease in risk of heart disease

I have read the foregoing information and understand it. Any questions which may have occurred to me have been answered to my satisfaction. I understand that I am free to withdraw from this program without prejudice at any time I desire. I am also free to deny answers to specific items or questions during interviews or when filling out questionnaires. The information which is obtained will be treated as privileged and confidential and will not be released or revealed to any person other than my physician without my expressed written consent. The information obtained, however, may be used for a statistical or scientific purpose with my right of privacy retained.

Participant's Signature _____

Date _____

Witness Signature _____

Date _____

qualified staff, and the participant voluntarily assumes risk as outlined in the consent form, the possibility of legal action is minimized.[1, 3]

Strategies for Reducing Liability Exposure

Rates for insurance premiums are rising quickly, reducing profit margins of club industries.[11] Fitness facilities are finding it more and more difficult to find insurance companies to cover them. There are several strategies for reducing liability exposure:[9, 12, 13]

1. Purchase as much insurance as you and your program can afford and include indemnity provisions in all contracts whenever possible.

2. Establish a risk management committee to review all policies and procedures from a safety and litigation perspective.

3. Establish written policies for: hiring and firing of personnel; training and competency assessment of instructors and supervisors; routine record keeping; in-service or continuing education; medical care; inspection, maintenance and use of equipment and facilities; insurance coverage; travel and transportation; contracts with outside entities; public relations; crowd control; accident reporting. Establish forms and checklists for each.

4. Provide opportunities for all staff to have training in CPR and first aid. In addition, all staff should obtain certification, preferably from the American College of Sports Medicine, to demonstrate competence. (See Sports Medicine Insight at the end of this chapter.)

5. Establish and publicize (post) procedures for injuries and emergencies. Rules and regulations and safety recommendations should be clearly posted in all areas.

6. Regularly analyze and critique effectiveness of staff in terms of safe leadership and participation.

7. Ensure that participants are at all times supervised. Make sure that supervisors know policies for stopping dangerous activities, and that safety rules are enforced. Make sure supervisors are competent and trained to perform their jobs.

8. Ensure that supervisors make frequent inspections of the equipment and facility, analyzing

them from a safety perspective, and that safety checklists have been published.[14]

9. Use nationally recognized screening, pretesting, and program procedures, preferably those of the American College of Sports Medicine.

10. Use accepted consent forms, supplemented with oral explanations.

11. Individualize information so that it is appropriate for individual participants.

Equipment-related injuries are a common cause of participant claims and litigation. Several principles should be followed that will help minimize the threat of these types of lawsuits:[15]

1. Equipment should be of good design and free from defects.

2. Equipment should be inspected when received and assembled in strict compliance with the manufacturer's instructions.

3. Equipment should be arranged appropriately within the facility so as to permit intended and safe participant use.

4. Equipment should be tested prior to being placed in service.

5. Warnings should be provided and displayed appropriately.

6. Clear, concise, and correct instruction should be given each participant before use.

According to Dr. Herb Appenzeller, author of six books on legal issues in sports and fitness, there are five general factors that influence liability:[9]

1. Ignorance of the law (simply not knowing the law).

2. Ignoring the law (doing something that you know is contrary to law).

3. Failure to act (knowing that you should do something, but failing to act).

4. Failure to warn (not making everyone sufficiently aware of the dangers).

5. Expense (failing to budget or spend money to further your safety objectives).

Thus, risk management strategy simply means that potential for litigation is minimized through routine inspection and maintenance of equipment and facilities, anticipation of foreseeable problem areas, reasonable administrative policies, and the exercise of common sense.[9]

Concepts and Purposes in Physical Fitness Testing

Reduced to its simplest terms, the function of measurement is to determine status.[16] Status needs to be determined before individualized exercise counseling can be conducted. The information from the physical fitness testing is used along with the medical test information to better meet the individual's needs.

When conducting physical fitness tests, several important test criteria should be considered:

1. **Validity**—refers to the degree to which the test measures what it was designed to measure. A valid test is one that measures accurately what it is used to measure.[17]

2. **Reliability**—deals with how consistently a certain element is measured by the particular test.[18] It is concerned with the repeatability of the test—if a person is measured two separate times by two different people, the result should be close to the same.

3. **Norms**—represent the achievement level of a particular group to which the measured scores can be compared.[18] Norms provide a useful basis for interpretation and evaluation of test results.

4. **Economy**—refers to ease of administration, the use of inexpensive equipment, the limitation of time needed to administer the test, and the simplicity of the test so that the person taking it can easily understand the purpose and results.[12, 16, 17]

So in other words, a good physical fitness test measures what it is supposed to accurately, can be consistently used by different people, produces results that can be compared to a data set, and is relatively inexpensive, simple, and easy to administer.

In a complete physical fitness program, testing of participants before, during, and after participation is important for several reasons:[19, 20]

1. To assess current fitness levels
2. To identify special needs for individualized counseling
3. To evaluate progress
4. To motivate

Test results are a means to an end.[21] They should not be considered as an end in themselves. Expensive, elaborate, and lengthy testing is seldom needed, and can detract from the exercise program itself. Scores on the various items of the simple and inexpensive test batteries noted at the end of this chapter are adequate to identify the strengths and weaknesses of participants, so that special attention can be given within individualized programs. If anything, it is better to undertest than overtest, so that more time and attention can be given to counseling and guiding each participant through the exercise program.

It is important to emphasize that the testing process should never be allowed to become a separate entity.[21] The testing process is merely the stepping stone in the progress towards better understanding, attitudes, and practices in health and fitness.

Physical Fitness Testing Batteries

The very process of administering a fitness test draws attention to what is considered worthy of special attention in a person's lifestyle. The test results can therefore be used to educate, motivate, and stimulate interest in exercise and other health-related topics.

Recommended Order for Fitness Evaluation Tests

The evaluation procedure has a recommended order for both safety and efficiency. In general, it is best for the participant to fill out the medical/health status questionnaire at home before coming to the testing center. The testing batteries listed at the end of this chapter usually take only 1-1/2 to 2 hours.

Precise instructions should be given to the participants before they come to the testing site. In general they should come in jogging attire (and bring a swim suit if necessary); should avoid eating or drinking for 3 hours before the test; should avoid alcohol, tobacco, and coffee for at least 3 hours before the test; avoid exercise the day of the test; try to get a good night's sleep; bring the medical/health status questionnaire.

If blood is to be analyzed, alcohol consumption and vigorous exercise should be avoided for 24 hours beforehand,[2] and a 12-hour fast is recommended. Diabetics should be allowed to keep their dietary habits and injections of insulin as regular as possible.

The organization of the testing session is important. It should begin with the quiet, resting tests (heart rate, blood pressure, blood drawing, all after a 5-minute rest). Body composition measures should follow next, then the graded exercise test for cardiorespiratory endurance. Finally, the musculoskeletal tests should be given.

This order is very important. If musculoskeletal tests precede the graded exercise test, the heart rate can be elevated, giving false information on fitness status, especially when submaximal tests are conducted.

Immediate feedback and counseling should follow the testing.

Follow-up evaluations should be conducted after 3 to 6 months, after 1 year of training, and yearly thereafter.[2]

Health-Related Fitness Testing Batteries

The YMCA, Fitness and Amateur Sport in Canada, the American Association of Health, Physical Education, Recreation and Dance (AAHPERD), and the Public Health Service have each developed physical fitness testing batteries that follow the recommended criteria of testing outlined earlier in this chapter. They are valid, reliable, economic, and have sound norms. In addition, they each follow a comprehensive "health-related" fitness approach, testing each of the five components.

The norms for the various tests within these batteries are found in Appendix B. Descriptions of how to conduct the tests are found in Part 2. A brief outline of each testing battery is listed below.

YMCA

The YMCA physical fitness testing battery is administered in the following order:[19]

- Standing height
- Weight
- Resting heart rate
- Resting blood pressure
- Skinfold tests for men and women (at three or four sites)
- Submaximal bicycle test for cardiorespiratory endurance (3-minute step test for mass testing)
- Sit-and-reach test for flexibility
- Bench press test (35 pounds, women; 80 pounds, men) at a rate of 30 times per minute for muscular endurance and strength
- One-minute timed sit-ups for abdominal muscular endurance

Fitness and Amateur Sport, Canada

In 1981, the Canada Fitness Survey (CFS) was initiated and funded by Fitness and Amateur Sport in Canada.[22] A major objective of the survey was to provide reliable statistics on physical activity patterns and fitness levels of the Canadian population. The survey sample consisted of 11,884 households that had been identified by Statistics Canada, and that were located in urban and rural areas of each province. Fifteen thousand five hundred and nineteen members of these households between the ages of 7 and 69 undertook the Canadian Standardized Test of Fitness. The CFS was the largest and most comprehensive study of physical activity and fitness ever undertaken. (See Appendix B.)

Wellsource, Inc., has developed a computer software program based on the Canadian Fitness Survey results.[23] The printout adds a "high-tech" touch that can help create a more favorable environment for motivating the participant. (See Figure 3.3.)

The Wellsource, Inc., computer software program includes the following:

- Resting heart rate
- Resting blood pressure
- Three-site skinfold test (chest, abdomen, and thigh for men; triceps, suprailium, and thigh for women)

The computer program will also accept results from hydrostatic weighing.*

- Canadian home fitness test for cardiorespiratory endurance (The computer program will also accept time to exhaustion on the Bruce's treadmill test, total time for the Cooper 1.5 mile running test, results from a submaximal bicycle test, or any distance over 1.5 miles run in best time.)
- Sit-and-reach test for flexibility
- Hand-grip dynamometer test (both hands) for muscular strength
- One-minute timed sit-ups for abdominal muscular endurance
- Push-ups (consecutively, without a time limit) for upper body muscular strength and endurance.

AAHPERD: Health-Related Fitness Test for College Students

AAHPERD released the results of their new testing program for college students in 1985.[24] The study

---

*The Canadian Standardized Test of Fitness included other anthropometric measurements, including girths of chest, waist, hip, and right thigh, and five skinfold measurements (triceps, biceps, subscapular, iliac crest, and medial calf).

population consisted of 5,158 young adults in colleges from all geographic regions of the United States. The data for the study were collected under the supervision of 24 coinvestigators. The test items in order are as follows:

- Two-site skinfold test (triceps and subscapular)

- Mile run or nine-minute run for cardiorespiratory endurance

- Sit-and-reach test for flexibility

- One-minute timed sit-ups for abdominal muscular endurance

AAHPERD released the instructions for and results of the new health-related testing program for children and youth in 1980. It marked the beginning of a new era for physical education in the United States. The test items were the same as the ones listed above for the college students.

Public Health Service: National Children and Youth Fitness Study

Recently the U.S. Public Health Service, in response to the landmark government report, *Promoting Health/Preventing Disease: Objectives for the Nation*, launched the National Children and Youth Fitness Study

---

FITNESS PROFILE

Report for: Brown, John   **Rec. #8**   **ID# 15460**   **M 38**   **08-30-1988**

Fitness Factors	Test Results	V. Low	Low	Avg	Good	Excel	Fitness Score
Body Composition							
Percent body fat (%)	14.5	******** *** *****	*** *****	*** ******	*** *** >		30/30
Present Weight (lbs.)	165	21	18	16	15		
Fat weight (lbs.)	24						
Ideal wt. based on 12%	160						
Musculoskeletal Fitness							
Grip Strength (Kg)	90	******** *** *****	*** >				5/10
Both hands combined		6	88	106	125		
Abdominal Strength	25	******** **** *****	** >				5/19
# situps in one min.		15	25	34	44		
Arm strength	20	******** *** **** *	*** *** >				5/10
# pushups in one min.		12	17	22	30		
Flexibility (in.)	12.0	******** *** *****	*** *** >				5/10
Sit and reach test		5	10	14	18		
Cardiovascular Fitness							
Resting pulse (b/min)	70	******** *** *****	*** ***** >				5/10
		88	78	68	58		
Resting BP systolic	140	******** >					1/10
		139	130	120	110		
Resting BP diastolic	83	******** *** *****	*** ***** >				5/10
		89	86	82	80		
Aerobic workouts/week	0	>					1/10
20–30+ minutes/session		2	3	4	5		
Aerobic power	43.6	******** **** *****	*** *** >				15/30
V̇O₂max (ml/kg min)		35	40	45	49		
Total Fitness Score	55	******** *** *****	*** ***** >				55/100
Recommended score of 60+		20	40	60	80		

Figure 3.3 Summary of results of Canadian Fitness Survey (CFS) results developed by Wellsource Inc. A fitness score is tabulated for each test item based on a comparison of test results with CFS norms. An exercise prescription based on exercise history and test results accompanies test results.

(NCYFS 1) to determine how fit and how active 1st through 12th-grade students actually are.[25] Data on 10- to 18-year-olds were collected from a random sample of 10,275 students from 140 public and private schools in 19 states between February and May, 1984. The NCYFS I was the first nationwide assessment of the physical fitness of American young people in nearly a decade, and the most rigorous study of fitness among our youth ever conducted.

Fitness norms were last developed on a national sample of school children in 1975. These norms reflect children's performance on the AAHPERD Youth Fitness Test, which is primarily a test of motor fitness (or athletic ability).[25]

The more recently developed AAHPERD Health-Related Physical Fitness Test (HRPFT),[21] released in 1980, measures aspects of fitness that are related to and predictive of health.

Unfortunately, the HRPFT used "convenience sample" norms (with students who were readily available in schools that had volunteered to assist in norms development) instead of nationally representative sample norms. The NCYFS norms are nationally representative. The HRPFT set more stringent standards for the mile run and sit-ups test because the less fit and less motivated students tended to be excluded.[25]

The NCYFS not only has better norms than the older 1980 AAHPERD HRPFT battery, but has also added one other test, chin-ups, to better measure upper body muscular strength and endurance. The norms are found in Appendix B. Descriptions of the tests are found in Part 2. Here is an outline of the testing battery, in the suggested order:

- Two-site skinfold test (triceps and subscapular)
- Mile run (for cardiorespiratory endurance)
- Sit-and-reach test for flexibility
- Chin-ups (for upper body muscular strength and endurance)
- One-minute timed sit-ups for abdominal muscular endurance

As described in Chapter 1, the second National Children and Youth Fitness Study (NCYFS II)[26] was launched to study the physical fitness and physical activity habits of 4,678 children ages six to nine. The study was the first to assess the fitness and activity patterns of six- to nine-year-olds.

Test items of the NCYFS II include:

- Triceps, subscapular, and medial calf skinfolds for body composition

- One-mile (age 8 or 9) or half-mile (age 6 or 7) walk/run for cardiorespiratory endurance
- Sit-and-reach test for lower back/hamstring flexibility
- Modified pull-up for upper body muscular strength and endurance
- One minute bent-knee sit-ups for abdominal strength/endurance

Physical Best from AAHPERD is a new, comprehensive, physical fitness education and assessment program that utilizes the testing procedures and norms developed from the NCYFS.[27] Physical Best is the first program to combine assessment of health-related fitness with practical classroom instructional materials that teach why and how to stay fit for a lifetime.

There are three components that make up the complete Physical Best program:

- A health-related fitness assessment
- An educational component, contained in a kit available from AAHPERD
- A set of awards, to reinforce positive behavior change and recognize personal achievement

Students are tested at the beginning of the school year to determine their current fitness level. Teachers then work with them to set intermediate and year-end goals which incorporate fitness activities, knowledge, and values. They then help the students develop specific activities based on their personal interests to help them meet the fitness goals, adding support from both inside and outside the classroom. Weekly logs are kept to help monitor progress. There is periodic reassessment, with award patches given for various types of goals.

Health-Related and Skill-Related Test for Children

As described in Chapter 1, the President's Council on Physical Fitness and Sports School Population Fitness Survey was conducted in 1985.[28] Data were collected to assess the physical fitness status of American public school children ages 6–17. A four-stage probability sample was designed to select approximately 19,200 boys and girls from 57 school districts and 187 schools.

The test was not designed to measure all of the health-related fitness components (body composition was not assessed), and several skill-related tests were included. The following nine test items were selected for both boys and girls (norms for these tests are included in Appendix B):

- one minute bent-knee sit-ups for abdominal strength/endurance
- pull-ups
- flexed-arm hang
- fifty yard dash
- standing long jump
- shuttle run
- sit-and-reach flexibility test
- one mile run/walk
- two mile walk

Sports Medicine Insight
Certification for Health and Fitness Professionals

Certification provides health/fitness professionals with public recognition of their knowledge, technical skills, and experience in their particular field. It certifies that the individual is qualified to practice in accordance with the standards deemed to be essential by the certifying body.[29]

The most prestigious health and fitness certification program is conducted by the American College of Sports Medicine. This Sports Medicine Insight provides a full description of their certification program.

American College of Sports Medicine (ACSM)

The American College of Sports Medicine is a national professional and scientific organization representing more than 40 medical and scientific specialties. ACSM members represent leadership in research, education and application in many fields, including exercise physiology, cardiac and respiratory rehabilitation, physical fitness, physical education, athletic training and physical therapy. ACSM is a nonprofit society dedicated to generating and disseminating knowledge concerning the motivation, responses, adaptations and health aspects of persons engaged in sport and exercise.

ACSM publishes scientific and educational information through books, an official journal, a quarterly news magazine, an annual science review series, official

Position Stands/Opinion Statements, and lay translation of the Position Stands/Opinion Statements.

Certification Objectives

The ACSM certification program, which currently includes six professional certifications, has evolved from a recognized concern in 1972 that there was a need to: (1) increase the competencies of individuals involved in preventive and rehabilitative exercise programs; and (2) establish means whereby the public consumer can recognize professional competence.

ACSM certifications are available to all professionals within the health and fitness and clinical fields who meet the established prerequisites. Candidates for ACSM certification need not be ACSM members.

Health/Fitness Instructor

There are two certification tracks:

1. The Health and Fitness Track (Health Fitness Director, Health Fitness Instructor, and Exercise Leader).
2. The Clinical Track (Preventive/Rehabilitative Program Director, Preventive/Rehabilitative Exercise Specialist, and Exercise Test Technologist).

The Health/Fitness Instructor certification is provided for those individuals who conduct exercise programs for people with controlled disease or without disease. These exercise programs should apply scientific principles of conditioning and motivation techniques for establishing an appropriate lifestyle which includes healthy exercise habits. The program should offer activities that will improve the participant's functional capacity. Positive attitudes toward work and play, as well as positive physical or psychological benefits, are the desired outcomes.

The Health/Fitness instructor must be able to evaluate the physiological and psychological effects of regular exercise and possess the ability to incorporate suitable and innovative activities for each individual.

Preventive exercise programs require that participants not only establish, but adhere to, long-range commitments to regular physical activity in order to maintain optimal levels of fitness. Programs need to include health appraisal, risk-factor identification, motivation, counseling, teaching and behavior modification techniques to emphasize current and valid health information and promote lifestyle changes.

Knowledge of the scientific principles of exercise and physical conditioning, and the ability to design safe, appropriate and enjoyable individualized exercise programs, are the primary objectives for a well-prepared and competent Health/Fitness Instructor.

Health/Fitness Instructor Certification Eligibility

The Health/Fitness Instructor certification provides recognition of professionals who have demonstrated the knowledge, skills and competence required to lead exercise and health-enhancement programs for apparently healthy individuals. In addition, a Health/Fitness Instructor must meet the following criteria:

1. Demonstration of an adequate knowledge of health-appraisal techniques, risk-factor identification, submaximal-exercise testing and evaluating physical performance to properly recommend an exercise program.
2. A baccalaureate degree in an allied health field or the equivalent.
3. A demonstrated understanding of appropriate techniques including motivation, counseling, teaching and behavior modification to promote lifestyle changes.
4. A knowlege of basic exercise science including exercise physiology, kinesiology, functional anatomy, nutrition and cardiorespiratory fitness.
5. Current certification in cardiopulmonary resuscitation.

Health/Fitness Instructor Workshop

A four-day workshop is conducted prior to the Health/Fitness Instructor certification. **The workshop is optional and is not a prerequisite for certification.** The primary focus of the workshop is to develop and enhance the knowledge base and practical skills of the Health/Fitness Instructor. Specific emphasis will be directed to scientific principles of exercise physiology, nutrition and weight control, exercise programming, emergency procedures, health appraisal and fitness evaluation techniques, exercise leadership, human-behavior psychology, human development/aging, func-

tional anatomy and kinesiology, and risk-factor identification.

Workshop Participant Qualifications

All workshop participants must have an active interest in the health profession. There are no absolute prerequisites for the workshop. However, participants without knowledge and background in the health and fitness profession should understand that the **workshop is not intended to provide the full experience and knowledge necessary for ACSM certification** as stated in the behaviorial objectives for Health/Fitness Instructor.

Participants should have prior experience and competence in monitoring heart rate and blood pressure both at rest and during exercise. Blood pressure training sessions are usually available from the local chapter of the American Heart Association, if additional training is warranted. Experience in leading an exercise class, basic counseling skills, functional anatomy and knowledge of exercise physiology are also expected prior to attendance. The workshop fee is $280.

Certification

The Health/Fitness Instructor certification is granted to candidates successfully completing separate written and practical examinations. The written and practical examinations can be taken during the same one-day certification session. Candidates must receive a passing grade on both the written and practical examinations to be granted certification. The certification fee is $170 for ACSM members, $220 for non-ACSM members.

The Written Examination

The written examination is a two-part multiple-choice format and is based upon the Behavioral Objectives as outlined in the ACSM publication: *Guidelines for Exercise Testing and Prescription,* fourth edition, 1991; Lea & Febiger, 200 Chester Field Parkway, Malvern, PA 19355 USA; $15 (U.S. funds only). To order, call: (800) 444-1785; outside the continental U.S., call (215) 251-2230 for foreign distributors and rates. In order to successfully complete the written portion of the Health/Fitness Instructor certification, candidates must receive a minimum score of 67% on each part of the written examination.

Fitness and Sports Medicine: An Introduction was written specifically to prepare students for both the written and practical exams, and is recommended by ACSM for this purpose.

The Practical Examination

The practical examination includes an assessment of each candidate at separate stations. Candidates must successfully complete each of the stations to receive a passing grade for the practical examination. Candidates will spend 15 minutes at each of the following stations:

1. *Body Composition/Flexibility* . . . The candidate should be able to:
   A. Identify the location and measure the anatomical sites for circumferential and skinfold assessments, employing the correct techniques.
   B. Administer a functional evaluation of flexibility (sit and reach test).

2. *Muscular Strength/Endurance* . . . The candidate should be able to:
   A. Administer functional evaluations of muscular strength (grip strength) and muscular endurance (bench press, sit-up, push-up).
   B. Administer, evaluate and suggest appropriate exercise intervention for specific muscle groups.

3. *Physical Work Capacity: Preparation* . . . The candidate should be able to prepare a client for a submaximal physical work capacity evaluation on either a motorized treadmill or a stationary bicycle ergometer. The candidate should be able to reasonably explain the procedures of the test, as well as to educate the individual on the proper use of the exercise equipment. The candidate will be required to measure resting heart rate and blood pressure.

4. *Physical Work Capacity: Demonstration* . . . The candidate should be able to administer a continuous, multi-staged physical fitness test to sub-maximal levels. The test will be performed on either a motorized treadmill or a stationary bicycle ergometer in accordance with a standard protocol which will be provided for the candidate. Various test termination criteria may be experienced by the candidate.

Certification Candidates Must Provide to the Certification Site . . .

1. Transcript Copies and Recommendations . . .

Degree Candidates—If you are a candidate with a **baccalaureate degree in an allied health field** (physical education, health education, nursing, medicine, physical therapy, exercise physiology or similar health-related areas), **a copy of your college transcript of degree completion and one recommendation must be sent directly to the certification site.**

It is preferred that the letter of recommendation be from an ACSM-certified professional. However, recommendations from a supervisor, faculty member or individual familiar with your knowledge base and experience is acceptable.

NOTE: If you have a degree in a non-health related area, or if a transcript is not available, follow the requirements for a non-degree candidate as stated:

Non-Degree Candidates—If you are a **non-degree candidate** with experience equivalent to academic preparation for a baccalaureate degree, **two letters of recommendation must be sent directly to the certification site.**

It is preferred that at least one of the letters of recommendation be from an ACSM certified professional. The second recommendation should come from a professional who has worked with you in a health-related field. Both recommendations must document experience equivalent to academic preparation for a baccalaureate degree in an allied health field, specifically, a minimum of 600 hours of work-related experience in the past two years.

2. CPR Verification . . .

Candidate must submit verification of current cardiopulmonary resuscitation certification. **Verification indicating an expiration date must be sent directly to the certification site.** (Call ACSM at 317-637-9200 for listing of sites.)

3. PAR Q & YOU . . .

Candidate must submit the completed PAR Q & YOU Form which must be **sent directly to the certification site.**

Summary

1. The American College of Sports Medicine takes the position that candidates for an exercise program or testing for physical fitness status be categorized as either "apparently healthy," "at higher risk," or "with disease."

2. A medical/health status questionnaire should be used for such ACSM classification.

3. All people planning to start an exercise program are advised to have a physical examination by a physician. While apparently healthy people under the age of 45 and those at higher risk under the age of 35 do not require a treadmill-EKG test, all others are advised to take one.

4. Various relative and absolute contraindications to exercise have been submitted by ACSM. Physicians are responsible for diagnosing the presence and significance of these factors for those planning to start an exercise program.

5. We live in an increasingly litigious society. Proper informed consent forms and the adoption of appropriate strategies for reducing liability exposure are needed.

6. The function of measurement is to determine status. Tests should be valid, reliable, have sound norms, and be economical in terms of money, time, and testing expertise.

7. Physical fitness tests have several purposes, including assessment of status, identification of special needs, evaluation of progress, and motivation.

8. Evaluation procedures should follow a certain order for both safety and efficiency.

9. The YMCA, Fitness and Amateur Sport, Canada, AAHPERD, and U.S. Public Health Service have all developed health-related physical fitness testing batteries.

References

1. American College of Sports Medicine. Guidelines for Exercise Testing and Prescription (4th Ed.). Philadelphia: Lea & Febiger, 1991.

2. Pollock ML, Wilmore JH, Fox SM. Exercise In Health and Disease: Evaluation and Prescription for Prevention and Rehabilitation. Philadelphia: WB Saunders and Co., 1984.

3. Froelicher VF. Exercise Testing and Training. Chicago: Year Book Medical Publishers, Inc., 1983.

4. Chisholm DM, Collis ML, Kulak LL, Davenport W, Gruber N. Physical Activity Readiness. Br Col Med J 17:375–378, 1975.

5. Shephard RJ. PAR-Q, Canadian Home Fitness Test and Exercise Screening Alternatives. Sports Med 5:185–195, 1988.

6. U.S. Department of Health and Human Services, Public Health Service, National Institutes of Health. Exercise and Your Heart, 1981. NIH Publication No. 83–1677, Superintendent of Documents, U.S. Government Printing Office, Washington, D.C., 20402.

7. Hage P. Exercise Guidelines: Which to Believe? Physician Sportsmed 10:23, 1982.

8. Sharkey BJ. Physiology of Fitness. Champaign, Illinois: Human Kinetics Publishers, 1979, p. 60.

9. Ross CT. Managing Risk. Athletic Business, June 1985, pp. 22–29.

10. American College of Sports Medicine. Policy Statement Regarding the Use of Human Subjects and Informed Consent. Med Sci Sports Exerc 17:v, 1985.

11. Brox A. Liability Insurance: Putting the Lid on Premiums. Club Industry, December, 1986, p. 33.

12. Stoltar DK. Liability In Recreation: Sound Risk Management Can Prevent Litigation. Athletic Business, August, 1984, pp. 48–50.

13. Stoltar DK. Taking Notice of Negligence. Corporate Fitness and Recreation, June/July 1986, pp. 41–46.

14. Olson JR. Safety Checklists: Does Your Facility Measure UP? Athletic Business, October 1985, pp. 47–52.

15. Herbert DL, Herbert WG. Frequent Claims and Suits in Equipment-Related Injuries. Fitness Management, February 1988, p. 22.

16. Clarke HH. Application of Measurement to Health and Physical Education. Englewood Cliffs: Prentice-Hall, Inc., 1967.

17. Johnson BL, Nelson JK. Practical Measurements for Evaluation in Physical Education. Minneapolis: Burgess Publishing Co., 1979.

18. Phillips DA, Hornak JE. Measurement and Evaluation in Physical Education. New York: John Wiley and Sons, 1979.

19. Golding LA, Myers CR, Sinning WE. The Ys Way to Physical Fitness. (3rd Ed.) Champaign IL., Human Kinetics Publishers, 1989.

20. Fischer S. Fitness Tests Can Screen Out Trouble. Athletic Business: December, 1985, pp. 18–22.

21. The American Alliance for Health, Physical Education, Recreation and Dance. Health-Related Physical Fitness Test Manual. 1900 Association Drive, Reston, Virginia 22091: AAHPERD, 1980.

22. Canadian Standardized Test of Fitness (CSTF) Operations Manual (3rd Ed.). (For 15 to 69 years-of-age). 1987. Published by authority of the Minister of State, Fitness and Amateur Sport. Journal Tower(s), 365 Laurier Avenue West, Ottawa, Ontario K1A0X6.

23. Wellsource, Inc., 15431 S.E. 82nd Dr., Suite F. Clackamas, OR 97015.

24. Pate RR. Norms for College Students: Health Related Physical Fitness Test, 1985. American Alliance for Health, Physical Education, Recreation and Dance. 1900 Association Drive, Reston, Virginia 22091.

25. Summary of Findings From National Children and Youth Fitness Study. JOPERD, January, 1985, pp. 44–90.

26. Ross JG, Pate RR. The National Children and Youth Fitness Study II: A Summary of Findings. JOPERD, November/December, 1987, pp. 51–56.

27. Physical Best: The American Alliance Physical Fitness Education & Assessment Program. The American Alliance for Health, Physical Education, Recreation, and Dance, 1988. 1900 Association Drive, Reston, Virginia 22091.

28. Youth Physical Fitness in 1985. The President's Council on Physical Fitness and Sports School Population Fitness Survey. President's Council on Physical Fitness and Sports. 450 Fifth St NW, Suite 7103, Washington, D.C. 20001.

29. Herbert WG. The Importance of Certification for Health/Fitness Directors. Fitness In Business, April 1988, pp. 173–177.

Physical Fitness Activity 3.1—Using the Medical/Health Status Questionnaire

Appendix A contains an employee wellness program medical/health status questionnaire used at the Loma Linda University Center for Health Promotion. In this Physical Fitness Activity, you will be filling out this questionnaire and then answering the following questions.

1. Based on your responses to the questions in the medical/health status questionnaire in Appendix A, in what ACSM classification would you put yourself?

   A. apparently healthy

   B. individual at higher risk

   C. patient with disease

2. Describe to the best of your knowledge your cardiovascular disease risk status. Use the six risk factors outlined by ACSM (Table 3.1) and information from Table 3.2.

   _____

   _____

   _____

   _____

   _____

   _____

3. Based on your ACSM classification, what medical evaluation and graded exercise testing recommendations would be necessary for you to begin an exercise program? (See Table 3.3).

   _____

   _____

   _____

   _____

   _____

   _____

   _____

Chapter 4

Assessment of Cardiorespiratory Fitness

"Cardiorespiratory fitness (CRF) reflects the functional capacities of the heart, blood vessels, blood, lungs, and relevant muscles during various types of exercise demands. Specifically, CRF affects numerous physiological responses: at rest; in response to submaximal exercise; in response to maximal exercise; during prolonged work. Cardiorespiratory fitness can be justified as an important component of physical fitness since it is related to health and can be affected by physical activity."[1]

The Assessment of $\dot{V}O_{2max}$

The laboratory test generally regarded as the best measure of heart and lung endurance is the direct measurement of oxygen uptake during maximal exercise.[1-4] The exercise is usually performed using a bicycle ergometer or treadmill, which allows the progressive increase in workload from light to exhaustive (maximal) exercise. The amount of oxygen consumed during the exercise test is measured using various methods (douglas bag collection of expired air, mixing box and gas flow meter, or computerized metabolic carts).[5] (See Figure 4.1.)

Maximal Oxygen Uptake ($\dot{V}O_{2max}$) is defined "as the greatest rate at which oxygen can be consumed during exercise at sea level."[1, 3, 4] ("$\dot{V}$" is the volume of oxygen used per minute, "O_2" is oxygen, and "max" represents maximal exercise conditions.) The maximal rate of oxygen uptake is the maximal rate at which oxygen can be taken up, distributed, and used by the body during physical activity.[5]

$\dot{V}O_{2max}$ is usually expressed in terms of milliliters of oxygen consumed per kilogram of body weight per minute ($ml \cdot kg^{-1} \cdot min^{-1}$). By factoring in body weight, it

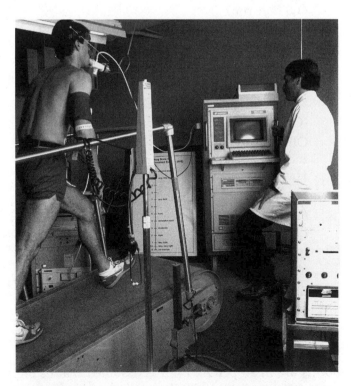

Figure 4.1 $\dot{V}O_{2max}$ is best measured in the laboratory during a maximal exercise test in which the oxygen consumed is measured by a computerized metabolic cart.

becomes possible to compare the $\dot{V}O_{2max}$ of people of varying size in different environments.

A high level of $\dot{V}O_{2max}$ depends upon the proper functioning of three important systems in the body:

1. the respiratory system, which takes up oxygen from the air in the lungs and transports it into the blood

2. the cardiovascular system, which pumps and distributes the oxygen-laden blood throughout the body

3. the musculoskeletal system, which uses the oxygen to convert stored carbohydrates and fats into ATP for muscle contraction and heat production.[5]

Laboratory measurement of $\dot{V}O_{2max}$ is expensive and time-consuming, requires highly trained personnel, and therefore is not practical for mass testing situations. Various tests have been developed as substitutes. The tests in parentheses represent those used in the physical fitness testing batteries presented in the previous chapter:

▪ **Field Tests of Cardiorespiratory Endurance**

(1 mile run)

(1.5 mile run)

Others: 1-mile walk, 9-minute run; 3-mile walking test; 12-minute cycling test; 12-minute swimming test.[9]

▪ **Step Tests**

(3-minute step test, YMCA)

(Canadian Aerobic Fitness Step Test)

Others: Nagle maximum step test; Astrand submaximum step test; McArdle submax step test; Harvard Step Test

▪ **Submaximal Laboratory Tests**

(YMCA Physical Working Capacity Bicycle Test)

Others: Astrand submaximal bicycle test; treadmill submaximal

▪ **Maximal Laboratory Tests**

Bicycle maximal tests (Storer and Davis, Astrand)

Treadmill maximal tests (Bruce, Balke)

Wingate anaerobic test

These various tests will be discussed in this chapter (the norms are in Appendix B). It is assumed that before these tests are conducted, the preliminary considerations outlined in the previous chapter have been attended to (medical/health status questionnaire, consent form, and for those at high risk, a physical examination by a physician, treadmill test, and possibly a blood lipid analysis). It is also assumed that the order outlined for each testing battery is followed, with subjects following the appropriate pre-test preparation routine (abstention from eating, drinking and smoking for 2–3 hours, proper hydration, and comfortable exercise clothes).

When conducting a bicycle or treadmill test, the tester should include blood pressure and electrocardiogram (ECG) monitoring on all high-risk individuals. The test can then be used for determination of both cardiorespiratory fitness and potential health problems such as high blood pressure and heart disease (as diagnosed by a physician). Although blood pressure and ECG monitoring is not necessary when testing apparently healthy subjects, some testing facilities do it as an extra precaution.

Resting and Exercise Blood Pressure and Heart Rate Determination

Resting Blood Pressure

Blood pressure is the force of blood against the walls of the arteries and veins created by the heart as it pumps blood to every part of the body. *Hypertension* is simply a condition in which the blood pressure is chronically elevated above optimal levels. The 1988 Joint National Committee on Detection, Evaluation, and Treatment of High Blood Pressure has established blood pressure classifications.[6] (See Table 4.1.)

Hypertension is diagnosed for adults when the average of two or more *diastolic* measurements (of blood pressure when the heart is resting) on at least two separate visits is 90 mm Hg or higher. If the *diastolic* blood pressure is below 90 mm Hg, *systolic* hypertension is diagnosed when the average of multiple systolic blood pressure (pressure when heart is pumping) measurements on two or more separate visits is consistently greater than 140 mm Hg.[6] Hypertension is severe when the diastolic blood pressure is greater than 115 mm Hg. Recommended follow-up procedures for hypertension testing are given in Table 4.2.

As many as 58 million people in the U.S. have elevated blood pressure of 140 mm Hg or greater and/or diastolic blood pressure of 90 mm Hg or greater, or are taking antihypertensive medication.[6] Prevalence increases with age, and is higher among blacks than

Table 4.1 Classification of Blood Pressure in Adults

BP Range, mm hg	Category
Diastolic Blood Pressure	
<85	Normal
85-89	High-normal
90-104	Mild hypertension
105-114	Moderate hypertension
≥115	Severe hypertension
Systolic Blood Pressure When Diastolic Blood Pressure is <90 mm Hg	
<140	Normal
140-159	Borderline isolated systolic hypertension
≥160	Isolated systolic hypertension

Note: Classification is based on the average of two or more readings on two or more occasions.

Source: 1988 Joint National Committee. The 1988 Report of the Joint National Committee on Detection, Evaluation, and Treatment of High Blood Pressure. Arch Intern Med 148:1023–1038, 1988.

whites. Health care professionals are urged to measure blood pressure at each patient visit.

To take the resting blood pressure, a sphygmomanometer and a stethoscope are needed.[7] The *sphygmomanometer* consists of an inflatable compression bag enclosed in an unyielding covering called the cuff, plus an inflating bulb, a manometer from which the pressure is read, and a controlled exhaust valve to deflate the system. The *stethoscope* is made of rubber tubing attached to a device that amplifies the sounds of blood passing through the blood vessels. (See Figure 4.2.) This equipment can be obtained in most drug stores for under $30, though more expensive blood pressure equipment is available.

Those taking blood pressure should be trained by qualified instructors. Blood pressure should be measured two or three times until consistency is achieved. A single blood pressure reading does not provide an accurate measure.[7] Several blood pressure readings by different observers, or on different occasions by the same observer, are recommended to check the validity of initially high values.

For best results in taking blood pressure:[6-10]

- Measurements should be taken with a mercury sphygmomanometer, a recently calibrated aneroid manometer, or a validated electronic device.
- Two or more readings should be averaged. If the first two readings differ by more than 5 mm Hg, additional readings should be obtained.
- Take the measurement in a quiet room with the temperature approximately 70 to 74 degrees Fahrenheit (21 to 23 degrees C).
- Having the upper arm bare makes it easier to adjust the cuff.
- With older people, because of potential arterial obstructions, it is best to take readings on both arms.
- Use the proper size cuff. The rubber bladder should encircle at least two thirds of the arm. The three most frequently used cuff sizes are child (13 to 20 cm), adult (17 to 26 cm) and large adult (32 to 42 cm). If the person's arm is large, the normal size cuff will be too small, making the reading larger than it actually should be (and vice versa).

Table 4.2 Recommended Follow-Up Testing Procedures for Initial BP Measurement

BP Range, mm hg	Recommended Follow-Up
Diastolic Blood Pressure	
<85	Recheck within two years
85-89	Recheck within one year
90-104	Confirm within two months
105-114	Evaluate or refer promptly to source of care within 2 weeks.
≥115	Evaluate or refer immediately to source of care
Systolic Blood Pressure when Diastolic Blood Pressure is <90 mm Hg	
<140	Recheck within two years
140-199	Confirm within two months
≥200	Evaluate or refer promptly to source of care within 2 weeks

Source: 1988 Joint National Committee. The 1988 Report of the Joint National Committee on Detection, Evaluation, and Treatment of High Blood Pressure. Arch Intern Med 148:1023–1038, 1988.

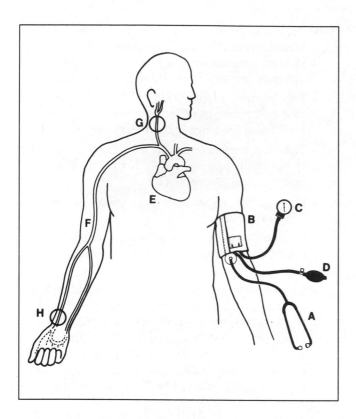

Figure 4.2 Blood pressure is taken with a stethoscope (A) and sphygmomanometer, which consists of an inflatable cuff (B) connected by rubber tubes to a manometer, which measures pressure in millimeters of mercury (C), and a rubber bulb that regulates air during the measurements (D). Blood pressure is the force of blood against the walls of the arteries and veins created by the heart (E) as it pumps. The blood pressure cuff fits over the brachial artery (F). The upper circle (G) represents the common carotid artery, and the lower circle (H) the radial artery, for sensing the heart rate.

- Between determinations, allow at least 30–60 seconds for normal circulation to return to the arm.

- The subject should be comfortably seated, with the arm straight (just slightly flexed), palm up, and the whole forearm supported at heart level on a smooth surface.

- Anxiety, emotional turmoil, food in the stomach, bladder distension, climate variation, exertion, and pain all may influence blood pressure, and when possible, should be controlled or avoided. Heavy exercise or eating should be avoided, and the individual being tested should sit quietly for at least five minutes before the test. One should also avoid smoking or ingesting caffeine for at least 30 minutes prior to measurement.

- Place the cuff (deflated) with the lower margin about 1 inch above the inner elbow crease (antecubital space). The rubber bag should be over the brachial artery (inner part of upper arm).

- The stethoscope should be applied lightly to the antecubital space. It has been determined recently that excessive pressure on the stethoscope head can erroneously lower diastolic readings.[8] The stethoscope should not touch clothing, the cuff, or the cuff tubing (to avoid unnecessary rubbing sounds).

- With the stethoscope in place, the pressure should be raised 20–30 mm Hg above the point at which the pulse sound disappears (listen carefully through the stethoscope as the cuff bladder is inflated. The pressure will close off the blood flow in the brachial artery, causing the pulse sound to stop).

- The pressure should be slowly released at a rate of 2 to 3 mm Hg/second. Do not go slower than this, however, because it can cause pain, and also raise blood pressure.

- As the pressure is released, the blood pressure sounds (the *Korotkoff's sounds*) become audible and pass through several phases. Phase One (the systolic pressure) is marked by the appearance of faint, clear tapping sounds, which gradually increase in intensity. This represents the blood pressure when the heart is contracting.

  To obtain the diastolic blood pressure, the following rules should be followed:

  At rest—diastolic blood pressure equals the disappearance of the pulse sound (also called the fifth sound).

  During exercise testing—sometimes the disappearance of sound drops all the way to zero. Therefore, the point at which there is an abrupt muffling sound (fourth phase) should be used for the diastolic blood pressure.

- A true systolic blood pressure cannot be obtained unless the Korotkoff's sounds are relatively sharp. Korotkoff's sounds can be made louder by having the person being tested open and clench his fist about 10 times during cuff inflation, inflating the cuff quickly, and elevating the arm before inflating the cuff.[11]

Exercise Blood Pressure

Blood pressure should be taken at least every three minutes during exercise testing on the treadmill or bicycle. (See Figure 4.3.) Several important principles should be followed when taking blood pressure readings during exercise:

- If the exercise stages are three minutes long (as in the Bruce treadmill protocol, for example), blood pressure readings should be taken at 2 minutes and 15 seconds into each stage. The cuff should be taped onto the person being tested for the entire test, but the inflating bulb should be removed between readings.

- It is best to stand on a stool and have the person being tested raise his arm to heart level while you support it. If you are using a mercury stand sphygmomanometer, the mercury column should be elevated to the person's heart level.

- Taking blood pressure during exercise is somewhat difficult because of the noise. It is best to raise the cuff pressure quickly until pulse sounds disappear (usually 200 mm Hg), and then, because the heart rate is higher than at rest, let the cuff pressure fall 5–6 mm Hg per second. Try to focus only on the pulse sounds through the stethoscope. Try to keep the various tubes from flapping and rubbing against objects. If you can't hear the pulse sounds, it may be necessary to stop the test for 15 seconds for a quick blood pressure determination.

- During exertion, the diastolic reading stays basically the same as the resting diastolic, whereas the systolic rises linearly with the increase in workload. (See Figure 4.4.)

- If the systolic rises above 250 mm Hg, or the diastolic rises above 120 mm Hg, the test should be terminated.

- During recovery, blood pressure should be taken every two to three minutes.[12]

Resting Heart Rate

The resting heart rate can be obtained through auscultation (using the bell of the stethoscope), palpation (feeling the pulse with your fingers), or EKG recordings.[10] When taking heart rate by auscultation, the bell of the stethoscope is placed to the left of the sternum just above the level of the nipple. The heart beats (lub-dub)

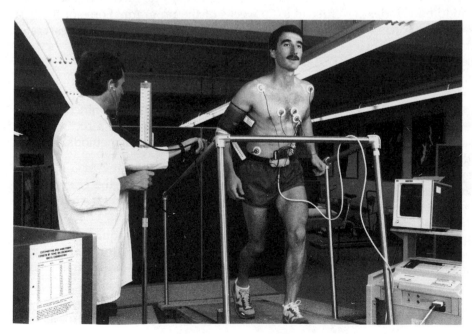

Figure 4.3 Blood pressure determination during exercise is a difficult skill, and requires considerable experience. Korotkoff sounds are easier to hear if the tubes are not allowed to rub or bump the subject or the treadmill. The stethoscope head should be attached to the subject's arm. The manometer should be at the level of the subject's heart.

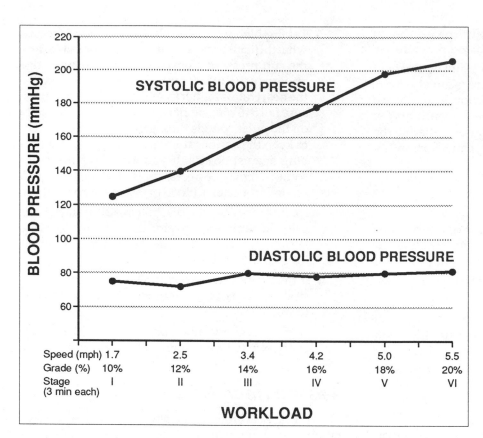

Figure 4.4 Pattern of systolic and diastolic blood pressures during graded exercise testing.

can be counted for 30 seconds, and then multiplied by two for beats per minute (bpm).

In using palpation techniques, the pulse is best determined during rest at the radial artery (lateral aspect of the palm side of the wrist in line with the base of the thumb). (See Figure 4.2.) The tip of the middle and index fingers should be used (not the thumb, which has a pulse of its own). Start the stopwatch simultaneously with the pulse beat. Count the first beat as zero. Continue counting for 30 seconds and then multiply by two to get total heart beats per minute.

During exercise, the carotid artery is easier to palpate because it is bigger than the radial. (See Figure 4.2.) When palpating the carotid (in the neck just lateral to the larynx), heavy pressure should not be applied, because pressure receptors (baroreceptors) in the carotid arteries can detect the pressure and cause a reflex slowing of the heart rate.[10]

The heart rate is a variable that fluctuates widely and easily due to the same factors that influence blood pressure. Resting heart rate is best determined upon awakening, averaged from measurements taken on at least three separate mornings. Lower heart rates are usually (but not always) indicative of a heart conditioned by exercise training, a heart able to push out more blood with each beat (having a larger stroke volume) and therefore needing fewer beats. (See Appendix B, Table 38.) Accordingly, the resting heart rate usually drops with regular exercise, decreasing approximately one beat every one or two weeks for the first 10 to 20 weeks of the program.[9] Some of the best endurance athletes in the world have resting heart rates as low as 35 to 45 beats per minute.

Exercise Heart Rate

Heart rate during exercise is best determined through the use of an *electrocardiogram* (EKG), a record of the electrical activity of the heart. Several methods are used:

- Using a heart rate ruler, count 2 or 3 R waves (depending on the ruler) from the reference arrow, and then read the heart rate from the ruler. (See Figure 4.5.)

- Counting the number of larger squares between R waves and dividing into 300 (for example, if 2 large blocks are between R waves, then the heart rate is 300/2 or 150 bpm).

- Counting the number of millimeters between 4 R waves, and dividing into 6000 (for example, if 40

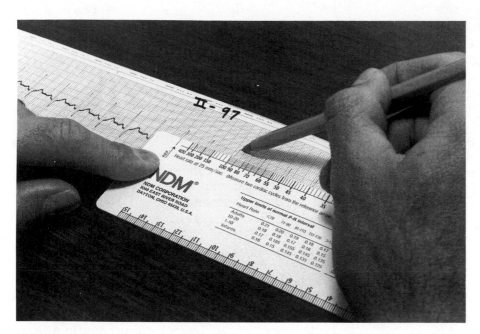

Figure 4.5 The heart rate can be determined from an EKG recording by using a heart rate ruler. With this particular ruler, heart rate is determined by reading the ruler after counting two heart rate cycles to the right of the reference arrow.

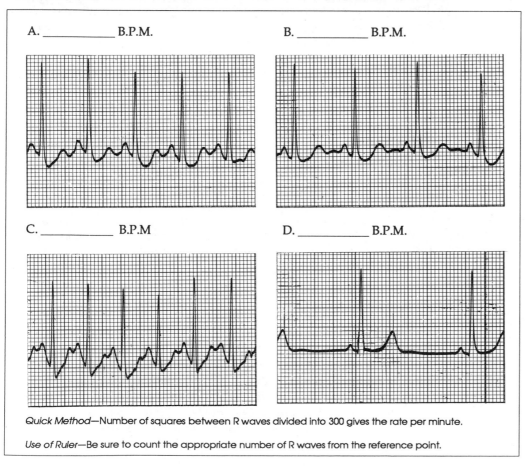

A. _____ B.P.M.

B. _____ B.P.M.

C. _____ B.P.M

D. _____ B.P.M.

Quick Method—Number of squares between R waves divided into 300 gives the rate per minute.

Use of Ruler—Be sure to count the appropriate number of R waves from the reference point.

Figure 4.6 Use this form to practice heart rate determination from EKG recording strips. Practice each of the three methods described in this section (EKG ruler, large square method, four-R method).

mm separate 4 R waves, then the heart rate is 6000/40 or 150 bpm).

Figure 4.6 is a form for practicing EKG heart rate determination.

Another method involves *auscultation* (the process of listening for sounds within the body) with the stethoscope. The blood pressure cuff can be filled, the systolic blood pressure taken, and then midway between the systolic and diastolic blood pressures (usually around 100 to 110 mm Hg), the release of pressure can be stopped and the pulse counted through the stethoscope for 10 seconds. (Often the pulse sounds are very loud when this method is used.) The pressure can then be released for diastolic blood pressure determination.

Box 4.1 Heart Rate Monitors

Several types of heart rate measuring devices have been developed. Researchers have determined that heart rate monitors using chest electrodes are very accurate, stable, and functional (13). Heart rate monitors using photocells to measure the opacity of blood flow (earlobe or fingertip) are not recommended. The best overall heart rate monitor identified in one study is the AMF Quantum XL (also known as the Sport Tester PE 3000, Vantage Performance Monitor, or CIC Heart Watch 8799). The CIC 8799 Deluxe Heartwatch can be ordered from the Computerized Instruments Corporation of Plymouth, Michigan. A telemetry device with permanent electrodes is attached to the chest, with the heart rate signal sent to a receiver worn on the wrist. Heart rate and elapsed time are displayed (the heart rate is updated every five seconds) and kept in memory for every minute for up to 16 hours. It costs about $250.

Field Tests for Cardiorespiratory Fitness

As was mentioned earlier, a number of performance tests such as maximal endurance runs on a track have been devised for testing large groups in field situations.[10] These tests are practical, inexpensive, less time-consuming than laboratory tests, easy to administer for large groups, and quite accurate when properly conducted.

Endurance runs should be of one mile or greater to test the aerobic system. For ease of administration, the one mile and 1.5 mile runs are most commonly used. Various set-timed runs such as the 9-minute run are hard to administer because exact distance determination is difficult. With the one-mile or 1.5-mile runs, those being tested simply run the set distance around a track (or exactly measured course) while their time is measured. The objective is to cover the distance in the shortest possible time.[14] The effort should be maximal, and only made by those properly motivated and experienced in running.[1]

The one-mile run is used in both the AAHPERD college student health-related physical fitness test, and also the Public Health Service National Children and Youth Fitness test. Norms for both are found in Appendix B (Tables 9, 10, 17, 21, 30). The 1.5-mile test can be used in the Wellsource, Inc., software computer package test, as discussed in Chapter 3.

Performance on distance running tests of one mile or longer has been shown to correlate significantly with maximal aerobic power.*

Recently, equations have been developed to predict $\dot{V}O_{2max}$ from one's ability to run various distances at maximal speed.[15] Table 4.3 summarizes these equations for various racing distances. Notice that the correlations of calculated values of $\dot{V}O_2$ with actual measured $\dot{V}O_2$ are very high (0.88 to 0.98).

These equations assume that the person being tested has run the distance at maximum speed. The average running speed is then computed in kilometers per hour (kmh). The equation can then be used to calculate the $\dot{V}O_{2max}$ in METS.

One *MET* is equal to the resting oxygen consumption of the reference "average human," which equals 3.5 $ml \cdot kg^{-1} \cdot min^{-1}$. To get $\dot{V}O_{2max}$ the number of METS is multiplied by 3.5 $ml \cdot kg^{-1} \cdot min^{-1}$. (See example in Table 4.3.)

Table 4.4 summarizes calculations from the equations in Table 4.3. Equivalent relationships between $\dot{V}O_{2max}$ and running performance for races ranging from 1.5 km to 42.195 km (marathon) are given. Notice, for example, that running a mile in 6:01 demands the same

---

*Correlation coefficients from most investigators have ranged from 0.54 all the way up to 0.90.[1,9]

Table 4.3 Estimation of $\dot{V}O_{2max}$ from Average Running Speed During Racing[15]

Racing Distance	Equation to calculate $\dot{V}O_{2max}$	Correlation
1.5 km	METS = 2.4388 + (0.8343× kmh)	0.95
1.6093 km (mile)	METS = 2.5043 + (0.8400× kmh)	0.95
3 km	METS = 2.9226 + (0.8900× kmh)	0.98
5 km	METS = 3.1747 + (0.9139× kmh)	0.98
10 km	METS = 4.7226 + (0.8698× kmh)	0.88
42.195 km m = (marathon)	METS = 6.9021 + (0.8246× kmh)	0.85

Note: kmn = average racing speed in competition in kilometers per hour.

Note: 1 MET = 3.5 ml · kg^{-1} · min^{-1}. To calculate total oxygen power, multiply number of METS times 3.5 ml · kg^{-1} · min^{-1}. For example, if you can run a 5-km race in 18:30 (which is 16.2 kmh, calculated by multiplying the number of kilometers in the race by 60, and then dividing by the race time in decimal form (5 × 60)/18.5 = 16.2 kmh), using the equation above, $\dot{V}O_{2max}$ in METS is equal to:

METS = 3.1747 + (0.9139 × 16.2) = 18 METS

$\dot{V}O_{2max}$ in ml · kg^{-1} · min^{-1} = 18 METS × 3.5 ml · kg^{-1} · min^{-1} = 63 ml · kg^{-1} · min^{-1}.

$\dot{V}O_{2max}$ (56 ml · kg^{-1} · min^{-1}) as running the 5 km in 21:23, the 10 km in 46:17, or the marathon in 3:49:28.

The maximal endurance run tests are only for the healthy (ACSM "apparently healthy" category). Cooper suggests that the 1.5–mile run test should not be taken unless one can already jog nonstop for fifteen minutes.[16] In addition, there always should be proper warm-up of slow jogging and calisthenics. After the test, there should be an adequate "warm-down" or "cool-down," with several minutes of walking, followed by flexibility exercises.

A one-mile walk test was developed recently.[17] Walking is safer than running and more easily performed by most Americans. Three hundred and forty-three males and females, 30 to 69 years of age, were tested using a one-mile walk test. They walked a mile as fast as possible, performing the test a minimum of two times, with heart rates monitored. They then were given a treadmill $\dot{V}O_{2max}$ test, and the one-mile walk results correlated very highly with actual measured $\dot{V}O_2$ (r = 0.93).

The following equation was developed to determine $\dot{V}O_{2max}$ from one-mile walk test results:

$\dot{V}O_{2max}$(L · min^{-1}) = 6.9652 + (0.0091 × body weight lb.) – (0.0257 × age) + (0.5955 × sex*) – (0.2240 × mile walk time in minutes) – (0.0115 × ending heart rate).

* Sex (1 = male, 0 = female)

For example, if a male subject weighs 150 pounds, is 30 years old, and can walk one mile in 12 minutes with an ending heart rate of 120 beats·min^{-1}:

$\dot{V}O_{2max}$ = 6.9652 + (0.0091 × 150 lb.) – (0.0257 × 30) + (0.5955 × 1) – (0.2240 × 12 min) – (0.0115 × 120 bpm) = 4.09 liters of oxygen per minute (L · min^{-1}).

To change the $\dot{V}O_{2max}$ units from liters per minute to milliliters per kilogram body weight (in order to use fitness classification tables), first multiply 4.09 L · min^{-1} by 1000 to get milliliters (4.09 L · min^{-1} × 1000 = 4090 ml · min^{-1}). Next divide the body weight (lb) by 2.2046 to get kilograms (150 lb/2.2046 lb/kg = 68.04 kg. Next divide the $\dot{V}O_{2max}$ by body weight (4090 ml · min^{-1}/68.04 kg = 60.1 ml · kg^{-1} · min^{-1}). Using the $\dot{V}O_{2max}$ norms in Appendix B (Table 44), this 30-year-old male would be classified as being in "athletic" cardiorespiratory shape.

Step Tests for Cardiorespiratory Endurance

There are two types of step tests—maximal and submaximal. A maximal, graded step test has been designed by Nagle, Balke, and Naughton[18] and is recommended

Table 4.4   Equivalent Performances for Various Distances

$\dot{V}O_{2max}$ (ml · kg⁻¹ · min⁻¹)	Performance Time for Various Distances			(hours:minutes:seconds)	
	1.5 km	Mile	5 km	10 km	42.2 km
28	13:30	14:46	56:49	2:39:14	31:41:25
31.5	11:27	12:29	47:04	2:02:00	16:35:05
35	9:56	10:49	40:10	1:38:53	11:13:52
38.5	8:46	9:33	35:02	1:23:08	8:29:26
42	7:51	8:33	31:04	1:11:43	6:49:30
45.5	7:07	7:44	27:54	1:03:03	5:42:21
49	6:30	7:03	25:20	0:56:15	4:54:07
52.5	5:59	6:29	23:11	0:50:47	4:17:48
56	5:32	6:01	21:23	0:46:17	3:49:28
59.5	5:09	5:36	19:50	0:42:30	3:26:44
63	4:50	5:14	18:30	0:39:33	3:08:06
66.5	4:32	4:55	17:20	0:36:33	2:52:34
70	4:17	4:38	16:18	0:34:10	2:39:23
73.5	4:03	4:23	15:23	0:32:12	2:28:05
77	3:50	4:09	14:34	0:30:12	2:18:16
80.5	3:39	3:57	13:50	0:28:33	2:09:41
84	3:29	3:46	13:10	0:27:04	2:02:06
87.5	3:20	3:36	12:34	0:25:44	1:55:21
SEE $\dot{V}O_2$	3.2%	2.3%	2.3%	4.8%	5.6%

Source: Tokmakidis SP, Léger L, Mercier D, Péronnet F, Thibault G. New Approaches to Predict $\dot{V}O_{2max}$ and Endurance from Running Performance. J Sports Med 27:401–409, 1987. SEE = Standard Error of Estimate.

by the American Heart Association.[19] An adjustable step is used that permits the height to be varied from 2 to 50 cm without interrupting the exercise. The step height is initially set at 3 cm. After two minutes, the height is raised 2 cm to 5 cm. Every minute thereafter, the height is raised 4 cm. The rhythm of stepping is regulated with a metronome at 30 steps per minute, using a four-count stepping procedure: one, two—up; three, four—down. The test is terminated when the person being tested is unable to maintain the required rhythm.

Heart rate and blood pressure can be monitored during maximal step testing. But the up and down stepping action can make measurement of blood pressure difficult; an effective means is to use a long stethoscope tube, with the head of the stethoscope attached to the exerciser's arm.

Steps are inexpensive compared to treadmills or bicycles. Bench stepping is the least desirable mode of maximal exercise testing, because of the large amount of body movement and the difficulty in adjusting the step heights.[10]

Submaximal Step Tests

The prediction of $\dot{V}O_{2max}$ also can be determined by a submaximal bench stepping test. With submaximal testing, physiological responses (usually heart rate) to submaximal exercise are measured.

The workload is usually fixed—for example, a particular grade and speed on a treadmill, a fixed rate and resistance on a bicycle *ergometer* (an apparatus for measuring the amount of work performed), or a fixed rate of stepping and height of bench in a step test. Usually heart rate is measured during and at the end of such exercise.

On the other hand, the physiological response may be fixed and the exercise required to reach the response measured (e.g., work required to reach a heart rate of 170). The reasoning underlying both types of submaximal tests is that the person with the higher $\dot{V}O_{2max}$ is able to accomplish a given amount of exercise with less effort (or more exercise at a particular heart rate).[20]

The submaximum exercise test makes three assumptions :[10, 20]

- that a linear relationship exists between heart rate, oxygen uptake, and workload,
- that the maximum heart rate at a given age is uniform, and
- that the mechanical efficiency (oxygen uptake at a given workload) is the same for everyone.

These assumptions are not wholly accurate, however, and can result in an error in estimating $\dot{V}O_{2max}$ of from 10 to 20 percent. Figure 4.7 shows that in most submaximal tests, heart rates at submaximal workloads are plotted, then extrapolated to an estimated maximum heart rate level, and then further extrapolated to an average oxygen consumption. These extrapolations can result in substantial error.

Your *maximum heart rate* is the fastest heart rate that can be measured when you are brought to total exhaustion during a graded exercise test.

A formula has been developed to represent the average maximum heart rate in humans:

$$\text{maximum heart rate} = 220 - \text{age}$$

The maximum heart rate varies substantially among different people of the same age, however. (One standard deviation is ± 12 bpm, which means that two-thirds of the population varies an average of plus or minus 12 heart beats from the average). If the line connecting submaximal heart rates is extrapolated to an average maximum heart rate level that is really 15 beats lower than the real maximum heart rate in an individual, the final extrapolation to the workload and esti-

mated oxygen consumption will underestimate the real cardiorespiratory fitness of the individual. (See Figure 4.7.)

Oxygen uptake at any given workload can vary 15 percent between different people.[21] In other words, people vary in the amount of oxygen they require to perform a certain exercise workload. Some are more efficient than others, and thus the average oxygen consumption associated with a given workload may vary significantly from one person to another.

For these reasons, $\dot{V}O_{2max}$ predicted by submaximum stress tests tends to be overestimated for those who are highly trained (who respond with a low heart rate to a given workload and are mechanically efficient), and underestimated for the untrained (those with a high heart rate for a given workload who are also inefficient).[10]

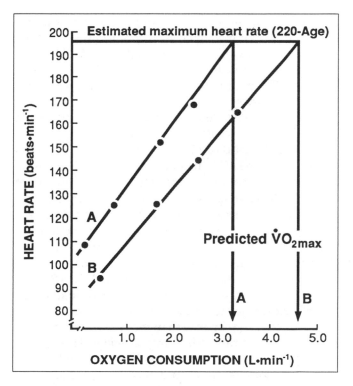

Figure 4.7 In most submaximal tests, heart rates at submaximal workloads are plotted (A or B), then extrapolated to an estimated maximum heart rate level, and then further extrapolated to an estimated workload that has been associated with an average oxygen consumption. These extrapolations can result in substantial error.

Nonetheless, submaximal exercise testing has its place in cardiorespiratory fitness determination.[20] Sometimes large populations are required to be tested, and the time, equipment, and skill needed to measure $\dot{V}O_{2max}$ is prohibitive. The measurement of $\dot{V}O_{2max}$ through maximal testing requires an all-out physical effort. For some people it can be hazardous, and at the very least often requires medical supervision and evaluation. Also, maximal testing, while definitely the most accurate way to determine fitness status, requires a high level of motivation.

Submaximal exercise testing, though not as accurate, can still give a somewhat accurate picture of fitness status without the expense, risk, and hard effort.

The Canadian Aerobic Fitness Test

The Canadian Aerobic Fitness Test (CAFT) is a practical, fairly accurate (correlation of 0.88 with directly measured $\dot{V}O_2$), inexpensive, and fun way to determine cardiorespiratory endurance.

The CAFT was developed in the mid-1970s when it was suggested by the federal government that many Canadians would be motivated to increase their habitual exercise if there were a simple exercise test that indicated their current physical condition.[22]

The CAFT was then developed using double steps, each eight inches high and wide, as in a domestic staircase. The double step is climbed to an age-and sex-specific rhythm set by a long-playing record. Fitness is assessed from test duration and the radial or carotid pulse count immediately following exercise.

Over a period of 14 years, the CAFT was used by an estimated one million people, with the only reported complications being a very small number of minor muscle pulls (caused by stumbling), and very rare episodes of dizziness or transient loss of consciousness (arising from preexisting conditions).[23, 24] The test has been well received and has achieved its prime objective of stimulating an interest in endurance exercise.

Researchers have found that using the CAFT with an electrocardiogram for heart rate determination has given a closer approximation to direct treadmill estimates of training response than the Astrand nomogram based on the Astrand-Rhyming bicycle test.[25] It is now being proposed that a properly administered CAFT, with post-exercise heart rate accurately recorded by electrocardiogram, offers a convenient submaximum tool for evaluating cardiorespiratory fitness, particularly in such settings as employee fitness programs.[26] With the relatively high correlation with directly measured maximum oxygen uptake (0.88), it provides a means of accurately testing large populations without sophisticated equipment.[22]

The Canadian Standardized Test of Fitness (CSTF), which includes all the instructions on how to take the CAFT test, plus the cassette tape and other fitness materials, can be obtained from:

Fitness and Amateur Sport Canada
365 Laurier Avenue West
Ottawa, Ontario K1A 0X6
Canada

As described in Chapter 3, the following items are included in the CSTF.

- Resting heart rate
- Resting blood pressure
- Three-site skinfold test (chest, abdomen, and thigh for men; triceps, supraillium, and thigh for women). *Note:* the Canadian Standardized Test of Fitness includes other anthropometric measurements including girths of chest, waist, hip, and right thigh, and five skinfold measurements including triceps, biceps, subscapular, iliac crest, and medial calf.
- Canadian home fitness test for cardiorespiratory endurance
- Sit-and-reach test for flexibility
- Hand-grip dynamometer test (both hands) for muscular strength
- One-minute timed sit-ups for abdominal muscular endurance
- Push-ups (consecutively, without a time limit) for upper body muscular strength and endurance

The CAFT is a modified step test performed on two 8-inch (20.3 cm) steps. (See Figure 4.8.) Based on the age of the person being tested, the record is set at a certain stepping tempo. The person then steps up and down the steps at the given rate for three minutes. The cassette gives instructions and time signals as to when to start and stop exercising, and for the counting of the 10-second measurement of the post-exercise heart rate.

The cassette contains a choice of seven exercise tempos with the total number of ascents varying from 11 per minute all the way up to 26 per minute. It also plays music that gives a 6-beat cadence for each cycle. Some people need a bit of coaching to get used to the rhythm of the beat.

The stepping procedure follows a six-count format:

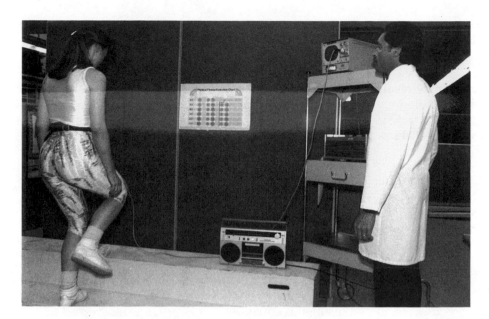

Figure 4.8 The Canadian Aerobic Fitness Test is a modified step test performed on two 8-inch (20.3 cm) steps.

1—(right foot on the first step); 2—(left foot on top of the second step); 3—(right foot on top of the second step along with the left); 4—(left foot down to the first step); 5—(right foot down to the floor); 6—(left foot down to the floor along with the right).

The pulse is taken immediately after the 3-minute stepping exercise, while the participant stands motionless, and the pulse count is compared with the norms. (See Figure 4.9.) If the pulse is low enough, another three-minute stepping exercise is undertaken at a slightly faster rate. For those in very good shape, a third three-minute cycle is performed.

The most important skill to master for the test is accurate pulse taking—on the radial or carotid artery for 10 seconds. Although one study showed that with proper training, exercisers could measure their own heart rates with an average variance of only 7 beats from the actual rate as determined with EKG,[22] the EKG is highly recommended. The CAFT should not be taken after a large meal, after performing vigorous exercise, after using alcohol, coffee, or tobacco, or in hot rooms.

In theory, the CAFT is designed to stop all participants before they exceed approximately 70–80 percent of $\dot{V}O_{2max}$. However, this is based on an extrapolation of

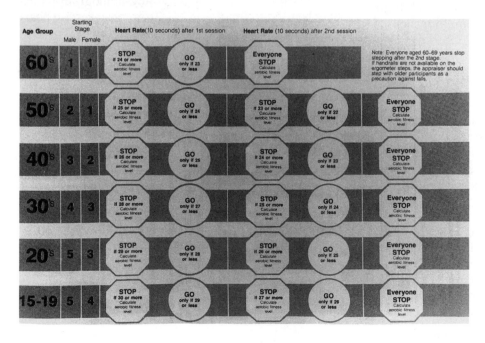

Figure 4.9 The Canadian Aerobic Fitness Test norms are based on 10-second pulse counts at the end of 3-minute stages of exercise.

the submaximal heart rate to an estimated maximal heart rate level—an imprecise method (and the major weakness of all submaximal testing, as explained earlier).

Predicted $\dot{V}O_{2max}$ can be calculated from the results of the step test by utilizing the following equation:

$$\dot{V}O_{2max} \text{ ml} \cdot \text{kg}^{-1} \cdot \text{min}^{-1} = 42.5 + (16.6 \times \dot{V}O_2) - (0.12 \times \text{Weight}) - (0.12 \times \text{Heart rate}) - (0.24 \times \text{Age}).$$

Use kilograms for body weight and the heart rate after the final stage of stepping in beats per minute. $\dot{V}O_2$ is the average oxygen cost of the last completed exercise stage in liters per minute which is taken from the following data listing:

Stage	Males	Females
1	1.1391	0.9390
2	1.3466	1.0484
3	1.6250	1.3213
4	1.8255	1.4925
5	2.0066	1.6267
6	2.3453	1.7867
7	2.7657	—

See the norms for $\dot{V}O_{2max}$ in Appendix B (Table 44) to determine the classification for aerobic fitness.

The YMCA Three-Minute Step Test

The YMCA uses the three-minute step test for mass testing of participants. (See norms, Appendix B, Table 41.)

The equipment involved includes: a 12-inch-high, sturdy bench; a metronome set at 96 bpm (four clicks of the metronome equals one cycle, up 1,2, down 3,4), which should be properly calibrated with a wrist watch; a timing clock for the 3-minute stepping exercise and 1-minute recovery; and preferably a stethoscope to count the pulse rate.[27]

It is important to first demonstrate the stepping technique to the person to be tested (four counts—right foot up onto the bench on 1, left foot up on 2, right foot down to the floor on 3, and left foot down on 4). The exerciser should have some preliminary practice, and should be well rested, with no prior exercise of any kind.

The test involves stepping up and down at the 24-steps-per-minute rate for 3 minutes, then immediately sitting down. Within 5 seconds the person testing should be counting the pulse with the stethoscope, and should *count for one full minute*. The person can take his own pulse at the same time by palpating the radial artery,

allowing each person involved in the testing to verify the other's count. The one-minute count limit reflects the heart's ability to recover quickly.

The total one-minute post-exercise heart rate is the score for the test and should be recorded. It can be affected by many factors other than fitness, such as emotion, tiredness, prior exercise, resting and maximum heart rates that differ from population averages, and miscounting.

Other Step Tests

McArdle in 192 devised a step test to predict $\dot{V}O_{2max}$ in which the subject steps at a rate of 22 steps per minute (females) or 24 steps per minute (males) for 3 minutes.[28] The bench height is 16.25 inches. After exercise, the subject remains standing, waits 5 seconds, and takes a 15-second heart rate count. The $\dot{V}O_{2max}$ is predicted using this equation:

Predicted $\dot{V}O_{2max} = 111.33 - (0.42 \times \text{heart rate})$ (for males)

Predicted $\dot{V}O_{2max} = 65.81 - (0.1847 \times \text{heart rate})$ (for females)

The standard error of prediction using this equation is within plus or minus 16 percent of the actual $\dot{V}O_{2max}$.

There are additional step tests described in the literature. The Harvard Step Test is for young men, who step 30 times per minute for 5 minutes on a 20-inch bench. A description of the test is given by Brouha.[29] There is also the Astrand-Rhyming nomogram which may be used to predict $\dot{V}O_{2max}$ from postexercise heart rate and body weight during bench stepping. The subject steps at a rate of 22.5 steps per minute for 5 minutes. The bench height is 33 cm for women and 40 cm for men. The postexercise heart rate is obtained by counting the number of beats between 15 and 30 seconds immediately after exercise (then multiplying by 4).[30]

ACSM Bench Stepping Equation

The American College of Sports Medicine has determined the energy expenditure for stepping in terms of METS.[12] (See Table 4.5.) There are two important terms that are used by the American College of Sports Medicine in their equations and calculations. These two terms are "METS" and kcal $\cdot$ min^{-1}. As explained earlier, one MET is equal to 3.5 ml $\cdot$ kg^{-1} $\cdot$ min^{-1} or the oxygen consumption during rest. One MET is also equal to one kcal $\cdot$ kg^{-1} $\cdot$ hour^{-1}. Thus the energy expenditure in kcal $\cdot$ min^{-1} can be determined by multiplying the MET value of the exercise by the body weight of the person tested in kilograms, and then dividing by 60 (minutes per hour). (See Box 4.2. See also Physical Fitness Activity 4.1 at the end of this chapter.)

Submaximal Laboratory Tests

The weaknesses and strengths of submaximal testing were discussed in the previous section.

Submaximal testing is done not only on steps, but also on the treadmill and bicycle.[10, 20] Submaximal testing on treadmills uses a cutoff point based on a predetermined heart rate, usually 85 percent of the predicted heart rate range, using the *Karvonen formula*. (See Chapter 8.)*

---

*The Karvonen formula will be explained in greater detail in Chapter 8, but is listed here for reference: Exercise Heart Rate = [(MHR - RHR) x percent INTENSITY] + RHR. (MHR = maximum heart rate; percent INTENSITY = percentage value ranging from 50 to 85 percent; RHR = resting heart rate).

Table 4.5 Energy Expenditure in METS During Stepping at Different Rates on Steps of Different Heights

Step Height		Steps Per Minute			
(CM)	(IN)	12	18	24	30
0	0	1.2	1.8	2.4	3.0
4	16	1.5	2.3	3.1	3.8
8	3.2	1.9	2.8	3.7	4.6
12	4.7	2.2	3.3	4.4	5.5
16	6.3	2.5	3.8	5.0	6.3
20	7.9	2.8	4.3	5.7	7.1
24	9.4	3.2	4.8	6.3	7.9
28	11.0	3.5	5.2	7.0	8.7
32	12.6	3.8	5.7	7.7	9.6
36	14.2	4.1	6.2	8.3	10.4
40	15.8	4.5	6.7	9.0	11.2

Source: American College of Sports Medicine. Guidelines for Graded Exercise Testing, 1986. Philadelphia: Lea & Febiger. Used with permission.

Box 4.2

Each MET is equal to 3.5 ml of oxygen per kilogram of body weight per minute (3.5 ml $\cdot$ kg^{-1} $\cdot$ min^{-1}). Total oxygen uptake can thus be determined by multiplying the MET value by 3.5 ml $\cdot$ kg^{-1} $\cdot$ min^{-1}. The data in this table are based on submaximal, steady-state exercise; thus, caution should be taken in extrapolating to $\dot{V}O_{2max}$ (data may overpredict $\dot{V}O_{2max}$ by 1 to 2 METS). This table is based on formulas derived from the ACSM as follows:

$\dot{V}O_2$ ml $\cdot$ kg^{-1} $\cdot$ min^{-1} = (height in meters $\cdot$ step^{-1} $\times$ steps $\cdot$ min^{-1} $\times$ 1.33 $\times$ 1.8 ml $\cdot$ kgm^{-1}) + $\dot{V}O_2$ of horizontal stepping. (*Note:* The $\dot{V}O_2$ of horizontal stepping is equal to steps $\cdot$ min^{-1} $\times$ 0.35 ml $\cdot$ kg^{-1} $\cdot$ min^{-1}/steps $\cdot$ min^{-1}).

For example, if a person is stepping 30 times per minute on a 10 cm bench, then the $\dot{V}O_2$ in ml $\cdot$ kg^{-1} $\cdot$ min^{-1} = (0.1 m $\cdot$ step^{-1} $\times$ 30 steps $\cdot$ min^{-1} $\times$ 1.33 $\times$ 1.8 ml $\cdot$ kgm^{-1}) + (10.5 ml $\cdot$ kg^{-1} $\cdot$ min^{-1}) = (7.18 ml $\cdot$ kg^{-1} $\cdot$ min^{-1} + 10.5 ml $\cdot$ kg^{-1} $\cdot$ min^{-1}) = 17.68 ml $\cdot$ kg^{-1} $\cdot$ min^{-1}. METS = 17.68 ml $\cdot$ kg^{-1} $\cdot$ min^{-1} /3.5 ml $\cdot$ kg^{-1} min^{-1} = 5 METS.

Since 1 MET = 1 kcal $\cdot$ kg^{-1} $\cdot$ hour^{-1}, energy expenditure in kcal $\cdot$ min^{-1} can be determined by multiplying the MET value by the body weight of the person in kilograms, and then dividing by 60 minutes per hour. For example, for a person weighing 65 kg:

5 METS = 5 kcal $\cdot$ kg^{-1} $\cdot$ hour^{-1} = 5 kcal $\cdot$ kg^{-1} $\cdot$ hour^{-1} $\times$ 65 kg $\cdot$ hour^{-1} = 325 kcal $\cdot$ hour^{-1} or 5.4 kcal $\cdot$ min^{-1}.

Often the Balke or Bruce protocol is used (see next section), with the test terminated when the heart rate reaches the cutoff point. Heart rate during exercise can be determined by using a heart rate ruler with an EKG recording, a heart rate monitor, or stethoscope auscultation as described earlier in this chapter. A well-conditioned person can perform longer on the treadmill before reaching the cutoff heart rate point.

As discussed previously, there are several problems with this method, especially the inaccuracy of the predicted maximal heart rate.

Submaximal bicycle ergometer tests can also be used to predict $\dot{V}O_{2max}$. These tests are once again based on the assumption that heart rate and oxygen uptake are linear functions of workload. The heart rate response to submaximum work loads is used to predict $\dot{V}O_{2max}$.[10, 20]

Bicycle and Treadmill Ergometers

Before discussing the YMCA submaximal bicycle test, a comparison of the advantages and disadvantages of treadmills vs. bicycles is helpful.[9, 31] (See Box 4.3.)

In general, the advantages of the treadmill outweigh the disadvantages. A national survey of 1,400 exercise testing facilities in America showed that 71 percent used treadmills for exercise testing, 17 percent used cycle ergometers, and 12 percent used steps.[32]

The most commonly used submaximal cycle ergometer tests include the multistage physical work capacity test developed by Sjostrand[33] and a single stage test by Astrand and Rhyming.[34] Both tests assume that because heart rate and $\dot{V}O_2$ are linearly related over a broad range, the submaximal heart rate at a certain workload can predict $\dot{V}O_{2max}$.

A Description of Bicycle Ergometers

Before describing the Sjostrand cycle test adapted by the YMCA,[27] a few facts on cycle ergometers need to be explained.

- There are two major types of bicycle ergometers—mechanically braked or electronically braked. (See Figure 4.10.) The mechanically braked cycle ergometers are very accurate in workload adjustment, and are not as expensive as the electronic versions. The mechanically braked cycle ergometers have a front flywheel braked by a belt running around the rim attached to a weighted pendulum. The workload is adjusted by tightening or loosening the brake belt. The pedaling rate has to be maintained by the person being tested in time to a metronome. The electronically braked ergometers use an electromagnetic braking force to adjust the workload (the resistance is variable in relation to the pedaling rate, so that a constant work output in watts is maintained). (*Note:* Because of the high expense of the electronically braked ergometer, the rest of this discussion will focus on mechanically braked cycle ergometers.)

- The mechanically braked bicycle ergometer should be accurate, easily calibrated, have constant torque, and have a range of 0–2100 kilogram-meters per

Box 4.3 Treadmills vs. Bicycle Ergometers

Advantages of Treadmills

1. Walking, jogging, or running are the most natural forms of locomotion. Most Americans are unaccustomed to bicycling (the treadmill was invented in America; the bicycle ergometer in Europe).

2. In general, subjects reach higher $\dot{V}O_{2max}$ values during treadmill tests than they do with the bicycle. $\dot{V}O_{2max}$ is usually 5 to 25 percent lower with bicycle tests than with treadmill tests, depending on the participant's conditioning and leg strength. Only elite cyclists can achieve $\dot{V}O_{2max}$ values on bicycles that equal treadmill values.

Disadvantages of Treadmills

1. Treadmills are more expensive than most bicycle ergometers.

2. The treadmill is less portable than the bicycle, requires more space, is heavy, and makes more noise.

3. The power (workload) of the treadmill cannot be measured directly in kgm·min⁻¹ or watts, so it must be calculated.

4. The workload on the treadmill depends on body weight. In longitudinal studies with body weight changes, the workload changes. The body weight has a much smaller effect on bicycle ergometer performance.

5. The danger of a fall is greater while running on a treadmill than while cycling on the bicycle ergometer.

6. Measurement of heart rate and blood pressure is more difficult when a person is exercising on a treadmill than when on a bicycle.

minute. Several ergometers meet these specifications (Bodyguard and Monark, for example—see equipment list in Appendix C.)

- The calibration of the bicycle should always be checked before testing. If using the Monark, be sure the red line on the pendulum weight is reading zero on the workload scale. An adjusting wing nut easily corrects malalignments. The calibration of the bike itself is done precisely at the factory and unless the adjusting screw on the pendulum weight has been tampered with, there is seldom a need for recalibration. The calibration can be checked by

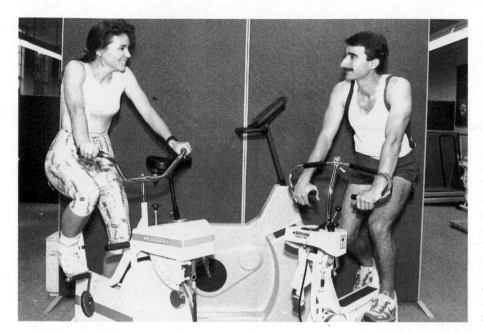

Figure 4.10 Mechanically braked cycle ergometers such as the Monark and Bodyguard models pictured here have a front flywheel braked by a belt running around the rim attached to a weighted pendulum. The workload is adjusted by tightening or loosening the brake belt. The pedaling rate has to be maintained by the exerciser in time to a metronome. Good mechanically braked models cost between $750 and $1,000. The electronically braked ergometers use an electromagnetic braking force to adjust the workload. The resistance is variable in relation to the pedaling rate, so that a constant work output in watts is maintained. However, electronically braked ergometers such as the Lifecycle pictured here cost over $2,500.

hanging a known 2- or 4-kilogram weight on the part of the strap that moves the pendulum weight. The pendulum weight should read exactly 2 or 4 kg. If the numbers don't agree, the adjusting screw on the pendulum weight should be adjusted.

- The seat height of the ergometer should be set to the leg length of the rider. With the pedal in its lowest position, if the heel of the foot is put onto the pedal, the leg should be straight. When the ball of the foot is put onto the pedal (as should be done during cycling), a slight bend of the leg at the knee should be apparent.

- The workload on the Monark or other mechanically braked bicycles is usually expressed in *kilogram-meters per minute* (kgm · min⁻¹) or in *watts* (one watt = 6 kgm · min⁻¹). The equation W = F × D (W = Work in kgm · min⁻¹; F = the force or resistance in kilograms; D = the distance traveled by the flywheel rim per pedal revolution) applies to the Monark and Bodyguard bicycle ergometers. On a Monark or Bodyguard bicycle, the flywheel travels 6 meters per pedal revolution. If the resistance is set with the front handwheel knob (which sets the weighted pendulum at 1 kilogram or 1 kilogram, 2 kilograms, etc.), the workload is easily figured out. If for example, the cycling rate is 50 revolutions per minute with the weighted pendulum set at 2 kilograms, then the workload is:

Work = 2 kg × 6 m · rpm⁻¹ × 50 rpm = 600 kgm · min⁻¹ (100 watts)

The YMCA Submaximal Bicycle Test

- For the YMCA test, set the metronome at 100 beats per minute, for a rate of 50 rpm (one beat for each foot down). Let the person being tested get used to the cadence, warming up for about 3–5 minutes.

- Next, set the workload, using Figure 4.11. The initial workload is set at 150 kgm · min⁻¹.

  The person exercising cycles at the first workload for 3 minutes, then stops, and his heart rate is counted immediately with a stethoscope for 10 seconds (and then multiplied by 6). If there is doubt as to the accuracy of the heart rate, let him cycle another minute at the same workload and try again. The objective is to get a steady state heart rate at this particular workload.

- Check Figure 4.11 to decide on the next workload setting. Workloads are adjusted on the basis of heart rate response.

- Regularly check the workload setting during each workload period. As the friction belt gets hot, the workload creeps upward, so continual readjustment during the early stages is necessary.

Guide to Setting Workloads on Bicycle Ergometer

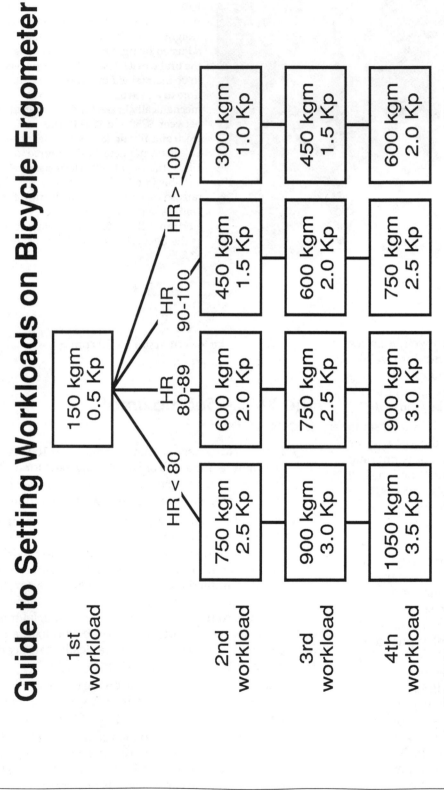

Directions:

1. Set the first workload at 150 kgm/min (0.5 Kp).
2. If the HR in the third min is
   - less than (<) 80, set the second load at 750 kgm (2.5 Kp);
   - 80 to 89, set the second load at 600 kgm (2.0 Kp);
   - 90 to 100, set the second load at 450 kgm (1.5 Kp);
   - greater than (>) 100, set the second load at 300 kgm (1.0 Kp).
3. Set the third and fourth (if required) loads according to the loads in the columns below the second loads.

Figure 4.11 Guide to setting workloads for males on the YMCA's submaximal bicycle ergometer test. *Source:* Reprinted from Y's Way to Physical Fitness (3rd Ed) 1989 with permission of the YMCA of the U.S.A., 101 N. Wacker Drive, Chicago, IL 60606.

- Again check the pulse after three or four minutes of cycling at the new workload. Determine the steady state pulse rate, and check Figure 4.11 to determine the third and final workload. (*Note:* If the first workload produced a heart rate greater than 110 bpm, the third workload is not necessary.)

- Throughout the test, watch for exertional intolerance or other signs of undue fatigue or unusual response. Explain to the participant that he/she should feel between 3 and 5 on the Borg scale.[35, 36] (See Figure 4.12.)

- The objective of the YMCA submaximal bicycle test is to obtain two heart rates between 110 and 150 bpm. There is a linear relationship between heart rate and workload between these two rates for most people. When the heart rate is less than 110, many external stimuli can affect the rate (talking, laughter, nervousness, etc.). However, once the heart rate climbs between 110 and 150, external stimuli no longer affect the rate, and there is a linear relationship. If the heart rate climbs above 150, the relationship becomes curvilinear. So the objective of this test is to obtain two heart rates between 110–150 bpm (steady state) at two different workloads, to establish linearity between heart rate and workload for the person being tested.

- To establish the line, two points are needed. It is important that the heart rates taken be true steady state values. To ensure this, it is better to let participants cycle beyond 3 minutes, especially during the second workload (the heart rate takes longer to plateau when the workload is harder).

- Once the test is completed, the two steady-state heart rates should be plotted against the respective workload in Figure 4.13. A straight line is drawn through the two points and extended to that participant's predicted maximal heart rate (220 – age). The point at which the diagonal line intersects the horizontal predicted maximal heart rate line represents the maximal working capacity for that participant. A perpendicular line should be dropped from this point to the baseline where the maximal physical workload capacity can be read in kgm · min⁻¹.

- The maximal physical workload capacity in kgm · min⁻¹ can then be used to predict a person's maximum oxygen uptake. These values are listed at the

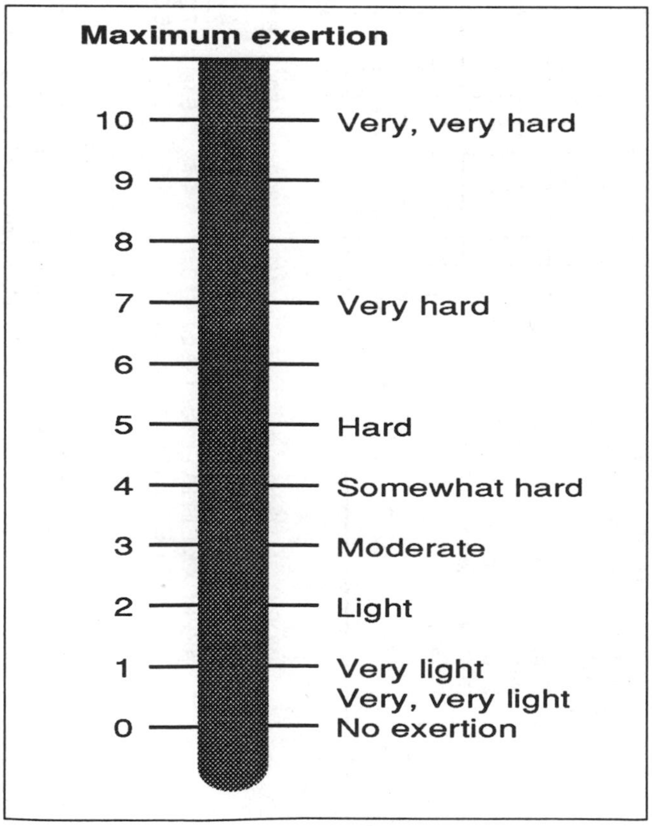

Figure 4.12 Borg Scale Rating of Perceived Exertion During exercise heart rates of 110-150, exercise for most people will feel "3-Moderate" to "5-Hard." If the exercise feels harder than this, the workload should be reassessed. *Source:* Jacobs I. Blood Lactate and the Evaluation of Endurance Fitness. *Sports: Science Periodical On Research and Technology In Sports, 1983.* The Coaching Association of Canada, 333 River Road, Ottawa, Ontario, K11 8B9. Used with permission.

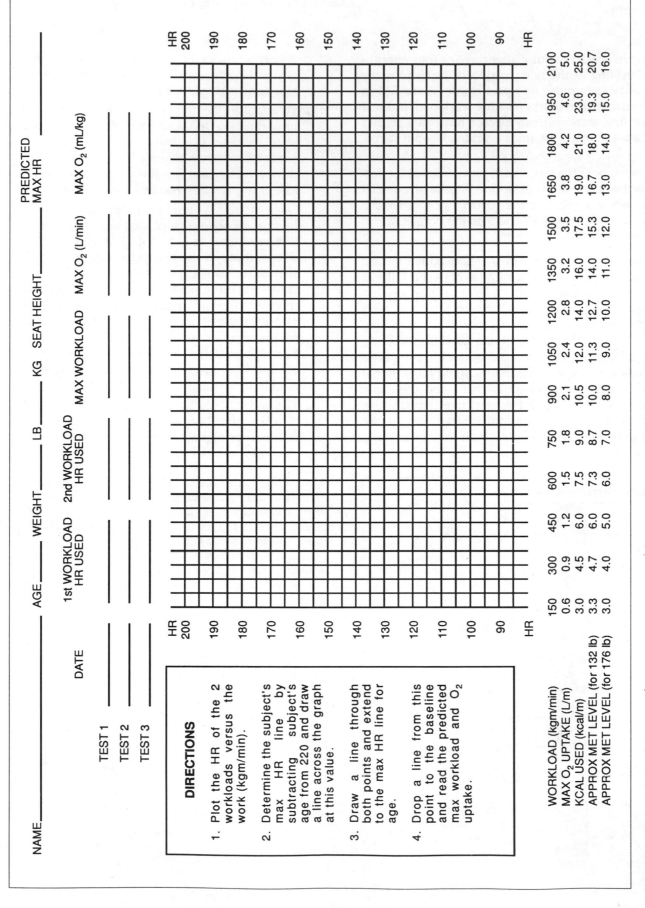

Figure 4.13 Graph for determining $\dot{V}O_{2max}$ from submaximal heart rates obtained during the YMCA's submaximal bicycle test.
Source: Reprinted from The Y's Way to Physical Fitness (3rd Ed. Champaign, Il, Human Kinetics Publisher, 1989), with permission of the YMCA of the U.S.A., 101 N. Wacker Drive, Chicago, IL 60606.

bottom of the graph. Use the norms in Appendix B (Tables 42 and 44) for interpretation. Remember that these results are predictions or estimates, not direct measurements, and are thus open to error (but usually within 15 percent of the actual value).

ACSM Bicycle Equation

▪ The American College of Sports Medicine has established tables and formulas to estimate the MET cost of bicycle ergometry.[12] Table 4.6 shows the MET energy expenditure values during bicycle ergometry.

Maximal Laboratory Tests

The graded exercise test (GXT) to exhaustion, with EKG monitoring, is considered the best substitute for the gold-standard test (direct $\dot{V}O_{2max}$ determination).[20] This diagnostic, functional capacity test is mandatory for all people in the high-risk category who want to start an exercise program.[9]

The maximal graded exercise test (usually done with a treadmill or bicycle ergometer) with EKG serves several purposes:[37]

▪ To diagnose overt or latent heart disease
▪ To evaluate cardiorespiratory functional capacity (heart and lung endurance)
▪ To evaluate responses to conditioning or cardiac rehabilitation programs

---

Box 4.4 Estimated Oxygen Demand Formula

The formula for estimating oxygen demands for cycle ergometer exercise is:

$\dot{V}O_2$ ml · min^{-1} = WORK RATE IN kgm · min^{-1} × 2 ml · kgm^{-1} + SITTING $\dot{V}O_2$ OF 3.5 ml · kg^{-1} · min^{-1} × KG (body weight)

To get $\dot{V}O_2$ in ml · kg^{-1} · min^{-1}, divide final answer by body weight in kilograms.

For example, if a 70 kg man cycles at a work rate of 900 kgm · min^{-1}, the $\dot{V}O_2$ in ml · min^{-1} is =[(900 kgm · min^{-1} × 2 ml · kgm^{-1}) + 245 ml · min^{-1}] = 2045 ml · min^{-1}.

To get $\dot{V}O_2$ in ml · kg^{-1} · min^{-1}, divide by body weight of 70 kg which is 2045 ml · min^{-1}/70 kg = 29.2 ml · kg^{-1} · min^{-1} or 8.3 METS.

▪ To increase individual motivation for entering and adhering to exercise programs.

Maximal Graded Exercise Treadmill Test Protocols

Figures 4.14 and 4.15 describe the most commonly used maximal treadmill protocols.[10, 16, 38] Of the treadmill protocols, the Bruce is by far the most commonly used, followed by the Balke. The Bruce has relatively large,

---

Table 4.6 Energy Expenditure in METS During Bicycle Ergometry

Body Weight		Exercise Rate in KGM · Min^{-1} and Watts						
KG	LBS	300 50	450 75	600 100	750 125	900 150	1050 175	1200 KGM · Min^{-1} 200 WATTS
50	110	5.1	6.9	8.6	10.3	12.0	13.7	15.4
60	132	4.3	5.7	7.1	8.6	10.0	11.4	12.9
70	154	3.7	4.9	6.1	7.3	8.6	9.8	11.0
80	176	3.2	4.3	5.4	6.4	7.5	8.6	9.6
90	198	2.9	3.8	4.8	5.7	6.7	7.6	8.6
100	220	2.6	3.4	4.3	5.1	6.0	6.9	7.7

Note: $\dot{V}O_2$ for zero load pedaling is approximately 550 ml · min^{-1} for 70 to 80 kg subjects.

Source: American College of Sports Medicine. Guidelines for Graded Exercise Testing and Prescription. Philadelphia: Lea and Febiger, 1986. Reprinted with permission.

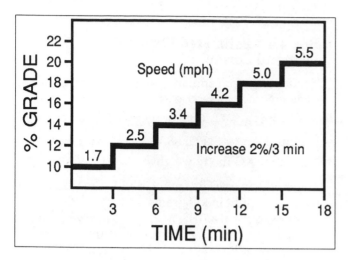

Figure 4.14 The Bruce maximal graded exercise test protocol. *Source:* Bruce RA. Kusumi F, Hosmer D: Maximal oxygen intake and nomographic assessment of functional aerobic impairment in cardiovascular disease. Am Heart J 85:546-562, 1973.

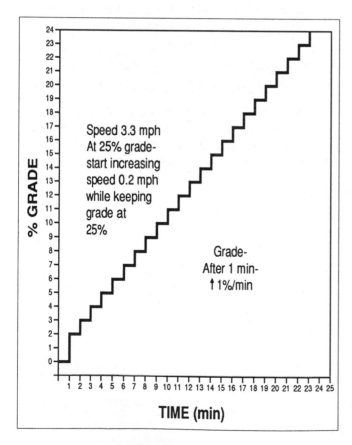

Figure 4.15 The Balke maximal graded exercise test protocol. *Source:* Cooper KH. The Aerobics Way. New York: M. Evans and Co., 1977.

abrupt increases in work load every three minutes, and some have criticized the test for this. Nonetheless, excellent maximal data can be obtained, and because the test is so widely used, there is an abundance of comparative data.[9] (See Appendix B, Table 43.)

The main criticism of the Balke test is its duration (nearly twice as long as the Bruce). In testing large numbers of people, the length of time needed for the Balke makes its use prohibitive. Ken Cooper uses the Balke protocol in his Aerobics Center in Dallas because he feels the Balke allows for a more gradual warm-up and is therefore safer. The Balke is basically an uphill walking test, while the Bruce starts out as an uphill walking test, and then in Stage 4 becomes an uphill running test.

In general, $\dot{V}O_{2max}$ can be estimated accurately from performance time on the treadmill. Maximal treadmill tests using performance time show very high correlations with laboratory-determined $\dot{V}O_{2max}$.[9] Thus actual measurement of $\dot{V}O_{2max}$ is not actually necessary if the person is taken to a "true max" which means:

- The person is allowed to practice one time before the maximal test to become "habituated" to the treadmill.

- He is *urged* to exercise until exhaustion is reached.

- When he is "maxed-out," there is no additional increase in heart rate despite an increase in workload, he shows signs of exertional intolerance (fatigue, staggering, inability to keep up with the work load, facial pallor), and reports going to #10 or above on the Borg scale. (See Figure 4.12.)

- During the test, he is not allowed to hang onto the treadmill bar in any way.

To ensure valid and reliable $\dot{V}O_{2max}$ values, the testing protocol should be very specific to the type of exercise the person is accustomed to.[39] The laboratory environment should be 20–23°C, 50% humidity. If follow-up testing is conducted, tests should be repeated at the same time of the day, using the exact same procedures.

The Bruce Treadmill Equation for Predicting $\dot{V}O_{2max}$

When the participant is allowed to exercise to maximal capacity in this way, $\dot{V}O_{2max}$ can be estimated very precisely. Appendix B, (Table 43) contains a table from Pollock[9] which accurately estimates $\dot{V}O_{2max}$ based on length of time until exhaustion with the Bruce or Balke protocol. Appendix B (Table 44) also contains norms for classifying $\dot{V}O_{2max}$.

Formulas have been developed for predicting the oxygen uptake of healthy men using the Bruce protocol.[40, 41] The best equation is as follows:[41]

$$\dot{V}O_{2max}\ ml \cdot kg^{-1} \cdot min^{-1} = 14.8 - 1.379(time) + 0.451(time^2) - 0.012(time^3)$$

Note: Time = total time to exhaustion during the Bruce maximal graded treadmill exercise test.

ACSM Equations for Estimating $\dot{V}O_2$ for Walking and Running

The American College of Sports Medicine has published steady-state $\dot{V}O_2$ values for running outdoors and on the treadmill, and also for walking.[12] This information is given in Tables 4.7, 4.8, and 4.9. The formula for graded treadmill exercise has been validated with a large number of people and found to be very accurate for adults.[42] Once again, these data are *steady-state* values, which means that if they are used to predict $\dot{V}O_{2max}$ data 2 to 4 minutes from the endpoint should be used. *Note:* 1 mph = 26.8 m · min⁻¹ = 1.6 kmh.

Maximal Graded Exercise Bicycle Test Protocols

There are two recommended maximal graded exercise bicycle test protocols, the Astrand and the Storer-Davis.

The Astrand Maximal Bicycle Protocol

For the Astrand maximal bicycle test, the initial work load is 300 kgm · min⁻¹ (50 watts) (1 kg at 50 rpm) for women, and 600 kgm · min⁻¹ (100 watts) (2 kg at 50 rpm) for men.[10] (See Figure 4.16.) After 2 minutes at this initial work load, it is increased every 2–3 minutes in increments of 150 kgm · min⁻¹ (25 watts or 1/2 kg) for women, and 300 kgm · min⁻¹ (50 watts or 1 kg) for men. The test is continued until the participant is exhausted or can no longer maintain the pedaling frequency of 50 rpm. A metronome should be used, with the tester carefully ensuring that the proper cadence is maintained.

The $\dot{V}O_{2max}$ for most people (except for elite cyclists) will be lower when derived from the maximal bicycle test than when derived from the Bruce's treadmill protocol.[9, 10] The ACSM bicycle formula can be used

---

Box 4.5 ACSM Energy Requirement Formulas

The American College of Sports Medicine formulas for these data are as follows:

Walking:

$\dot{V}O_2\ ml \cdot kg^{-1} \cdot min^{-1}$ = speed m · min⁻¹ × 0.1 ml · kg⁻¹ · min⁻¹/m·min⁻¹ + 3.5 ml · kg⁻¹ · min⁻¹.

Example: For 80 m · min⁻¹ (3 mph): 80 m · min⁻¹ × 0.1 + 3.5 = 11.5 ml · kg⁻¹ · min⁻¹ (METS = 11.5 / 3.5 = 3.3)

Grade Walking:

Use above equation plus:

$\dot{V}O_2\ ml \cdot kg^{-1} \cdot min^{-1}$ = percent grade × speed m · min⁻¹ x 1.8 ml · kgm · min⁻¹ /m · min⁻¹.

Example: if person walks at 80 m · min⁻¹ up 13 percent grade, then $\dot{V}O_2$ is equal to 11.5 ml · kg⁻¹ · min⁻¹ (see above) plus: (0.13 × 80 m · min⁻¹ × 1.8 ml · kgm⁻¹ = 18.72) =11.5 + 18.72 = 30.22 ml · kg⁻¹ · min⁻¹ (8.64 METS).

Jogging and Running (Speeds over 5 MPH):

$\dot{V}O_2\ ml \cdot kg^{-1} \cdot min^{-1}$ = speed m · min⁻¹ × 0.2 ml · kg⁻¹ · min⁻¹/ m · min⁻¹ +3.5 ml · kg⁻¹ · min⁻¹.

Example: For 200 m · min⁻¹ (7.5 mph):

$\dot{V}O_2\ ml \cdot kg^{-1} \cdot min^{-1}$ = 200 m · min⁻¹ × 0.2 ml · kg⁻¹ · min⁻¹/ m · min⁻¹ + 3.5 ml · kg⁻¹ · min⁻¹ = 43.5 (METS = 43.5/3.5 = 12.4).

Note: For speeds in units of kmh, the MET requirement is approximately equal to the speed (10 kmh = 10 METS; 16 kmh = 16 METS).

Inclined Running

Use the equation for running, plus:

On Treadmill: $\dot{V}O_2\ ml \cdot kg^{-1} \cdot min^{-1}$ =speed in m · min⁻¹ × percent grade × 1.8 ml · kgm · min⁻¹ / m · min⁻¹ × 0.5

Note: Since the oxygen cost of grade running off the treadmill (running outdoors up hills) may not be reliably predicted, the equation does not apply to this activity.

Table 4.7 Energy Requirements in METS for Horizontal and Uphill Jogging/Running

Outdoors on Solid Surface

% Grade	MPH M · Min⁻¹	5 134	6 161	7 188	7.5 201	8 215	9 241	10 268
0		8.6	10.2	11.7	12.5	13.3	14.8	16.3
2.5		10.3	12.3	14.1	15.1	16.1	17.9	19.7
5.0		12.0	14.3	16.5	17.7	18.8		
7.5		13.8	16.4	18.9				
10.0		15.5	18.5					

Source: American College of Sports Medicine. Guidelines for Graded Exercise Testing and Prescription. Philadelphia: Lea & Febiger, 1986. Reprinted with permission.

Table 4.8 Energy Requirements in METS for Horizontal and Uphill Jogging/Running

On the Treadmill

% Grade	MPH M·Min⁻¹	5 134	6 161	7 188	7.5 201	8 215	9 241	10 268
0		8.6	10.2	11.7	12.5	13.3	14.8	16.3
2.5		9.5	11.2	12.9	13.8	14.7	16.3	18.0
5.0		10.3	12.3	14.1	15.1	16.1	17.9	19.7
7.5		11.2	13.3	15.3	16.4	17.4	19.4	
10.0		12.0	14.3	16.5	17.7	18.8		
12.5		12.9	15.4	17.7	19.0			
15.0		13.8	16.4	18.9				

Note: Differences in energy expenditures between treadmill and outdoor running are accounted for by the effects of wind resistance. *Source:* American College of Sports Medicine. Guidelines for Graded Exercise Testing and Prescription. Lea & Febiger, 1986. Reprinted with permission.

Table 4.9 Approximate Energy Requirements in METS for Horizontal and Grade Walking

% Grade	MPH M·Min⁻¹	1.7 45.6	2.0 53.7	2.5 67.0	3.0 80.5	3.4 91.2	3.75 100.5
0		2.3	2.5	2.9	3.3	3.6	3.9
2.5		2.9	3.2	3.8	4.3	4.8	5.2
5.0		3.5	3.9	4.6	5.4	5.9	6.5
7.5		4.1	4.6	5.5	6.4	7.1	7.8
10.0		4.6	5.3	6.3	7.4	8.3	9.1
12.5		5.2	6.0	7.2	8.5	9.5	10.4
15.0		5.8	6.6	8.1	9.5	10.6	11.7
17.5		6.4	7.3	8.9	10.5	11.8	12.9
20.0		7.0	8.0	9.8	11.6	13.0	14.2
22.5		7.6	8.7	10.6	12.6	14.2	15.5
25.0		8.2	9.4	11.5	13.6	15.3	16.8

Source: American College of Sports Medicine. Guidelines for Graded Exercise Testing and Prescription. Philadelphia: Lea & Febiger, 1986. Reprinted with permission.

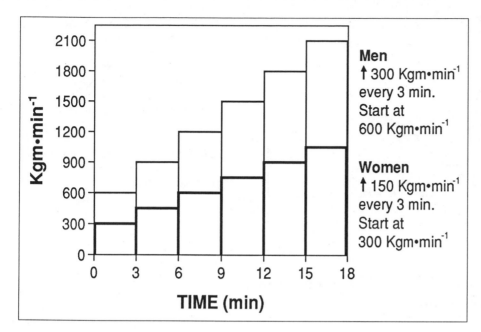

Figure 4.16 The Astrand maximal graded bicycle exercise test protocol. The metronome should be set at 100, with a cycling rate of 50 rpm (one foot down with each click of the metronome). With the pedaling speed at 50 rpm, 300 kgm/min is achieved with the bicycle ergometer belt tension set at 1 kg, 600 kgm/min at 2 kg, 900 kgm/min at 3 kg, etc. *Source:* Heyward VH. Designs for Fitness. Minneapolis: Burgess Publishing Co., 1984.

to estimate $\dot{V}O_{2max}$. (See Table 4.6.) However, the ACSM bicycle formula assumes that a steady-state has been achieved, and for the normal population, it has been shown that $\dot{V}O_2$ often plateaus one to three minutes before the test is completed (if the participant is taken to a "true max"). Steady-state $\dot{V}O_2$ tables will thus over-predict $\dot{V}O_{2max}$, unless steady-state values 2 to 4 minutes from the endpoint are used.[10, 12] In addition, the ACSM formulas may not be accurate for workloads over 200 watts. For people with high fitness levels, direct measurement of $\dot{V}O_{2max}$ is necessary.

The Storer-Davis Maximal Bicycle Protocol

Since there had been no precise equation for predicting $\dot{V}O_{2max}$ from cycle ergometer testing, the Storer-Davis equation was developed to make maximal bicycle testing more practical and accurate. This equation was developed after testing 115 males and 116 females, ages 20 to 70.[43] The protocol provides for a 4-minute warm-up at 0 watts. The workload is then increased by 15 watts per min, with a recommended rate of 60 rpm. On a mechanically braked ergometer, the kg setting should be increased 1/4 kg each minute. (See Figure 4.17.)

The equation uses the final workload in watts.

Males $\dot{V}O_{2max}$ (ml · min^{-1}) = (10.51 × watts) + (6.35 × kg) − (10.49 × age) + 519.3

Females $\dot{V}O_{2max}$ (ml · min^{-1}) = (9.39 × watts) + (7.7 × kg) − (5.88 × age) + 136.7

For males, the correlation with measured oxygen consumption is very high ($r = 0.94$). The standard error of estimate is low for both males (±212 ml · min^{-1}), and for females ($r = 0.93$) (SEE = ±145 ml · min^{-1}).

These SEEs are lower than they are with the Bruce treadmill equation.

Figures 4.18 and 4.19 are two nomograms that make the use of these equations much easier. (See the instructions in the legends.)

The Wingate Anaerobic Test

The maximal treadmill and bicycle protocols described thus far test maximal cardiorespiratory capacity. A different type of test has been developed to test *maximal anaerobic power*. Anaerobic power is the ability to exercise for a short time at high power levels, and is important for various sports where sprinting and power movements are common (e.g., football).

The test requires pedaling or arm cranking on a bicycle ergometer for 30 seconds at maximal speed against a constant force.[44] Power in watts is determined by counting pedal revolutions (watts = kp × rpm).

Three indices are measured: (1) peak power (the highest mechanical power in watts elicited during the test, usually within the first 10 seconds); (2) mean power (the average power sustained throughout the 30-second

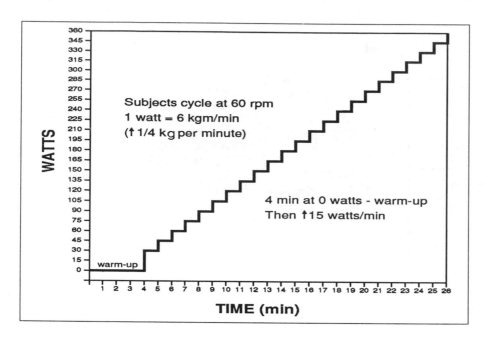

Figure 4.17 The Storer-Davis maximal bicycle protocol. In the protocol, subjects cycle for 4 min at 0 watts to warm-up. The workload is then increased 15 watts per min, at a recommended rate of 60 rpm. On a mechanically braked ergometer, the kg setting should be increased 1/4 kg each minute. *Source:* Storer TW, Davis JA, Caiozzo VJ. Accurate Prediction of $\dot{V}O_{2max}$ in Cycle Ergometry. Med Sci Sports Exerc 19:S64, 1987.

period); (3) rate of fatigue (peak power divided by the lowest power).

A predetermined force is used to ensure that a supramaximal effort is given. As a general guideline, with the Monark ergometer, a force of 0.090 kg/kg body weight should be used with adult nonathletes and of 0.100 kg/kg with adult athletes. The use of toe stirrups increases performance by 5 to 12 percent. Some tentative norms have been developed.[44] (See Table 4.10.)

Table 4.10 Norms for Wingate Anaerobic Test

Specialty (Watts/Kg)	Peak Power (Watts/Kg)	Mean Power
Males		
Power lifters	12.7	9.5
Gymnasts	12.3	9.1
Wrestlers	12.0	9.4
10 km runners	11.4	9.3
Ultra-marathoners	11.3	8.9

Source: Bar-Or O. The Wingate Anaerobic Test: An Update on Methodology, Reliability, and Validity. Sports Med 4:381–394, 1987.

When to Terminate the Maximal GXT-EKG Test

Cooper has reported that in his first 16,000 maximal GXT-EKG tests, he had four emergencies with no fatalities (personal communication). Bruce has reported no mortalities in 20,000 tests with less than 0.1 percent morbidity. A survey of clinical exercise facilities has shown that in general, GXT-EKG is a safe procedure with approximately one death and five nonfatal complications per 10,000 tests. Evidence suggests that maximum effort stress tests are no more dangerous than submaximum tests.[10] However, the risk is substantially higher for anyone who is coronary prone (6–12 times normal) and for coronary disease patients (60 times normal).[45]

To safely conduct a maximal GXT-EKG test, various criteria should be carefully adhered to, and emergency drugs and equipment, along with an attending physician, should be available.[12]

In a maximum graded exercise stress test, the exercise usually continues until the participant voluntarily terminates the test because of exhaustion. However, if the exercise technician and attending physician notice any of the signs or symptoms in the following list, the test should be stopped immediately.[12] (*Note:* Interpretation of most of the stress test termination points listed below should be made by a physician. Exercise technicians are not expected to be able to diagnose these problems.)

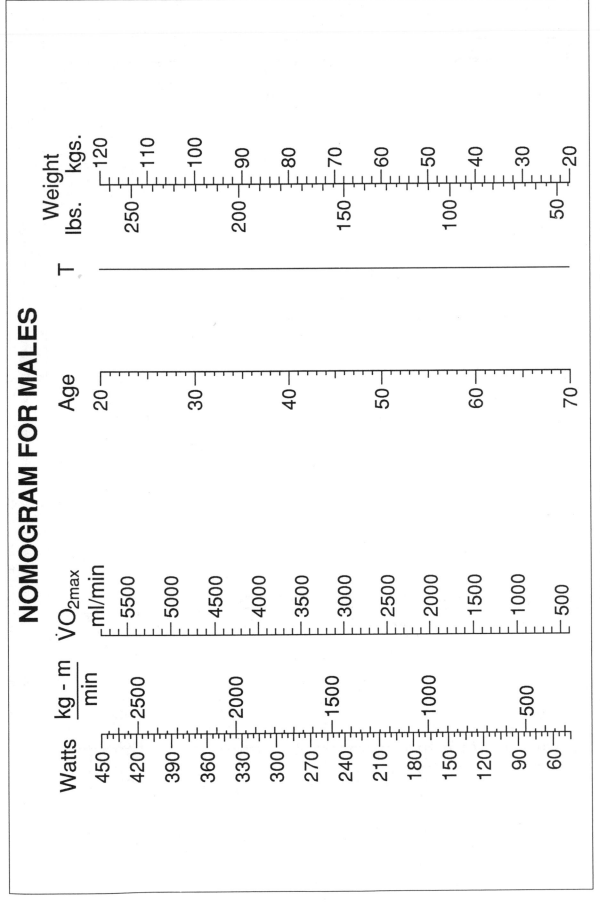

Figure 4.18 Nomogram for males, Storer-Davis maximal bicycle protocol. To use the nomogram, first put dots on the lines representing the participant's weight and age. Use a ruler and connect these two dots. Mark another dot on the "T" line where the connecting line crosses it. Finally put a dot on the "watts" representing the final workload achieved during the maximal bicycle text. Connect the dot on the "T" line with the "watts" line with a ruler. Mark another dot where this connecting line crosses the $\dot{V}O_{2max}$ line. This final dot represents the $\dot{V}O_{2max}$ in ml·min⁻¹. To calculate the $\dot{V}O_{2max}$ in ml·kg⁻¹·min⁻¹, divide by body weight in kilograms. *Source:* nomogram developed by Dr. Jerry Lee, School of Public Health, Loma Linda University.

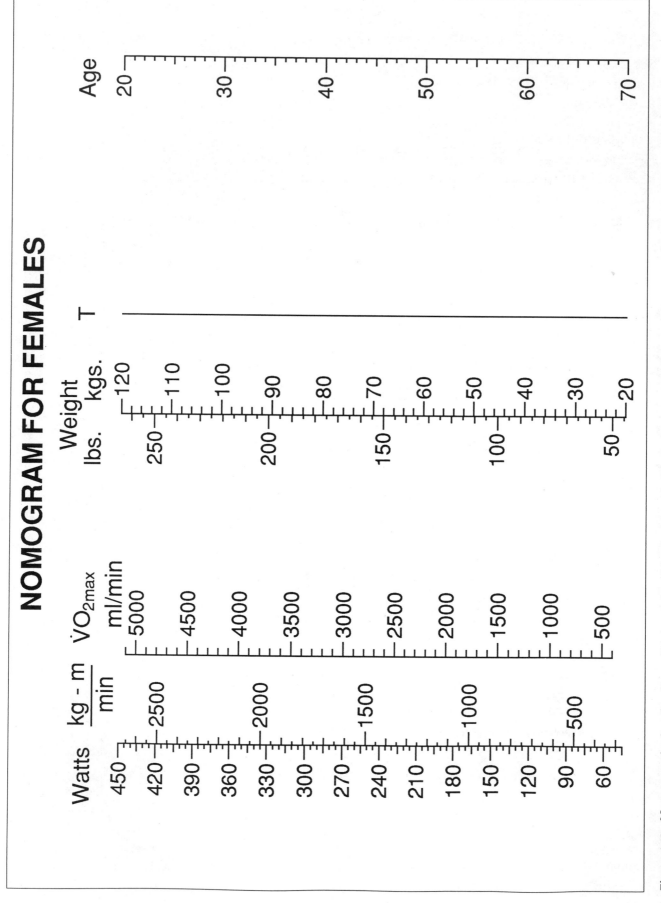

Figure 4.19 Nomogram for females, Storer-Davis maximal bicycle protocol. (See instructions for Figure 4.18.) *Source: nomogram developed by Dr. Jerry Lee, School of Public Health, Loma Linda University.

1. Subject asks to stop
2. Failure of the monitoring system
3. Progressive angina
4. Early onset, deep (74 mm) horizontal or down-sloping ST depression or elevation.
5. Sustained supraventricular tachycardia
6. Ventricular tachycardia
7. Exercise induced left bundle branch block
8. Any significant drop (20 mm Hg) of systolic blood pressure, or failure of the systolic blood pressure to rise with an increase in exercise load after the initial adjustment period
9. Lightheadedness, confusion, ataxia, pallor, cyanosis, nausea, or signs of severe peripheral circulatory insufficiency
10. Excessive blood pressure rise: Systolic greater than 250 mm Hg; diastolic greater than 120 mm Hg
11. Increasing ventricular ectopy, multiform PUCs, or R on T PUCs.
12. Increase in heart rate that is < 25 beats/min below age-predicted normal value.
13. Onset of second or third degree A-V heart block

Emergency Procedures

The American College of Sports Medicine advises the following:[12]

1. All personnel concerned with an exercise testing program should be trained in cardiopulmonary resuscitation.
2. The exercise program director or laboratory supervisor when possible should be trained in Advanced Cardiac Life Support.
3. Emergency equipment and drugs must be available in the immediate areas or through a mobile emergency unit and telephone call system. (See Table 4.11.)
4. Telephone numbers for emergency assistance should be clearly posted at all telephones.
5. Evacuation plans should be established and posted. Every staff person should be thoroughly familiar with all specific duties and evacuation procedures required in an emergency.

6. Procedures (code team drills) should be practiced on a regularly scheduled basis. (See Table 4.12.)

Although the supervising physician should be responsible for screening the participant before testing regarding medications, the exercise technician should have a basic working knowledge of the effects of various drugs on exercise performance as listed in Table 4.13.

Personnel

The ACSM[12] advises that ACSM-certified personnel administer the graded exercise test. When low risk participants are being tested, a physician need not be in attendance (but a qualified physician should be the overall director of any testing program, and consulted concerning protocols and emergency procedures). When testing people classified as high risk, a physician should be in the testing area, but not necessarily in visual contact with the person being tested. All other tests should be conducted with the physician in visual contact.

Sports Medicine Insight
Interpreting the
Electrocardiogram

Learning to interpret the electrocardiogram (EKG) takes special training under the guidance of experienced health professionals. Nevertheless, many experts feel that health and fitness leaders should be familiar with basic EKG principles. In addition, treadmill or bicycle ergometer operators are expected to be able to know when abnormal EKG patterns are appearing on the oscilloscope (and to call the attending physician, or if necessary terminate the test). The following description should be reviewed with an instructor familiar with EKG interpretation.

The EKG

The EKG presents a visible record of the heart's electrical activity, by means of a stylus that traces the activity on a continuously moving strip of special heat sensitive paper.[46-49] All heartbeats appear as a similar pattern, equally spaced, and consist of three major units (See Figures 4.6 and 4.20):

- *P Wave* (transmission of electrical impulse through the atria)
- *QRS Complex* (impulse through the ventricles)
- *T Wave* (electrical recovery or repolarization of the ventricles)

Heart cells are charged or *polarized* in the resting state (negative ions inside the cell, positive outside), but when electrically stimulated, they DEPOLARIZE (positive ions go inside the heart cell, negative ions go outside) and contract. Thus when the heart is stimulated, a wave of depolarization passes through the heart (an advancing wave of positive charges within the cells). As the positive wave of depolarization within the heart cells moves toward a positive skin electrode, there is a positive upward deflection recorded on the EKG.

Table 4.11   Emergency Equipment and Drugs

Equipment

1. Defibrillator with electrode paste
2. Airway
3. Oxygen
4. Intravenous sets including fluids, canulas, stands
5. Syringes and needles in multiple sizes
6. Adhesive tape
7. AMBU bag with pressure release valve
8. Suction equipment

Drugs

1. Aromatic ammonia
2. Metaraminol (Aramine)
3. Furosemide (Lasix
4. Epinephrine
5. Atropine

6. Isoproterenol (Isuprel)
7. Calcium chloride
8. Sodium bicarbonate
9. Lidocaine
10. Amyl nitrate ampule
11. Digoxin—I.V. and tablets
12. Nitroglycerin tablets
13. Verapamil (Isoptin)
14. I.V. Propranolol (Inderal)
15. I.V. Diazepam (Valium)
16. Dopamine
17. I.V. Nitroglycerin

Source: American College of Sports Medicine. Graded Exercise Testing and Prescription. Philadelphia: Lea & Febiger, 1986. Used with permission.

Table 4.12   Exercise Related Cardiovascular Emergencies[7]

Basic Causes	Emergency Procedures
1. Cardiac Arrest (ventricular fibrillation or cardiac standstill)	Physician defibrillates
2. Low Cardiac Output States (inadequate venous return with low BP, pallor, dizziness.	Put victim in supine position with legs elevated. Physician starts IV. Monitor BP and victim closely.
(arrhythmias like tachycardia or bradycardia or PACs, PVCs)	Physician administers medications. If needed, administer oxygen.
(drug induced lowering of HR and blood pressure from beta blockers, diuretics)	
3. Ischemic Status (chest pain, severe ST segment depression or EKG evidence of MI, cerebral ischemia with dizziness, ataxia, nausea, vomiting, impaired consciousness)	Stop exercise, place in supine resting position, and administer oxygen. Physician administers appropriate drugs. Monitor BP.

Table 4.13   Effects of Various Drugs on Exercise Performance[12]

1. Beta Blockers

The beta-blocking agents lower both exercise heart rate and blood presuure, and have a mixed effect on performance, tending to ↑performance in patients with angina.

2. Nitrates

Tend to increase heart rate, but decrease blood pressure during exercise, improving exercise performance in patients with angina or congestive heart failure.

3. Antiarrhythmic Agents: (e.g., Procaina-mide, Disopyramide, Quinidine, Phenytoin, Tocainide, Disopyramide

During exercise, may increase or have no effect on heart rate, with no effect on exercise performance. Quinidine may cause "false-negative" test results while Procainamide may cause "false-positive" test results.

4. Diuretics

Diuretics may decrease exercise blood pressure, but have no effect on exercise heart rate or performance.

5. Digitalis

This drug may produce ST segment depression during exercise, leading to a false-positive test. Tends to increase heart rate if given in toxic amounts, or to reduce it if it blocks the AV node. Exercise performance tends to be enhanced in some patients.

6. Other Agents:

Tranquilizers and Depressants:	(may increase HR during exercise, decrease BP, and cause T wave changes that may cause a false-positive test)
Nicotine:	(may increase both HR and BP during exercise)
Bronchodilators:	(may increase both HR and BP during exercise)
Antihistamines:	(have no effect on HR and BP during exercise)
Thyroid Drugs:	(increase both HR and BP during exercise)
Cold Remedies:	(may increase both HR and BP during exercise)
Alcohol:	(chronic use may increase BP and provoke arrhythmios)

Source: Adapted from the American College of Sports Medicine. Guidelines for Exercise Testing and Prescription (4th ed). Philadelphia: Lea & Febiger, 1991.

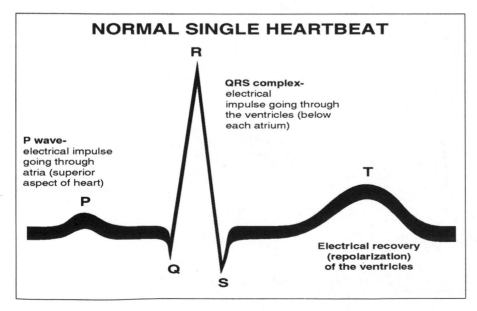

NORMAL SINGLE HEARTBEAT

R

QRS complex- electrical impulse going through the ventricles (below each atrium)

P wave- electrical impulse going through atria (superior aspect of heart)

P

T

Q

S

Electrical recovery (repolarization) of the ventricles

Figure 4.20   All heartbeats consist of three major units, the P wave, the QRS complex, and the T wave, which represent the transmission of electrical impulses through the heart.

The P wave (atrial wave) begins in the SA node (the normal physiological pacemaker) located near the top of the atrium. The impulse reaches the AV node located in the superior aspect of the ventricles. There is a 1/10 second pause, allowing blood to enter the ventricles from the contracting atria. (See Figure 4.21.)

The QRS complex (ventricular wave) begins in the AV node. After the 1/10-second pause, the AV node is stimulated, initiating an electrical impulse that starts down the AV Bundle called the *Bundle of HIS* into the *Bundle Branches* and finally into the *Purkinje Fibers*. The neuromuscular conduction system of the ventricles is composed of specialized nervous material which transmits the electrical impulse from the AV Node into the ventricular heart cells.

The EKG is recorded on ruled paper. The smallest divisions are one millimeter squares. On the horizontal line, one small block represents 0.04 second (one large block of 5 small blocks is 0.20 second). On the vertical axis, one small block represents 1/10 of a millivolt (10 small blocks vertically or two large blocks is 1 millivolt). (See Figure 4.22.)

The standard EKG is composed of 12 separate leads:

Limb leads:	I, II, III
Augmented Unipolar leads:	AVR, AVL, AVF
Chest Leads:	V1, V2, V3, V4, V5, V6

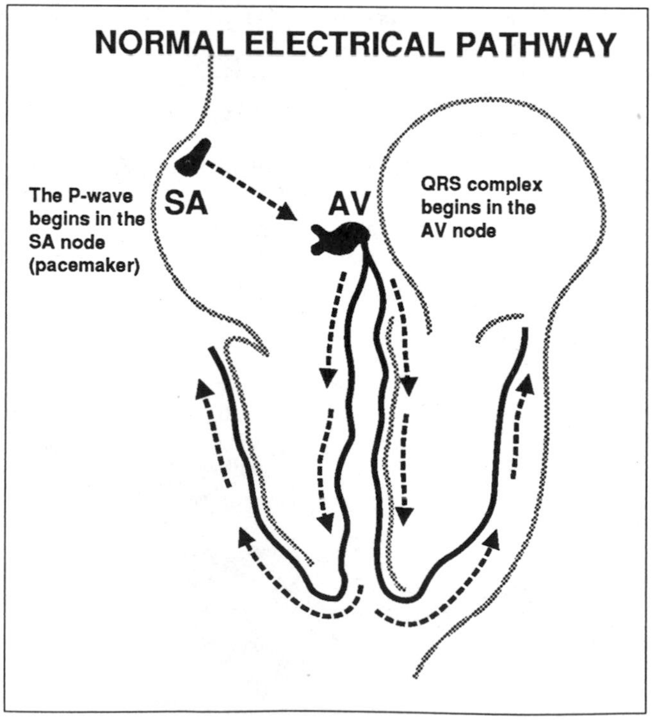

An *EKG lead* is a pair of electrodes placed on the body and connected to an EKG recorder. An axis is an imaginary line connecting the two electrodes. The electrodes for the three limb leads are placed on the right arm, left arm, and left leg. The ground electrode is placed on the right leg. This is electronically equivalent to placing the electrodes at the two shoulders and the symphysis pubis. From these three electrodes (with the ground), the EKG recorder can make certain electrodes positive and others negative to produce six leads (I, II, III, AVR, AVL, AVF). (See Figure 4.23.)

It is not the purpose of this book to give details on how to interpret the EKG. The exercise technician can administer the resting 12-lead EKG, but a qualified physician (especially cardiologists and internists) should interpret the results. The resting 12-lead EKG should be administered to high-risk patients before the treadmill-EKG to help screen out those with various contraindications to exercise.

Exercise Test Electrode Placement

The diagnostic GXT should be performed with a multiple-lead electrocardiographic system. The best possible GXT-EKG test is one in which all 12 leads are monitored. The *Mason-Likar* 12-lead exercise EKG system should be used, in which the six precordial electrodes are placed in their usual positions: the right and

NORMAL ELECTRICAL PATHWAY

The P-wave begins in the SA node (pacemaker)

SA   AV   QRS complex begins in the AV node

Figure 4.21 The P wave (atrial wave) begins in the SA node (normal physiological pacemaker) located near the top of the atrium. The QRS complex (ventricular wave) begins in the AV node.

left arm electrodes are placed on the shoulders at the distal ends of the clavicles; and the right and left leg electrodes are positioned at the base of the torso, just medial to the anterior illiac crests.[50] (See Figure 4.23.)

However, the majority of abnormal EKG responses to exercise can be picked up by lead V5 alone.[9] The

American College of Sports Medicine advises that during the GXT-EKG, V5 should always be recorded.[12] When only V5 is monitored, the CM5 electrode placement system is generally used, in which the second electrode (the negative) is placed on the top third of the sternum (RA electrode), and the third electrode (the

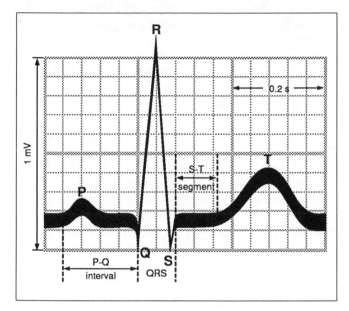

Figure 4.22 On the horizontal line, one small block represents 0.04 second or one millimeter. One large block of 5 small blocks is 0.20 second. On the vertical axis, one small block represents 1/10 of a millivolt. Ten small blocks vertically or two large blocks is 1 millivolt.

Standard or bipolar limb leads	Electrodes connected	Marking code		Recommended positions for multiple chest leads (Line art illustration of chest positions)
Lead 1	LA & RA	· '		V[1] Fourth intercostal space at right margin of sternum — ·
Lead 2	LL & RA	··		V[2] Fourth intercostal space at left margin of sternum — ··
Lead 3	LL & LA	···		V[3] Midway between position 2 and position 4 — ···
Augmented unipolar limb leads				V[4] Fifth intercostal space at junction of left midclavicular line — ···· ·
a VR	RA & (LA-LL)	—		V[5] At horizontal level of position 4 at left anterior axillary line — ···· ··
a VL	LA & (RA-LL)	— —		V[6] At horizontal level of position 4 at left midaxillary line — ··· ···
a VF	LL (RA-LA)	— — —		
Chest or precordial leads				
V	C & (LA-RA-LL)	(see data on right)		

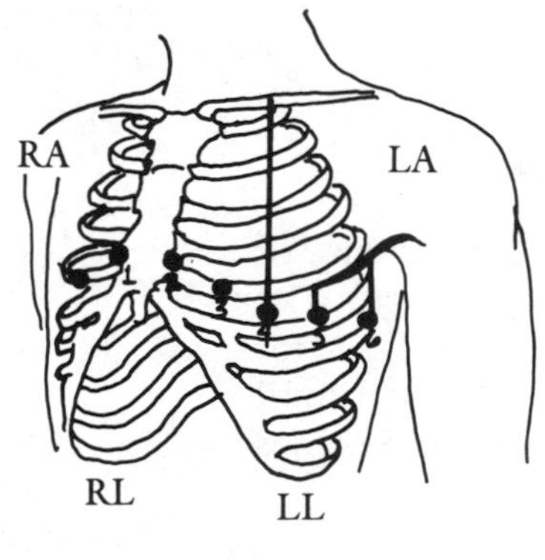

Figure 4.23 Ten electrode positions form 12 leads for the routine electrocardiogram. Electrodes should be placed in the exact anatomical position noted so that the physician can compare the EKG with appropriate standards.

ground) is placed on the right side of the chest in the V5 position (RL electrode)[50,51] The V5 electrode (LA) is put in its normal position.

All leads should be continuously monitored by oscilloscope and recordings taken at the end of each minute of exercise or when significant EKG changes or abnormalities are noted on the screen. During recovery, this should continue every one or two minutes for the 8-minute post-exercise test.

During the early part of the recovery period, the participant should exercise at low intensity (2 mph, 0 percent grade on the treadmill).[12] The EKG and blood pressure should be recorded every one to two minutes for at least 8 minutes of recovery (or longer if there are abnormalities). The participant should not be allowed to stand still or sit still immediately following the exercise test. After approximately 2 minutes of cool-down, he can sit down and continue to move his feet for several more minutes.

The newer disposable electrodes (now available for about 25 cents each) stick on the body very well despite the accumulation of sweat, and conduct the electrical impulses from the body to the electrocardiograph with little or no movement artifact interference. These are much more convenient and effective than the older, nondisposable, silverplated electrodes.

Proper skin preparation is essential for the best EKG recordings. The resistance of the skin should be lowered by first cleansing thoroughly with an alcohol-saturated gauze pad, and then removing the superficial layer of the skin by rubbing vigorously with fine-grain emery paper or the equivalent.[50] Shaving of the skin is not necessary.[12]

Basic Principles in Arrhythmia Determination

An *arrhythmia* is any disturbance of rate, rhythm, or conduction of electrical impulses in the heart.[46] The following criteria should be systematically analyzed for each EKG strip (while watching the oscilloscope), until such analysis to pick out abnormal EKGs becomes automatic.

1. **R to R intervals:** evenly spaced (maximum allowable difference between R waves is 3 small squares)

2. **P Waves:**
   a. within the 3 × 3 small square box
   b. positive
   c. same consistent, rounded shape

3. **P-R interval:** 3 to 5 small squares (.12 to .20 seconds)

4. **P to QRS ratio:** always 1:1 ratio

5. **QRS duration:** less than 2 1/2 small squares (.10 seconds)

The exercise technician should be able to monitor the screen and pick out any abnormal PQRST wave complex, and be alert to call the supervising physician for an interpretation. However, the exercise technician does not necessarily need to know how to interpret abnormal EKGs during exercise. (One of the most common EKG abnormalities during the exercise test is the *premature ventricular contraction* (PVC). (See Figure 4.24 for examples of PVCs.)

One of the major purposes in giving a treadmill EKG stress test is to load the heart muscle beyond normal demands to see if any obstruction to blood flow in the coronary arteries can be picked up on the EKG.[51,52] During the maximal exercise test, coronary blood flow increases five-fold. If the coronary blood vessel is restricted approximately two-thirds, the ST segment of the PQRST wave complex may be depressed.

ST segment depression is determined if all of the following criteria are present (See Figure 4.24 for examples):

- 1 mm or more depressed (below baseline)
- at least 0.08 sec. (2 small squares) in length
- flat or downsloping
- 3 or more consecutive complexes

When ST segment depression is recorded, there is a "positive" test for coronary heart disease. When ST segment depression is not present, the test is called "negative."

Summary

1. While the direct measurement of $\dot{V}O_{2max}$ is the best measure of heart and lung endurance, for various practical reasons other tests have been developed as substitutes. These include field tests (mainly running tests), step tests (YMCA 3-minute step test, Canadian Home Fitness Step Test), submaximal laboratory tests (YMCA physical working capacity bicycle tests), and maximal laboratory tests (both bicycle and treadmill).

2. This chapter provides a detailed description of these tests. Maximal treadmill testing with EKG is explained in detail because of its great value

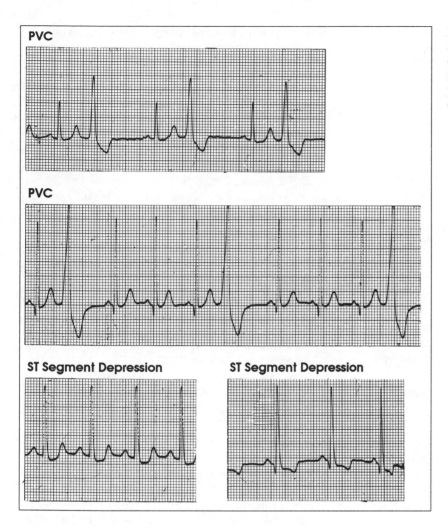

Figure 4.24 One of the most common arrhythmias is the premature ventricular contraction (PVC). ST segment depression may occur when coronary blood vessels are partially restricted, decreasing blood flow during exercise.

in diagnosing overt or latent heart disease, evaluating cardiorespiratory functional capacity, evaluating responses to conditioning or cardiac rehabilitation programs, and increasing individual motivation for entering and adhering to exercise programs.

3. Resting and exercise blood pressure and heart rate determination are reviewed. The diagnosis of adult hypertension is confirmed when the average of two or more diastolic measurements on at least two separate visits is 90 mm Hg or higher.

4. Principles for taking blood pressure measurements are listed. At rest, diastolic blood pressure equals the disappearance of the pulse sound (fifth Korotkoff's sound). During exercise testing, however, both the fourth (abrupt muffling of sound) and the fifth phases should be recorded.

5. Heart rate can be determined through several methods, including the use of heart rate rulers, auscultation with the stethoscope, or heart rate monitors.

6. A number of performance tests such as maximal endurance runs on a track have been devised for testing large groups in field situations. Equations for predicting $\dot{V}O_{2max}$ from one's ability to run various distances at maximal speed have been developed. Recently, a one-mile walk test was developed to more safely test American adults.

7. Both maximal and submaximal step tests have been developed for predicting $\dot{V}O_{2max}$. Of these, the Canadian Aerobic Fitness Test and the YMCAs three-minute step test have been most widely used.

8. The American College of Sports Medicine has developed equations for predicting oxygen

consumption during bench stepping, bicycling, walking, and running. Two important terms are used by the American College of Sports Medicine in their equations and calculations— "METS" and kcal · min^{-1}. One MET is equal to 3.5 ml · kg^{-1} · min^{-1} or the oxygen consumption during rest. One MET is also equal to one kcal · kg^{-1} · hour^{-1}.

9. Both treadmill and bicycle ergometers are utilized in testing cardiorespiratory fitness. In this country, most facilities use treadmills for exercise testing, because walking, jogging, or running are more familiar to Americans, who generally are unaccustomed to bicycling. In addition, most people reach higher $\dot{V}O_{2max}$ values during treadmill tests than they do with the bicycle.

10. A complete description of bicycle ergometers is presented. The workload on the Monark or other mechanically braked bicycles is usually expressed in kilogram-meters per minute (kgm · min^{-1}) or in watts (one watt = 6 kgm · min^{-1}). Work = kg setting × 6 m · rpm^{-1} × rpm = kgm · min^{-1}.

11. One of the best submaximal bicycle protocols is the one used by the YMCA is their testing program. The objective of the YMCA submaximal bicycle test is to obtain two heart rates between 110 and 150 bpm, and then extrapolate these to an estimated maximal oxygen consumption.

12. The most commonly used maximal treadmill protocols are the Bruce and Balke. $\dot{V}O_{2max}$ can be estimated accurately from performance time to exhaustion during these protocols. A practical plan for using the Bruce protocol is described in detail.

13. There are two recommended maximal graded exercise bicycle test protocols, the Astrand and the Storer-Davis.

14. The maximal treadmill and bicycle protocols described above test maximal cardiorespiratory capacity. A different type of test, the Wingate anaerobic test, has been developed to test maximal anaerobic power. The Wingate anaerobic test requires pedaling or arm cranking on a bicycle ergometer for 30 seconds at maximal speed against a constant force.

15. Emergency procedures are outlined, including recommended equipment and drugs, and action plans.

16. The Sports Medicine Insight reviewed basic principles for interpreting electrocardiograms.

References

1. AAHPERD. Technical Manual: Health Related Physical Fitness (1984). The American Alliance for Health, Physical Education, Recreation and Dance. 1900 Association Drive, Reston, CA 22091.

2. Fox El. Matthews DK. The Physiological Basis of Physical Education and Athletics. New York: Saunders College Publishing, 1981.

3. Wasserman K, Hansen JE, Sue DY, Whipp BJ. Principles of Exercise Testing and Interpretation. Philadelphia: Lea & Febiger, 1987.

4. Skinner JS. Exercise Testing and Exercise Prescription for Special Cases. Philadelphia: Lea & Febiger, 1987.

5. American College of Sports Medicine. Resource Manual for Guidelines for Exercise Testing and Prescription. Philadelphia: Lea & Febiger, 1988.

6. 1988 Joint National Committee. The 1988 Report of the Joint National Committee on Detection, Evaluation, and Treatment of High Blood Pressure. Arch Intern Med 148:1023–1038, 1988.

7. American Heart Association. Recommendations for Human Blood Pressure Determination by Sphygmomanometers. Dallas: American Heart Association (National Center, 7320 Greenville Avenue, Dallas, TX 75231), 1967.

8. Londe S, Klitzner TS. Auscultatory Blood Pressure Measurement—Effect of Pressure on the Head of the Stethoscope. West J Med 141:193–195, 1984.

9. Pollock ML, Wilmore JH, Fox SM. Exercise In Health and Disease. Philadelphia: WB Saunders Co., 1984.

10. Heyward VH. Designs for Fitness. Minneapolis: Burgess Publishing Co., 1984.

11. Constant J. Accurate Blood Pressure Measurement. Postgrad Med 81:73–86, 1987.

12. American College of Sports Medicine. Guidelines for Exercise Testing and Prescription (4th edition). Philadelphia: Lea & Febiger, 1991.

13. Léger L, Thivierge M. Heart Rate Monitors: Validity, Stability, and Functionality. Physician Sportsmed 16(5):143–151, 1988.

14. AAHPERD. Norms for College Students: Health Related Physical Fitness Test (1985). American Alliance for Health, Physical Education, Recreation and Dance. 1900 Association Drive, Reston, VA 22091.

15. Tokmakidis SP, Léger L, Mercier D, Péronnet F, Thibault G. New Approaches to Predict. $\dot{V}O_{2max}$ and Endurance from Running Performance. J Sports Med 27:401–409, 1987.

16. Cooper KH. The Aerobics Way. New York: M. Evans and Co., 1977.

17. Kline GM, Porcari JP, Hintermeister R, et al. Estimation of $\dot{V}O_{2max}$ from a One-Mile Track Walk, Gender, Age, and Body Weight. Med Sci Sports Exerc 19:253–259, 1987.

18. Nagle FS, Balke B, Naughton JP. Gradational Step Tests for Assessing Work Capacity. J Appl Physiol 20:745–748, 1965.

19. Ellestad MH, Blomqvist CG, Naughton JP. Standards for Adult Exercise Testing Laboratories. Circulation 59:421A–430A, 1979.

20. Montoye HJ, Ayen T, Washburn RA. The Estimation of $\dot{V}O_{2max}$ from Maximal and Sub-Maximal Measurements in Males, Age 10–39. Res Quart Exerc Sport 57:250–253, 1986.

21. Cavanagh PR, Kram R. The Efficiency of Human Movement—A Statement of the Problem. Med Sci Sport Exerc 17:304–308, 1985.

22. Shephard RJ. Development of the Canadian Home Fitness Test. Can Med Assoc J 114:675–679, 1976.

23. Shephard RJ. Present Views on the Canadian Home Fitness Test. Can Med Assoc J 124:875–879, 1981.

24. Shephard RJ. PAR-Q, Canadian Home Fitness Test and Exercise Screening Alternatives. Sports Med 5:185–195, 1988.

25. Jette M, Mongeon J, Shephard RJ. Demonstration of a Training Response by the Canadian Home Fitness Test. Eur J Appl Physiol 49:143–150, 1982.

26. Jette M. Technical Report. Standardized Test of Fitness in Occupational Health. Fitness and Amateur Sports. Ottawa: Department of National Health and Welfare, 1978.

27. Golding LA, Myers CR, Sinning WE. The Y's Way to Physical Fitness (3rd Edition) Champaign, IL. Human Kinetics Publishers, 1989.

28. Katch FI, McArdle WD. Nutrition, Weight Control, and Exercise. Philadelphia: Lea and Febiger, 1983.

29. Brouha L. The Step Test: A Simple Method of Measuring Physical Fitness for Muscular Work in Young Men. Res Quart Exerc Sport 14:31–36, 1943.

30. Astrand PO, Rhyming I. A Nomogram for Calculation of Aerobic Capacity (Physical Fitness) From Pulse Rate During Submaximal Work. J Appl Physiol 7:218–221, 1954.

31. Smodlaka VN. Treadmills vs Bicycle Ergometers. Physician Sportsmed 10:75–80, 1982.

32. Stuart RJ, Ellestad MH. National Survey of Exercise Stress Testing Facilities. Chest 77:94–97, 1980.

33. Sjostrand T. Changes in Respiratory Organs of Workmen at an Ore Melting Works. Acta Med Scand. (Suppl) 196:687–695, 1947.

34. Astrand PO, Rhyming I. A Nomogram for Calculation of Aerobic Capacity From Pulse Rate During Submaximal Work. J Appl Physiol 7:218–221, 1954.

35. Jacobs I. Blood Lactate and the Evaluation of Endurance Fitness. Sports: Science Periodical On Research and Technology In Sport (September, 1983). The Coaching Association of Canada. 333 River Road, Ottawa, Ontario, K11 8B9.

36. Noble B, Borg GAV, Jacobs I, Ceci R, Kaiser P: A category-ratio perceived exertion scale: relationship to blood and muscle lactates and heart rate. Med Sci Sports Exerc 15:523–528, 1983.

37. American Heart Association. The Committee on Exercise. Exercise Testing and Training of Apparently Healthy Individuals: A Handbook for Physicians (1972). American Heart Association, 7320 Greenville Avenue, Dallas, TX 75231.

38. Bruce RA, Kusumi F, Hosmer D: Maximal oxygen intake and nomographic assessment of functional aerobic impairment in cardiovascular disease. Am Heart J 85:546–562, 1973.

39. McConnell TR. Practical Considerations in the Testing of $\dot{V}O_{2max}$ in Runners. Sports Med 5:57–68, 1988.

40. Liang MTC. The Accuracy of the Bruce Equation for Predicting Oxygen Uptake in Healthy Young Men. Med Sci Sports Exerc 16:151, 1984.

41. Foster C, Jackson AS, Pollock ML, et al. Generalized Equations for Predicting Functional Capacity From Treadmill Performance. Am Heart J 108:1229–1234, 1984.

42. Montoye HJ, Ayen T, Nagle F, Howley ET. The Oxygen Requirement for Horizontal and Grade Walking on a Motor-Driven Treadmill. Med Sci Sports Exerc 17:640–645, 1985.

43. Storer TW, Davis JA, Caiozzo VJ. Accurate Prediction of $\dot{V}O_{2max}$ in Cycle Ergometry. Med Sci Sports Exerc 19:S64, 1987 (abstract).

44. Bar-Or O. The Wingate Anaerobic Test: An Update on Methodology, Reliability, and Validity. Sports Med 4:381–394, 1987.

45. Froelicher VF. Exercise Testing and Training. Chicago: Year Book Publishers, Inc., 1983.

46. Dubin D. Rapid Interpretation of EKGs. Tampa: Cover Publishing Co., 1974.

47. How to Read An ECG. RN Journal, January, 1973, pp. 36–45.

48. Bing OHL. Clinical EKG Guide (1981). (48 Westland Avenue, Winchester, Massachusetts 01890).

49. Amsterdam EA, Wilmore JH, DeMaria AN. Exercise In Cardiovascular Health and Disease. New York: Yorke Medical Books, 1977.

50. Froelicher VF. Exercise Testing and Training. Chicago: Year Book Publishers, Inc., 1983.

51. Ellestad MS. Stress Testing Principles and Practice. Philadelphia: FA Davis Co., 1980.

52. Ellestad MH. Multiple Variables in Exercise Testing. Practical Cardiology 11:130–143, 1985.

Physical Fitness Activity 4.1— Practical Use of the ACSM Equations

The American College of Sports Medicine equations presented in this chapter are highly useful for health and fitness instructors. However, the use of these equations can be initially confusing to some students. It is highly recommended that one practice using the equations many times over, applying them to varying situations to gain a full understanding of them. In the ACSM Health/Fitness Instructor Certification program, the ACSM equations are an integral part of the process.

Here are some sample questions to help you learn how to use the equations. Correct answers are noted with an " * ". Consult your instructor to help clarify use of the equations. However, all the information you need to solve these problems is in this chapter.

1. If a person is cycling at 60 rpm with the bicycle ergometer set at 2 kp, the workload in watts is:

    A. 200

    B. 120*

    C. 150

    D. 180

    E. none of the above

2. If a 60-g man runs 9 mph for 45 minutes, how many kcal will he expend?

    A. 750

    B. 857

    C. 1142

    D. 665*

    E. 443

3. If a 100-kg man is expending 5 METS during exercise, how many kcal/min is this:

    A. 7.5

    B. 4.8

    C. 5.8

    D. 6.2

    E. 8.3*

4. If a 60-kg woman is cycling at a work rate of 600 kgm · min^{-1}, the energy expenditure in METS is:

    A. 6.7*

    B. 6.2

    C. 7.0

    D. 5.3

    E. 4.0

5. If a person walks at 5.0 mph, what is the energy expenditure in METS:
   A. 2.3
   B. 4.8*
   C. 5.3
   D. 3.0
   E. 6.9

6. If the person in the previous question weighs 70 kg, how many kilo-calories would he burn if he walked for 30 minutes:
   A. 100
   B. 284
   C. 154
   D. 168*
   E. 220

7. The oxygen cost of running on the level at 300 meters/min would be about:
   A. 6 METS
   B. 8 METS
   C. 10.5 METS
   D. 12.5 METS
   E. 18.1 METS*

8. If a person is cycling at 50 rpm with the bicycle ergometer set at 4 kp, the workload in kgm · min^{-1} is:
   A. 200
   B. 1200*
   C. 1500
   D. 2200
   E. none of the above

9. If a 50-kg man is expending 10 METS during exercise, how many kcal per hour is this:
   A. 500*
   B. 600
   C. 650
   D. 750
   E. none of the above

10. If a 72-kg man is cycling at a work rate of 600 kgm · min^{-1}, the energy expenditure in ml · kg^{-1} · min^{-1} is:
    A. 15
    B. 20.2*
    C. 34
    D. 48
    E. none of the above

11. If an 80-kg person walks at 2.0 mph, how many kilocalories will be expended after two hours:

    A. 405*

    B. 502

    C. 609

    D. 650

    E. none of the above

12. The oxygen cost in $ml \cdot kg^{-1} \cdot min^{-1}$ of running on the level at 8 mph would be:

    A. 34.2

    B. 46.4*

    C. 53.9

    D. 56.7

    E. 65.0

Questions 13 to 18 apply to Mr. Smith's graded exercise test on a bicycle ergometer (3 min stages, 80 rpm). This was conducted without a physician present because Mr. Smith is an athlete training for national competition, is 22 years old, weighs 65 kg, and is apparently healthy.

Stage	Work Rate	Heart Rate	Blood Pressure	RPE
1	50 watts	100	125/70	2
2	100 watts	135	140/72	3
3	150 watts	150	150/70	4
4	200 watts	164	160/73	5
5	250 watts	178	172/70	6
6	300 watts	190	185/73	8
7	350 watts	200	190/72	9
8	400 watts	205	195/75	10

13. The final workload in kilogram-meters per minute is approximately:

    A. 1,200

    B. 2,400*

    C. 1,500

    D. 3.500

    E. none of the above

14. What was the final approximate "kg" setting (if test was conducted on Monark mechanically braked bike):

    A. 5.0*

    B. 3.5

    C. 4.4

    D. 6.4

    E. none of the above

15. What was the energy expenditure in METS during Stage 7 (assume he reached close to a steady state):

    A. 15.6

    B. 17.4

    C. 19.5*

    D. 20.2

    E. none of the above

16. What is his energy expenditure in kcal·min^{-1} during Stage 5:

    A. 15.4*

    B. 10.4

    C. 11.5

    D. 8.6

    E. none of the above

17. What is his energy expenditure in METS during Stage 3:

    A. 5.4

    B. 8.9*

    C. 9.5

    D. 10.8

    E. 12.4

18. What is his energy expenditure in L·min during Stage 6:

    A. 3.83*

    B. 4.23

    C. 5.67

    D. 5.8

    E. none of the above

Physical Fitness Activity 4.2—
Cardiorespiratory Endurance Testing

In this chapter, detailed information is given for several tests of cardiorespiratory endurance $\dot{V}O_{2max}$), including the following:

- One mile run
- YMCA 3-minute step test
- Canadian aerobic fitness step test
- YMCA physical working capacity bicycle test
- Storer-Davis maximal bicycle test
- Bruce maximal treadmill test

Under the supervision of your instructor or a local fitness center director, using the directions outlined in the chapter and the norms outlined in Appendix B, take each of these six tests and fill in the cardiorespiratory test worksheet. Be sure to follow the precautions outlined in this chapter. If you are not categorized as "apparently healthy" using the ACSM guidelines, these tests should not be taken unless under the direct supervision of a physician. (See Chapter 3.)

After taking these tests, answer the following questions.

1. Did the estimated $\dot{V}O_{2max}$ vary widely for the six different tests? (Define "widely" as more than 25% from the Bruce treadmill maximal test result).

   A. Yes

   B. No

2. If you answered "yes" on Question #1, list at least five reasons below as to why you feel $\dot{V}O_{2max}$ varied so widely.

   A. _____

   _____

   B. _____

   _____

   C. _____

   _____

   D. _____

   _____

   E. _____

   _____

Worksheet for Cardiorespiratory Endurance Testing

Test	Your Score	Classification
One mile run		
YMCA three-minute step test		
Canadian aerobic fitness test		
YMCA submaximal bicycle test		
Storer-Davis maximal bicycle test		
Bruce maximal treadmill test		

Note: Record all scores in $ml \cdot kg^{-1} \cdot min^{-1}$, except for YMCA Three-minute step test. Use $\dot{V}O_{2max}$ norms for Appendix B for classification.

For the one-mile run, use the estimating equation from Table 4.3. For the YMCA three-minute step test, record 60-second recovery pulse, and then use norms in Appendix B (Table 41). For the Canadian aerobic fitness test, use the $\dot{V}O_{2max}$ estimating equation described in the text. For the YMCA submaximal bicycle test, use Figure 4.13. For the Storer-Davis maximal bicycle test, use nomograms from Figures 4.18 and 4.19. For the Bruce maximal treadmill use the equation described in the text.

Chapter 5

Body Composition Measurement

"Quantification of body fat is needed to study the nature and treatment of obesity, to assess nutritional status, and to determine the response of patients to a range of metabolic disorders."[1]

Assessment of Body Composition— Understanding the Concept

Interest in measurement of body composition has grown tremendously during the last 20 years. Elite athletes, people seeking to reach or maintain optimal body weight, and patients in hospitals have all benefited from the increased popularity and accuracy of body composition measurement.

Research to establish ways of determining body composition through indirect methods began during the 1940s.[2] Since then, a wide variety of methods have been developed. These methods will be described with emphasis on the most practical techniques.

Most body composition analyses are based on seeing the body as consisting of two separate compartments, fat and fat-free.[2] Thus, *body composition* is often defined as the ratio of fat to fat-free mass.

The density of fat is 0.90 g/cc. It contains no water and is nearly 100 percent free of potassium. As Figure 5.1 shows, the fat-free compartment consists of bone, muscle, and other tissues that are chemically made up of water, protein, and bone minerals. The density of the fat-free mass varies among humans depending on age, gender, race, and degree of fitness, but it is assumed to have an average density of 1.1 g/cc, with a water content of 72–74 percent and a potassium content of 60–70 mmol/kg for men and 50–60 mmol/kg for women.

The more traditional body composition measurement methods, such as skinfold testing and underwater

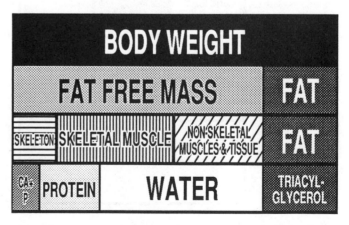

Figure 5.1 There are two body composition models currently in use: the two-compartment model (fat-free mass and fat) and the four-compartment model (bone mineral, protein, water, and fat).

weighing, are based on the two-compartment model. Some of the newer techniques (which are described in the Sports Medicine Insight section of this chapter) attempt to measure the four compartments of the human body—water, protein, bone mineral, and fat. As research continues, the accuracy of these newer methods will no doubt improve.

Methods for Measuring Body Composition

Obesity is generally defined as an excess of body fat.[3] Figure 5.2 shows that weight measurement alone cannot always accurately determine the body fat status of a person. Weight measurement does not differentiate *lean body weight,* or between fat-free mass and fat mass. In other words, some people with *mesomorphic* or athletic, muscular body types (such as football players) can have normal or low body fat even though they are overweight according to standard charts. Some people who are *ectomorphic* (or lean, thin, and linear) with low amounts of fat-free mass can be underweight according to the weight charts, but be overly fat when their fat tissue is measured.

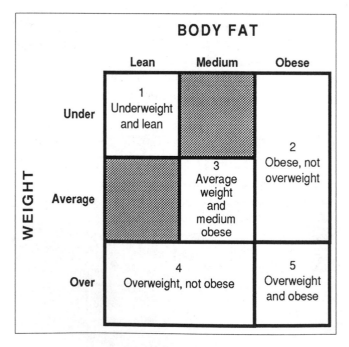

Figure 5.2 The relationship between three categories of body weight and body fat can be described in five different ways. Weight measurement alone cannot always accurately determine the body fat status of a person.

The following common body composition methods for measuring obesity are listed in order from the least accurate to the most precise: height-weight charts; body mass index; skinfold measurement; and underwater weighing.

The Height-Weight Tables

Historical Review

Since the 1940s, tables have been developed by the Metropolitan Life Insurance Company for "ideal" and "desirable" weights.[4–8] They were derived from the 1959 Build and Blood Pressure Study, based on the combined experience of 26 life insurance companies in the United States and Canada from 1935 to 1954, involving observation of nearly 5 million insured people for periods of up to 20 years. Height and weight were measured with street shoes and indoor clothing. The study excluded those with heart disease, cancer, or diabetes. In the resulting 1959 Metropolitan Life Insurance Co. "Desirable Weights for Men and Women," "desirable weights" were those associated with the lowest mortality.[7]

These 1959 tables set forth weight ranges for small, medium, and large-frame men and women of differing heights. (See Table 5.1.) Unfortunately, the method of determining frame size was not given.[5, 7]

In 1973 a table of "recommended weights" in relation to heights was prepared for the Fogarty International Center Conference on Obesity. The data in this chart are simply the 1959 Metropolitan weight table data recalculated to express heights without shoes and weights without clothes. Both average weights and ranges of weight were given for men and women of various heights. (See Table 5.2.) (The mean weights from those tables were used in developing the 1980 Recommended Dietary Allowances issued by the Food and Nutrition Board.)

On March 1, 1983, the Metropolitan Life Insurance Company issued new height-weight tables derived from the 1979 Build Study.[7] (See Table 5.3.) It utilized data from 25 insurance companies reporting the U.S. and Canadian mortality experience from 1954 to 1972 for over four million insured, again excluding applicants with major diseases.

In these most recent tables, weights associated with lowest mortality are no longer called "desirable" or "ideal." Also, this time, a method for determining *frame size* by utilizing elbow breadth measurement was included. (See Table 5.4.) These frame size measurements are based on the National Health and Nutrition

Table 5.1   Desirable Weights for Men and Women Age 25 and Over
(In Pounds by Height and Frame, in Indoor Clothing)

Men (In shoes, 1-inch heels)				Women (In shoes, 2-inch heels)			
Height (inches)	Frame			Height (inches)	Frame		
	small	medium	large		small	medium	large
62	112-120	118-129	126-141	58	92- 98	96-107	104-119
63	115-123	121-133	129-144	59	94-101	98-110	106-122
64	118-126	124-136	132-148	60	96-104	101-113	109-125
65	121-129	127-139	135-152	61	99-107	104-116	112-128
66	124-133	130-143	138-156	62	102-110	107-119	115-131
67	128-137	134-147	142-161	63	105-113	110-122	118-134
68	132-141	138-152	147-166	64	108-116	113-126	121-138
69	136-145	142-156	151-170	65	111-119	116-130	125-142
70	140-150	146-160	155-174	66	114-123	120-135	129-146
71	144-154	150-165	159-179	67	118-127	124-139	133-150
72	148-158	154-170	164-184	68	122-131	128-143	137-154
73	152-162	158-175	168-189	69	126-135	132-147	141-158
74	156-167	162-180	173-194	70	130-140	136-151	145-163
75	160-171	167-185	178-199	71	134-144	140-155	149-168
76	164-175	172-190	182-204	72	138-148	144-159	153-173

Source: New Weight Standards for Men and Women. Stat Bull Metropol Life Insur Co. 40:1, 1959. Courtesy of the Metropolitan Life Insurance Company.

Examination Survey (NHANES I and II) data, and are so devised that 50 percent of the population falls within the medium-frame area, 25 percent fall within the small-frame area, and 25 percent within the large-frame area.[3]

The NIH conference panel adapted these 1983 Metropolitan weight tables following the format of the Fogarty Tables.[3] (See Table 5.5.) This makes the tables easier to use (no shoe heel or clothing weight adjustments are necessary). Comparison with the Fogarty Tables is easier. As with the Fogarty tables, weight ranges are given for each height, instead of categories arranged according to frame size. The NIH conference panel felt that superimposing NHANES frame size data on Metropolitan weight data might not be appropriate.

However, using the frame size data to help determine whether one should use the weights given at the high or low end of the weight range for each height is helpful. (Also, those with an athletic, mesomorphic body type should use the high end of each weight range to adapt for increased muscle weight.)

Giving a wide range of weights for each height actually helps users to understand that many factors affect "ideal weight" and that weighing yourself (without other more sophisticated measurements) does not enable you to determine whether you are at an "ideal weight" by reading a chart.

There are several considerations to bear in mind in using either the 1959 or 1983 weight tables (even after the adaptations of the Fogarty and NIH conferences):[3, 6-9]

- The 1983 weight tables present weight ranges that are 2–13 percent higher than the 1959 tables.[6,7] (See Figure 5.4.) These upward revisions, however, are not uniformly distributed throughout the height categories; the largest increases are for the shorter men and women.

- The tables are based on specific populations that are not representative of the whole population. The data for the 1959 and 1983 tables were drawn from people who were able to purchase nongroup insurance (excluding those who purchased group insurance), and who were 25 to 59 years of age (excluding the elderly). Thus insurees were predominantly white, middle-class adults. Blacks,

Table 5.2   1973 Fogarty Height-Weight Table
(Height Without Shoes; Weight Without Clothing)

Height inches)	Weight Men	Women
58		92-121
59		95-124
60		98-127
61	105-134	101-130
62	108-137	104-134
63	111-141	107-138
64	114-145	110-142
65	117-149	114-146
66	121-154	118-150
67	125-159	122-154
68	129-163	126-159
69	133-167	130-164
70	137-172	134-169
71	141-177	
72	145-182	
73	149-187	
74	153-192	
75	157-197	

Source: Adapted from: New Weight Standards for Men and Women.
Stat Bull Metropol Life Insur Co. 40:1 1959. Courtesy of the Metropolitan Life Insurance Company.

Asians, and low-income and other population groups were not represented proportionally. Also, people with serious chronic diseases or acute illnesses were not included.

■ No consideration was made for cigarette smoking. Cigarette smoking is associated with lower weight and shorter life span. Including smokers in the data thus skewed the "ideal weights" upward.[10]

■ The height-weight tables are based on the lowest mortality, and do not take into account the health problems that are often associated with obesity. Such disease conditions as cardiovascular disease, cancer, hypertension, high blood cholesterol levels, and many other health problems are more prevalent among the obese. For these reasons, the American Heart Association and others have urged the populace to use the weight tables as a "mere gross estimate,"[6] and to use the 1959 tables instead

of the 1983 tables because they are more conservative.

■ Measurement of frame size was never defined for the 1959 Metropolitan weight tables. Using NHANES data for small, medium, and large frames is probably not appropriate.[3]

■ Only initial weights were used in the determination of ideal weight. People taking out insurance policies had their weights measured, but no further data were collected on weight or development of disease after the policy was initially purchased. If weight changed between issuance of the policy and death, this was not taken into account.[6]

■ Finally, weight tables do not provide information on actual body composition. As stated previously, what really matters is the quality of the weight, not the quantity. "Ideal body weight" is not ideal for

Table 5.3   Height-Weight Tables Metropolitan 1983
(In Pounds by Height and Frame in Indoor Clothing,
Men—5 lbs, 1-inch Heel; Women—3 lbs, 1-inch Heel)

Men				Women			
Height (inches)	Frame small	medium	large	Height (inches)	Frame small	medium	large
62	128-134	131-141	138-150	58	102-111	109-121	118-131
63	130-136	133-143	140-153	59	103-113	111-123	120-134
64	132-138	135-145	142-156	60	104-115	113-126	122-137
65	134-140	137-148	144-160	61	106-118	115-129	125-140
66	136-142	139-151	146-164	62	108-121	118-132	128-143
67	138-145	142-154	149-168	63	111-124	121-135	131-147
68	140-148	145-157	152-172	64	114-127	124-138	134-151
69	142-151	148-160	155-176	65	117-130	127-141	137-155
70	144-154	151-163	158-180	66	120-133	130-144	140-159
71	146-157	154-166	161-184	67	123-136	133-147	143-163
72	149-160	157-170	164-188	68	126-139	136-150	146-167
73	152-164	160-174	168-192	69	129-142	139-153	149-170
74	155-168	164-178	172-197	70	132-145	142-156	152-173
75	158-172	167-182	176-202	71	135-148	145-159	155-176
76	162-176	171-187	181-207	72	138-151	148-162	158-179

Source: Reprinted with permission from the Metropolitan Life Insurance Company, New York.

everyone at a given height because of bone and muscle differences.

So in summary, height-weight tables are merely gross estimates. Other methods, such as anthropometric measures, should be used to refine the estimate of proper weight.

Relative Weight

Obesity has been defined as being 20 percent overweight, using the concept of relative weight.[3] *Relative weight* uses the ratio or percentage of actual weight to desirable weight. Most researchers use as the point of reference the midpoint value of the weight range for the subject's height. A man who is 70 inches tall and weighs 180 pounds, for example, would have the following relative weight using the midpoint value of the range given in the 1983 tables (Table 5.5):

relative weight =

body weight / midpoint value of weight range =
180 / 160 = 1.125

In other words, this person is 12.5 percent overweight (20 percent overweight is generally considered obese). If the 1959 tables are used as adapted by the Fogarty conference (Table 5.2), then the relative weight would be:

180/ 154.5 =1.165 (or 16.5 percent overweight)

Measuring Body Weight

Body weight should be measured on a physician's balance beam scale, with minimal clothing, preferably shorts and light T-shirt, and no shoes, or better yet, a disposable paper gown.[11] (See Figure 5.5.) The beam scale should have movable weights, with the scale readable from both sides. Balance beam scales are available from various companies. (See Appendix C.)

The scale should be positioned on a level, solid floor (not carpet), so that the measurer can stand behind the beam, facing the person being measured, and can move the beam weights without reaching around him. The scale should be calibrated each time before use by putting the beam weight on zero, and seeing if the beam

Table 5.4 Height and Elbow Breadth for Men and Women

Men

Height (inches, no shoes)	Small Frame (elbow breadth in inches)	Medium Frame	Large Frame
61-62	<2-1/2	2-1/2 – 2-7/8	>2-7/8
63-66	<2-5/8	2-5/8 – 2-7/8	>2-7/8
67-70	<2-3/4	2-3/4 – 3	>3
71-74	<2-3/4	2-3/4 – 3-1/8	>3-1/8
75	<2-7/8	2-7/8 – 3-1/4	>3-1/4
Women			
57-58	<2-1/4	2-1/4 – 2-1/2	>2-1/2
59-62	<2-1/4	2-1/4 – 2-1/2	>2-1/2
63-66	<2-3/8	2-3/8 – 2-5/8	>2-5/8
67-70	<2-3/8	2-3/8 – 2-5/8	>2-5/8
71	<2-1/2	2-1/2 – 2-3/4	>2-3/4

Source: Reprinted with permission from Metropolitan Life Insurance Company, New York.
Note: tables adapted to represent height without shoes.
Note: to measure the elbow breadth, extend the arm, and then bend the forearm upwards at a 90 degree angle, fingers straight up, palm turned toward the body. Measure with a sliding caliper the width between the two prominent bones on either side of the elbow (measure the widest point). (See Figure 5.3). Make sure that the arm is positioned correctly, and that the upper arm is parallel to the ground. The elbow breadth frame gauge ($5) is available from: Metropolitan Life Insurance Company, Health and Safety Education Division, One Madison Avenue, New York, N.Y. 10010.

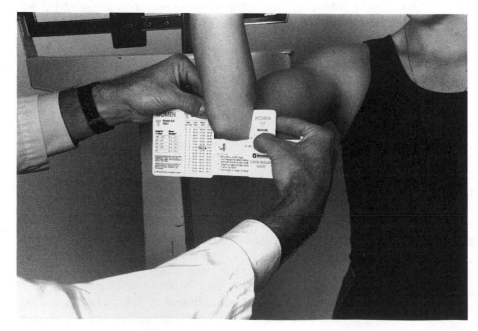

Figure 5.3 The elbow breadth measurement is used for determining frame size. With the arm in this position, the sliding caliper is used to measure the widest point at the elbow.

Table 5.5   NIH Consensus Panel Weight Table
(Height Without Shoes; Weight Without Clothing)

Height (inches)	Weight Men	Weight Women
58		100-131
59		101-134
60		103-137
61	123-145	105-140
62	125-148	108-144
63	127-151	111-148
64	129-155	114-152
65	131-159	117-156
66	133-163	120-160
67	135-167	123-164
68	137-171	123-167
69	139-175	129-170
70	141-179	132-176
71	144-183	135-176
72	147-187	
73	150-192	
74	153-197	
75	157-202	

Source: Adapted from the 1983 Height-Weight Tables, Metrpolitan. Courtesy of the Metropolitan Life Insurance Company.

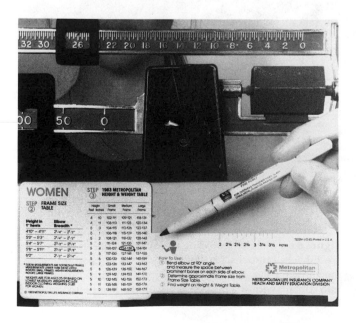

Figure 5.4   In 1983, the Metropolitan Insurance Company released their newest version of the height-weight tables. The 1983 weight tables include weight ranges that are 2–3 percent higher than the 1959 tables.

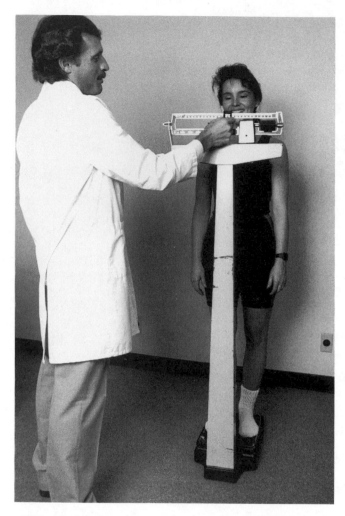

Figure 5.5 Body weight should be measured on a physician's balance beam scale, with minimal clothing.

scale balances out. If not, a screwdriver can be used on the movable tare weight to adjust the beam weight. The weight should be read to the nearest 0.25 pound.

If the objective is to assess changes in weight, great care should be taken to repeat measurement of weight under the same conditions and at the same time of day.[12] The weight of an average adult varies approximately 4 to 5 pounds (2 kg) within one day.

Measuring Height

The measurement of height (or stature) requires a vertical ruler with a horizontal headboard that can be brought into contact with the highest point on the head.[11] The headboard and ruler taken together are called a *stadiometer.*

When measuring height, have the person being measured stand without shoes, heels together, back as straight as possible, heels, buttocks, shoulders, and head touching the wall, and looking straight ahead. Weight should be distributed evenly on both feet, arms hanging freely by the sides of the body. Just before measurement, the person being measured should inhale deeply, and hold the breath, while the headboard is brought onto the highest point on the head, with sufficient pressure to compress the hair.[11, 12]

Fixed and portable stadiometers are available from various companies. (See Appendix C.) Plans for building a stadiometer are available from: Field Services Branch, Division of Nutrition, Centers for Disease Control, Atlanta, Georgia 30333.

If a professional stadiometer is not available, a measuring ruler should be affixed to the wall, and a right angle measuring block (such as a clipboard on edge) used, measuring straight back from the crown of the head.[11,12] A wall should be chosen that does not have a baseboard, and a floor without a carpet should be used. (See Figure 5.6.) Measurement of height while

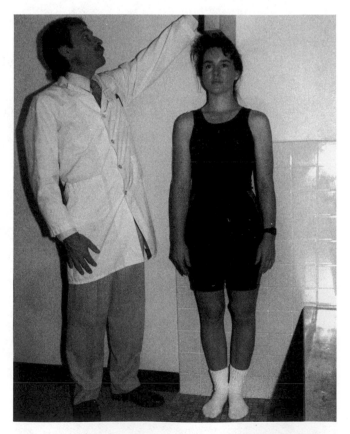

Figure 5.6 Height should be measured while standing erect, heels, buttocks, back of shoulders, and head touching the vertical ruler. A right-angle object should be brought into contact with the highest point on the head after a deep inhalation and holding of breath.

standing on a physician balance beam scale is **not** recommended—it invites substantial error.

Measuring Frame Size

As discussed above, frame size is most commonly determined by measuring the width of the elbow. Other measures have been proposed as estimates of frame size, including bony chest diameter and wrist circumference,[13] but national norms are not yet available for these measurements.

When measuring the width of the elbow, the person being measured should stand erect, with his right arm extended forward perpendicular to his body. His arm is then flexed until the elbow forms a 90-degree angle, with fingers up, palm facing him.[14] (See Figure 5.3.) The measurer should first feel for the widest bony width of the elbow, and put the caliper heads at those points.

A sliding caliper should be used[12] (Figure 5.7), with pressure firm enough to compress soft tissue over the bone. Table 5.4 summarizes how the data are used to determine frame size. Sliding calipers are available from various companies. (See Appendix C.)

Body Mass Index

In large population studies of obesity, a commonly used measure of obesity is the *body mass index*.[16] A number of body mass indices (BMI) have been developed, all derived from body weight and height measurements. The more popular BMIs include the weight-height ratio W/H, Quetelet index W/H^2, and Khosla-Lowe index W/H^3. These BMIs are widely used in large population studies because of their simplicity of measurement and calculation, and low-cost.

The *Quetelet index* or kg/m^2 (body weight in kilograms divided by height in meters squared) is the most widely accepted BMI.[16, 17] Studies have shown that the Quetelet index correlates rather well ($r = 0.70$) with actual measurement of body fat from hydrostatic weighing—better than it does with relative weight calculations or height-weight tables and body fat.[16]

The following example can be used to learn how to calculate the Quetelet index. For example, a man weighing 154-pounds (or 70 kilograms—divide weight in pounds by 2.2), standing 68 inches tall (or 1.73 meters tall—multiply height in inches by 0.0254) has a Quetelet index of:

$$\text{Quetelet index} = 70 \text{ kg} / (1.73 \text{ m})^2 =$$
$$70/2.99 = 23.4 \text{ kg}/m^2.$$

The Quetelet index of 23.4 puts this man in the desirable range. Figure 5.8 makes calculation of the Quetelet index easy through use of a nomogram.

Some experts feel that the major limitation of the body mass index is that it is difficult to interpret to patients, and to relate to needed weight loss.[3] It does have the advantage of being more precise than weight

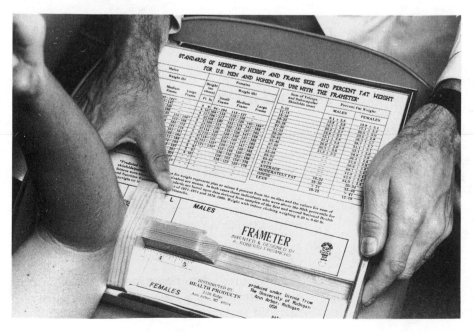

Figure 5.7 The elbow breadth, which is used as a measure of frame size, can be measured with an instrument developed by Frisancho.[13] *Source:* Frisancho AR. Frameter (1985). Health Products, 2126 Ridge, Ann Arbor, Michigan 48104.

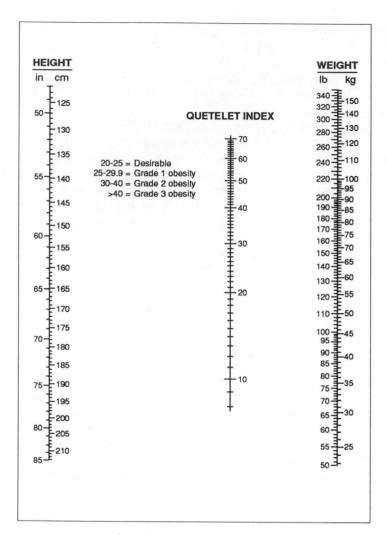

Figure 5.8 The Quetelet index (kg/m²) is calculated from this nomogram by reading the central scale after a straight edge is placed between height and body weight.

tables, and of permitting comparison of populations. However, skinfold measurements correlate more highly with data from hydrostatic weighing, measuring percent body fat, and are thus more accurate for fat-related classification than the Quetelet index.[16] For example, someone with a large fat-free mass (e.g., a football player) would be classified by the Quetelet index as obese, though not to the same extent as he would with relative weight or the height-weight tables.

Researchers from The Panel on Energy, Obesity, and Body Weight Standards have recommended that the following table be used when using the Quetelet index for obesity classification:[18]

> 20–25 kg/m² —desirable range for adult men and women
> 25–29.9 kg/m²—Grade 1 obesity
> 30–40 kg/m²—Grade 2 obesity
> >40 kg/m² —Grade 3 obesity (morbid obesity)

The health risks associated with obesity begin in the range of 25–30 kg/m².[18] (See Chapter 11.)

Skinfold Measurements

The most widely used method for determining obesity is based on the thickness of skinfolds. *Skinfold measurements* correlate well with the gold standard underwater weighing method and have several advantages:

1. The necessary equipment is inexpensive and needs little or no space.

2. The measures can be obtained quickly and easily.

3. The measures when performed correctly have a high correlation ($r = 0.80+$) with body density. Skinfold variables provide more accurate

estimates of body fat than the various height-weight ratios do.[19]

Rules for Taking Skinfolds:[17, 19, 22, 23]

Many researchers in the United States (including those performing the large national surveys of the U.S. population that form the basis for normative data worldwide) take skinfold measurements on the right side of the body.[24] European investigators, on the other hand, tend to take measurements on the left side of the body. Most research, however, reveals that it matters little on which side measurements are taken.[24] It is the opinion of this author, however, that students in the United States should be taught to take all skinfold measurements on the right side, to coincide with the efforts of most U.S. researchers.

1. As a general rule, those with little experience in skinfold measurement should mark the site to be measured with a black felt pen. A flexible steel tape can be used with sites when it is necessary to locate a bodily midpoint. With experience, however, the sites can be located without marking.[22]

2. The measurer should feel the site prior to measurement, to familiarize himself and the person being measured with the area where the skinfold will be taken.

3. The skinfold should be firmly grasped by the thumb and index finger of the left hand and pulled away from the body. While this is usually easy with thin people, it is much harder with the obese, and can be somewhat uncomfortable for the person being tested. The amount of tissue pinched up must be enough to form a fold with approximately parallel sides. The thicker the fat layer under the skin, the wider the necessary fold (and the more separation needed between thumb and index finger).

4. The caliper is held in the right hand, perpendicular to the skinfold and with the skinfold dial facing up and easily readable. The caliper heads should be placed 1/4–1/2 inch away from the fingers holding the skinfold, so that the pressure of the caliper will not be affected.

5. The skinfold caliper should not be placed too deep into the skinfold or too far away on the tip of the skinfold. Try to visualize where a true double fold of skin thickness is, and place the caliper heads there. It is good practice to position the caliper arms one at a time—first the

fixed arm on one side, and then the lever arm on the other.

6. The dial is read approximately 4 seconds after the pressure from your hand has been released on the lever arm of the caliper jaw.

7. A minimum of two measurements should be taken at each site. Measurements should be at least 15 seconds apart to allow the skinfold site to return to normal. If consecutive measurements vary by more than 1 mm, more should be taken, until there is consistency.

8. Maintain the pressure with the thumb and forefinger throughout each measurement.

9. When measuring the obese, it may be impossible to elevate a skinfold with parallel sides, particularly over the abdomen. In this situation, try using both hands to pull the skinfold away while a partner attempts to measure the width. If the skinfold is too wide for the calipers, underwater weighing or another technique will have to be used.

10. Measurements should not be taken when the skin is moist because there is a tendency to grasp extra skin, obtaining inaccurately large values. Also measurements should not be taken immediately after exercise or when the person being measured is overheated, because the shift of body fluid to the skin will inflate normal skinfold size.

11. It takes practice to be able to grasp the same amount of skinfold consistently at the same location every time. Accuracy can be tested by having several technicians take the same measurements and comparing results. It may take up to 20–50 practice sessions to become proficient.

Calipers* should be accurately calibrated and have a constant pressure of 10 g/mm² throughout the full measurement range.[24, 25] (See Figure 5.9.) (See Appendix C for a listing of companies that sell skinfold calipers.)

The accuracy of skinfold measurements can be reduced by many factors, including measurement at the wrong sites, inconsistencies among different calipers

---

*The Lange skinfold caliper is highly recommended and has been used by many U.S. researchers in developing their prediction equations or norm tables.[19] Some researchers have suggested that the use of cheaper calipers can often give accurate results.[27, 28] The inexpensive plastic Slimguide caliper has been shown to be quite accurate. (See Figure 5.9.) (See Appendix C for address.) More information is needed on long-term durability and accuracy.

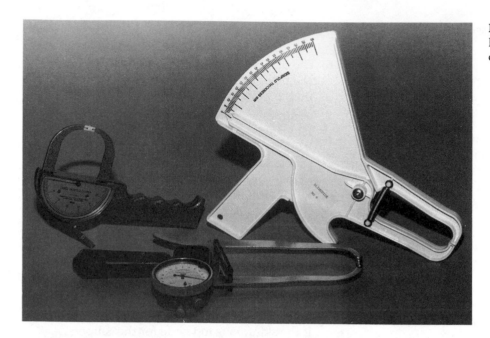

Figure 5.9 Pictured are the Lange, Harpenden, and Slimguide skinfold calipers.

and testers, and the use of inconsistent equations.[29] However, when testers practice together and take care to standardize their testing procedures, inconsistencies among testers can usually be held under one percent. The source of largest error is the nonstandardization of sites, with consequent differences in site selection.[30]

Eight skinfold sites are described below.[17,19,22,31,32] They are in accordance with the Airlie Consensus Conference that resulted in the publication of the *Anthropometric Standardization Reference Manual* (Champaign, Illinois: Human Kinetics Publishers, Inc., 1988).

To reduce error, skinfold sites should be precisely determined and verified by a trained instructor before measurement. The measurements should be made carefully, in a quiet room, and without undue haste.

Figures 5.10 to 5.17 depict the correct site marking and method of measurement for each site. If the reader has not had an anatomy course, Appendix E can be of help in finding the various anatomic sites used in skinfold testing.

- **Chest**—the chest or pectoral skinfold is measured using a skinfold with its long axis directed to the nipple. The skinfold is picked up just next to the anterior axillary fold (front of armpit line). The measurement is taken one-half inch from the fingers. The site is approximately one inch from the anterior axillary line towards the nipple. The measurement is the same for both men and women.

- **Abdomen**—a horizontal fold is picked up slightly more than one inch (3 cm) to the side of and one-half inch below the naval.

- **Thigh**—a vertical fold on the front of the thigh, midway between the hip (inguinal crease) and the nearest border of the patella or knee cap. The person being tested should first flex his hip to make it

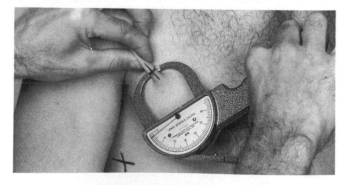

Figure 5.10 Measurement of the chest or pectoral skinfold.

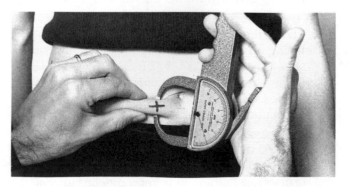

Figure 5.11 Measurement of the abdominal skinfold.

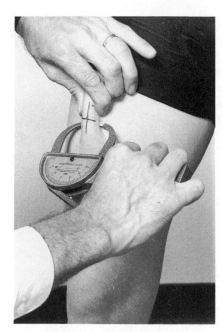

Figure 5.12 Measurement of the thigh skinfold.

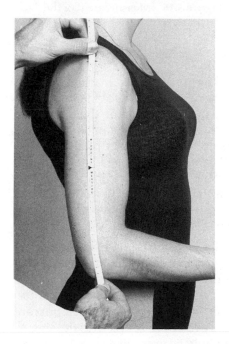
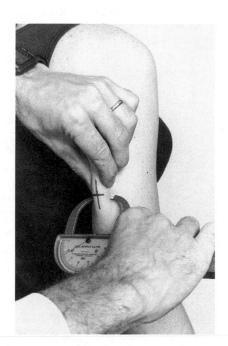

Figure 5.13 (a & b) Measurement of the triceps skinfold.

easier to locate the inguinal crease. Be sure to pick a spot on the hip crease that is exactly above the midpoint of the front of the thigh. The closest border of the knee cap should be located while the knee is extended. When measuring the thigh skinfold, the body weight should be shifted to the other foot, while the leg on the side of the measurement is relaxed with the knee slightly flexed and the foot flat on the floor.

∎ **Triceps**—a vertical fold on the rear midline of the upper arm, halfway between the lateral projection of the acromion process of the scapula (bump on back side of shoulder) and the inferior part of the olecranon process (the elbow). The site should first be marked by measuring the distance between the lateral projection of the acromial process and the lower border of the olecranon process of the ulna, using a tape measure, with the elbow

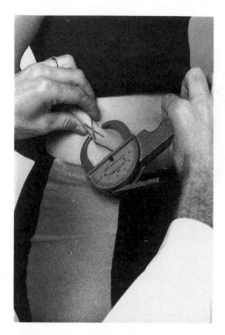

Figure 5.14 Measurement of the suprailiac skinfold.

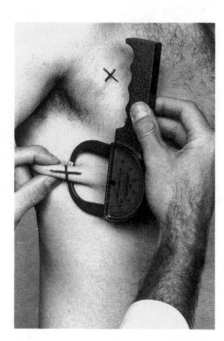

Figure 5.15 Measurement of the midaxillary skinfold.

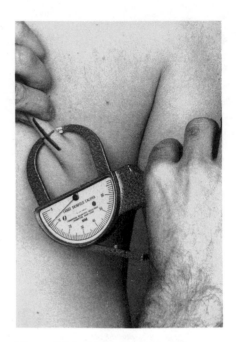

Figure 5.16 Measurement of the subscapular skinfold.

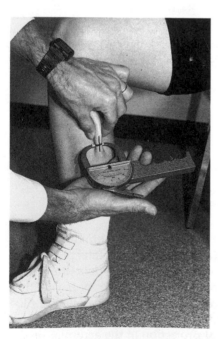

Figure 5.17 Measurement of the medial calf skinfold.

flexed to 90. The midpoint is marked on the lateral side of the arm. The skinfold is measured with the arm hanging loosely at the side. The measurer stands behind the person being measured and picks up the skinfold site on the back of the arm, with the thumb and index finger directed down towards the feet. The triceps skinfold is picked up with the left thumb and index finger, approximately one-half inch above the marked level where the tips of the caliper are applied.

■ **Suprailiac**—a diagonal fold above the crest of the ilium at the spot where an imaginary line would come down from the mid-axillary line. The person being measured should stand erect with feet together. The arms should hang by the sides, but can be moved slightly to improve access to the site. A diagonal fold should be grasped just to the rear of the midaxillary line, following the natural cleavage lines of the skin. The skinfold caliper jaws should be applied about one-half inch from the fingers.

■ **Midaxillary**—a horizontal fold on the midaxillary line at the level of the xiphi-sternal junction (bottom of the sternum where the xiphoid process begins). The arm of the person being measured can be moved slightly backward during measurement to allow easy access to the site.

- **Subscapular**—The site is just below the lowest angle of the scapular. A fold is taken on a diagonal line directed at a 45-degree angle towards the right side. To locate the site, the measurer should feel for the bottom of the scapula. In some cases it helps to place the arm of the person being measured behind his back.

- **Medial Calf**—For the measurement of the medial calf skinfold, the person being measured sits with his right knee flexed to about 90 degrees, sole of the foot on the floor. The level of the maximum calf circumference is marked on the inside (medial) of the calf. Facing from the front, the measurer raises a vertical skinfold, and measures at the marked site.

One-Site Skinfold Test

The triceps skinfold site has been used most often in large population group studies. The percentile breakdowns of triceps skinfold thicknesses (in millimeters) for various age groups is given in Appendix B (Table 50).[15] The data were derived from the first and second National Health and Examination Surveys (NHANES I and II) for 1971–1974 and 1976–1980.

These surveys involved a multistage, stratified sampling of the noninstitutionalized civilians of the United States, which excluded those who tested above the 85th age- and sex-specific percentile (6,088 out of 29,208). Thus the triceps skinfold norms in Appendix B present reference percentile values based upon a sample that is not obese. Optimal values are thus at the 50th percentile.

Care should be taken when classifying as to obesity with the use of just one skinfold site. No equations for body fat estimation have been developed using just the triceps skinfold, and individual values must therefore be compared to tables developed from national norms. Some people have a higher proportion of their body fat distributed on the backs of their upper arms than others, which could lead to an overestimation of their degree of obesity. Therefore, the single-site skinfold test should only be used as a rough approximation of total body fat percentage.

Two-Site Skinfold Test for Children, Youth, and Those of College Age

The two-site skinfold test, using the triceps and subscapular sites, has been the most commonly used body composition test for young people age 6 through college.[33-35] Recently, norms utilizing the sum of triceps

and medial calf skinfolds have been developed.[36,37] The American Alliance for Health, Physical Education, Recreation and Dance (AAHPERD) promotes the use of the triceps and medial calf skinfold sites in their "Physical Best" assessment program.[38] Norms for the various skinfold tests for young people are found in Appendix B (Tables 1, 2, 11, 12, 13) and in Figures 5.18 and 5.19.

The choice of the triceps and subscapular sites over other commonly measured sites (medial calf, abdomen, suprailiac, thigh, etc.) was originally made for several reasons:[31]

- Correlations between these sites and other measures of body fat have been consistently among the highest in many studies.

- These sites are more reliably and objectively measured than most other sites.

- There are available national norms for these sites.

Recently, however, use of the subscapular site has been questioned.[30,37] Some parents of school-aged children are concerned that the modesty of their children is infringed upon when the physical educator raises the shirt of the child to gain access to the subscapular site. The medial calf skinfold site is more easily accessible, and recent studies have found it to be valid and reliable.[37]

Figures 5.18 and 5.19 outline recently developed skinfold and body fat standards for children and youth, ages 6 to 17.[37] Girls at all ages carry more fat than boys. Average body fat percent values for different age groups by gender are outlined in Table 5.6. Based on these average values, the optimal range of percent body fat has been defined as 10 to 20 percent for males, and 15 to 25 percent for females.[37] These percent body fat ranges account for age differences and individual preference, and are associated with little or no health risk from fatness-related diseases.

Table 5.6 Average Body Fat Percent Values

Age Range	Average Body Fat Males	Average Body Fat Females
6- 8	13-15%	16-18%
14-16	10-12%	21-23%
18-22	11-15%	22-26%

Source: Adapted from: Lohman TG. The Use of Skinfold to Estimate Body Fatness on Children and Youth. JOPERD/November- December, 1987, pp. 98-102.

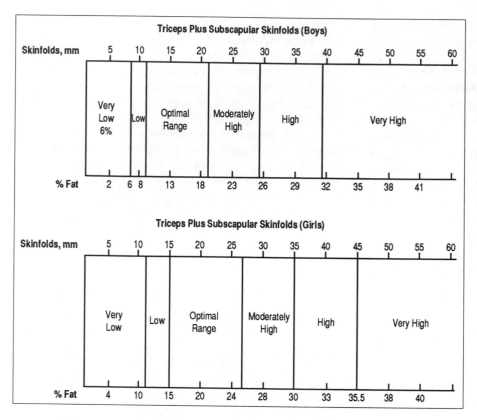

Figure 5.18 Body fat standards for children and youth (ages 6 to 17) using the triceps and subscapular skinfolds. *Source:* Lohman TG. The Use of Skinfold to Estimate Body Fatness on Children and Youth. JOPERD, November—December, 1987, pp. 98—102. Reprinted with permission from the Journal of Physical Education, Recreation & Dance, a publication of the American Alliance for Health, Physical Education, Recreation and Dance, 1900 Association Drive, Reston, VA 22091.

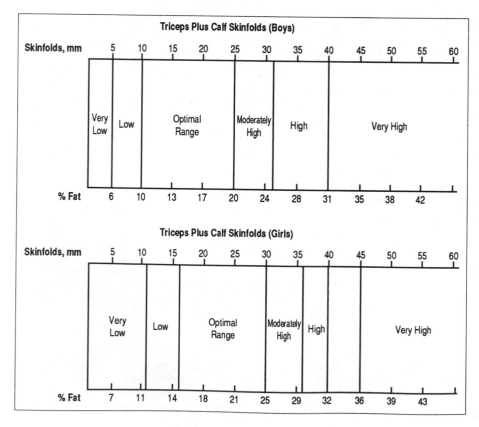

Figure 5.19 Body fat standards for children and youth (ages 6 to 17) using the triceps and medial calf skinfolds. *Source:* Lohman TG. The Use of Skinfold to Estimate Body Fatness on Children and Youth. JOPERD, November—December, 1987, pp. 98—102. Reprinted with permission from the Journal of Physical Education, Recreation & Dance, a publication of the American Alliance for Health, Physical Education, Recreation and Dance, 1900 Association Drive, Reston, VA 22091.

The relation between skinfold thicknesses and percent body fat is well established for adults, but until recently had not been well established for children and youth.[37] Children have a higher water and lower bone mineral content than adults, and as a result, percent body fat is overestimated when using the underwater weighing technique. Figures 5.18 and 5.19 represent the results from new equations that have been developed for children and youth. Using Figures 5.18 and 5.19, obesity for children and youth is defined as a body fat percent greater than 25 percent for males and 32 percent for females.[37]

To assist educators in making accurate skinfold measurements, an audiovisual tape has been developed by the American Alliance for Health, Physical Education, Recreation, and Dance with Human Kinetics Books. (Write to: Human Kinetics, Box 5076, Champaign, Illinois 61820 or to AAHPERD, 1900 Association Drive, Reston, Virginia 22091).

Teachers are also encouraged to attend workshops where training is offered on the skinfold measurement technique. It is recommended that skinfold measurements be taken for all children at least once a year, with records kept to track children from year to year.

Multiple Skinfold Tests for Adults

Since 1951, more than 100 body composition regression equations using anthropometric techniques (skinfold measurements and circumference and diameter measures) have been published.[19] Most of these equations have been developed for specific types of people (athletes or young men or elderly women, etc.), and are thus limited to the groups they were developed for.[23]

The more recent trend has been to develop generalized rather than population-specific equations. These equations have been developed using regression models that take into account data from many different research projects. The main advantage is that one generalized equation replaces several population-specific equations without a loss in prediction accuracy for a wide range of people.[19]

Jackson and Pollock have published generalized equations for both adult men and women.[17, 19, 23, 32, 40, 41] (See Table 5.7.) The three-site equations utilizing triceps, suprailiac, and abdomen skinfolds for adult females, and chest, abdomen, and thigh skinfolds for adult males have been most widely used. The Jackson and Pollock equations have performed well in various studies.[42-44]

Notice that the equations in Table 5.7 predict either body fat percent or body density. The body density formulas require an additional step to estimate percent body fat, using either the Siri or the Brozek equations:[16]

Brozek: % body fat = (457 / body density) − 414
Siri: % body fat = (495 / body density) − 450

For ease of determination, a nomogram has been developed to calculate percentage body fat using age and the sum of three skinfolds for both men and women.[45] (See Figure 5.20.) The nomogram is based on the three-site skinfold equations listed in Table 5.7 that use the

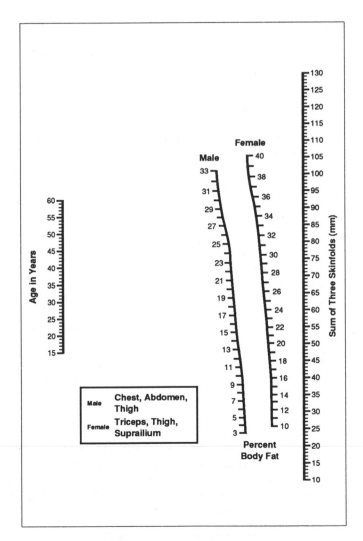

Figure 5.20 To use the nomogram, place a straight edge connecting the age and sum of three skinfolds. The percent body fat is read at the point where the straight edge crosses the line representing the gender of the subject. *Source:* Baun WB, Baun MR, Raven PB. Res Quart Exerc Sport 52:380—384, 1981. Used with the permission of Dr. W. B. Baun.

Table 5.7   Generalized Body Composition Equations

Males

7-Site Formula

Body Density = 1.11200000 − 0.00043499 (*Sum of Seven Skinfolds*) + 0.00000055 (*Sum of Seven Skinfolds*)² − 0.00028826 (*Age*) (chest, midaxillary, triceps, subscapular, abdomen, suprailiac, thigh)

4-Site Formula

Percent Body Fat = 0.29288 (*Sum of Four Skinfolds*) − 0.0005 (*Sum of Four Skinfolds*)² + 0.15845 (*Age*) − 5.76377 (abdomen, suprailiac, tricep, thigh)

3-Site Formulas

Body Density = 1.1093800 − 0.0008267 (*Sum of Three Skinfolds*) + 0.0000016 (*Sum of Three Skinfolds*)² − 0.0002574(*Age*) (chest, abdomen, thigh)

Body Density = 1.1125025 − 0.0013125 (*Sum of Three Skinfolds*) + 0.0000055 (*Sum of Three Skinfolds*)² − 0.0002440 (*Age*) (chest, triceps, subscapular)

Percent Body Fat = 0.39287 (*Sum of Three Skinfolds*) − 0.00105 (*Sum of Three Skinfolds*)² + 0.15772 (*Age*) − 5.18845 (abdomen, suprailiac, triceps)

Women

7-Site Formula

Body Density = 1.0970 − 0.00046971 (*Sum of Seven Skinfolds*) + 0.00000056 (*Sum of Seven Skinfolds*)² − 0.00012828 (*Age*) (chest, midaxillary, triceps, subscapular, abdomen, suprailiac, thigh)

4-Site Formula

Percent Body Fat = 0.29669 (*Sum of Four Skinfolds*) − 0.00043 (*Sum of Four Skinfolds*)² + 0.02963 (*Age*) + 1.4072 (abdomen, suprailiac, tricep, thigh)

3-Site Formula

Percent Body Fat = 0.41563 (*Sum of Three Skinfolds*) − 0.00112 (*Sum of Three Skinfolds*)² + 0.03661 (*Age*) + 4.03653 (triceps, abdomen, suprailiac)

Body Density = 1.0994921 − 0.0009929 (*Sum of Three Skinfolds*) + 0.0000023 (*Sum of Three Skinfolds*)² − 0.0001392 (*Age*) (triceps, suprailiac, thigh)

Note: The researchers who developed these equations used vertical instead of horizontal skinfolds at the abdominal and midaxillary sites.

Source: Jackson AS, Pollock ML. Practical Assessment of Body Composition. Phys Sportsmed 13:76-90, 1985. Golding LA, Myers CR, Sinning WE. The Y's Way to Physical Fitness (3rd edition), 1989. Champaign, IL: Human Kinetics Publishers, Inc.

chest, abdomen, and thigh sites for males, and the triceps, suprailiac, and thigh skinfolds for women.

A sample skinfold testing form is outlined in Figure 5.21. In making the calculations for fat, lean body weight (fat-free mass), and ideal body weight, the following formulas should be used:

pounds of fat = total weight × body fat %
lean body weight = total weight − fat weight
ideal weight = [present lean body weight/
(100%−desired fat %)]

For example, if a subject weighs 200 pounds and is 25 percent body fat, and desires to be 15 percent body fat:

body fat = 200 × 0.25 = 50 pounds
lean body weight = 200 − 50 = 150 pounds
ideal weight = 150/0.85 = 176 pounds

Notice that the ideal weight formula assumes that the lean body weight stays the same during weight loss. Excess body weight, however, has been determined to be 75 percent body fat and 25 percent lean body weight (fat-free mass). For some people, therefore, a reduction in lean body weight is actually desirable, and should be represented in the equation by subtracting 25 percent of the excess weight (e.g., 25% of 12 excess pounds, or 3 pounds) from the present lean body weight.

SKINFOLD MEASUREMENTS

NAME _____ DATE _____

AGE _____ SEX _____ HEIGHT _____ WEIGHT _____

MEASUREMENTS(mm)

_____ CHEST   _____ SUPRAILIAC

_____ ABDOMINAL   _____ MID AXILLARY

_____ THIGH   _____ SUBSCAPULAR

_____ TRICEPS   _____ MEDIAL CALF

CALCULATIONS
(USE APPROPRIATE FORMULA)

_____ TOTAL SKINFOLDS (mm)

_____ BODY FAT PERCENT

_____ POUNDS OF FAT
(TOTAL WT x BODY FAT %)

_____ POUNDS OF LEAN BODY WEIGHT
(TOTAL WT - FAT WT)

_____ CLASSIFICATION
(SEE NORMS)

_____ IDEAL BODY WEIGHT
[LBW / (100% - DESIRED FAT %)]

Figure 5.21 Skinfold testing form.

Norms for body fat are listed in Table 5.8. Athletes involved in sports where the body weight is supported, such as canoeing, kayaking, and swimming, tend to have higher body fat values than athletes involved in sports such as running, that are very anaerobic (sprinting) or very aerobic (marathoning).[46, 47]

It is important to recognize that every measurement method has defined sources of error. Researchers have estimated that the standard error of estimate for percent body fat when using the underwater weighing technique (with residual volume measured accurately) is 2.7 per cent.[17, 48] Generalized equations using skinfolds add only about one percent to this measurement error.[17] In other words, if on the basis of the seven-site skinfold equation, a person is calculated to have 15 percent body fat, two-thirds of the time the actual percent body fat will range within ±4 percent of that estimated 15 percent (11 percent to 19 percent body fat).

Underwater Weighing[1, 2, 16, 49–55]

The most widely used laboratory procedure for measuring body density is *underwater weighing*. In this procedure, whole body density is calculated from body volume according to Archimedes' Principle of Displacement, which states that an object submerged in water is buoyed up by the weight of the water displaced.[2]

The protocol requires weighing a person underwater as well as on land. The densities of bone and muscle tissues are higher than water, while fat is less dense than water. Thus a person with more bone and muscle mass will weigh more in water and thus have a higher body density and lower percentage of body fat.

By using a standard formula, the volume of the body is calculated and the individual's body density determined. From body density, percent body fat can be calculated using the Siri or Brozek formulas as described earlier in this chapter.[1, 2, 17, 31]

As discussed previously, the human body can be divided into fat and fat-free components.[1, 2] The density (D) of the fat mass is quite constant and easily measured (0.900 gm/cc). The density of the fat-free mass cannot be measured accurately, but will depend on the relative contributions of bone mineral (D = 3.00 gm/cc), protein (D = 1.34 gm/cc), and water (D = 0.993 gm/cc). If it is assumed that the fat-free mass is composed of protein (20.5%), water (72.4%), and bone mineral (7.1%), the density of the fat-free mass can be calculated as 1.10 gm/cc.[54]

To determine body density from underwater weighing, the following equation has been developed:[48]

$$\text{body density} = \frac{WA}{\frac{(Wa-Ww)}{Dw} - (RV + 100 \text{ ml})}$$

Wa = body weight out of water; Ww = weight in water; Dw = density of water; RV = residual volume. (100 ml is the estimated air volume of the gastrointestinal tract.)

Equipment

The equipment is simple and relatively inexpensive. (See Figure 5.22.) The scale and chair can be suspended from a diving board or an overhead beam into a pool, small tank, or hot tub that is four to five feet deep. The water should be warm enough to be comfortable (85–92° F), and undisturbed by wind or the motions of other people during the time of the test. The water should be filtered and chlorinated.

The scale is a 9-kilogram Chatillon autopsy scale with 10-g divisions.*

Table 5.8   Percent Body Fat Classifications

Classification	Male	Female
Lean	<8%	<13%
Optimal	8-15%	13-20%
Slightly overfat	16-20%	21-25%
Fat	21-24%	26-32%
Obese (overfat)	≥25%	≥32%
Long distance runners	4- 9%	6-15%
Wrestlers	4-10%	—
Gymnasts	4-10%	10-17%
Body builders (elite)	6-10%	10-17%
Swimmers	5-11%	14-24%
Basketball athletes	7-11%	18-27%
Canoers/kayakers	11-15%	18-24%
Tennis players	14-17%	19-22%

Sources: Adapted from: Lohman TG. The Use of Skinfold to Estimate Body Fatness on Children and Youth. JOPERD/November-December, 1987, pp. 98–102; Fleck SJ. Body Composition of Elite American Athletes. Am J Sports Med 11:398, 1983; Wilmore JH. The Physiological Basis of the Conditioning Process. Boston: Allyn and Bacon, Inc., 1982.

---

*This can be obtained for approximately $560 (part number 12500-124) from: V.W.R. Scientific Company, P.O. Box 6016, Cerritos, CA 90702 (213) 404-0770)

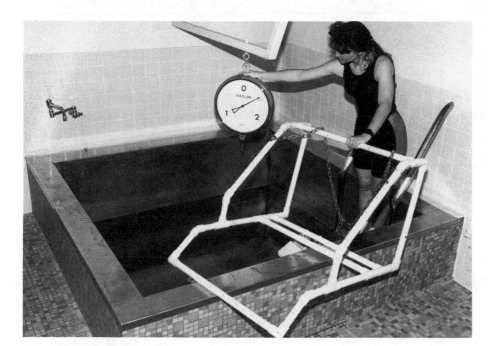

Figure 5.22 Equipment for underwater weighing includes a tank of sufficient size and shape for total human submersion, an accurate scale for measuring weight with 10-g divisions, a method of measuring water temperature so that water density can be corrected, and a chair that has been weighted to prevent flotation.

The chair can be constructed of 3/4–1 inch plastic pipe, which can be cut and assembled easily. The direct cost is only about $30 in materials (the plastic pipe and glue). Figure 5.22 gives an example of one type of underwater weighing chair. A simple cradle can also be used.[1]

The back height of the chair in Figure 5.22 is 24 inches, and the width, 32 inches. Other joints and dimensions need not be precise, and can be estimated from the figure. It is important that the chair be assembled so that the person being weighed can sit underwater with legs slightly bent, and the water at shoulder level. Very small or large people will have to adapt their sitting position.

Holes should be drilled in the plastic pipe to avoid air entrapment. The chair should be weighted down with skin diving weights or barbell weights to ensure that the weight of the chair underwater (tare weight) is at least 3 kg for normal-weight people being weighed, and 4–6 kg for obese people.

Procedures[1, 2, 16]

1. **Obtain basic data**—Name, date, age, sex, height, weight. The form in Figure 5.23 can be used to record this data. Weight should be taken wearing only a swimming suit and after an opportunity to go to the bathroom. The person being weighed should not eat or smoke for 2–3 hours before the test, and should try to avoid foods that can cause excessive amounts of intestinal gas. Care should be taken to expel any trapped air from the swim suit.

2. **Take Skinfolds**—Because some people have difficulty in blowing out all the air from their lungs underwater, it is a good idea to have skinfold data to help verify the results.

3. **Give basic instructions.**

   A. **How to sit in chair**—Sit in the chair with seat on the back bars, feet on the forward bar in the corners, legs slightly bent, hands gripping the lower side bars. (See Figure 5.24.)

   B. **Underwater position**—After making a full exhalation of air from the lungs, slowly lean forward until the head is underwater. Continue to press all air out of the lungs. When all air is out, count for 5 to 7 seconds, then come up. (See Figure 5.25.) The test will be repeated 4–10 times until a consistent reading is obtained.

      Note: When the person goes under water, keep one hand on the scale to steady it. Try to keep the water as calm as possible to get a good reading on the scale needle. The person being weighed should be as still as possible underwater during the 5–7 second count.

BODY COMPOSITION WORKSHEET

NAME _____ DATE _____

AGE _____ SEX _____ HEIGHT (shoes off) _____ inches

SKINFOLDS (mm)

MALE		FEMALE	
_____ CHEST		TRICEPS _____	
_____ ABDOMEN		SUPRAILLIUM _____	
_____ THIGH		THIGH _____	
_____ TOTAL		_____	

HYDROSTATIC MEASUREMENTS

_____ BODY WEIGHT IN AIR (pounds)

_____ NET BODY WEIGHT IN WATER (kg) (subtract tare from gross weight)

_____ GROSS WEIGHT IN WATER (kg)

_____ TARE WEIGHT (weight of apparatus - kg)

_____ H_2O DENSITY (see table) _____ _____ _____

_____ RESIDUAL VOLUME (L) _____ _____ _____

(use equation or measure directly)   (take 4-6 determinations until steady)

CALCULATIONS

_____ BODY FAT % = (495/density) - 450

$$\text{Density} = \text{dry wt.} / \left[\left(\frac{\text{dry wt. - net underwater wt.}}{\text{Density water}} \right) - (RV + 100ml) \right]$$

_____ FAT WEIGHT (pounds) (dry body weight x fat %)

_____ LEAN BODY WEIGHT (pounds) (dry body weight - fat weight)

_____ FAT % CLASSIFICATION (see norms)

RECOMMENDATIONS

_____ ESTIMATED IDEAL WEIGHT [LBW / (100% - desired fat %)]

_____ _____ _____

_____ POUNDS OF FAT YOU NEED TO LOSE

_____ POUNDS OF LEAN BODY WEIGHT YOU NEED TO GAIN

Figure 5.23

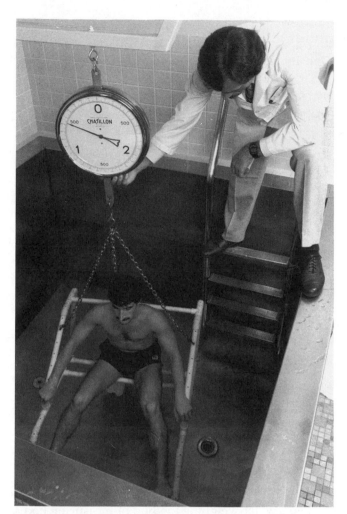

Figure 5.24 The position of the person being weighed before underwater weighing.

4. **Record the consistent underwater weight.** The underwater weight should be recorded as the "gross weight in water (kg)," and then the tare weight (weight of chair apparatus alone) should be subtracted from it to obtain the "net body weight in water." It is important to be exact in determining the gross underwater weight. A 100-gram error can result in close to a one percent body fat error.[17]

   Many testers have trouble with the oscillations of the scale needle. To minimize this, use a small tank, keep the water as calm as possible, and teach the person being tested to move as slowly as possible. Testers should practice reading the scale with known weights attached.

5. **Determine the water density.** Measure the temperature of the water, and then consult Table 5.9 for the water density.

6. **Determine the residual volume.** The residual volume is the amount of air left in the lungs after a maximal expiration.[17] The residual volume can be measured or estimated. Measurement of residual volume can be conducted using nitrogen washout, helium dilution, or oxygen dilution. Considerable controversy exists regarding whether measurement of residual volume should take place while the person being weighed is in or outside the tank.[1, 50–52]

   Whenever possible, residual volume should be measured directly. When residual volume is estimated, hydrostatically determined percent body fat has been no more accurate than it was with skinfolds, because of the large amount of error in residual volume estimation formulas.[50]

   When necessary, the following formulas can be used to estimate residual volume:[53]

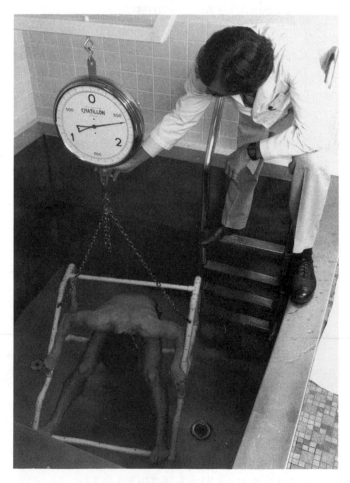

Figure 5.25 The position of the person being weighed during underwater weighing.

Table 5.9   Density of Water at Different Temperatures

Water Temp (°C)	Density H_2O	Water Temp (°C)	Density H_2O
23	.997569	31	.995372
24	.997327	32	.995057
25	.997075	33	.994734
26	.996814	34	.994403
27	.996544	35	.994063
28	.996264	36	.993716
29	.995976	37	.993360
30	.995678		

Source: Handbook of Chemistry and Physics. Cleveland: Chemical Rubber Company, 1967. Reprinted with permission from CRC Press, Inc., Boca Raton, FL 33431.

males: (0.017 AGE) + (0.06858 × height in inches) – 3.447

females: (0.009 AGE) + (0.08128 × height in inches) – 3.9

7. **Calculate percent body fat.** Below is an example of how to use the formula (putting the formula into a programmable calculator saves time):

Body density = body weight/body volume

body volume = [(body wt kg – underwater wt kg) / density of H_2O] – (RV + 100 ml)

relative fat percent = (495 / density) – 450

fat weight = body weight × relative fat percent

lean weight = body weight – fat weight

ideal weight = present lean body weight / (100% – desired fat %)

Example: Male, 18 years of age, weighs 180 lb (81.8 kg), has a net underwater weight of 3.8 kg. Estimated RV is 1.660 (adding 100 ml for GI trapped air = 1.760), based on his height of 70 inches, age, and sex. The density of the water is 0.995678 based on a water temperature of 30 degrees Centigrade.

body volume = (81.8–3.8/0.995678) – 1.760 = 76.579

body density = 81.8 / 76.579 = 1.0682

relative fat % = (495/1.0682) – 450 = 13.4%

fat weight = (180 lb × 0.134) = 24.1 lb

lean body weight = 180 – 24.1 = 155.9

ideal weight if a person wants to get to 10% body fat (often for athletic reasons) = 155.9 / (100% – 10%) = 155.9 / 0.9 = 173.2 lb (needs to lose 9 lb fat)

Weaknesses

The underwater weighing method of measuring body composition is less practical for testing large numbers of people. Ten to 20 percent of people who try it find it difficult to be weighed underwater. The procedure requires special equipment, experience, and financial investment. In most situations, skinfold thickness measurement is more practical.

Recently the whole concept of body density determination has been questioned.[1,2,17] While the density of human body fat is relatively constant within and between individuals (0.90 gm/cc), and is independent of sex, age, or location within the body, the density of the lean component appears to be quite variable, tending to vary depending on age, sex, activity, and race.[55]

For example, athletes have denser bones and muscles than nonathletes, which leads to an underestimation of their body fat. Similarly, osteoporosis among the elderly reduces bone density and results in an overestimation of body fat.

Also, research on body density has utilized cadavers, which have not represented the normal population—especially the children, youth, and the elderly.[31] More

CORP AUTHOR   United States Gymnastics Safety Association.
TITLE   Gymnastics safety manual : the official manual of the United
              States Gymnastics Safety Association / contributors to text,
              Norman Barnes ... [et al.] ; Eugene Wettstone, editor, with the
              assistance of Raleigh DeGeer Amyx ... [et al. ; drawings in
              text by C. K. Bingham].
EDITION   2d ed.
IMPRINT   University Park : Pennsylvania State University Press, 1979.
DESCRIPT   147 p. : ill. ; 23 cm.
BIBLIOG.   Bibliography: p. 142-144.

    LOCATION   CALL #   STATUS
1 > Riverside Main Stack   GV 461 U53 1979   CHECK SHELVES
2 > Riverside Main Stack   GV 461 W4   CHECK SHELVES
3 > Riverside Main Stack   GV 461 U53 1979 C.2   CHECK SHELVES

AUTHOR   Brown, James Rollar, 1939-
TITLE   Teaching and coaching gymnastics for men and women / James R.
              Brown, David B. Wardell.
              New York : Wiley, c1980.

TMPRTNT

```
DESCRIPT      xiv, 441 p. : ill. ; 24 cm.
BIBLIOG.      Includes bibliographical references and index.
SUBJECT       Gymnastics.
              Gymnastics. --Coaching.
ALT AUTHOR    Wardell, David B., 1941-
ISBN          0471107980 :
     LOCATION             CALL #                STATUS
1 > Riverside Main Stack   GV 461 B72           CHECK SHELVES
                                                Record 2 of 9

AUTHOR        Loken, Newton C.
TITLE         Complete book of gymnastics [by] Newton C. Loken [and] Robert J.
              Willoughby.
EDITION       2d ed.
IMPRINT       Englewood Cliffs, Prentice-Hall [1967]
DESCRIPT      xiii, 274 p. illus. 26 cm.
BIBLIOG.      "Selected list of reference materials and visual aids": p. 261-
              267.
SUBJECT       Gymnastics.
ALT AUTHOR    Willoughby, Robert J.
     LOCATION             CALL #                STATUS
1 > Riverside Main Stack   GV 461 L6 1967       CHECK SHELVES
```

research is needed to develop more refined equations for predicting percentage of body fat among all groups.

Nonetheless, hydrostatic weighing at this time remains the laboratory standard, especially when residual volume is measured directly. As with all testing procedures, there are weaknesses, and the goal should be to adapt for these weaknesses in the best way possible.

One special situation is pregnancy, when there is a relative excess of body water.[54] For this reason, general equations for estimated body fat mass are not accurate, and new equations for pregnant women during different phases of gestation have been developed. (See Table 5.10.)

Bioelectrical Impedance

Several articles have recently appeared in the literature evaluating the effectiveness of electrical impedance methods (impedance plethysmography).[1,2,56-65] A harmless 50-KHz current (800 microamps maximum) is generated and passed through the person being measured. (See Figure 5.26.) The measurement of electrical conductance (or impedance) is detected as the resistance to electrical current. Electrical impedance is greatest in fat tissue (14–22 percent water) because the conductive pathway is directly related to the percentage of water (which is greatest in the fat-free tissue).

The total body water can be detected, therefore, as shifts in total body impedance. Once total body water is known, various formulas are used to calculate the lean body mass and fat components.

In general, most of the studies show that bioelectrical impedance is accurate in measuring total body water, but in extrapolating to lean body mass and fat mass, there is a loss of accuracy. The manufacturers of the commercial impedance devices accept that the method is only as good as the regression equations and are constantly modifying them as the data base increases.[1] In general, with the formulas now being used, body composition results are no more accurate than with accurate skinfold measurements.

The especially lean and obese are especially susceptible to inaccurate measurement. The daily fluctuation in water content from exercise, dehydration, eating, and drinking all need to be standardized to obtain the best results.

In the future, better formulas based on a broader sample may improve the accuracy of bioelectrical impedance in determining body composition. The technique is very convenient, rapid, noninvasive and safe, and correlates rather well with the more cumbersome body composition techniques.

Topography of Human Body Fat

Research evidence is accumulating that the pattern of human fat distribution is an important predictor of the health hazards of obesity.[66] This issue will be discussed in greater detail in Chapter 11. Briefly, three types of obesity have been identified.

Table 5.10 Equations for Underwater Weighing of Pregnant Women

General equation	WFM = WB/100 × [(100/DB-100/DFFM) /(1/DFM-1/DFFM)]
Siri's equation assumes	DFM=0.900 gm/cc and DFFM = 1.10 gm/cc
	WFM = WB/100 × [(495/DB-450)]
No edema or leg edema only	
	WFM = WB/100 × [(496/DB-452)] 10 wk gestation
	WFM = WB/100 × [(502/DB-458)] 20 wk gestation
	WFM = WB/100 × [(511/DB-468)] 30 wk gestation
	WFM = WB/100 × [(523/DB-481)] 40 wk gestation
WB, WFM	weight of body, weight of fat mass
DB, DFM, DFFM	density of body, fat mass, and fat-free mass (kg) (gm/cc)

Source: van Raaij JM, Peek MEM, Vermaat-Miedema SH, et al. New Equations for Estimating Body Fat Mass in Pregnancy From Body Density or Total Body Water. Am J Clin Nutr 48:24-29, 1988.

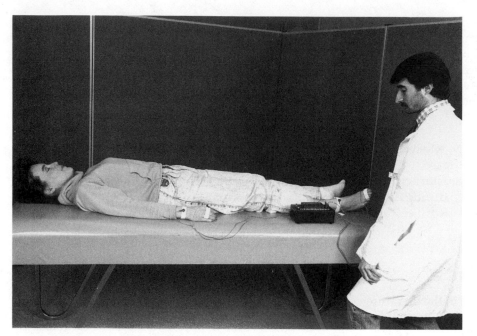

Figure 5.26 Bioelectrical impedance procedures are relatively simple. The person lies on a table with his limbs not touching his body. Electrodes are placed on his right hand and his right foot, and a harmless 50 KHz current (800 microamps maximum) is passed through him. The measurement of electrical conductance (or impedance) is detected as the resistance to electrical current. Several types of bioelectrical impedance measuring devices are available.

The male (*android* or apple shape) type of obesity is characterized by a predominance of body fat in the upper half of the body. In contrast, the female (*gynoid* or pear shape) form of obesity is characterized by excess body fat in the lower half of the body, especially the hips, buttocks, and thighs.[66] The third type of obesity is the intermediate form, characterized by both upper and lower body fat predominance.

The male type of obesity, which can occur in both genders, is associated with many of the health problems of obesity, including hypertension, high serum cholesterol levels, cardiovascular disease, and diabetes.

A number of the researchers have found that the ratio of *waist to hip circumference* (WHR) is an accurate and convenient method of determining the type of obesity present. Circumferences should be measured while wearing only nonrestrictive briefs or underwear, or a light smock over the underwear.

Waist or abdominal circumference is defined as the smallest waist circumference below the rib cage and above the umbilicus, while standing with abdominal muscles relaxed (not pulled in). The measurer faces the person being measured and places an inelastic tape in a horizontal plane, at the level of the natural waist (the narrowest part of the torso, as seen from the rear). If there appears to be no "smallest" area around the waist, the measurement should be made at the level of the navel.

Hip or gluteal circumference is defined as the largest circumference of the buttocks-hip area while the person is standing. The measurer should squat at the person's side so he can see where the buttocks circumference is the greatest, and places an inelastic tape around the buttocks and hips in a horizontal plane at that point without compressing the skin. An assistant is needed to help position the tape on the opposite side of the body.

The WHR is calculated by dividing the waist circumference by the hip circumference. For example, the idealized beauty contest female with a waist of 24 inches and hips of 36 inches would have a WHR of 0.67. In one study of 44,820 women who were members of TOPS Clubs, Inc. (Take Off Pounds Sensibly), the WHR varied between 0.39 and 1.45.[67] Women with higher WHRs were at greater risk for diabetes, hypertension, gallbladder disease, and oligomenorrhea (irregular menses).

More research is needed to establish more precise norms for the WHR. At present, the risk of disease increases steeply when the WHR of men rises above 0.9, and of women, above 0.8.[66]

A nomogram for determining the WHR is given in Figure 5.27, with preliminary norms outlined in Figure 5.28.[68]

Sports Medicine Insight
Other Methods of Determining Body Composition

This chapter has reviewed some of the more practical and standard methods for determining body composi-

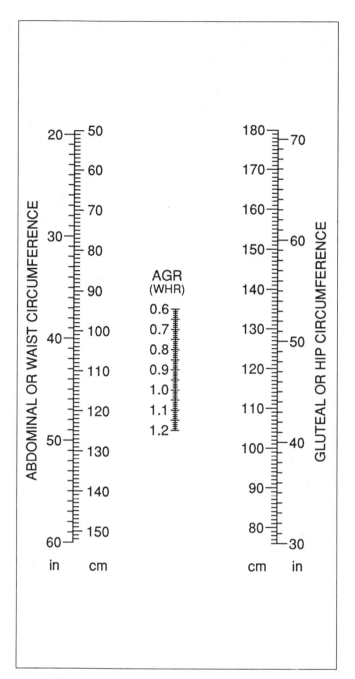

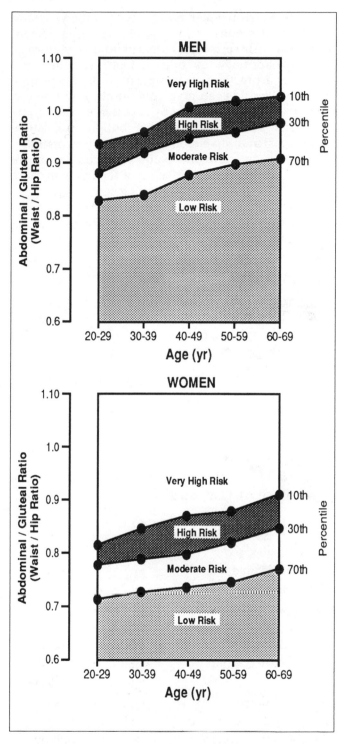

Figure 5.27 The abdominal (waist) to gluteal (hips) ratio (AGR or WHR) can be determined by placing a straight edge between the column for waist circumference and the column for hip circumference and reading the ratio from the point where this straight edge crosses the AGR or WHR line. The waist or abdominal circumference is the smallest circumference below the rib cage and above the navel, and the hips or gluteal circumference is taken as the largest circumference at the posterior extension of the buttocks. *Source:* Bray GA, Gray DS. Obesity: Part 1—Pathogenesis. West J Med 149:429—441, 1988. Reprinted by permission of the Western Journal of Medicine.

Figure 5.28 The percentiles for the ratio of abdominal circumference to gluteal circumference (or waist to hips) are shown for men (top figure) and women (bottom figure). These are preliminary norms. *Source:* Bray GA, Gray DS. Obesity: Part 1—Pathogenesis. West J Med 149:429—441, 1988. Reprinted by permission of the Western Journal of Medicine.

tion, for which the standard is hydrostatic weighing. However, it requires relatively expensive equipment, and requires direct measurement of residual volume for optimum accuracy. In contrast, Quetelet's Index is a simple and practical measurement of degree of overweight. Skinfolds can give an accurate assessment of body fat levels when done by experienced health professionals. For regional fat distribution, calculations using waist and hip circumferences are very useful.

However, new and better methods are on the way;[69] a comparison with some of the older methods will show the promise of an exciting new era for laboratory research in this area.[1, 2, 68, 70] Table 5.11 summarizes the relative costs, ease of use, and accuracy of the different techniques.

Ultrasound

Ultrasonic methods directly measure the depth of adipose tissue and muscle. Studies have been done mainly on pigs, though recent research has been done on humans.[71] With lean males, ultrasonic methods are as effective as skinfold calipers in predicting body fat percent.[72, 73] For the obese, ultrasound has proved to be superior to the caliper technique in measuring subcutaneous fat.[74] There is a lightweight body composition meter (Ithaco Corp., Ithaca) which provides a portable system with a digital measure of tissue thickness.[1]

The ultrasound meter operates by emitting high frequency sound waves that penetrate the skin surface and pass through the adipose tissue to be reflected off the fat-muscle interface. The time taken for the echo to return to the ultrasound receiver is converted to a distance score. In contrast with skinfold measurement, where the varing compressibility of skinfolds among different people can cause error, ultrasound involves no pressure on the skin surface, and may thus be more accurate, especially for the obese.

Total Body Water

Typically, the body of a man weighing 70 kg will contain 42 kg of water (60 percent body weight). Water is not present in stored triglyceride (part of fat storage), but is present in a relatively constant fraction (73.2%) of the fat-free mass.[2]*

---

*This water compartment is relatively easy to measure, since a tracer dose of water, labeled isotopically (^3H_2O or tritium, D_2O or deuterium oxide, or ^{18}O or isotope oxygen),[75] will reach equilibrium with virtually all body water in 3 to 4 hours.

Table 5.11   Comparison Between Body Composition Methods: Cost, Ease of Use, and Accuracy in Estimating Body Fat

Method	Cost	Ease of Use	Accuracy
Quetelet Index	low	easy	low
3 to 7 site skinfold tests	low	moderate	moderate
Hydrostatic weighing	moderate	difficult	high
Electrical impedance	moderate	easy	moderate
TOBEC	very high	easy	high
Total body water	moderate	moderate	moderate
Total body potassium	high	difficult	moderate
Creatinine	low	moderate	low
3-Methyhistidine	low	moderate	moderate
Dual photon absorptiometry	high	difficult	moderate
Computed tomography	very high	difficult	moderate
Ultrasound	moderate	moderate	moderate
Infrared interactance	high	moderate	moderate

Sources: Adapted from: Lukaski HC. Methods for the Assessment of Human Body Composition: Traditional and New. Am J Clin Nutr 46:537–556, 1987. Bray GA, Gray DS. Obesity: Part 1—Pathogenesis. West J Med 149:429–441, 1988.

The problem with this method is that the fat free mass does not have a constant water content (the more adipose tissue a person carries, the higher will be the water content of fat-free tissue).[76] Also, it requires expensive equipment (for example, gas chromatography, mass spectrometry, or fixed-filter infrared absorption) needed to analyze the isotopic label in biological fluids.[77]

Excretion of Muscle Metabolites

The excretion of creatinine or 3-methyl histidine in urine can be measured in a 24-hour urine sample. The basis of the creatinine excretion method is that creatinine is the only metabolite of creatinine which is largely located in muscle (98% of the body creatinine pool). Creatinine excretion in the urine, however, has been found to have large day-to-day variability.[1]

On the other hand, assessment through measurement of 3-methylhistidine holds much future promise.[78] 3-Methylhistidine is an amino acid that is found almost exclusively in muscle protein.[1] When muscle protein is broken down, 3-methylhistidine is released and excreted in the urine without being reused by the body and has been found to correlate highly with fat free mass.[79]

Total Body Electrical Conductivity (TOBEC)

Lean tissues conduct electricity much better than fat. TOBEC operates on the principle than an object placed in an electromagnetic field will perturb the field, and the degree of perturbation is dependent on the quantity of conducting material (primarily electrolytes in lean body mass).[1] Since 1971, the lean tissues of farm animals have been measured by putting them in a box that emits electrical impulses and measures responses.[80, 81]

The TOBEC system for human use consists of a large solenoid coil into which the person being measured is slid on a stretcher. The coil (driven by a 5-mHz radio frequency current) induces a current within the person's body in proportion to the mass of the conductive tissues. The instrument measures ten total body conductivity readings in about 10 seconds. Studies show a very high correlation with hydrostatic weighing ($r = 0.93$).[1] TOBEC has also been found to be very sensitive to small changes in lean body mass[82] and total body water.[83] The major limitation of this technique is the high cost of the equipment.

Total Body Potassium

Total body potassium is an indication of lean tissue mass because more than 90 percent of body potassium is within non-fat cells.[1] Potassium contains a natural radioactive tracer, 40K, which emits a high-energy gamma ray. The measurement technique depends on counting the radiation using a whole-body radiation counter.

If fat-free tissue had a constant potassium content, it would be possible to calculate fat-free mass and body fat from a measurement of total body potassium. However, controversy exists over the accuracy of the values used for the ratio of body potassium to fat-free mass. The obese, for example, have fat-free tissue with a lower than normal potassium content.[77]

Computed Tomography

With this method a computed tomography (CT) scanner is used to produce a cross-sectional image of the distribution of x-ray transmission.[1] The person being measured is placed next to an x-ray tube, which directs a collimated beam of x-ray photons toward a scintillation detector.

Computed tomography can readily distinguish adipose tissue from adjacent skin, muscles, bones, vascular structures, and intra-abdominal and pelvic organs, because fat transmits poorly.[84] The cross-sectional CT images can be obtained at any level within the body. Computed tomography can thus noninvasively quantify body fat distribution at various sites—particularly useful is CT's ability to give a ratio of intra-abdominal to extra-abdominal fat.[68]

Summary

1. This chapter discussed the various methods of measuring obesity, starting with the least precise and progressing toward the more accurate (weight tables, body mass index, skinfolds, underwater weighing). The chapter ended with a brief discussion of some of the newer laboratory methods of evaluating body composition.

2. In general, in light of the various factors, validity, reliability, economy, and good norms, the various skinfold tests are probably most practical and useful. With proper training and practice, testers can learn to assess body composition quickly and accurately. However, careful

selection of specific anatomic sites, and observance of rules for measuring are important.

3 Height-weight tables only provide a rough estimate of ideal weight. Frame size can be determined by measuring the width of the elbow. Use of the Quetelet Index (kg/m²) produces a higher correlation with actual body composition than does use of the height-weight tables.

4. Underwater weighing remains the laboratory standard, but the time, expense, and expertise needed is prohibitive for many clinical settings.

5. More research is needed to develop some of the newer techniques. As better equations are developed, bioelectrical impedance should prove to be a most convenient, safe, accurate, and rapid method of body composition analysis.

6. Fat distribution on the body has been shown recently to be an important predictor of the health-consequences of obesity. A number of the researchers have found that the ratio of waist-to-hip circumference (WHR) is an accurate and convenient method for determining type of obesity. When the ratio is above 0.9 for men and 0.8 for women, obesity-associated risks rise sharply.

References

1. Brodie DA. Techniques of Measurement of Body Composition Part I. *Sports Med* 5:11–40, 1988. Part II. Sports Med 5:74–98, 1988.

2. Lukaski HC. Methods for the Assessment of Human Body Composition: Traditional and New. Am J Clin Nutr 46:537–556, 1987.

3. National Institutes of Health. Consensus Development Conference Statement. Health Implications of Obesity. February 11–13, 1985. Ann Intern Med 103:981–1077, 1985.

4. Simopoulos AP. The Health Implications of Overweight and Obesity. Nutr Rev 43:33–40, 1985.

5. Weigley ES. Average? Ideal? Desirable? A Brief Overview of Height-Weight Tables in the United States. J Am Diet Assoc 84:417, 1984.

6. Robinette-Weiss N, et al. The Metropolitan Height-Weight Tables: Perspectives for Use. J Am Diet Assoc 84:1480–1481, 1984.

7. Abraham S. Height-Weight Tables: Their Sources and Development. Clin Consult Nutr Support 3:5–8, 1983. Reprinted in: Shils ME, Young VR. Modern Nutrition in Health and Disease. Philadelphia: Lea & Febiger, 1988, pp. 1509–1513.

8. Simopoulos AP. Obesity and Body Weight Standards. Annu Rev Public Health 7:481–492, 1986.

9. Harrison GG. Height-Weight Tables. Ann Intern Med 103:989–994, 1985.

10. Garrison RJ, et al. Cigarette Smoking As A Confounder of the Relationship Between Relative Weight and Long-term Mortality. JAMA 249:2199–2203, 1983.

11. Gordon CC, Chumlea WC, Roche AF. Stature, Recumbent Length, and Weight. In: Anthropometric Standardization Reference Manual (Lohman TG, Roche AF, Martorell R (eds). Champaign, Illinois: Human Kinetics Books, 1988.

12. Frisancho AR. New Standards of Weight and Body Composition by Frame Size and Height for Assessment of Nutritional Status of Adults and the Elderly. Am J Clin Nutr 40:808–819, 1984.

13. Himes JH, Frisancho RA. Estimating Frame Size. In: Anthropometric Standardization Reference Manual Lohman TG, Roche AF, Martorell R (eds). Champaign, Illinois: Human Kinetics Books, 1988.

14. Wilmore JH, Frisancho RA, Gordon CC, Himes JH, Martin AD, Martorell R, Seefeldt VD. Body Breadth Equipment and Measurement Techniques. In: Anthropometric Standardization Reference Manual Lohman TG, Roche AF, Martorell R (eds). Champaign, Illinois: Human Kinetics Books, 1988.

15. Frisancho AR. Frameter (1985). Health Products, 2126 Ridge, Ann Arbor, Michigan 48104.

16. Revicki DA, Israel RG. Relationship Between Body Mass Indices and Measures of Body Adiposity. Am J Public Health 76:992–994, 1986.

17. Pollock ML, Wilmore JH, Fox SM. Exercise In Health and Disease. Philadelphia: W.B. Saunders Co., 1984.

18. Jéquier E. Energy, Obesity, and Body Weight Standards. Am J Clin Nutr 45:1035–1047, 1987.

19. Jackson AS, Pollock ML. Practical Assessment of Body Composition. Physician Sportsmed 13:76–90, 1985.

20. Welham WC, Behnke AR. The Specific Gravity of Healthy Man. Body Weight, Volume and Other Physical Characteristics of Exceptional Athletes and Of Naval Personnel. JAMA 118:498–501, 1942.

21. Hubert HB, Feinleib M, McNamara PM. Obesity As An Independent Risk Factor for Cardiovascular Disease: A 26-Year Follow-up of Participants in the Framingham Heart Study. Circulation 67:968–977, 1983.

22. Harrison GG, Buskirk ER, Carter JEL, Johnston FE, Lohman TG, Pollock ML, Roche AF, Wilmore J. Skinfold Thicknesses and Measurement Technique. IN: Anthropometric Standardization Reference Manual (Lohman TG, Roche AF, Martorell R (eds). Champaign, Illinois: Human Kinetics Books, 1988.

23. Jackson AS. Practical Methods of Measuring Body Composition. In: Evaluation and Treatment of Obesity (Stor-

lie J, Jordan HA, eds.). New York: Medical and Scientific Books, Spectrum Publications, Inc., 1984.

24. Martorell R, Mendoza F, Mueller WH, Pawson IG. Which Side to Measure: Right or Left? In: Anthropometric Standardization Reference Manual (Lohman TG, Roche AF, Martorell R (eds). Champaign, Illinois: Human Kinetics Books, 1988.

25. MacDougall JD, Wenger HA, Green HJ. Physiological Testing of the Elite Athlete. Canadian Association of Sports Sciences, 1982.

26. Wright RA. Nutritional Assessment. Boston: Blackwell Scientific Publications, Inc., 1984.

27. Leger LA, et al. Validity of Plastic Skinfold Caliper Measurements. Hum Biol 54:667–675, 1982.

28. Hawkins JD. An Analysis of Selected Skinfold Measuring Instruments. JOPERD, 54:25–27, 1983.

29. Lohman TG, Pollock ML, et al. Methodological Factors and the Prediction of Body Fat in Female Athletes. Med Sci Sports Ex 16:92–96, 1984.

30. Morrow JR, Fridye T, Monaghen SD. Generalizability of the AAHPERD Health Related Skinfold Test. Res Quart Exerc Sport 57:187–195, 1986.

31. AAHPERD. Technical Manual: Health-Related Physical Fitness. Reston, Virginia: AAHPERD, 1984.

32. Golding LA, Myers CR, Sinning WE. The Y's Way to Physical Fitness, (3rd Edition) 1989. Champaign IL: Human Kinetics Publishers, Inc.

33. AAHPERD. Health Related Physical Fitness Test Manual. Reston, Virginia: AAHPERD, 1980.

34. AAHPERD. Norms for College Students: Health-Related Physical Fitness Test. Reston, Virginia: AAHPERD, 1985.

35. Public Health Service. Summary of Findings from National Children and Youth Fitness Study. JOPHER, January 1985, pp. 44–90.

36. Ross JG, Pate RR, Delpy LA, Gold RS, Svilar M. New Health-Related Fitness Norms. JOPERD, November-December, 1987, pp. 66–70.

37. Lohman TG. The Use of Skinfold to Estimate Body Fatness on Children and Youth. JOPERD, November-December, 1987, pp. 98–102.

38. Physical Best: The American Alliance Physical Fitness Education & Assessment Program. Reston, Virginia: The American Alliance for Health, Physical Education, Recreation and Dance, 1988.

39. Luna-Raffy P, Lee JW, Nieman DC. Predicting Body Fatness in Children Using a Multiple Regression Equation. (in publication review).

40. Jackson AS, Pollock ML, Ward A. Generalized Equations for Predicting Body Density of Women. Med Sci Sport Exerc 12:175–182, 1980.

41. Jackson AS, Pollock ML. Generalized Equations for Predicting Body Density of Men. Br J Nutr 40:497–504, 1978.

42. Sinning WE, Wilson JR. Validity of "Generalized" Equations for Body Composition Analysis in Women Athletes. Res Quart Exerc Sport 55:153–160, 1984.

43. Thorland WG, et al. Validity of Anthropometric Equations for the Estimation of Body Density in Adolescent Athletes. Med Sci Sport Exerc 16:77–81, 1984.

44. Pollock Ml, Jackson AS. Research Progress in Validation of Clinical Methods of Assessing Body Composition. Med Sci Sport Exerc 16:606–613, 1984.

45. Baun WB, Baun MR, Raven PB. A Nomogram for the Estimate of Percent Body Fat from Generalized Equation. Res Quart Exerc Sport 52:380–384, 1981.

46. Fleck SJ. Body Composition of Elite American Athletes. Am J Sports Med 11:398, 1983.

47. Wilmore JH. The Physiological Basis of the Conditioning Process. Boston: Allyn and Bacon, Inc., 1982.

48. Lohman TG. Skinfolds and Body Density and Their Relation to Body Fatness: A Review. Hum Biol 53:181–225, 1981.

49. Brozek J, Grande F, Anderson JT, Keys A. Densiometric Analysis of Body Composition: Revision of Some Quantitative Assumptions. Ann New York Academy Sciences 110:113–140, 1963.

50. Morrow JR, Jackson AS, Bradley PW, Hartung GH. Accuracy of Measured and Predicted Residual Lung Volume On Body Density Measurement. Med Sci Sports Exerc 18:647–652, 1986.

51. Weltman A, Katch V. Comparison of Hydrostatic Weighing at Residual Volume and Total Lung Capacity. Med Sci Sports Exerc 13:210–213, 1981.

52. Nelson AG, Stuart DW, Fisher AG. The Effect of Hydrostatic Weighing Protocols on Body Density Measurement. Med Sci Sports Exerc 17:246, 1985.

53. Goldman HI, Becklake MR. Respiratory Function Tests. Am Rev Tuberc Pulm Dis 79:457–467, 1959.

54. van Raaij JM, Peek MEM, Vermaat-Miedema SH, et al. New Equations for Estimating Body Fat Mass in Pregnancy From Body Density or Total Body Water. Am J Clin Nutr 48:24–29, 1988.

55. Buskirk ER, Mendez J. Sports Science and Body Composition Analysis: Emphasis on Cell and Muscle Mass. Med Sci Sports Exerc 16:584–593, 1984.

56. Lukaski HC, et al. Assessment of Fat-Free Mass Using Bioelectrical Impedance Measurements of the Human Body. Am J Clin Nutr 41:810–817, 1985.

57. Hodgdon JA, Lawlor MR. Comparison of Whole Body Impedance, Body Circumferences, and Skinfold Thicknesses In the Prediction of Lean Body Mass. Med Sci Sports Exerc 17:271, 1985.

58. Lawlor MR, et al. Bioelectrical Impedance Analysis As A Method to Assess Body Composition. Med Sci Sports Exerc 17:271, 1985.

59. Keller B, Katch FI. Validity of Bioelectrical Resistance Impedance for Estimation of Body Fat in Lean Males. Med Sci Sports Exerc 17:272, 1985.

60. Segal KR, et al. Estimation of Human Body Composition by Electrical Impedance Methods: A Comparative Study. J Appl Physiol 58:1565–1571, 1985.

61. Cohn SH. How Valid Are Bioelectric Impedance Measurements in Body Composition Studies? Am J Clin Nutr 42:889–890, 1985.

62. Nash HL. Body Fat Measurement: Weighing the Pros and Cons of Electrical Impedance. Phys Sportsmed 13:124–128, 1985.

63. Segal KR, Van Loan M, Fitzgerald PI, et al. Lean Body Mass Estimation by Bioelectrical Impedance Analysis: A Four-Site Cross-Validation Study. Am J Clin Nutr 47:7–14, 1988.

64. Chumlea WC, Baumgartner RN, Roche AF. Specific Resistivity Used to Estimate Fat-Free Mass From Segmental Body Measures of Bioelectric Impedance. Am J Clin Nutr 48:7–15, 1988.

65. Jackson AS, Pollock ML, Graves JE, Mahar MT. Reliability and Validity of Bioelectrical Impedance in Determining Body Composition. J Appl Physiol 64:529–534, 1988.

66. Van Itallie TB. Topography of Body Fat: Relationship to Risk of Cardiovascular and Other Diseases. In: Anthropometric Standardization Reference Manual. Lohman TG, Roche AF, Martorell R (eds). Champaign, Illinois: Human Kinetics Books, 1988.

67. Rimm AA, Hartz AJ, Fischer ME. A Weight Shape Index for Assessing Risk of Disease in 44,820 Women. J Clin Epidemiol 41:459–465, 1988.

68. Bray GA, Gray DS. Obesity: Part 1—Pathogenesis. West J Med 149:429–441, 1988.

69. Wilmore JH. A Reaction to the Manuscripts of Roche and Buskirk. Med Sci Sports Exerc 16:594–595, 1984.

70. Roche AF. Body Composition Assessments in Youth and Adults. Report of the Sixth Ross Conference on Medical Research. Columbus, Ohio: Ross Laboratories, 1985.

71. Fannelli MY, et al. Ultrasound As An Approach to Assessing Body Composition. Am J Clin Nutr 39:703–709, 1984.

72. Ultrasonic Measurement of Depth of Adipose Tissue and Muscle Area in Swine. Nutr Rev 42:331, 1984.

73. Volz PA, Ostrove SM. Evaluation of a Portable Ultrasonoscope in Assessing the Body Composition of College-Age Women. Med Sci Sports Exerc 16:97–102, 1984.

74. Kuczmarski RJ, Fanelli MT, Koch GG. Ultrasonic Assessment of Body Composition in Obese Adults: Overcoming the Limitations of the Skinfold Caliper. Am J Clin Nutr 45:717–724, 1987.

75. Whyte RK, et al. The Measurement of Whole Body Water by $H_2^{18}O$ Dilution in Newborn Pigs. Am J Clin Nutr 41:801–809, 1985.

76. Lukaski HC, Johnson PE. A Simple, Inexpensive Method of Determining Total Body Water Using A Tracer Dose of D^2O and Infrared Absorption of Biological Fluids. Am J Clin Nutr 41:363–370, 1985.

77. Garrow JS. New Approaches to Body Composition. Am J Clin Nutr 35:1152–1158, 1982.

78. Buskirk ER, Mendez J. Sports Science and Body Composition Analysis: Emphasis On Cell and Muscle Mass. Med Sci Sports Exerc 16:584–593, 1984.

79. Mendez J, Lukaski HC, Buskirk ER. Fat-Free Mass As A Function of Maximal Oxygen Consumption and 24-Hour Urinary Creatinine, and 3-Methylhistidine Excretion. Am J Clin Nutr 39:710–715, 1984.

80. Harrison GG, Van Itallie TB. Estimation of Body Composition: A New Approach Based on Electromagnetic Principles. Am J Clin Nutr 35:1176–1179, 1982.

81. Presta E, et al. Measurement of Total Body Electrical Conductivity: A New Methods for Estimation of Body Composition. Am J Clin Nutr 37:735–739, 1983.

82. Van Loan MD, Belko AZ, Mayclin PL, Barbieri TF. Use of Total-Body Electrical Conductivity for Monitoring Body Composition Changes During Weight Reduction. Am J Clin Nutr 46:5–8, 1987.

83. Cochran WJ, Wong WW, Fiorotto ML, et al. Total Body Water Estimated by Measuring Total-Body Electrical Conductivity. Am J Clin Nutr 48:946–950, 1988.

84. Grauer WO, et al. Quantification of Body Fat Distribution In the Abdomen Using Computed Tomography. Am J Clin Nutr 39:631–637, 1984.

Physical Fitness Activity 5.1— Measurement of Body Composition

In this activity, you will be measuring the body composition of at least one individual using several different methods. It is highly recommended that you duplicate the worksheet from this activity and measure three or more individuals.

The body composition methods for this activity have been fully described in this chapter, and you should review each description before administering the test. Ideally, you should first learn the techniques while in a class laboratory under experienced supervision. Misclassification of the body composition status of an individual can lead to undue anxiety.

Body Composition Worksheet

Name_____   Date_____   Gender   M   F

Age _____   Ht _____(in   Wt _____ (lbs)

Method	Measurement	Classification
Relative Weight (from 1973 Fogarty Tables	_____	_____
Frame size (elbow width)	_____ (in)	_____
Quetelet Index (kg/m²)	_____	_____
Triceps skinfold	_____ (mm)	_____
Percent body fat (from 3-site skinfold)	_____	_____

_____ body fat (lbs) (body wt × % body fat)

_____ lean body weight (lbs) (body wt – fat wt)

_____ ideal body wt [(lean body wt/100% – desired fat %)]

Chapter 6

Assessment of Musculoskeletal Fitness

"In our subjects, 83 percent had acute back pain because of weak and/or tense muscles, and not from any specific lesion, disease, or structural problems."—Kraus and Weber[11]

Introduction

As outlined in Chapter 2, musculoskeletal fitness has three elements:

- **Muscular Strength:** the maximal one-effort force that can be exerted against a resistance.
- **Muscular Endurance:** the ability of the muscles to apply a submaximal force repeatedly or to sustain a muscular contraction for a certain period of time.
- **Flexibility:** the functional capacity of the joints to move through a full range of movement.

The purpose of this chapter is to describe the various types of tests that measure each of these three elements, concentrating on the tests that were outlined in the testing batteries at the end of Chapter 3.

Elaborate and expensive musculoskeletal fitness testing equipment is available, and many books have been written describing it, including the use of *isokinetic* equipment (e.g., the Cybex) for testing muscular strength and endurance.[1, 2, 3] The purpose of both this book and chapter, however, is to concentrate more on the physical fitness tests that are widely available, inexpensive (yet valid and reliable), and health-related.

Health-Related Benefits of Musculoskeletal Fitness

Most of the health-related benefits of musculoskeletal fitness have focused on the contribution of abdominal muscle strength and endurance and lower-back-hamstring flexibility to the prevention of low back pain.[4]

Prevention and Treatment of Low Back Pain

Low back pain (LBP) and tension are significant health problems for the American population.[4, 5] LBP is the number one symptomatic complaint expressed by patients 25–60 years old seeing office based physicians, and is the most costly medical problem in our society for the 30–60 age group.[5, 6] Data from the National Center for Health Statistics reveal that impairment of the back and spine is the most common cause of chronic limitation of activity among people under 45, and ranks third after cardiovascular disease and arthritis for those 45–64.[7]

But despite this prevalence, the correct treatment of LBP remains a mystery. Bed rest and analgesics seem to be the most effective means of therapy at present.

In all, 60–80 percent of the population will experience at least one episode of acute back pain. Acute LBP is a self-limited disorder, with 50 percent of patients pain-free by the first week, 80 percent by second week, and 90 percent by two months, regardless of therapy.[6]

LBP is a major problem for industry, where it is second only to upper respiratory illness as a cause of lost work time. Every year, 93 million work days are lost from LBP. There are an estimated 75 million Americans with recurring back problems, with two million of these unable to hold jobs as a result.[8, 9]

At the Kodak Company, for example, LBP develops in 35 percent of sedentary workers and 47 percent of manual material handlers, with only 15 percent of cases being related to a definite injury.[6] According to the American Medical Association, in 1983 seven million Americans were undergoing treatment for chronic back problems; 2 million more are added annually to this list.[8]

Clinical evidence, although often presenting a confusing image (with much more research needed), appears to point towards lack of flexibility in the lower back/hamstring muscle groups, combined with relatively weak abdominal wall muscles as the causes of a majority of low back pain cases.[10] Many therapists link the high incidence of low back problems with a corresponding lack of exercise.[4] Theoretically, weak muscles that are easily fatigued cannot support the spine in proper alignment. The groups primarily involved include the spinal (erector spinae), abdominal, hip flexors (psoas/ileopsoas), hip extensors (gluteals), and hamstrings. (See Appendix E.)

When a person is standing, weak abdominals and inflexible posterior thigh muscles allow the pelvis to tilt forward, causing *lordosis*, or curvature in the lower back. This places increased stress on the vertebral column, and a greater load on other postural muscles, leading to their fatigue—and the "low back pain syndrome."[4]

There has been very little controlled research to see whether musculoskeletal exercise of the hip and thigh area can prevent and relieve low back pain. The few available studies, however, provide interesting data. A study of 3000 adult patients with chronic and acute back pain concluded that in 83 percent of the cases the pain was the result of weak and/or tense muscles, and not any specific lesion, disease, or structural problem.[11, 12] When the participants in the study were treated with musculoskeletal exercises, 26 percent rated results as "fair," 65 percent as "good," and only 9.2 percent as "poor".[11, 12]

The YMCA conducted a pilot study in the early 1970s, testing exercise as a means of relieving LBP. Better than 82 percent of 312 people who completed the course reported reduction or complete elimination of pain.[13] As a result of this study, the YMCA started offering the program nationally (the "Y's Way to a Healthy Back Program"). By 1982, results were reported for 11,809 participants—with over 80.7 percent experiencing improvement.[11]

The Y's Way to a Healthy Back is a musculoskeletal program designed for those who have experienced occasional or persistent backache or discomfort.[14] Participants meet twice weekly and are taught appropriate exercises. They are urged to exercise daily at home. New exercises are added weekly and recommendations for outside reading are given. Classes may start with only 20 minutes of exercise, and then build up to 45 minutes.

The management of back pain requires a thorough history and physical examination to determine proper therapy. The physician should be aware that muscle deficiency (insufficient strength and inadequate elasticity) is often a cause of muscle strain and back pain.[15]

Exercise programs for rehabilitation begin with relaxation, progress to limbering and stretching of the lower back and hamstring areas, and culminate in abdominal strengthening, with all exercises performed slowly and each movement repeated several times. Exercise movements should then be performed in reverse order, followed by a cooling-off period with relaxation exercises to end the session.

Figure 6.1 depicts four of the exercise movements used in most back pain programs. Figure 6.2 summarizes four categories of movements used in popular exercise routines that can cause or aggravate low back problems: hyperextension, repetitive flexion, overstretching, and jumping stress.[16] Exercise leaders should screen these types of exercise movements out of exercise programs.

Thus clinical and research experience support the thesis that good abdominal muscle strength/endurance, and low back/hamstring flexibility reduce the risk of developing low back pain.[4, 5, 17] Accordingly, AAHPERD, the YMCA, and many other testing organizations have included within their testing batteries the one-minute, bent-knee sit-up test for abdominal muscle strength/endurance, and the sit-and-reach test for lower back/posterior thigh flexibility. These are the two most important of the musculoskeletal tests, because of their potential ability to predict susceptibility to low back pain.

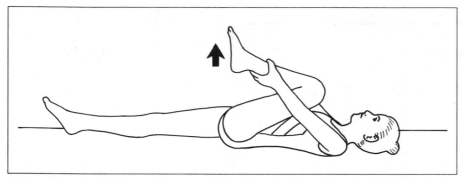

A. Hamstring Stretch

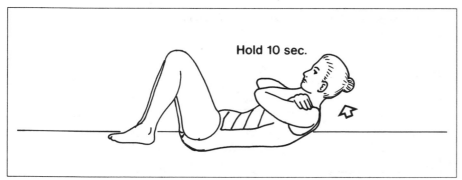

Hold 10 sec.

B. Bent-Knee Sit-ups

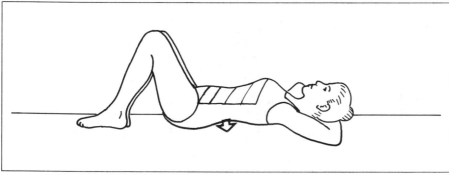

C. Pelvic Tilt

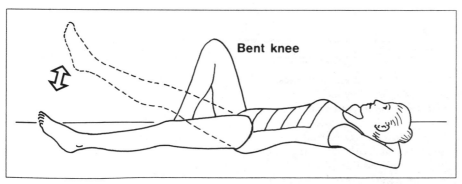

Bent knee

D. Leg Lift

Figure 6.1 Exercise for Treatment and Prevention of Lower Back Pain Many clinicians agree that one of the best techniques for relieving or preventing back pain is regular conditioning exercise for the muscles that support the back. Four important calisthenics include the following: *A. Hamstring stretch:* Lie on your back with one leg straight in front of you and the other bent so that your thigh is resting on your chest. Hold onto the ankle of your bent leg and slowly try to straighten your leg. Keep the lower back on the floor as you straighten your leg. Hold for 10 to 30 seconds, making sure that the stretch does not feel painful. Switch to the other leg, and do the same. Repeat 5 times. *B. Bent-knee sit-ups:* Lie on your back as shown, with knees bent and feet and lower back on the floor. Place your arms across your chest with the fingertips of each hand touching the shoulders. Slowly raise your head and shoulders slightly off the ground, using your stomach muscles. Hold for 10–15 seconds, then relax. Repeat the sequence 5 to 10 times, increasing the number of repetitions as your fitness level improves. *C. Pelvic tilt:* Lie as shown with knees bent and feet flat on the floor. Slowly tighten your stomach and buttocks muscles as you press your lower back onto the floor. Hold 10 seconds and then relax. Repeat 5 to 10 times. *D. Leg lift:* Lie on the floor with one leg straight in front of you and the other bent as shown. Slowly raise your straightened leg as far up as you can. Hold for 10 seconds. Then, slowly lower your leg to the floor. Repeat 5 times. Relax. Switch leg positions and repeat the same sequence with the other leg.

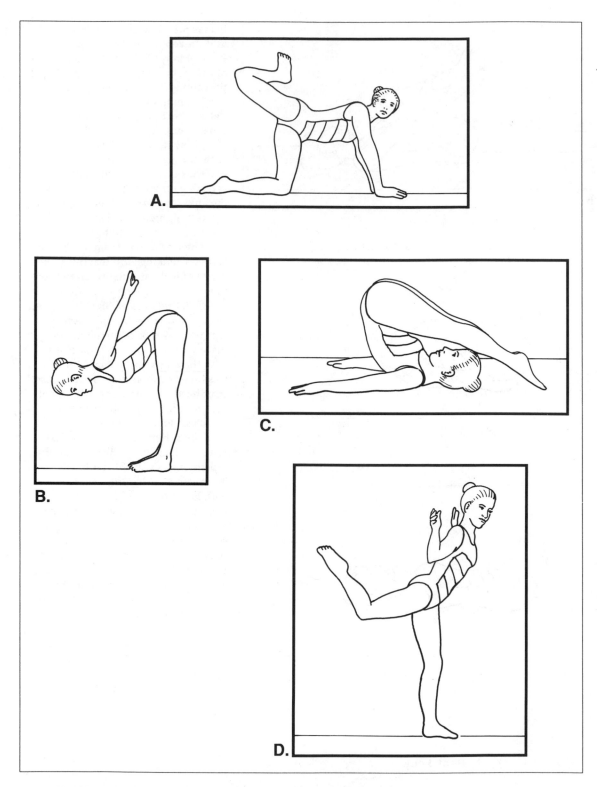

Figure 6.2   Exercise Movements that Can Cause or Aggravate Lower Back Pain   *A. Hyperextension exercises:* exercises such as the "donkey kick" can cause or aggravate low back problems. *B. Repetitive flexion:* repetitive flexion exercises can cause degenerative changes, most commonly at the lower back area, because of the hinge action at this site. *C. Overstretching:* overstretching exercises such as the yoga "plow" position can irritate nerve tissue. *D. Jumping stress:* jumping on one leg with the spine in an extended position places a shearing stress on the lower back area. *Source:* Goodman CE. Low Back Pain in the Cosmetic Athlete. Phys Sportsmed 15(8):97–104, 1987.

Tests for Muscular Endurance and Strength

Muscular strength and endurance are specific to each muscle group.[1] Therefore, no single test can be used to evaluate total body muscle strength and endurance. It is recommended that the strength/endurance battery include measures for the upper body, mid-body, and lower body.

One-Minute Timed, Bent-Knee Sit-Ups

The purpose of this test is to evaluate abdominal muscle strength and endurance.[18, 19] Although widely used, it has aroused considerable controversy and dissatisfaction. (This will be the topic of the Sports Medicine Insight at the end of this chapter.) The sit-up test procedures described here are based on guidelines established for the National Children and Youth Fitness Study.[19, 20] (See Figure 6.3.)

- One starts on his back with knees flexed, feet on floor, with the heels 12–18 inches from the buttocks.
- The arms are crossed on the chest with the hands on the opposite shoulders. The arms must be folded across and flat against the chest.
- The feet are held by the partner to keep them firmly on the ground.
- During the sit-up, arm contact with the chest must be maintained. This is critically important. An-

other important rule is that the buttocks must remain on the mat, no more than 18 inches from the heels.

- In the up position, the elbow-forearm must touch the thighs (without the arms pulling away from the chest).
- In the down position, the midback makes contact with the floor.
- The number of correctly executed sit-ups performed in 60 seconds is the score. See Appendix B for norms for all age groups (Tables 5, 6, 14, 15, 20, 29.)

Pull-Ups

The purpose of this test is to measure the muscular strength and endurance of the arms and shoulder girdle.[21] The procedures outlined here were used in the National Children and Youth Fitness Study.[19, 22] For children ages 10 to 18, the traditional pull-up was used; for those 6 to 9, a modified pull-up test was used. Procedures for both of these tests are summarized below. The test is performed exactly the same way for both boys and girls.

The Traditional Pull-Up

The traditional pull-up requires the following procedures: (see Figure 6.4.)

- The person being tested starts in a hanging position, with arms straight, hands in an *underhand* position (palms inward).

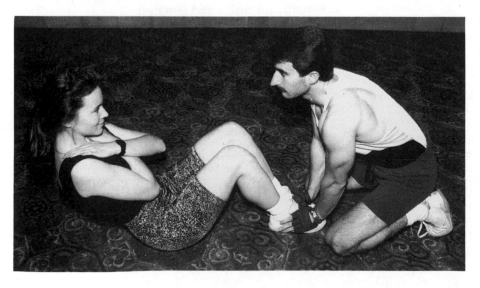

Figure 6.3 One-minute, Timed, Bent-knee Sit-ups The purpose of this test is to evaluate abdominal muscle strength and endurance.

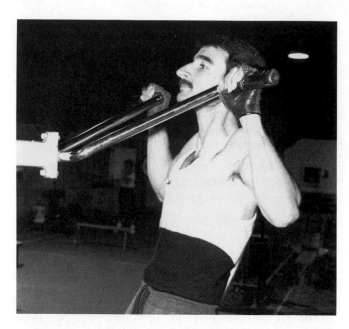

Figure 6.4 Traditional Pull-ups The purpose of this test is to measure the muscular strength and endurance of the arms and shoulder girdle in pulling the body upward.

- The body is pulled upward until the chin is *over* the bar.
- After each pull-up, the person returns to a fully extended hanging position.
- Swinging and snap-up movements are to be avoided.
- A partner should hold an extended arm across the front of the person's thighs to prevent swinging. The knees should stay straight during the entire test.
- The score is the total number of pull-ups until exhaustion. (See norms in Appendix B, Tables 3, 4, 18, 27.)

The Modified Pull-Up for Children Ages 6–9

Experience has revealed certain problems with the traditional pull-up and the flexed-arm hang.[22] Performance is markedly affected by body weight.

In 1985, the President's Council on Physical Fitness and Sports School Population Fitness Survey revealed that 70 percent of all girls tested could not do more than one pull-up, with 55 percent not being able to do even one.[23] Forty percent of boys ages 6 to 12 could not do more than one pull-up, and twenty-five percent could not do any. Fifty-five percent of all girls could not hold their chins over a raised bar for more than 10 seconds. Forty-five percent of boys 6 to 14 could not hold their chins over a raised bar for more than 10 seconds.

A better test of upper body muscular strength/endurance may be a modification of the traditional pull-up. This modified pull-up was used in the National Children and Youth Fitness Study II for children ages 6 to 9, but it can be used for all age groups. (See Appendix B, Table 14.)

- The child is positioned on his back with shoulders directly below a bar that is set at a height one or two inches beyond his reach.
- An elastic band is suspended across the uprights parallel to and about seven to eight inches below the bar.
- In the start position, the child is suspended from the bar, his buttocks off the floor, arms and legs straight, and only his heels in contact with the floor.
- The bar is held with an overhand grip (palm away from the body), with thumbs around the bar.
- A pull-up is completed when the chin is hooked over the elastic band. The movement should be accomplished using only the arms, with the body kept rigid and straight.

Push-Ups

The purpose of the push-up test is to assess upper body (triceps, anterior deltoids, and pectoralis major) muscle strength and endurance. This test is a part of the Canadian Standarized Test of Fitness.[24] It is accomplished differently for males and females:

Males

- The person being tested assumes the standard position for a push-up, with the body rigid and straight, toes tucked under, and hands approximately shoulder-width apart and straight under the shoulders.
- A partner places his fist on the floor beneath the person's chest, who lowers himself until his chest touches the fist, keeping his back perfectly straight; he then raises himself back up to the starting position. (See Figure 6.5.)
- The most common performance error is not keeping the back rigid and straight throughout the entire push-up.

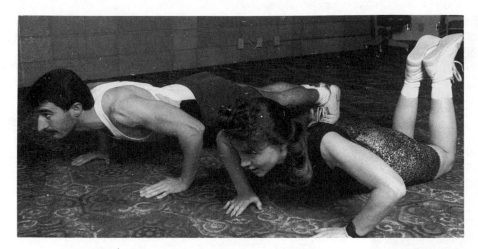

Figure 6.5 Push-ups The purpose of the push-up test is to assess upper body (triceps, anterior deltoids, and pectoralis major) muscle strength and endurance.

- Rest is allowed in the up position only.
- The score is the total number of push-ups to exhaustion. (See norms in Appendix B, Table 53.)

Females

- Everything is the same as for the males, except that the test is performed from the bent-knee position. (See Figure 6.5.) In addition, the person being tested should make sure that her hands are slightly ahead of her shoulders in the up position, so that her hands are directly under her shoulders in the down position.
- A common error for females also is not keeping the back rigid.
- The score is the total number of push-ups to exhaustion. (See norms in Appendix B, Table 53.)

Grip Strength Test with Hand Dynamometer

This test is used in the Canadian Standarized Test of Fitness.[24] Both the right and left hands should be measured. (See norms in Appendix B, Table 54.)

The hand-grip *dynamometer* should be adjustable for any hand size.[25] A maximum reading pointer should be available to hold the reading until it is manually reset. The Smedley handgrip dynamometer is recommended, and can be obtained for $155 to $165 from: Quinton Instrument Co., 2121 Terry Avenue, Seattle, WA 98121.

The purpose of the hand grip dynamometer test is to measure the static strength of the grip squeezing muscles. The hand grip test is easy to administer, relatively inexpensive, portable, and highly reliable.

To perform the test (see Figure 6.6):

- The person being tested should first dry and if practical chalk both hands.
- The dynamometer should be adjusted and placed comfortably in the hand to be tested. The second joint of the hand should fit snugly under the handle, which should be gripped between the fingers and the palm at the base of the thumb.[26]
- The person should assume a slightly bent forward position, with the hand to be tested out in front of her body. Her hand and arm should be free of her body, not touching anything. Her arm can be slightly bent.
- The test involves an all-out gripping effort for 2–3 seconds. No swinging or pumping of the arm is allowed. The dial can be visible for motivational purposes.
- The score is the sum of the test of both hands, based on the best of 2–4 trials for each. The scale is read in kilograms.

Bench Press Strength and Endurance Tests

Bench Press 1-RM Test for Strength

The muscular strength of the major muscle groups can be measured with the one-repetition maximum test (1-RM) (the greatest weight that can be lifted once for a muscle group).[27] Researchers have shown that the best single weight lift for predicting total dynamic strength safely is the 1-RM bench press test.[28]

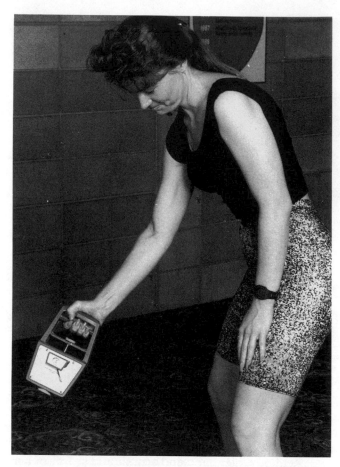

Figure 6.6   Grip Strength Test with Hand Dynamometer
Both the right and left hands should be measured. The
purpose of the hand grip dynamometer test is to measure
the static strength of the grip squeezing muscles.

The objective of the 1-RM bench press test is to test
the strength of the muscles involved in arm extension
(triceps, pectoralis major, anterior deltoid).

The test is performed as follows[21] (see Figure 6.7):

▪ The person being tested should first be allowed to
become familiar with the bench press test by practicing a few lifts with light weights. For the test, the
person lies on his back on a bench, with his arms
extended and hands gripping the bar, approximately shoulder width apart. The bar is lowered
until it touches the chest, and then is pushed
straight up with maximum effort until the arms
are locked once again. The person breathes in as
the weight is being lowered, and breathes out
during the weight lifting phase. (This helps to
prevent the *Valsalva's Maneuver*—the high buildup
of blood pressure and decrease of blood flow to
the brain owing to the high pressures that are built
up in the chest during weight lifting.)

▪ Free weights should be used with a spotter. The
use of machine weights (Universal, Paramount,
Nautilus, etc.) is unfair because the machines vary
the resistance to adapt for weak points in the lift.

▪ As many trials are allowed as it takes to achieve a
true maximum effort. Each trial requires maximum effort for one repetition. Allow 1–3 minutes
between trials.

▪ The best lifting score is divided by the person's
weight to derive a ratio. (See Appendix B, Table 57
for the norms.)

YMCA Bench Press Test for Muscular Endurance

There are several types of weight lifting tests used to test
muscular endurance. One test of muscular endurance
uses a fixed percentage of the person's body weight as
the resistance, with the test score being the number of
times this weight can be lifted.

Another method utilizes a fixed percentage (preferably 70 percent) of one's 1-RM or absolute strength for
the resistance. Good norms have yet to be established,
however, for these types of tests. On the basis of limited
data,[27] 12–15 repetitions at 70 percent of 1-RM are optimal for most people; athletes should aim for 20–25
repetitions.

The YMCA has developed a bench press test for
muscular strength and endurance using an absolute
weight. The advantage of this is that for certain occupations (firefighting, construction, etc.), being able to work
with absolute weights is very important. The disadvantage of such a test is that lighter people are discrimi-
nated against.

The YMCA bench press test[14] uses the following
steps (see Figure 6.8):

▪ Use a 35-pound barbell for women and an 80-
pound barbell for men.

▪ Set a metronome for 60 beats per minute.

▪ The person being tested lies on a bench with feet
on the floor.

▪ A spotter hands the weight to the person. The
down position is the starting position (elbows
flexed, hands shoulder width apart, hands gripping the barbell, palms facing up).

▪ The person presses the barbell upward using free
weights (with careful spotting) to fully extend the

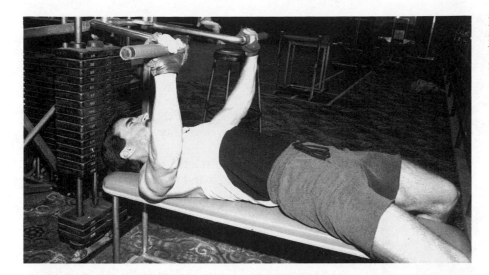

Figure 6.7 Bench Press 1-RM Test for Strength Muscular strength can be measured with the one-repetition maximum test (1-RM).

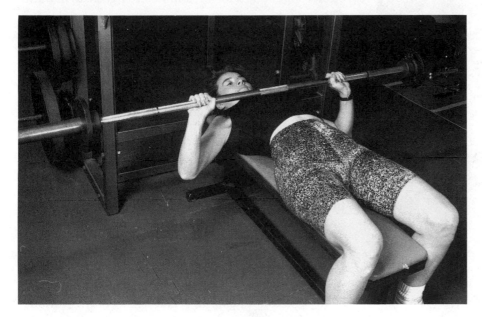

Figure 6.8 YMCA Bench Press Test for Muscular Endurance The YMCA has developed a bench press test for muscular strength and endurance using an absolute weight (35 pounds for females, 80 pounds for males).

elbows. After each extension, the barbell is returned to the original down position, the bar touching the chest. The rhythm is kept by the metronome, each click representing a movement up or down (30 lifts per minute).

▪ The score is the number of successful repetitions. (See Appendix B, Table 56 for the norms.) The test is terminated when the person is unable to reach full extension of the elbows or breaks cadence and cannot keep up with the rhythm of the metronome. Emphasize proper breathing technique (breathe in as weight comes down to chest, breathe out as weight is pushed up).

Parallel Bar Dips

This test is for measuring the muscular strength and endurance of the arms and shoulder girdle (triceps, deltoid, pectoralis major and minor).

To perform the test, follow these steps[21] (see Figure 6.9):

▪ The person being tested should assume a straight arm support position between parallel bars with legs straight.
▪ The body should be lowered until the elbows form a right angle, with the upper arm (humerus) par-

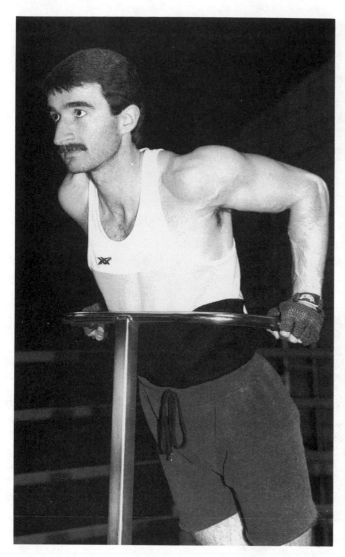

Figure 6.9 Parallel Bar Dip This test is for measuring the muscular strength and endurance of the arms and shoulder girdle (triceps, deltoid, pectoralis major and minor).

allel to the floor. The tester should indicate to the person when the proper position is attained.

- The person should then push back up to a straight arm support and continue the exercise for as many repetitions as possible.

- Rest is permitted in the up position. No swinging or kicking is allowed during the test.

- The score is the total number of bar dips until exhaustion. (See norms in Appendix B, Table 59.)

Flexibility Testing

As stated in Chapter 2, flexibility is the capacity of a joint to move fluidly through its full range of motion.[1] The

major limitation to joint flexibility is tightness of soft tissue structures (joint capsule, muscles, tendons, ligaments). The muscle is the most important and modifiable structure in terms of improving flexibility.

Flexibility is related to age and physical activity.[1] As a person ages, flexibility decreases, although this is due more to inactivity than the aging process itself. Exercises to increase flexibility will be discussed in Chapter 8.

Nearly all health-related physical fitness testing batteries now use the sit and reach test for a measure of flexibility. The sit and reach test is singled out because it has been noted in clinical settings that people with low back problems often have a restricted range of motion in the hamstring muscles and the lower back. The sit and reach test requires reaching forward and extension of the hamstring and lower back muscles. An inability to stretch far enough forward indicates tightness in these muscles.[4]

Contrary to popular opinion, the flexibility scores on the sit and reach test are largely unaffected by varying leg lengths, arm lengths, and their ratios.[4] The major limitation to joint flexibility is soft tissue restriction.

Flexibility of a certain joint does not necessarily indicate flexibility in other joints,[26] and there is no general flexibility test for total body flexibility.[27] The sit and reach test is selected because of its important bearing on the American problem of low back pain. The purpose of the sit and reach flexibility test is to evaluate the flexibility of the low back and posterior leg muscles.[18, 29]

Figure 6.10 shows the flexibility testing box that can be purchased or constructed before administering the test. It is 12 inches high, and has an overlap in front so that minus readings can be obtained when the person being tested is unable to reach her feet. The various testing batteries use different measuring scale settings at the footline. For standardization purposes, the footline can be set at zero, with plus or minus readings in inches or centimeters measured from the zero line. (See norms in Appendix B, Tables 7, 8, 16, 22, 31, 55.)

If a box is not available, a 12-inch bench with a ruler taped onto it can be used.

To perform the sit and reach test for flexibility (see Figure 6.10):[14, 27]

- The person being tested should first warm up, using static stretching exercises (discussed in Chapter 8). A brisk walking or cycling warmup is also advisable (on a treadmill or ergometer, if available). Warm muscles can stretch more safely.

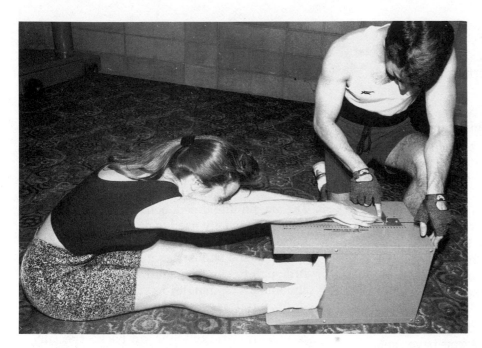

Figure 6.10 The purpose of the sit and reach flexibility test is to evaluate the flexibility of the low back and posterior leg muscles. A flexibility box is required that is 12 inches high, and has an overlap toward the person being tested; they can be purchased or constructed.

- To start, the persons being tested remove their shoes and sit facing the flexibility box, with knees fully extended, feet four inches apart. The feet should be flat, heels touching, against the end board.

- To perform the test, the arms are extended straight forward with the hands placed on top of each other, finger tips perfectly even. The person reaches directly forward, palms down, as far as possible along the measuring scale extending forward maximally four times, and then holds the position of maximum reach for one to two seconds.

- The score is the most distant point reached on the fourth trial measured to the nearest centimeter (or quarter of an inch). The test administrator should remain close to the scale and note the most distant line touched by the fingertips of both hands. If the hands reach unevenly, the test should be readministered. The tester should place one hand lightly on the person's knees to ensure that they remain locked.

Many other methods are used in addition to the sit and reach test for measuring flexibility.[1] Various tests have been devised to measure the range of motion of each major body joint using the goniometer (a protractor-like device with arms that are attached to body segments using the joint as a fulcrum) and Leighton flexometer (360-degree dial with weighted pointer).

Sports Medicine Insight
Testing the Abdominal Muscles

The abdominal muscles counteract the erector spinae muscles, which parallel the spine and which must contract with sufficient force to hold the trunk upright. (See Appendix E for illustrations of body muscles.) If the abdominal muscles are weak, the continual contraction of the erector spinae muscles may result in an exaggerated pelvic tilt or swayback, which often leads to periodic episodes of low back pain.[30]

Although the sit-up test is almost universally described as a test of abdominal strength and endurance, there has been, and still is, dissatisfaction with it.[31] Research has indicated that the abdominals (spinal flexors) are active during a sit-up, but hip flexor muscles are also involved. The use of the hip flexor muscles during the sit-up is potentially harmful to the low back, especially when the feet are held down, because there is increased stress on lumbar vertebrae.

Modifications to the sit-up, including the bent knee posture, do not appear to eliminate stress to the low back. Therefore, for safety and validity reasons, the continued use of the sit-up as the measure of abdominal fitness is questionable.

Trunk curling exercises are helpful for increasing the strength and endurance of the abdominal muscles. However, it is important that the feet not be held down (increasing the probability that the hip flexor muscles rather than the abdominal muscles will be challenged, potentially increasing pelvic tilt).

A curl-up has been suggested as an alternative to a sit-up motion.[31] Procedures for performing the curl-up are as follows (see Figure 6.11):

- The person to be tested starts back on the floor, arms by the sides, palms down on the floor, elbows locked, fingers straight, and without foot restraint. The knees are bent with the feet 12 to 18 inches away from the buttocks (knees at 90-degree angle).

- The person then curls her head and upper back upward, keeping the arms stiff, reaching forward along the floor to touch a line that is 3 inches away from the longest fingertip of each hand, then curls back down so that the upper back touches the floor. During the entire curl-up, the fingers, feet, and buttocks stay on the floor.

- The test score is the number of complete touches on the line within 60 seconds. Norms have yet to be developed for this new test.

Summary

1. This chapter focused on the various musculoskeletal tests that are economical in terms of time, money, and ease of administration, and are effectively health-related. Musculoskeletal testing centers around the flexibility of the lower back and the muscular strength/endurance of the abdominals because of the widespread prevalence of low-back pain in the United States. Although more research is needed, exercises that can improve the musculoskeletal fitness of the lower trunk area in particular appear to help prevent low back pain and rehabilitate it. Close to 80 percent of all low back pain is due to musculoskeletal insufficiency.

2. The musculoskeletal tests described in this chapter are based on the testing batteries outlined in Chapter 3, with the norms listed in Appendix B.

3. The one-minute timed, bent-knee sit-up test has been traditionally used to evaluate abdominal muscle strength and endurance. However, there has been, and still is, dissatisfaction with it. Although research has indicated that the abdominals (spinal flexors) are active during a sit-up, hip flexor muscles are also involved. The use of the hip flexor muscles during the sit-up is potentially harmful to the low back, especially when the feet are held down. Bending the knees does not appear to avoid this problem. Trunk curling exercises are helpful in increasing the strength and endurance of the abdominal muscles, and a new test using a curl-up motion has been developed.

4. The pull-up is used to measure the muscular strength and endurance of the arms and shoulder girdle. Because many children and youth cannot do a pull-up, a modified pull-up test has been developed.

5. Push-ups are used to assess upper body muscle strength and endurance; separate tests have been developed for men and women.

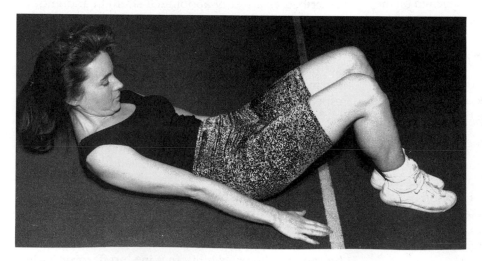

Figure 6.11 The Curl-up Test for Abdominal Endurance/Strength A curl-up has been suggested as an alternative to the sit-up. Although the sit-up test is almost universally described as a test of abdominal strength and endurance, there has been, and still is, dissatisfaction with it. The curl-up optimizes use of the abdominal muscles, avoiding use of the strong hip flexor muscles, and thus eliminating hyperextension of the low back. Therefore, for safety and muscle specificity reasons, the curl-up is preferable to the sit-up.

6. The grip strength test with the hand dynamometer measures the static strength of the grip squeezing muscles. However, because strength is specific to each muscle group, it is recommended that additional strength tests be administered.

7. The bench press exercise can be used for a test either of strength (greatest amount of weight that can be lifted just once) or endurance (number of successful repetitions using an absolute weight).

8. The sit and reach test has been developed to measure the flexibility of the low and back and posterior leg muscles.

References

1. Heyward VH. Designs for Fitness. Minneapolis: Burgess Publishing Co., 1984.

2. MacDougall JD, Wenger HA, Green HJ. Physiological Testing of the Elite Athlete. Canadian Association of Sport Sciences: Mutual Press Limited, 1982.

3. Davies GJ. A Compendium of Isokinetics in Clinical Usage and Rehabilitation Techniques. (3rd edition). Onalaska, Wisconsin: S & S Publishers, 1987.

4. AAHPERD. Technical Manual: Health-Related Physical Fitness, 1984. 1900 Association Drive, Reston, VA 22091.

5. Mayer TG, Gatchel RJ, Mayer H, et al. A Prospective Two-Year Trial of Functional Restoration in Treating Industrial Low Back Injuries. JAMA 258:1763–1767, 1987.

6. Reuler JB. Low Back Pain. West J Med 143:259–265, 1985.

7. Anonymous. Low Back Pain: What Is the Best Conservative Management. Data Centrum 2:15–29, 1985.

8. Shaw DA. Back to Back Fitness. Corporate Fitness and Recreation 2(1):31–37, 1983.

9. Kornfeld J. Getting Aggressive About Conservative Therapy for Back Pain. Medical World News, July 5, 1982, pp. 68–88.

10. Blair SN, Falls HB, Pate RR. A New Physical Fitness Test. Physician Sportsmed 11:87–95, 1983.

11. Melleby A. The Y's Way to a Healthy Back. Piscataway, New Jersey: New Century Publishers, 1982.

12. Kraus H, Raab W. Hypokinetic Disease. Springfield, Illinois: Charles C. Thomas, 1961.

13. Kraus H, Glover R, Melleby A. The Y's Way To a Healthy Back. Journal of Physical Education 21:335–340, 1976.

14. Golding LA, Myers CR, Sinning WE. The Y's Way to Physical Fitness. (3rd Edition) Champaign, IL. Human Kinetics, Publishers, Inc. 1989.

15. Rachlin ES, Kraus H. Management of Back Pain. Internal Medicine 8(3):216–237, 1987.

16. Goodman CE. Low Back Pain in the Cosmetic Athlete. Physician Sportsmed 15(8):97–104, 1987.

17. Leino P, Aro S, Hasan J. Trunk Muscle Function and Low Back Disorders: A Ten-Year Follow-Up Study. J Chronic Dis 40:289–296, 1987.

18. AAHPERD. Norms for College Students: Health Related Physical Fitness Test, 1985. 1900 Association Drive, Reston, VA 22091.

19. Public Health Service. Summary of Findings from National Children and Youth Fitness Study. JOPERD, January, 1985, pp. 44–90.

20. Ross JG, Pate RR. The National Children and Youth Fitness Study II: A Summary of Findings. JOPERD, November/December 1987, pp. 51–56.

21. Johnson BL, Nelson JK. Practical Measurements for Evaluation in Physical Education. Minneapolis: Burgess Publishing Co., 1979.

22. Pate RR, Ross JG, Baumgartner TA, Sparks RE. The National Children and Youth Fitness Study II. The Modified Pull-Up Test. JOPERD, November/December, 1987, pp. 71–73.

23. Youth Physical Fitness in 1985. The President's Council on Physical Fitness and Sports School Population Fitness Survey. President's Council on Physical Fitness and Sports. 450 Fifth St NW, Suite 7103, Washington, D.C. 20001. .

24. Canadian Standardized Test of Fitness (CSTF) Operations Manual (3rd edition). (For 15 to 69 years-of-age). 1987. Published by authority of the Minister of State, Fitness and Amateur Sport. Journal Tower(s), 365 Laurier Avenue West, Ottawa, Ontario K1A0X6.

25. Phillips DA, Hornak JE. Measurement and Evaluation in Physical Education. New York: John Wiley and Sons, 1979.

26. Larson LA. International Committee for the Standardization of Physical Fitness Tests. Fitness, Health, and Work Capacity: International Standards for Assessment. New York: Macmillan Publishing Co., Inc., 1974.

27. Pollock ML, Wilmore JH, Fox SM. Exercise In Health and Disease. Philadelphia: W.B. Saunders Company, 1984.

28. Berger RA. Applied Exercise Physiology. Philadelphia: Lea and Febiger, 1982.

29. Johnson BL. Practical Flexibility Measurement With the Flexomeasure. Portland, TX: Brown and Littleman Co., 1977.

30. Humphrey D. Abdominal Muscle Strength and Endurance. Phys Sportsmed 16(2):201–202, 1988.

31. Robertson LD, Magnusdottir H. Evaluation of Criteria Associated with Abdominal Fitness Testing. Res Quart Exerc Sport 58:355–359, 1987.

Physical Fitness Activity 6.1— Musculoskeletal Fitness Testing

Select a partner from class, and conduct the following musculoskeletal tests on each other. Use the procedures outlined in this chapter, being careful to follow each detail. After taking each test, record your score, and then use the norms in Appendix B to classify your results.

Assessment of Musculoskeletal Fitness

Test	Your Score	Classification
60-sec sit-up test		
Traditional pull-up		
Push-ups		
1-RM bench press test		
Parallel bars (males)		
Sit and reach flexibility test		
YMCA bench press endurance test		
Handgrip (sum of both hands, kg)		

Part 3

Conditioning for Physical Fitness

Chapter 7

The Acute and Chronic Effects of Physical Activity

"In the process of training, the getting wind, as it is called, is largely a gradual increase in the capability of the heart . . .

The large heart of athletes may be due to the prolonged use of their muscles, but no man becomes a great runner or oarsman who has not naturally a capable if not a large heart."—W. Osler, M.D., 1892[1]

Introduction

You are reading this textbook, and suddenly you notice black smoke rising from your friend's apartment complex, one mile away. If you were to run to your friend's aid, you would notice several immediate changes in body function.

Your breathing rate would quicken, as you breathe in larger quantities of air with each breath, supplying more vital oxygen to your body. You might observe that your heart is pounding faster as it pumps more blood to your active leg muscles. If your pace is too quick, you may feel a burning sensation in your legs as the lactic acid concentration increases. These sudden, temporary changes in body function caused by exercise are called *acute responses to exercise*, and they disappear shortly after the exercise period is finished.

On the other hand, if you were to run one or two miles at a hard pace every day, after a few weeks you might discern some changes in the way your body functioned during both rest and exercise. You might notice that your heart beats more slowly while you sit and study, as well as during your run. The amount of air you breathe in during each mile of your run might decrease, and you might feel less of a burning sensation in your legs. These persistent changes in the structure and function of your body following regular exercise training are called *chronic adaptations to exercise*—changes that apparently enable the body to respond more easily to exercise.

This chapter will include a brief description of the acute and chronic effects of exercise. Only the very basic and important material will be covered. For a deeper discussion of exercise physiology, the reader is referred to the excellent textbooks available on this topic.[2-9] In addition, see Appendix E for diagrams of the various body systems, and Chapter 9 for a discussion of energy metabolism.

Physiological Responses to Acute Exercise

The acute responses to exercise are influenced by a number of factors, including the level of training or fitness status of the participant, sufficiency of sleep, coffee intake, alcohol, tobacco, and general anxiety.[2, 5] For example, a person who is anxious about the treadmill test can have higher than normal heart rates during the first and second stages. Those who are fit usually have lower acute responses to certain levels of exercise than those who are unfit. These factors must be considered when interpreting the following list of acute effects.

Increase of Heart Rate

Figure 7.1 summarizes several important points relative to the way heart rate responds to increasing levels of exercise, such as during a graded treadmill exercise test (e.g., the Bruce protocol).

- The pre-exercise heart rate may be elevated owing to the *anticipatory response*. In one study of nearly 1,000 college students by the author (unpublished data), the average resting heart rate, measured in the student's dorm rooms upon waking for three mornings in a row and then averaged, was 67 beats per minute. However, when sitting before a treadmill before a maximal graded exercise test, the average "resting" heart rate of these same students was 95. (This pre-exercise increase is controlled by the limbic system, a system in the brain that regulates our emotions.)[8]

- During the graded exercise test, heart rate will increase in direct proportion to the intensity of the exercise. In other words, the heart rate rises in a linear fashion with increasing workload.

- At exhaustion, the rise in heart rate will flatten out. This is called the *maximal heart rate*. When the heart rate increases little if at all after a stage change during a graded exercise test, this is a good indication that the maximal heart rate has been reached.

  The average maximal heart rate is equal to 220 minus one's age (in years). This equation, however, is the average found in large groups of people. People for a given age vary widely, with a standard deviation of plus or minus 10 to 12 beats per minute. In other words, the average maximal heart rate for a 20-year-old person is 220 minus 20, or 200 beats per minute. However, two-thirds of the people this age vary between 190 and 210 beats per minute, and 95 percent vary between 180 and 220 beats per minute.

- At submaximal levels of exercise, when the workload is held steady, the heart rate will increase for one to three minutes, and then level off at a steady-state value. The harder the submaximal workload, the longer the heart rate will take to level off. For example, as you look at Figure 7.1, notice that in Stages 1 and 2, the heart rate plateaus relatively early in the stage, while in Stage 5, a more difficult stage, there is little indication of a plateau even after three minutes.

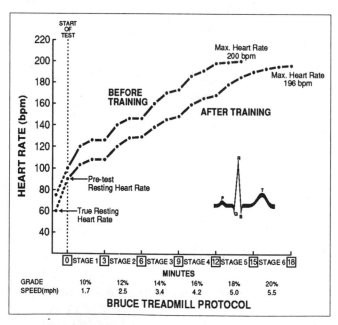

Figure 7.1 Heart rate results during the graded exercise test of a 20-year-old before and after exercise training. Notice that his pre-test exercise heart rate is much higher than his true resting heart rate. The exercise heart rate increases in a linear fashion with increase in workload until the maximal heart rate is reached, when it plateaus.

Increase of Stroke Volume

The *stroke volume* is the quantity of blood pumped out of the heart per heart beat.[8] Stroke volume is regulated by several factors, including the amount of venous blood that is returned to the heart, the force of contraction of the heart muscle, and sympathetic nervous stimulation. Figure 7.2 summarizes several important points regarding the change in stroke volume from rest to exercise exhaustion.

- The change in stroke volume during graded exercise does not follow the pattern of change in the heart rate. Instead of rising linearly with increase in workload, stroke volume increases strongly only up to a workload of 40 to 50 percent of $\dot{V}O_{2max}$. Beyond this intensity level, increasing workload brings only small increases in stroke volume.

- Resting stroke volume values for sedentary people range between 60 and 70 ml of blood per heartbeat. Those who are highly trained may have resting stroke volume values as high as 100 ml.

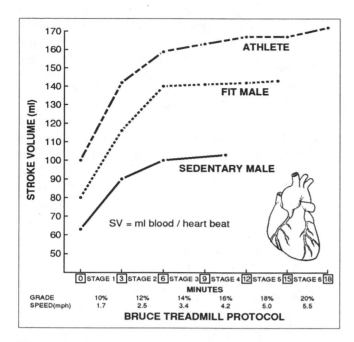

Figure 7.2 Stroke volume represents the amount of blood pumped per beat of the heart. Instead of rising linearly with increase in workload, stroke volume increases strongly up to a workload of 40 to 50 percent of $\dot{V}O_{2max}$. There is little change beyond this level, despite increasing workload.

Submaximal and maximal stroke volumes are also much higher for fit than for sedentary people. Stroke volumes of elite world-class runners have been measured as high as 180 ml per heart beat.

▪ When you go from lying down to standing, there is an immediate drop in your stroke volume, because of the influence of gravity and a corresponding increase in heart rate to maintain the flow of blood out of your heart (i.e., cardiac output, which equals stroke volume times heart rate). When exercise is performed in a horizontal position (as in swimming), the stroke volume is larger and the heart rate lower than when the same level of upright exercise is performed (as in running). Therefore, heart rate during exercises like swimming will be lower for a given percent of $\dot{V}O_{2max}$ than for running. Exercise training heart rates should thus be adjusted downward about 10 to 15 beats per minute when exercising in a horizontal position.

Increase in Cardiac Output

Cardiac Output (also designated "$\dot{Q}$" by exercise physiologists) is equal to the stroke volume (SV) times the heart rate (HR) $\dot{Q} = SV \times HR$). In other words, cardiac output represents the quantity of blood pumped out of the heart each minute. At rest, average cardiac output is approximately 5 liters per minute; it can rise to 20–40 liters per minute during maximal exercise, the amount depending on individual fitness status and size. (See Figure 7.3.)

Figure 7.3 demonstrates that:

▪ Cardiac output rises linearly with increasing workload, and plateaus slightly at exercise exhaustion.

▪ During the initial stages of exercise, the increase in cardiac output is due to increases in both heart rate and stroke volume. During upright exercise, when the intensity reaches 40–60 percent $\dot{V}O_{2max}$, any further increase in cardiac output is due primarily to an increase in heart rate.

Increased Arteriovenous Oxygen Difference

The *arteriovenous oxygen difference* ($\bar{a} - \bar{v}O_2$) is the difference between the amount of oxygen carried in the arterial blood and the amount in the mixed venous blood. Thus the $\bar{a} - \bar{v}O_2$ reflects the amount of oxygen extracted by the tissues of the body.

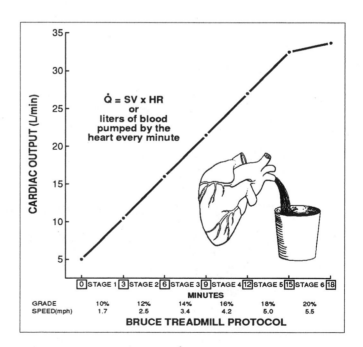

Figure 7.3 Cardiac output ($\dot{Q}$) follows a pattern similar to that of the heart rate. With increasing workload, cardiac output rises linearly, and plateaus slightly at exercise exhaustion.

- At rest, the oxygen content of arterial blood is approximately 20 ml of oxygen per 100 ml of blood, compared to an oxygen content of 15 ml/100 ml blood for the mixed venous blood. Thus the resting $\bar{a} - \bar{v}O_2$ is 5 ml/100 ml blood.

- During very intense exercise, the venous oxygen content can drop to 2 to 4 ml/100 ml blood. Thus the $\bar{a} - \bar{v}O_2$ can increase nearly threefold to 16–18 ml/100 ml blood.

Increase in $\dot{V}O_2$

In Chapter 4, maximal oxygen uptake $\dot{V}O_{2max}$ was defined as "the greatest rate at which oxygen can be consumed during exercise at sea level." $\dot{V}O_{2max}$ is usually expressed in terms of milliliters of oxygen consumed per kilogram of body weight per minute (ml · kg^{-1} · min^{-1}). With this allowance for body weight, the $\dot{V}O_{2max}$ of people of varying size and in different environments can be compared. $\dot{V}O_{2max}$ can also be expressed as liters per minute, representing the oxygen consumption of the entire body. (See Figure 7.4.)

During graded exercise, active muscle tissue needs more and more oxygen to burn the carbohydrates and fats needed for energy production. For every liter of oxygen that the body consumes during exercise, approximately 5 kilocalories of energy are produced. Figures 7.5, 7.6, and 7.7 demonstrate that:

- With increasing workload, oxygen consumption increases up to the last stage of exercise. At this point, $\dot{V}O_2$ plateaus, and is called the $\dot{V}O_{2max}$. If the person being tested is willing to push hard enough, a small decrease in $\dot{V}O_2$ can be seen just prior to exhaustion (as demonstrated in Figure 7.5). Many people, however, do not achieve a true $\dot{V}O_2$ plateau, and for this reason some exercise physiologists prefer the term "peak $\dot{V}O_2$." $\dot{V}O_{2max}$ values are greatly influenced by size, age, heredity, sex, and level of fitness. (See next section.)

- Figure 7.6 shows that if the cardiac output and $\bar{a} - \bar{v}O_2$ are known, oxygen consumption can be calculated using the formula: $\dot{V}O_2 = \dot{Q} \times \bar{a} - \bar{v}O_2$. In other words, if measurement of arterial and mixed

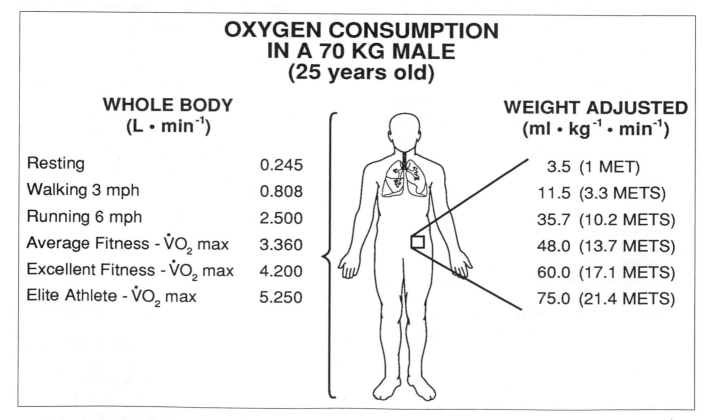

OXYGEN CONSUMPTION IN A 70 KG MALE (25 years old)

WHOLE BODY (L · min^{-1})		WEIGHT ADJUSTED (ml · kg^{-1} · min^{-1})
Resting	0.245	3.5 (1 MET)
Walking 3 mph	0.808	11.5 (3.3 METS)
Running 6 mph	2.500	35.7 (10.2 METS)
Average Fitness - $\dot{V}O_2$ max	3.360	48.0 (13.7 METS)
Excellent Fitness - $\dot{V}O_2$ max	4.200	60.0 (17.1 METS)
Elite Athlete - $\dot{V}O_2$ max	5.250	75.0 (21.4 METS)

Figure 7.4   Oxygen consumption ($\dot{V}O_2$) can be expressed in units of L·min^{-1} for the entire body, or in units of ml·kg^{-1}·min^{-1} to represent the oxygen consumption for each kilogram of body weight.

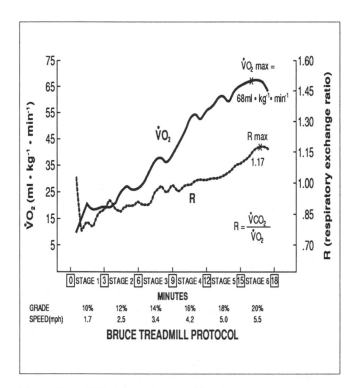

Figure 7.5 With increasing workload, oxygen consumption increases up to the last stage of exercise. At this point, $\dot{V}O_2$ plateaus, and is called the $\dot{V}O_{2max}$.

venous blood shows that for every liter of blood passing through the tissues, 150 milliliters of oxygen are being consumed, and that 20 liters of blood/minute are passing through those tissues, total oxygen consumption is easily determined by multiplying 150 ml $O_2 \cdot$ liter^{-1} by 20 liters $\cdot$ min^{-1}, which equals 3,000 ml $O_2 \cdot$ min^{-1}.

▪ *Oxygen debt* refers to the volume of oxygen consumed during the recovery period following exercise in excess of the volume normally consumed at rest. (See Figure 7.7.) This debt pays back the *oxygen deficit* built up during the initial minutes of exercise, on account of the body adjusting to the exercise, plus other metabolic factors built up during the exercise bout itself.

For example, if you were to start running at a 7-minute-per-mile pace, approximately 3.46 liters of oxygen per minute would be required immediately. However, because your body takes approximately 2 to 3 minutes to adjust to this workload, anaerobic sources of ATP (stored ATP and glycolysis) are utilized, building up an oxygen deficit. During recovery, you will breathe harder than during rest, to help restore this deficit and allow your body systems to return to normal.

Increased Systolic BP; Diastolic BP Unchanged

Blood pressure (BP) response during exercise was reviewed in Chapter 4, with an emphasis on accurate measurement. (See Figure 4.4.) Important concepts include:

▪ The systolic blood pressure increases in direct proportion to the increase in aerobic exercise intensity, with resting values of 120 mm Hg often rising to 200 mm Hg or greater at exhaustion.

▪ The diastolic blood pressure changes little if any during aerobic exercise.

▪ The exercise-induced increase in systolic blood pressure is related to the increase in cardiac output. The increase in blood pressure would be much higher except that arterial blood vessels in the active muscles dilate, reducing peripheral resistance.[8] *Total peripheral resistance* is the sum of all the forces that oppose blood flow in the body's blood vessel system. During exercise, total peripheral resistance decreases because the blood vessels in the active muscles dilate.

▪ Cycling with arms (arm ergometry), increases systolic and diastolic blood pressures 15 percent, compared to cycling with legs. This probably occurs because of the smaller muscle mass in the arms, which offers a greater resistance to blood flow than the larger muscles in the legs.

▪ Weight lifting or isometric contractions cause large increases in both systolic and diastolic blood pressures. This will be discussed in more detail in Chapter 8.

▪ Some researchers like to report the *mean arterial pressure*. This represents the average pressure exerted by the blood against the inner walls of the arteries. An estimate of mean arterial pressure is obtained by using the equation:

Mean arterial pressure =
1/3 (systolic blood pressure –
diastolic blood pressure) +
diastolic blood pressure.

For example, if during Stage 3 of the Bruce treadmill test, the systolic blood pressure is 150 mm Hg and the diastolic blood pressure is 80 mm Hg, then the mean arterial pressure equals one-third of the difference between systolic and diastolic blood pressures (0.33×70 mm Hg), or 23 mm Hg, plus the diastolic blood pressure ($23 + 80$), or 103 mm Hg. Maximal exercise mean arterial pressures approximate 130 mm Hg.

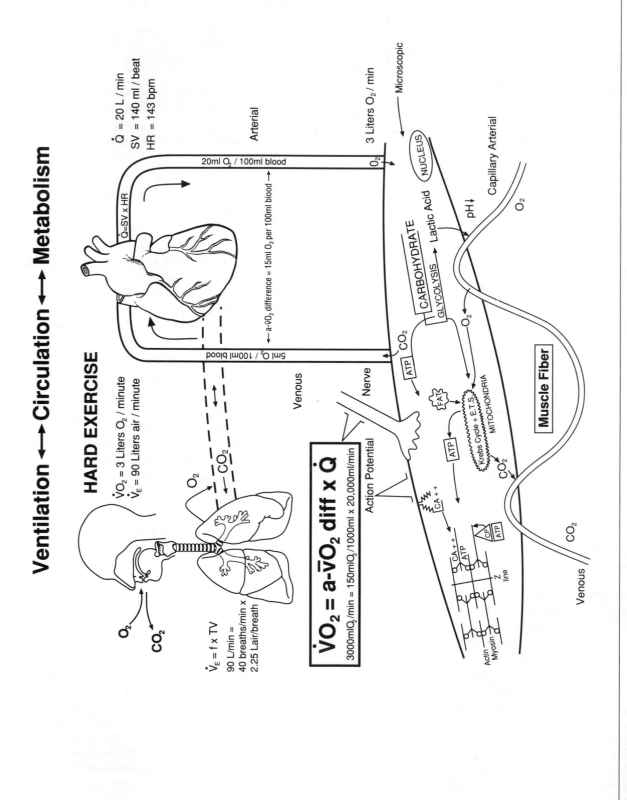

Figure 7.6 This figure summarizes the acute effects of exercise. The body coordinates ventilation, circulation, and metabolism to meet the demands of exercise. If the cardiac output and $\bar{a} - \bar{v}O_2$ are known, oxygen consumption can be calculated using the formula: $\dot{V}O_2 \times \dot{Q} \times \bar{a} - \bar{v}O_2$.

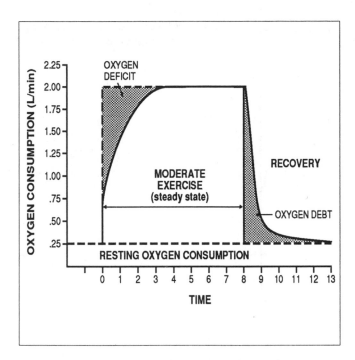

Figure 7.7 Oxygen debt refers to the volume of oxygen consumed during the recovery period following exercise in excess of the volume normally consumed at rest.

Increase in Minute Ventilation

Minute ventilation is the volume of air that is breathed into the body each minute. Minute ventilation is usually determined by measuring the volume of air breathed out or expired ($\dot{V}_E$), and then correcting this for *BTPS*, the volume of air at the temperature and pressure of the body, and 100 percent water vapor saturation (as in the human lung). The minute ventilation is equal to the *tidal volume* (TV) times the *frequency* (f) of breaths. At rest, the tidal volume is usually 0.5 liters of air per breath, and the frequency is about 12 breaths per minute, resulting in a minute ventilation of 6 liters of air per minute.

Figure 7.8 gives the various terms used by respiratory and exercise physiologists when reporting research or clinical findings. The tidal volume (TV) is the amount of air breathed into or out of the lung while at rest. The TV usually ranges between 0.4 and 1.0 liters of air per breath.[7] *Inspiratory reserve volume* (IRV) is the amount of air that can be breathed into the lung on top of a resting inspired tidal volume (2.5 to 3.5 liters). *Expiratory reserve volume* (ERV) is the amount of air that can be pushed out of the lung following an expired resting tidal volume (1.0 to 1.5 liters). *Residual volume* (RV) is the amount of air left in the lung after the expiratory reserve volume (1 to 2 liters). *Functional residual capacity* (FRC) is the com-

bined expiratory reserve volume and residual volume. *Forced vital capacity* (FVC) is the total amount of air that can be breathed into the lung on top of the residual volume (usually 3 to 4 liters for women, 4 to 5 liters for men). The *total lung capacity* (TLC) represents the total amount of air in the lung.

Figure 7.9 summarizes changes in minute ventilation during graded exercise testing.

- During graded exercise, minute ventilation increases in a curvilinear pattern from a resting value of 6 liters · min^{-1} to 60–120 liter · min^{-1} for females, and 100–200 liters · min^{-1} for males, depending on size and fitness status. Below 50 percent $\dot{V}O_{2max}$, minute ventilation increases in a linear fashion with increasing workload. At higher intensities, however, the relationship is curvilinear, with ventilation rising strongly relative to the workload.

- The insert in Figure 7.9 shows that at higher intensities, an increase in minute ventilation is produced primarily from increased breathing rates. The tidal volume tends to plateau at higher intensities.

- During graded exercise, the residual volume increases slightly, with the vital capacity decreasing slightly, keeping the overall total lung volume the same.

- The movement of air in and out of the lung during exercise requires considerable amounts of energy for the respiratory muscles. At rest, the energy cost of ventilation is 1 ml of oxygen per liter of air breathed, or 2 percent of the total oxygen being consumed at rest. During maximal exercise this can rise to 10 percent.

- *Lung diffusion* refers to the rate at which gases diffuse from the lung air sacs (*alveoli*) to the blood in the pulmonary capillaries. Diffusion capacity during exercise can increase three-fold from a resting value of 25 ml $O_2 \cdot$ min$^{-1} \cdot$ mm Hg^{-1} to 75 ml $O_2 \cdot$ min$^{-1} \cdot$ mm Hg^{-1} at max.

Increased Blood Flow to Active Muscle Areas

- During exercise, blood is redirected away from areas where it is not needed (e.g., organs) and to the muscles. At rest, only 15–20 percent of the cardiac output goes to the muscles, compared to as much as 88 percent during exhaustive exercise (See Table 7.1.)

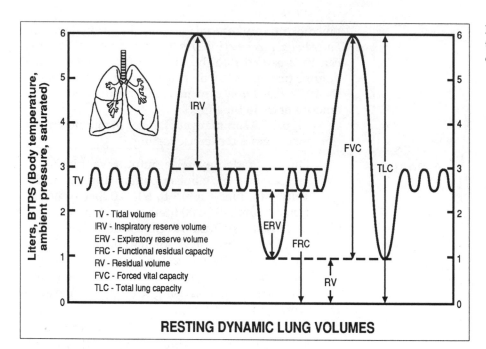

Figure 7.8 Terms used to represent the dynamic lung volumes and capacities.

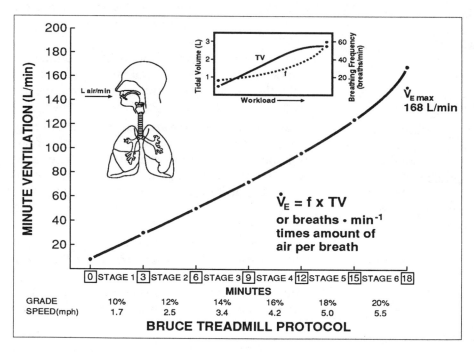

Figure 7.9 Minute ventilation increases in a curvilinear fashion during graded maximal exercise. The frequency of breathing also follows this pattern, while tidal volume plateaus during intense exercise.

▪ As the body heats up, an increasing amount of blood is directed to the skin, to conduct heat away from the body core. The primary means by which the body loses heat during exercise is through evaporation of sweat on the skin. (See Chapter 9.) The sweat glands will use fluid from the cells and from the blood to produce the sweat, which can reach 2 to 3 liters per hour during hard exercise in humid heat. If the sweat rate is high, blood volume will decrease, ultimately to the point of heat injury.

▪ During endurance exercise, plasma volume shifts to the muscles. During graded exercise testing, 12 to 16 percent of the plasma volume leaves the blood and enters the active muscle tissue.[9] This

Table 7.1 Distribution of Cardiac Output During Light, Moderate, and Strenuous Exercise

Tissue	Amount of Blood (ml · min⁻¹) and % Cardiac Output		
	Light exercise	Moderate exercise	Maximal exercise
Abdominal organs	1,100 (12%)	600 (3%)	300 (1%)
Kidneys	900 (10%)	600 (3%)	250 (1%)
Brain	750 (8%)	750 (4%)	750 (3%)
Heart	350 (4%)	750 (4%)	1,000 (4%)
Muscle	4,500 (47%)	12,500 (71%)	22,000 (88%)
Skin	1,500 (15%)	1,900 (12%)	600 (2%)
Other	400 (4%)	400 (3%)	100 (1%)
Total cardiac output	9,500	17,500	25,000

Source: Modified from: McArdle WD, Katch FI, Katch VL. Exercise Physiology: Energy, Nutrition, and Human Performance. Philadelphia: Lea & Febiger, 1986.

plasma volume shift, combined with the fluid loss from sweating, leads to an increase in the thickness of blood called *hemoconcentration.*

Changes in Respiratory Exchange Ratio

During exercise the muscles use oxygen (O_2) to burn carbohydrates and fats, producing carbon dioxide (CO_2) and ATP. Ventilation increases to help bring in more O_2 and to expel CO_2. Exercise physiologists use the *respiratory exchange ratio* (R) to help determine the type of fuel (primarily fat and carbohydrate) being used by the muscles. The respiratory exchange ratio is the ratio between the amount of carbon dioxide produced and the amount of oxygen consumed by the body during exercise ($R = \dot{V}CO_2/\dot{V}O_2$).

The R value will vary depending on what fuel the muscles are using. When only fats are being used, R = 0.71; when only carbohydrates are being used, R = 1.0.

With hard exercise, the R value approaches 1.0 because carbohydrate is the preferred fuel with heavy exercise. At rest, the R value is usually 0.75 to 0.81. Just prior to exercise, the R value can rise above 1.0, due to pretest anxiety, which causes hyperventilation (which "blows off" CO_2). During recovery, the R value can rise above 1.5, due to the buffering of lactic acid and carbon dioxide production. When R values rise to 1.15 or greater during exercise, this is usually a sign of maximal exertion, with the body relying on anaerobic metabolism.

- Figure 7.5 shows that as the intensity of exercise increases, R increases, meaning that more and more CO_2 is being produced relative to the O_2 being consumed. This indicates that more and more carbohydrate is being used by the muscles as the intensity of exercise increases.

- At rest, the blood pH is 7.4. When the exercise intensity of unconditioned people rises above 50 percent $\dot{V}O_{2max}$, or above 70–90 percent for conditioned people, the pH will drop, owing to lactic acid build up. Blood pH values can drop to 7.0 with maximal exercise; tissue pH levels can drop to 6.5. Blood lactate levels range from 10 mg/100 ml at rest (1.1 millimoles per liter of blood) to 200 mg/100 ml (22 millimoles per liter blood) within five minutes following exhaustive exercise.

- During graded maximal exercise, the *anaerobic threshold* is the point at which blood lactate concentrations start to rise above resting values.[10–13] The anaerobic threshold can be expressed as a percent of $\dot{V}O_{2max}$. Some of the best athletes in the world have anaerobic thresholds of between 80 and 90 percent $\dot{V}O_{2max}$; unfit people average 40–60 percent $\dot{V}O_{2max}$.

Although a discussion of the measurement of anaerobic threshold is beyond the scope of this book, Figure 7.10 shows that anaerobic threshold can be determined when the ratio of minute ventilation to oxygen consumption $\dot{V}_E/\dot{V}O_2$) rises sharply while the ratio of minute ventilation to carbon dioxide consumption $\dot{V}_E/\dot{V}CO_2$) remains

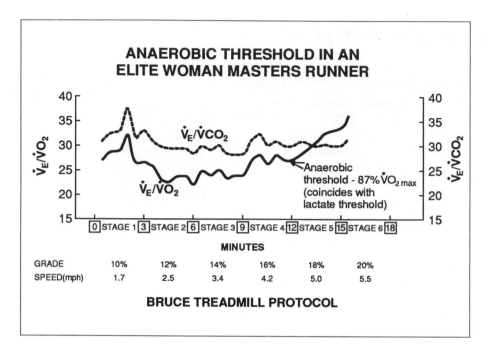

Figure 7.10 Anaerobic threshold represents the point at which lactic acid begins to build up in the blood. This can be measured indirectly by looking at the rise in $\dot{V}_E/\dot{V}O_2$ relative to $\dot{V}_E/\dot{V}CO_2$.

constant. Figure 7.10 reflects the measurement of an elite woman masters runner who holds several world records for ultramarathon distances. Her anaerobic threshold of 87.6 percent $\dot{V}O_{2max}$ is very high, allowing her to run at an intensity close to her capacity without lactic acid buildup. (See Sports Medicine Insight at the end of this chapter.)

Chronic Adaptations to Regular Exercise

As discussed earlier in this chapter, the persistent changes in the structure and function of the body following regular exercise training are called chronic adaptations to exercise.[2-8]

What quantity of exercise training is necessary to produce chronic adaptations? Do different body systems adapt to exercise training at different rates?

Several of the cardiorespiratory and metabolic responses of exercise appear to adapt very rapidly to exercise training.[14-16] Within the first 1–3 weeks of intensive cardiorespiratory training, the following adaptations have been reported (40 to 60 minutes per session, six sessions per week, 70–90 percent $\dot{V}O_{2max}$):

- Increase in $\dot{V}O_{2max}$. (In fact, several studies have shown that the maximal oxygen uptake of young people can increase 5–8 percent with just one week of intense training.)[15]

- Decrease in maximal and submaximal exercise heart rates.

- Decrease in blood lactate levels during submaximal exercise.

- Decrease in *catecholamine* (epinephrine and norepinephrine) concentrations during exercise.

Some adaptations to aerobic exercise, however, take longer. For example, the increase in number of capillaries per muscle fiber may take several months or years.[16]

Interestingly, exercise-induced changes are lost just as rapidly as they are gained. This (the effects of inactivity) will be discussed in the next section of this chapter.

The magnitude of the chronic adaptations of regular exercise training depend on the frequency, intensity, and duration of training, the mode of activity, and the initial fitness status. For example, overweight middle-aged people who have been inactive for many years have the potential for dramatic improvements in cardiorespiratory fitness (e.g., a 100-percent increase in $\dot{V}O_{2max}$) with weight loss and a few months of regular aerobic exercise. Relatively active college students, on the other hand, can expect only smaller improvements (e.g., a 10–20 percent increase in $\dot{V}O_{2max}$).

Changes that Occur in Skeletal Muscles as a Result of Aerobic Training

Exercise physiologists have had an ongoing debate for several decades regarding the relative importance of "central" versus "peripheral" adaptations to regular cardiorespiratory exercise. Figure 7.6 shows that ventilation and circulation (central elements) work closely with the muscle cells (peripheral elements) to allow physical activity to take place. While most researchers have reported that the circulation, specifically the stroke volume and cardiac output, are the prime limiting factors during intense exercise,[17] some feel that factors within the muscle cells are more important.[7, 18]

In response to regular aerobic training, many significant changes take place in the muscle cells.[2–8, 18]

- An increase in *myoglobin* content. Myoglobin aids in the delivery of oxygen from the blood to the *mitochondria* (organelles in the muscle cell which produce ATP for energy). (See Figure 7.6.)
- An increase in the number (+120 percent) and size (+14–40 percent) of mitochondria.
- An increase in the concentration of important enzymes in the mitochondria, specifically those of the *Krebs cycle* and the *electron transport system*. These enzymes are involved in the production of ATP.
- An increase in the amount of glycogen stored in the muscle (up to 250 percent).
- An increase in the amount of muscle triglycerides (up to 150 percent).
- An increased capacity to oxidize fat (primarily from muscle fat stores, but also from adipose tissue stores).[19,20] The trained person thus oxidizes more fat and less carbohydrate during cardiorespiratory exercise, which means less glycogen depletion, less lactic acid accumulation, and therefore less muscle fatigue and greater endurance.
- An increase in the area of *slow-twitch fibers*. The aerobic-type muscle fibers are called Type I (red, tonic, slow twitch); the anaerobic type fibers are called Type II (white, glycolytic, fast-twitch). People vary widely in their proportions of slow-twitch and *fast-twitch fibers*. This proportion is set at birth, and remains constant throughout life.[7]

The fast-twitch muscle cells are capable of producing high amounts of ATP through *glycolysis*, a process that does not require oxygen (*anaerobic*). Fast-twitch muscle cells are important in activities that require sprinting and jumping. Slow-twitch muscle cells generate ATP in the presence of oxygen (aerobically), and have high numbers of mitochondria and a good capillary supply.

Endurance athletes usually have a high proportion of slow-twitch muscle fibers, sprinters a high proportion of fast-twitch muscle fibers. For example, trained cross country skiers average 70 to 80 percent slow-twitch fibers, and long distance runners, 60 to 70 percent slow-twitch fibers; sprinters, on the other hand, average only 40 percent slow-twitch fibers.[21,22] Blacks have been found to have a higher percentage of fast-twitch fibers than Caucasians, helping to explain why they excel in sports requiring sprinting and jumping.[23]

With regular aerobic training, the size of the slow-twitch fibers can be increased. Some researchers have reported that some fast-twitch muscle cells can be changed into slow-twitch muscle cells through regular aerobic training over a long time period.[24, 25] However, the ability of slow-twitch fibers to change into fast-twitch fibers appears to be of minor importance.

Major Cardiorespiratory Changes from Exercise Training When at Rest

Several major cardiorespiratory changes at rest follow exercise training:

- An increase in heart size.[1] The size of the left and right ventricular cavities increases, with proportional increases in the thicknesses of the heart muscle walls and septum.[26] These changes occur gradually over months or years of training.[8]
- A decrease in resting heart rate. The resting heart rate decreases approximately one beat per minute for every 1–2 weeks of aerobic training for about 10 to 20 weeks.

In one study of nearly 1000 college students by the author (unpublished data), the average college male's resting heart rate decreased from 67 bpm to 60 bpm after seven weeks of regular aerobic training (five sessions per week, 30 minutes per session, 70–80 percent $\dot{V}O_{2max}$). Female college students on the same program decreased their resting heart rates from 69 bpm to 62 bpm after seven weeks. Endurance athletes who have trained for years often have resting heart rates below 50 bpm.

The decrease in resting heart rate is attributable to an increase in *parasympathetic* control (through the vagus nerve which slows the heart rate).[8] This results in:

- An increase in stroke volume, with more blood pumped per beat. This allows the resting heart rate to decrease.
- The resting cardiac output staying about the same.[8]
- An increase in the total blood volume. Although both plasma volume and hemoglobin increase, the increase in plasma volume is greater, leading to a slightly decreased *hematocrit* or red blood cell count per 100 ml blood. This increase in the plasma volume is directly related to the increase in stroke volume.[27, 28] The increased blood volume is approximately 500 ml, through the expansion of the plasma volume. This adaptation is gained after only a few bouts of exercise, and is quickly reversed when training ceases.[27]
- An increase in capillary density. Untrained human muscle has about 1.5 to 2.0 capillaries per muscle fiber, while elite endurance athletes have 2.5 to 3.0 capillaries per muscle fiber.[29]

In general, pulmonary function characteristics (total lung capacity, forced vital capacity residual volume) are not changed by training.[30] Some may experience a slight increase in vital capacity and a slight decrease in residual volume.[7] Resting minute ventilation is not affected by training.

Major Cardiorespiratory Changes During Submaximal Exercise

What cardiorespiratory changes during submaximal exercise can be expected following exercise training? Tables 7.2 and 7.3 summarize data from a study conducted by the author.[31] This study was conducted on 20 males, nine of whom were sedentary, and 11 experienced runners. All were tested in the laboratory using the Balke maximal graded exercise test, with cardiorespiratory variables measured every five minutes to complete exhaustion. During the three previous years, the athletes had averaged 42.5 ± 4.0 miles per week of running, with an average personal marathon record of 3.1 ± 0.1 hours.

Maximal oxygen uptake and ventilation were 63 percent and 39 percent higher, respectively, for the athletes than for the nonathletes, with percent body fat nearly 50 percent lower.

Important differences in submaximal exercise parameters between the sedentary and trained males can be summarized as follows:

- There were no significant differences in oxygen consumption during any of the three submaximal

workloads. When adjusted for weight changes, training does not appear to decrease oxygen consumption during submaximal exercise. However, between individuals, the amount of oxygen utilized during any given workload can vary widely. Notice in Table 7.3 that oxygen consumption varied from 16 percent to 36 percent depending on the workload.

- Heart rates of the trained males were significantly lower than those of the sedentary males. This was due to a higher stroke volume—cardiac output was not different for the two groups. The cardiac output remained constant as stroke volume increased and heart rate decreased.[32] (See also Figures 7.1 and 7.2.)
- Ventilation was significantly lower for the trained males than it was for the sedentary males during each stage. They ventilated less air while achieving the same oxygen consumption.

  The trained body is much more efficient in the transport and utilization of oxygen. The $\bar{a} - \bar{v}O_2$ difference is slightly higher, meaning that the muscle cells are extracting more oxygen. The heightened extraction of oxygen is due to the increased capillary density around each muscle cell.

- The respiratory exchange ratio (R) was much lower for the athletes. As discussed earlier, when the R is lower, this is an indication that the muscle cells are utilizing more fat and less glycogen for fuel. This decreases the concentration of lactic acid, increasing the anaerobic threshold. This allows one to exercise at a higher intensity without interference from lactic acid. (These benefits result primarily from the exercise-training-induced increase in the number and size of mitochondria.)[19]

Major Cardiorespiratory Changes During Maximal Exercise

During graded exercise testing, those tested are taken to complete exhaustion. What changes during maximal exercise can be expected after regular exercise training? Table 7.2 shows the following differences:

- Training provides a significantly higher maximal aerobic power ($\dot{V}O_{2max}$). This means a greater amount of oxygen can be consumed during maximal exercise. Figure 7.4 outlines some of the increases in $\dot{V}O_{2max}$ that can be expected in response to increasing levels of training.

Table 7.2   Differences Between Sedentary and Trained Males During a Balke Treadmill Graded Exercise Test (resting and maximal exercise parameters)

Parameter	Sedentary males (N=9)	Trained males (N=11)
Age (years)	44.2	42.7
Weight (lb)	185	171
Percent body fat (%)	24.5	12.5
Resting heart rate (bpm)	66.8	52.5
$\dot{V}O_{2max}$ (ml·kg^{-1}·min^{-1})	33.3	54.2
Ventilation, max (L·min^{-1})	119	165
Heart rate, max (bpm)	188	177

Table 7.3   Differences Between Sedentary versus Trained Males During a Balke Treadmill Graded Exercise Test [mean (range)]

Time Speed Grade	5 min 3.3 mph 5%	10 min 3.3 mph 10%	15 min 3.3 mph 15%
$\dot{V}O_2$ (ml·kg^{-1}·min^{-1})			
Sedentary males	18.4	24.8	32.1
	(16.0–21.8)	(22.4–28.2)	(29.6–34.4)
Trained males	19.7	26.7	34.0
	(17.2–22.8)	(25.1–30.1)	(31.3–38.5)
Heart rate (bpm)			
Sedentary males	123	152	177
	(100–139)	(128–175)	(164–197)
Trained males	88	107	126
	(77–96)	(98–120)	(112–138)
Ventilation (L·min^{-1})			
Sedentary males	42	63	88
	(35–54)	(47–88)	(62–106)
Trained males	37	52	66
	(30–47)	(44–64)	(57–85)
Respiratory exchange ratio			
Sedentary males	0.95	1.08	1.24
	(0.90–1.09)	(1.01–1.23)	(1.12–1.46)
Trained males	0.87	0.95	0.99
	(0.78–1.00)	(0.87–1.02)	(0.92–1.06)

In a study of nearly 1000 college students by the author (unpublished findings), male students had an average $\dot{V}O_{2max}$ of 49.0 ml·kg^{-1}·min^{-1} before, and 55.0 ml·kg^{-1}·min^{-1} after seven weeks of regular aerobic exercise (5 sessions per week, 30 minutes per session, 70–80 percent $\dot{V}O_{2max}$). Female college students averaged 36.0 ml·kg^{-1}·min^{-1} before training, and 41.0 ml·kg^{-1}·min^{-1} after training.

The 12–14 percent increase in $\dot{V}O_{2max}$ realized by these young adults after seven weeks of training is typical.[7] The 36-percent difference in $\dot{V}O_{2max}$ between genders has also been reported by others.[33] (See subsection on gender differences.)

- The increase in $\dot{V}O_{2max}$ is primarily attributable to a greater cardiac output and a greater oxygen extraction by the muscle cells.

The major limiting factor to performance is cardiac output, and the ability to achieve a large stroke volume.[17, 34] The single biggest difference, according to most researchers, is the increase in stroke volume that comes with training. It is directly related to the training-induced increase in plasma volume.[27]

(As discussed previously, some researchers feel that the "weak link" in maximal exercise performance is the inability of the working muscle to utilize the oxygen provided by the circulation.[35] However, there is little support for this contention.)

- Trained athletes have a higher maximal ventilation. This means that trained people can ventilate more air during maximal exercise. Their maximal tidal volume and frequency are also higher. Lung diffusion capacity also improves with training, meaning that oxygen can diffuse from the lung alveoli to the blood more readily.
- Maximum heart rate usually changes little with training. The maximum heart rate of adults under the age of 30 may decrease a few beats per minute with exercise training, but more research is needed to establish this relationship.

Other changes that occur during maximal exercise with training include:

- An increase of blood flow to the active muscles, with better constriction of blood vessels in inactive areas and *vasodilatation* in active muscle areas.[36]
- An increased ability to tolerate higher lactic acid levels at max.

Table 7.4 summarizes the changes in cardiorespiratory parameters that occur during rest, submaximal exercise, and maximal exercise following endurance training.

Other Physiological Changes with Aerobic Exercise

Other changes that occur in response to regular cardiorespiratory exercise include:

- A small decrease in total body fat, and a slight increase in lean body weight. (See Chapter 11.)
- An increase in HDL cholesterol, a decrease in triglycerides, but little or no change in total serum or LDL cholesterol. (See Chapter 10.)
- Greater ability to exercise in the heat. (See Chapter 9.)
- An increase in the density and breaking strength of bone, ligaments, and tendons, and an increase in the thickness of cartilage in the joints. (See Chapter 12.)

Changes that Occur in Muscles Due to Strength Training

What changes in the skeletal muscle occur in response to strength training? (See Figure 7.11 for an overview of the structure of muscle.)

- *Hypertrophy* (increase in size) of muscle cells, especially the fast-twitch fibers. The fibers of untrained muscle vary considerably in diameter. Strength training brings the smaller muscle fibers up to the size of the larger ones. This hypertrophy is caused by an increase in the number and size of myofibrils per muscle cell, increased total protein (especially myosin), increased capillary density, and increased amounts and strength of connective, tendinous, and ligamentous tissues.
- Contrary to some reports, there is no strong evidence that training leads to an increase in the number of muscle cells.[19,36,37] Similarly, there is no support for the theory that extensive weight training enables one to convert slow-twitch fibers to fast-twitch fibers.[8]
- There is a selective hypertrophy of fast-twitch fibers, however, with an associated increase in the ratio of fast-twitch to slow-twitch muscle fiber area. Therefore, people born with a high percentage of fast-twitch fibers can "bulk up" more easily than those with a high percentage of slow-twitch fibers.

Table 7.4 Summary of Changes in Cardiorespiratory Parameters with Endurance Training

Cardiovascular Parameter	Resting	Submax Exercise	Maximal Exercise
Oxygen consumption	No change	No change	Increase
Heart rate	Decrease	Decrease	No/slight change
Stroke volume	Increase	Increase	Increase
Cardiac output	No change	No change	Increase
Active muscle blood flow	No change	Increase	Increase
Ventilation	No change	Decrease	Increase
$\bar{a} - \bar{v}O_2$ difference	No change	Slight increase	Increase
Lactic acid levels	No change	Decrease	Increase

■ The normal inhibitory nervous impulses from the brain are lessened. During the first 3 to 5 weeks of strength training, substantial gains in strength occur without concomitant increases in muscle mass.[38]

Many experts feel that the nervous system adapts to regular weight training, resulting in a *disinhibition* of the muscle. With these adaptations, more *motor units* (motor nerve and attached muscle cells) can be activated, and there is a better recruitment pattern and synchronization of motor units. Thus the increase in strength is not due to an increase in size of muscle cells alone.

■ The biochemical changes are small and inconsistent. Traditional weight training programs do not appear to improve either oxidative or glycolytic enzyme activity.

■ Most studies have shown that weight training programs will increase lean body mass and decrease the percentage of body fat.[38] Weight training programs of from 7 to 24 weeks generally increase the lean body mass by between 0.5 and 3.0 percent.

■ $\dot{V}O_{2max}$ is not effectively increased by strength training programs.[38] There may be small increases in cardiorespiratory fitness after *circuit resistance training* (weight lifting with little pause between a series of different stations). However, these improvements are relatively minor (5 to 8 percent) compared to those typical in aerobic programs.

The heart adapts to the stresses (especially the rise in blood pressure) imposed during weight training by increasing the thickness of the left ventricle wall without an increase in the volume.

Interestingly, weight training to increase leg strength has been shown to improve short-term (4–8 min) cycling or running endurance, and long-term cycling, but not long-term running endurance.[39] The increase in leg strength increases the participation of slow-twitch fibers, postponing the contribution of fast-twitch fiber recruitment, thereby delaying fatigue.

The Effects of Gender, Age, and Heredity

Do females adapt to regular exercise differently than males? Do middle-aged and elderly people adjust differently than younger adults? Are there special considerations for children and teenagers? How much is the ability to improve $\dot{V}O_{2max}$ due to heredity?

The Influence of Gender

Although there are wide differences in performance between genders in the general population, many of these differences narrow or disappear when sexes are matched for various characteristics.[40-42] Men and women experience similar relative strength gains when training under the same program. However, there appears to be less muscle hypertrophy and associated strength improvement among women.

Data suggest that there are no differences between genders in central or peripheral cardiovascular adaptations to aerobic training. There seem to be no differences in relative increases in $\dot{V}O_{2max}$ for men and women when

STRUCTURE OF SKELETAL MUSCLE

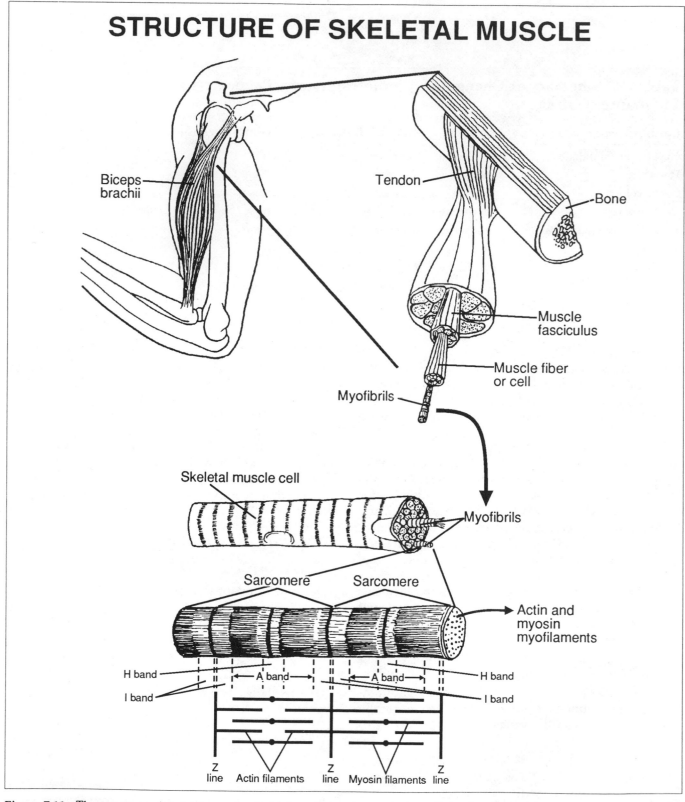

Figure 7.11 The structure of skeletal muscle. *Skeletal muscle* is composed of parallel cells (also called fibers). The number and type of muscle cells (slow-twitch or fast-twitch) is set at birth.

Each muscle cell contains groups of *actin* and *myosin* protein *myofilaments* called *myofibrils*. Skeletal muscle cells have alternating dark and light bands, caused by the overlap of the myosin and actin myofilaments, the basic contractile proteins of skeletal muscle. The smallest functional skeletal muscle subunit capable of contraction is the *sarcomere*, which extends from Z-line to Z-line. Skeletal muscle contraction takes place as the myofilaments slide past each other, and the actin and myosin form and reform bonds.

they train with the same intensity, frequency, and duration.

Women in general, however, have a reduced oxygen carrying capacity (less hemoglobin in the blood) and more body fat than men. Differences in the performances of similarly trained male and female distance runners are due largely to percentage body fat, less to cardiorespiratory fitness, and even less to running economy. Men and women who are capable of similar performances (in a 15-mile race) do not differ in body composition or cardiorespiratory or metabolic response.

Women appear to experience less change in their total cholesterol-high density lipoprotein ratio with aerobic training than men do, but this is due to their higher initial levels of high-density lipoprotein. Generally, menstrual cycle phase makes no difference to the performance of women. World records have been set during all phases of the menstrual cycle.[40]

The Influence of Age

The influence of the aging process on chronic adaptations to exercise will be covered in more detail in Chapter 12. With aging, the ability to engage intensively in physical exercise declines, with a reduction of maximal aerobic power.[23] Aerobic power normally decreases 8–10 percent per decade after 30 years of age.[44-46] Data suggest that the overall rate of loss is similar for active and inactive people, but that at any given age the active conserve more function. Most researchers have shown that the cardiorespiratory trainability of the elderly does not differ greatly from that of younger adults when groups are compared on a percentage but not absolute basis.[43-49]

For children and teenagers, researchers have in general concluded that when programs satisfy adult-related criteria for intensity and duration, children demonstrate a similar physiological training effect.[50] However, the aerobic systems of active children appear to be more responsive to training than their anaerobic systems (which may be utilized more often in their daily activities).

Children tend to have higher maximum oxygen uptake values than young adults, when adjusted for weight. One study showed that 20 prepubertal boys had average $\dot{V}O_{2max}$ values of 57.9 ml·kg⁻¹·min⁻¹ as compared with 48.3 ml·kg⁻¹·min⁻¹ for males age 23–33 years.[49] Although children may have higher $\dot{V}O_{2max}$ values than adults, however, the amount of oxygen they use during a given workload is higher.[49]

The American Academy of Pediatrics has contended that weight training should not be attempted by prepubertal boys because they do not have sufficient levels of circulating male hormones.[51-53] However, researchers have found that weight training programs increase strength for this group as much as they do for adult males. Interestingly, boys tend to increase muscular strength in the absence of muscular hypertrophy; the increases in strength are probably the result of neural adaptations.[52]

The Influence of Heredity

Studies reporting the influence of heredity on aerobic performance have had conflicting results.[54-58] Several twin studies have suggested that $\dot{V}O_{2max}$ and work capacity were almost entirely inherited, while others have reported little genetic effect. Many of these studies have failed to control for age, sex and other factors.

In one study,[56] these various factors were controlled in a study of 42 brothers, 66 dizygotic twins of both sexes, and 106 monozygotic twins of both sexes. They were given various exercise performance tests, including maximal bicycle tests and tests of total work output during a 90-minute, high-intensity bicycle test. The magnitude of the genetic effect was determined to be 40 percent for $\dot{V}O_{2max}$, 50 percent for maximal heart rate, 60 percent for maximal ventilation, and 70 percent for 90 minute work output. These results are in sharp contrast with those of other twin studies in which it was reported that the heritability of $\dot{V}O_{2max}$ was about 90 percent of the total variance.

There is in general large variability in trainability.[58] For example, in one 20-week cycle ergometer training program, the increase in $\dot{V}O_{2max}$ for 25 participants varied from 7 to 87 percent.

Researchers have concluded that sensitivity of $\dot{V}O_{2max}$ improvement to exercise training is largely dependent on hereditary.[54, 55, 57, 58] In one study[55] of ten pairs of monozygotic twins, results showed a large variety of responses to the exercise program (a range of 0–41 percent $\dot{V}O_{2max}$ improvement with all subjects cycling 40 minutes, 4–5 times per week, at 80 percent $\dot{V}O_{2max}$), but the members of each twin-pair reacted approximately the same way to the exercise program. In general, sensitivity to long-term training appears to be largely inherited.

Prior endowment, and an adequate training program will produce exceptionally high performance. From a practical point of view, because of heredity it is almost impossible to accurately predict an individual response to a given training program.

Table 7.5 is a review of the chronic effects that can take place with regular aerobic training. See also Figure 7.6 for a review of the terms used.

Table 7.5 Comparison of Hypothetical Physiological and Body Composition Changes from an Endurance Training Program for a Sedentary, Normal Person and a World Class Endurance Runner of the Same Age

Variable	Sedentary Normal Pre-*	Post-*	World Class Athlete
Cardiovascular			
Resting HR (bpm)	71	59	36
Max HR (bpm)	185	183	174
Resting SV (ml)	65	80	125
Max SV (ml)	120	140	200
Rest $\dot{Q}$ (L/min)	4.6	4.7	4.5
Max $\dot{Q}$ (L/min)	22.2	25.6	34.8
Heart volume (ml)	750	820	1200
Blood volume (L)	4.7	5.1	6.0
Systolic BP (mmHg)	135	130	120
Diastolic BP (mmHg)	78	76	65
Respiratory			
Resting $\dot{V}_E$ (L/min)	7	6	6
Max $\dot{V}_E$ (L/min)	110	135	195
Rest F (breaths/min)	14	12	12
Max F (breaths/min)	40	45	55
Rest TV (L/breath)	0.5	0.5	0.5
Max TV (L/breath)	2.75	3.0	3.5
Vital capacity (L)	5.8	6.0	6.2
Residual volume (L)	1.4	1.2	1.2
Metabolic			
$\bar{a} - \bar{v}O_2$ difference (ml/dL)	6.0	6.0	6.0
Max $\bar{a} - \bar{v}O_2$ difference (ml/dL)	14.5	15.0	16.0
$\dot{V}O_{2max}$ (ml · kg^{-1}· min^{-1})	40.5	49.8	76.7
Max lactate (ml/dL)	110	125	185
Body Composition			
Weight (lbs)	175	170	150
Fat weight (lbs)	28	21.3	11.3
Lean weight (lbs)	147	148.7	138.7
Relative fat (%)	16.0	12.5	7.5

*= six-month training program, jogging 3–4 times per week, 30 min/day, at 75 percent $\dot{V}O_{2max}$.

Source: Wilmore JH, Norton AC. The Heart and Lungs at Work. Schiller Park, IL: Beckman Instruments, 1974. Used with permission of Sensor Medics Corporation, 1630 South State College Blvd., Anaheim, CA 92806.

HR = heart rate; SV = stroke volume; $\dot{Q}$ = cardiac output; BP = blood pressure; $\dot{V}_E$ = ventilation; F = frequency; TV = tidal volume

The Effects of Inactivity

Prolonged inactivity has many detrimental effects on the human body.[59, 60] Disuse adversely affects all body tissues and all body functions. For example, limbs in casts lead to stiff and atrophied muscles, bed rest leads to a muscle protein loss of 8 grams per day, a bone calcium loss of 1.54 grams per week, and a 10–15 percent decrease in plasma volume within several days.[60]

Detraining Physiological Effects

Few humans undergo prolonged bed rest. However, nearly all people have exercised for a certain period of time and then for various reasons reduced or terminated formal exercise while continuing normal day-to-day activities. This period of *detraining* leads to many changes in physiological function.

Dr. Edward Coyle from the University of Texas at Austin has been a leading researcher of the physiological effects of detraining.[61–64] In one study, Dr. Coyle studied the effects of 84 days of no formal exercise on athletes who had been training hard for 10 years.[63, 64]

During this long detraining period, the various systems of the body reacted differently. In the first three weeks after training ceased, runners quickly lost most of their cardiovascular conditioning, primarily due to a rapid decline in stroke volume. The maximal stroke volume declined 10–14 percent below the trained level in just 12 days, and dropped to a level no different from sedentary controls by the end of the study. $\dot{V}O_{2max}$ declined 7 percent in the first 21 days, and stabilized after 56 days at a level 16 percent below the trained level. At the end of eight weeks, the oxidative enzyme levels in the muscles had dropped 40 percent from the trained levels.

Other researchers have also found that the activities of mitochondrial enzymes are markedly reduced with the cessation of physical training.[65]

Muscle capillarization, however, dropped only 7 percent below trained levels after 84 days. Although maximal cardiac output and stroke volume declined to untrained levels, $\dot{V}O_{2max}$ levels in the detrained athletes remained 17 percent above untrained levels, primarily because of an elevation of maximal arteriovenous $\bar{a} - \bar{v}O_2$ difference.

Eighty-four days of detraining also affected responses to submaximal exercise (74 percent $\dot{V}O_{2max}$, trained state).[64] Within eight weeks, most of the negative adaptations occurred, including an 18-percent increase in oxygen consumption (using the same workload), a 17-percent increase in heart rate (158 when trained vs 185 when detrained), a 24-percent increase in ventilation, a 6-percent increase in the respiratory exchange ratio (R), and a 34-percent increase in the rating of perceived exertion (as measured on the Borg scale). Within eight weeks, the rise in lactate in response to the same workload was nearly sixfold.

Even after detraining for twelve weeks, however, the athletes still had high muscle capillary densities and a mitochondrial enzyme level 50 percent above that of the sedentary controls. These represent persistent adaptations resulting from many years of hard training, and helped to partially preserve their exercise performance ability.

These studies support the argument that physical activity must be continued on a regular basis if one is to retain the benefits. As noted previously, when athletes detrain after many years of intense training, they display large reductions in cardiorespiratory fitness during the first 12 to 21 days of inactivity. The decline in stroke volume appears to be largely a result of reduced plasma volume, which also drops 12 percent within 12 to 21 days.[62] Interestingly, Dr. Coyle has shown that if an athlete who has detrained for 2 to 4 weeks expands the blood volume back to that of the trained state, using 6 percent dextran solution in saline, stroke volume and $\dot{V}O_{2max}$ can be increased to within 2–4 percent of trained values.[62, 67]

As stated previously, researchers have shown that the rise in aerobic power with training is just as rapid as its fall without it.[16] Studies also show that most of the improvements in $\dot{V}O_{2max}$ occur within 3 weeks of beginning intense cardiorespiratory training. In addition, researchers have shown that once the desired $\dot{V}O_{2max}$ is achieved, it is possible to maintain it by reducing the frequency while maintaining the intensity of training.[66, 67]

In one study, twelve participants bicycled and ran for 40 minutes, 6 days per week, following an intensive interval training regimen.[66] After 10 weeks, they continued to train at the same intensity and daily duration, but the frequency was lowered to 2 days per week for half of them, four days for the others. After five weeks, the $\dot{V}O_{2max}$ in both groups remained at the 25 percent improved level attained at the end of the first 10 weeks of training.

In other words, it appears to take more energy expenditure to increase $\dot{V}O_{2max}$ than to maintain it. It also appears that training intensity is an essential requirement for maintaining the increased $\dot{V}O_{2max}$ and performance ability gained from hard aerobic training.

Sports Medicine Insight
Factors Affecting Performance

If a group of people are asked to run five miles as fast as possible, would it be possible to predict the top finishers? What factors are most important in cardiorespiratory endurance performance?

There are three major physiological factors that affect cardiorespiratory endurance performance:[68-77]

1. $\dot{V}O_{2max}$
2. Anaerobic Threshold
3. Exercise Oxygen Economy

If a group of people varying widely in activity patterns (sedentary to elite athlete) were examined in the laboratory, $\dot{V}O_{2max}$ would be the most important variable predicting ability to engage in cardiorespiratory endurance events. On the other hand, great variations in $\dot{V}O_{2max}$ have been found among runners with similar performance capabilities.[68]

Although important, $\dot{V}O_{2max}$ is only one of several factors that determine success in running. There can be a large variation in performance between runners of equal $\dot{V}O_{2max}$.[68] Relatively low $\dot{V}O_{2max}$ values have been reported among some top-class marathon runners. Derek Clayton, former world record holder in the marathon (2:08.33), had a $\dot{V}O_{2max}$ of only 66.8 ml · kg⁻¹ · min⁻¹. Stahl, presently one of the best master runners in the world, also has a $\dot{V}O_{2max}$ of 66.8 ml · kg⁻¹ · min⁻¹.

Joan Benoit Samuelson, one of the best female marathon runners in the world (2:21) has a $\dot{V}O_{2max}$ of 78 ml · kg⁻¹ · min⁻¹, a value much higher than that of Clayton's and Stahl's, yet her marathon time is much slower. Obviously, other factors play an important role in cardiorespiratory endurance performance.

Exercise oxygen economy is the oxygen cost of exercise, usually expressed as $\dot{V}O_2$ at a certain running or exercise pace. It is a well established fact that $\dot{V}O_2$ at a certain workload or running speed can vary considerably among different runners.[68, 69, 72] (See Figure 7.12.) Some of the best performers have low oxygen requirements at specific running velocities. While it is not possible to explain this variation precisely, biomechanical, physiological, psychological, and biochemical factors probably all play a part.

Perhaps the most important factor influencing athletic performance is the anaerobic threshold. Anaerobic threshold is highly correlated with endurance performance ($r = 0.94$ to 0.98).[10-13, 68] If a performer can exercise at a high percent of $\dot{V}O_{2max}$ before lactic acid builds up in the blood stream, it provides a great advan-

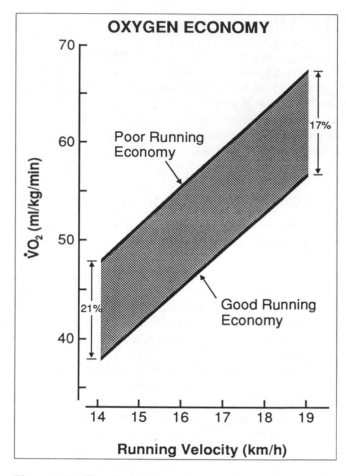

Figure 7.12 The shaded area represents the entire range in the oxygen cost of running at different velocities for good and elite runners. *Source:* Adapted from: Sjodin B, Svedenhag J. Applied Physiology of Marathon Running. Sports Med 2:83–99, 1985. Used with permission by ADIS Press Limited, Auckland, New Zealand.

tage. Such a capacity is built up through long years of training, with an emphasis on interval training.

The best correlation with running performance is the speed at which a runner can run just below the point at which lactate accumulates in the blood. For example, if a runner's lactate threshold occurs at a running pace of 8 minutes per mile, a predicted 15-mile race time would be approximately 2 hours.

Other factors, nonphysiological in nature, also play an important role in cardiorespiratory endurance capacity. In one study of 4358 runners, the most important predictors of 16-km race time in order were: weekly training distance, age, body mass index, years of regular running, and weekly training frequency.[77] Other studies have also consistently shown weekly training distance to provide the highest correlation with endurance race performance.[68]

Table 7.6 summarizes the physical and physiological characteristics of different categories of endurance runners.[68]

Summary

1. This chapter summarized the acute responses and chronic adaptations that occur with exercise.

2. The acute responses include: increases of heart rate, stroke volume, cardiac output, blood flow to active muscles, systolic blood pressure, arteriovenous oxygen difference, ventilation, lung diffusion capacity, oxygen uptake, and a decrease in blood pH and plasma volume (RBC count rises).

3. Chronic adaptations include: biochemical changes in skeletal muscles (increased myoglobin, mitochondria, enzymes, fuels, slow-twitch fiber area); resting cardiorespiratory changes (increase in heart size, stroke volume, blood volume, and capillary density, with a decrease in resting heart rate); submaximal exercise changes (increase in anaerobic threshold and stroke volume, with a decrease in lactic acid production, heart rate, and cardiac output); maximal exercise changes (increase in $\dot{V}O_{2max}$, stroke volume, blood flow to active muscles, ability to tolerate higher lactic acid levels,

ventilation, and lung diffusion capacity, plus a variable effect on maximal heart rate); and other assorted changes (decrease in total body fat, blood lipids, and recovery heart rate, with an increase in heat acclimatization and the density and strength of bone and connective tissues).

4. Although there are wide differences in performance between genders in the general population, many of these differences narrow or disappear when sexes are matched for various characteristics. Most researchers have shown that cardiorespiratory trainability of the elderly does not differ greatly from that of younger adults when groups are compared on a percentage (not absolute) basis. For children and teenagers, researchers have in general concluded that when programs satisfy adult-related criteria for intensity and duration, children demonstrate a similar physiological training effect.

5. The genetic effect has been determined as 40 percent for $\dot{V}O_{2max}$. There is large variability in trainability, and researchers have concluded that the sensitivity of $\dot{V}O_{2max}$ improvement to exercise training largely depends on hereditary factors. Therefore an exceptionally high performance level will be the result of prior endowment, an adequate training program, and genetic characteristics associated with the status of a high responder to training.

Table 7.6 Physical and Physiological Characteristics of Different Categories of Endurance Runners

	Elite runners	Good runners	Slow runners
Age (years)	26	30	36
Weight (kg)	66	67	71
Type I fibers (%)	76	64	56
Years of training	7	4	2
Average weekly distance (km)	145	115	57
$\dot{V}O_{2max}$ (ml·kg^{-1}·min^{-1})	72	66	59
$\dot{V}O_2$ at 15 km/hr	45	49	51
Anaerobic threshold*	88	88	85

* Percent $\dot{V}O_{2max}$ when lactic acid is at a concentration of 4 mmol/L.

Source: Adapted from: Sjodin B, Svedenhag J. Applied Physiology of Marathon Running. Sports Med 2:83–99, 1985.

6. Inactivity (through bedrest) affects virtually every physiological system. Early responses involve the fluid, electrolyte, and blood pressure control systems, with significant muscular atrophy and decreases in bone density occurring somewhat later.

7. Detraining (termination of exercise training, but not bed rest) effects the different systems variously, with stroke volume being affected quickly (decreasing to control levels within one month), and muscle capillarization dropping only 7 percent after 84 days of detraining. The respiratory capacity of trained muscles (mitochondrial enzymes) decreases by 50 percent after one week of inactivity. To prevent these detraining effects, maintaining the intensity of exercise is more important than the frequency of exercise.

8. Factors affecting performance include $\dot{V}O_{2max}$, anaerobic threshold, and exercise oxygen economy. While $\dot{V}O_{2max}$ is most important when evaluating the performance ability of a heterogeneous group, the anaerobic threshold and exercise oxygen economy are most important when comparing athletes of similar ability.

References

1. Huston TP, Puffer JC, Rodney WM. The Athletic Heart Syndrome. N Engl J Med 313:24–31, 1985.

2. Lamb DR. Physiology of Exercise. New York: Macmillan Publishing, 1984.

3. Fox EL, Mathews DK. The Physiological Basis of Physical Education and Athletics. Philadelphia: Saunders College Publishing, 1981.

4. Fox EL. Sports Physiology. New York: CBS College Publishing, 1984.

5. Wilmore JH. Training for Sports and Activity. Boston: Allyn and Bacon, Inc., 1982.

6. Lamb DR, Murray R. Perspectives in Exercise Science and Sports Medicine. Volume 1: Prolonged Exercise. Indianapolis: Benchmark Press, Inc., 1988.

7. McArdle WD, Katch FI, Katch VL. Exercise Physiology: Energy, Nutrition, and Human Performance. Philadelphia: Lea & Febiger, 1986.

8. American College of Sports Medicine. Resource Manual for Guidelines for Exercise Testing and Prescription. Philadelphia: Lea & Febiger, 1988.

9. Senay LC, Pivarnik JM. Fluid Shifts During Exercise. Exerc Sport Sci Rev 13:335–387, 1985.

10. Tanaka K, Matsuura Y. Marathon Performance, Anaerobic Threshold, and Onset of Blood Lactate Accumulation. J Appl Physiol 57:640–643, 1984.

11. Davis JA. Anaerobic Threshold: Review of the Concept and Directions for Future Research. Med Sci Sports Exerc 17:6–18, 1985.

12. Davis JA, et al. Does the Gas Exchange Anaerobic Threshold Occur at a Fixed Blood Lactate Concentration of 2 or 4 mM? Int J Sports Med 2:89–93, 1983.

13. Yoshida T, Chida M, Ichioka M, Suda Y. Blood Lactate Parameters Related to Aerobic Capacity and Endurance Performance. Eur J Appl Physiol 56:7–11, 1987.

14. Gaesser GA, Poole DC. Lactate and Ventilatory Thresholds: Disparity in Time Course of Adaptations to Training. J Appl Physiol 61:999–1004, 1986.

15. Rogers MA, Yamamoto C, Hagberg JM, et al. Effect of 6 d of Exercise Training on Responses to Maximal and Sub-Maximal Exercise in Middle-Aged Men. Med Sci Sports Exerc 20:260–264, 1988.

16. Hickson RC. Time Course of the Adaptive Responses of Aerobic Power and Heart Rate to Training. Med Sci Sports Exerc 13:17–20, 1981.

17. Blomqvist CG, Saltin B. Cardiovascular Adaptations to Physical Training. Annu Rev Physiol 45:169–189, 1983.

18. Moore RL, Thacker EM, Kelley GA, et al. Effect of Training/Detraining on Submaximal Exercise Responses in Humans. J Appl Physiol 63:1719–1724, 1987.

19. Matoba H, Gollnick PD. Response of Skeletal Muscle to Training. Sports Med 1:240–251, 1984.

20. Jansson E, Kaijser L. Substrate Utilization and Enzymes in Skeletal Muscle of Extremely Endurance-Trained Men. J Appl Physiol 62:999–1005, 1987.

21. Nieman DC, Carlson KA, Brandstater ME, Naegele RT, Blankenship JW. Running Endurance in 27-h-Fasted Humans. J Appl Physiol 63:2502–2509, 1987.

22. Bergh U. Maximal Oxygen Uptake and Muscle Fiber Types in Trained and Untrained Humans. Med Sci Sports Exerc 10:151, 1978.

23. Ama PFM, Simoneau JA, Boulay MR, et al. Skeletal Muscle Characteristics in Sedentary Black and Caucasian Males. J Appl Physiol 61:1758–1761, 1986.

24. Pette D. Activity-Induced Fast to Slow Transitions In Mammalian Muscle. Med Sci Sports Exerc 16:517–528, 1984.

25. Howard H, Hoppeler H, Cloassen H, et al. Influences of Endurance Training On the Ultrastructural Composition of the Different Muscle Fiber Types In Humans. Pflugers Arch 403:369–376, 1985.

26. Cohen JL, Segal KR. Left Ventricular Hypertrophy In Athletes: An Exercise-Echocardiographic Study. Med Sci Sports Exerc 17:695–700, 1985.

27. Hopper MK, Coggan AR, Coyle EF. Exercise Stroke Volume Relative to Plasma-Volume Expansion. J Appl Physiol 64:404–408, 1988.

28. Nadel ER. Physiological Adaptations to Aerobic Training. Amer Sci 73:334–343, 1985.

29. Costill DL, Fink WJ, Flynn M, Kirwan J. Muscle Fiber Composition and Enzyme Activities in Elite Female Distance Runners. Int J Sports Med 8 (suppl):103–106, 1987.

30. Martin DE, May DF. Pulmonary Function Characteristics in Elite Women Distance Runners. Int J Sports Med 8 (suppl):84–90, 1987.

31. Nieman DC, Tan SA, Lee JW, Berk LS. Complement and Immunoglobulin Levels in Athletes and Sedentary Controls. Int J Sports Med 10:124–128, 1989.

32. Pate RR, Sparling PB, Wilson GE, Cureton KJ, Miller BJ. Cardiorespiratory and Metabolic Responses to Submaximal and Maximal Exercise in Elite Women Distance Runners. Int J Sports Med 8 (suppl):91–95, 1987.

33. Vogel JA, Patton JF, Mello RP, Daniels WL. An Analysis of Aerobic Capacity in a Large United States Population. J Appl Physiol 60:494–500, 1986.

34. Hammond HK, Froelicher VF. The Physiologic Sequelae of Chronic Dynamic Exercise. Med Clinics N Amer 69:21–39, 1985.

35. Farhi LE. Physiologic Requirements to Perform Work. Am Rev Respir Dis 129 (suppl):54–55, 1984.

36. Martin WH, Montgomery J, Snell PG, et al. Cardiovascular Adaptations to Intense Swim Training in Sedentary Middle-Aged Men and Women. Circulation 75:323–330, 1987.

37. Taylor NAS, Wilkinson JG. Exercise-Induced Skeletal Muscle Growth: Hypertrophy or Hyperplasia? Sport Med 3:190–200, 1986.

38. Kraemer WJ, Deschenes MR, Fleck SJ. Physiological Adaptations to Resistance Exercise: Implications for Athletic Conditioning. Sports Med 6:246–256, 1988.

39. Hickson RC, Dvorak BA, Gorostiaga EM, Kurowski TT, Foster C. Potential for Strength and Endurance Training to Amplify Endurance Performance. J Appl Physiol 65:2285–2290, 1988.

40. Lewis DA, Kamon E, Hodgson JL. Physiological Differences Between Genders: Implications for Sports Conditioning. Sports Med 3:357–369, 1986.

41. Graves JE, Pollock ML, Sparling PB. Body Compositions of Elite Female Distance Runners. Int J Sports Med 8 (suppl):96–102, 1987.

42. Pate RR, Sparling PB, Wilson GE, Cureton KJ, Miller BJ. Cardiorespiratory and Metabolic Responses to Submaximal and Maximal Exercise in Elite Women Distance Runners. Int J Sports Med 8 (suppl):91–95, 1987.

43. Shephard, R., Sidney, K.: Exercise and aging. Exerc Sport Sci Rev 2:1–57, 1978.

44. Asmussen, E., Fruensgaard, K, Norgaard, S.: A follow-up longitudinal study of selected physiologic functions in former physical education students—after forty years. J Am Geriat Soc 23:442–450, 1975.

45. Astrand, I.: Aerobic work capacity in men and women with special reference to age. Acta Physiol Scand 49(suppl 169):1–92, 1960.

46. Astrand, I.: Reduction in maximal oxygen uptake with age. J Appl Physiol 35:649–654, 1973.

47. Heath, G., Hagberg, J., Ehsani, A., Holloszy, J.: A physiological comparison of young and older endurance athletes. J Appl Physiol 51:634–640, 1981.

48. Hossack, K., Bruce, R.: Maximal cardiac function in sedentary normal men and women: comparison of age-related changes. J Appl Physiol 53:799–804, 1982.

49. Sidney, K., Shephard, R.: Frequency and intensity of exercise training for elderly subjects. Med Sci Sports Exerc 10:125–131, 1978.

50. Rowland TW. Aerobic Response to Endurance Training in Prepubescent Children: A Critical Analysis. Med Sci Sports Exerc 17:493–497, 1985.

51. Rowland TW, Auchinachie JA, Keenan TJ, Green GM. Int J Sports Med 8:292–297, 1987.

52. Weltman A, Janney C, Rians CB, et al. The Effects of Hydraulic Resistance Strength Training in Pre-Pubertal Males. Med Sci Sports Exerc 18:629–638, 1986.

53. Docherty D, Wenger HA, Collis ML. The Effects of Resistance Training on Aerobic and Anaerobic Power of Young Boys. Med Sci Sports Exerc 19:389–392, 1987.

54. Bouchard C, Lortie G. Heredity and Endurance Performance. Sports Med 1:38–64, 1984.

55. Prud'Homme D, Bouchard C, et al. Sensitivity of Maximal Aerobic Power to Training is Genotype-Dependent. Med Sci Sports Exerc 16:489–493, 1984.

56. Bouchard C, Lesage R, Lortie G, et al. Aerobic Performance in Brothers, Dizygotic and Monozygotic Twins. Med Sci Sports Exerc 18:639–646, 1986.

57. Hamel P, Simoneau JA, Lortie G, Boulay MR, Bouchard C. Heredity and Muscle Adaptation to Endurance Training. Med Sci Sports Exerc 18:690–696, 1986.

58. Bouchard C, Boulay MR, Simoneau JA, Lortie G, Pérusse L. Heredity and Trainability of Aerobic and Anaerobic Performances: An Update. Sports Med 5:69–73, 1988.

59. Greenleaf JE. Physiological Responses to Prolonged Bed Rest and Fluid Immersion in Humans. J Appl Physiol 57:619–633, 1984.

60. Bortz WM. The Disuse Syndrome. West J Med 141:691–694, 1984.

61. Coyle EF. Detraining and Retention of Training-Induced Adaptations. In: American College of Sports Medicine. Resource Manual for Guidelines for Exercise Testing and Prescription. Philadelphia: Lea & Febiger, 1988, pp 83–89.

62. Coyle EF, Hemmert MK, Coggan AR. Effects of Detraining on Cardiovascular Responses to Exercise: Role of Blood Volume. J Appl Physiol 60:95–99, 1986.

63. Coyle EF, Martin WH, Sinacore DR, et al. Time Course of Loss of Adaptations After Stopping Prolonged Intense Endurance Training. J Appl Physiol 57:1857–1864, 1984.

64. Coyle EF, Martin WH, Bloomfield SA, et al. Effects of Detraining on Responses to Submaximal Exercise. J Appl Physiol 59:853–859, 1985.

65. Costill DL. Metabolic Characteristics of Skeletal Muscle During Detraining From Competitive Swimming. Med Sci Sports Exerc 17:339–343, 1985.

66. Hickson RC, Rosenkoetter MA. Reduced Training Frequencies and Maintenance of Increased Aerobic Power. Med Sci Sports Exerc 13:13–16, 1981.

67. Hickson RC, et al. Reduced Training Intensities and Loss of Aerobic Power, Endurance, and Cardiac Growth. J Appl Physiol 58:492–499, 1985.

68. Sjodin B, Svedenhag J. Applied Physiology of Marathon Running. Sports Med 2:83–99, 1985.

69. Morgan DW, Baldini FD, Martin PE, Kohrtlum. Ten Kilometer Performance and Predicted Velocity at $\dot{V}O_{2max}$. Among Well-Trained Male Runners. Med Sci Sports Exerc 21:78–83, 1989.

70. Hagan RD, et al. Marathon Performance in Relation to Maximal Aerobic Power and Training Indices. Med Sci Sports Exerc 13:185–189, 1981.

71. Mahler DA, Loke J. The Physiology of Marathon Running. Physician Sportsmed 13:85–97, 1985.

72. Cavanagh PR, Kram R. The Efficiency of Human Movement—A Statement of the Problem. Med Sci Sports Exerc 17:304–308, 1985.

73. Noakes TD. Implications of Exercise Testing for Prediction of Athletic Performance: A Contemporary Perspective. Med Sci Sports Exerc 20:319–330, 1988.

74. Londeree BR. The Use of Laboratory Test Results with Long Distance Runners. Sports Med 3:201–213, 1986.

75. Scrimgeour AG, Noakes TD, Adams B, Myburgh K. The Influence of Weekly Training Distance on Fractional Utilization of Maximal Aerobic Capacity in Marathon and Ultramarathon Runners. Eur J Appl Physiol 55:202–209, 1986.

76. Miller FR, Manfredi TG. Physiological and Anthropometrical Predictors of 15-Kilometer Time Trial Cycling Performance Time. Res Quart Exerc Sport 58:250–254, 1987.

77. Marti B, Abelin T, Minder CE. Relationship of Training and Life-Style to 16-km Running Time of 4000 Joggers: The '84 Berne "Grand-Prix" Study. Int J Sports Med 9:85–91, 1988.

Physical Fitness Activity 7.1— Labeling Figures that Depict Acute and Chronic Responses to Exercise

Figure 7.13 illustrates eight different resting dynamic lung volumes, and acute and chronic changes associated with exercise. As explained in this chapter, the *acute responses to exercise* are the sudden, temporary changes in body function caused by exercise, which disappear shortly after the exercise period is finished. The *chronic adaptations to exercise* are the persistent changes in the structure and function of your body following regular exercise training, which apparently enable the body to respond more easily to subsequent exercise bouts.

Your assignment is to label each illustration with one of the listings given below. In some of the illustrations, the solid line represents the response of an untrained person; the dashed line represents the response of a trained person.

Match these answers with the appropriate figure (A through H).

1. Respiratory exchange ratio
2. $\dot{V}O_{2max}$
3. Minute ventilation
4. Heart rate differences of trained and untrained people
5. Tidal volume
6. Stroke volume differences of trained and untrained people
7. Oxygen deficit
8. Cardiac output differences of trained and untrained people

PHYSICAL FITNESS ACTIVITY 7.1

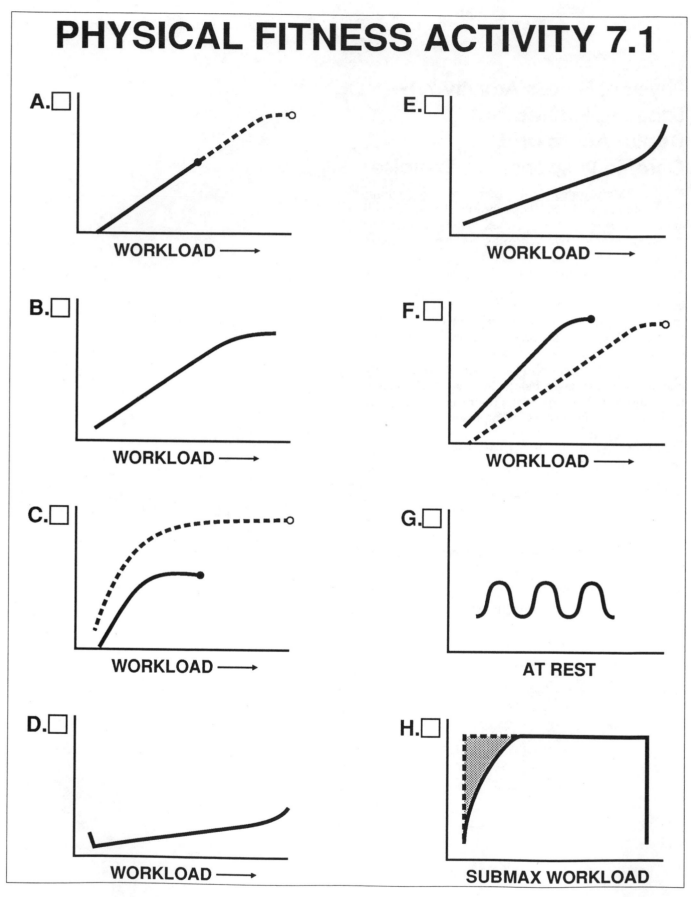

Figure 7.13

Chapter 8

Individualized Exercise Prescription

"My present prescription for exercise is as follows: Daily—at least 60 minutes of physical activity, not necessarily vigorous, nor all at the same time. Weekly—at least two or three periods of 30 minutes of intermittent or sustained activity at a submaximal rate of work are necessary for maintaining good cardiovascular fitness."—Dr. Per Olaf Astrand.[1]

A Public Health Approach to Exercise Prescription

As discussed in Chapters 2, 4, and 7, maximal physical working capacity is also called maximal aerobic power $\dot{V}O_{2max}$ or cardiorespiratory fitness. $\dot{V}O_{2max}$ is not only important for fitness, it is also a health parameter, in that it has been associated with other health variables such as blood pressure, blood lipids, and obesity.

In addition, $\dot{V}O_{2max}$ is directly related to the ability to function during the course of daily living. Current living conditions for most Americans seldom challenge the limits of their $\dot{V}O_{2max}$. The more fit person has a greater capacity to enjoy more active leisure time activities, has more resources to perform required household or occupational tasks, and can perform these activities without becoming exhausted. Many people who suffer from nonspecific, general fatigue have no particular medical condition, they are simply so unfit that the ordinary tasks of daily living leave them exhausted.[2]

The American College of Sports Medicine (ACSM) has recommended since 1975 that intensity of exercise range from 50 to 80 percent of $\dot{V}O_{2max}$, that duration be 20 to 60 minutes, and frequency a minimum of three days per week.[3]

The F.I.T. model promoted by ACSM has been of great benefit to both researchers and the exercising public; however, it has a few potential problems. Most of the research in support of this model has been short term (10 to 20 weeks). Therefore, it has actually served to predict short-term change of $\dot{V}O_{2max}$, with an emphasis on intensity of exercise.[2]

Research on the benefits of informal, lower intensity exercise spread throughout the day is needed. For example, if a nurse in a medical center uses the stairs instead of the elevator, and averages at least 15 minutes a day of brisk stair climbing, can this exercise promote fitness and health despite its discontinuous nature? Two reports from Finland suggest that intermittent stairclimbing spread throughout the day provides a suitable on-the-job physical activity program.[4, 5]

Emphasizing $\dot{V}O_{2max}$ above other components of physical fitness such as body composition and musculoskeletal fitness may be unwarranted. Several studies are suggesting that low-intensity physical activity may benefit health and promote leanness despite having little effect on $\dot{V}O_{2max}$.[2] In addition, the intensity range recommended by ACSM for improving $\dot{V}O_{2max}$ may be too high, increasing the risk of musculoskeletal injury for many people. Well-designed studies are now showing that intensities as low as 42 percent of functional capacity can promote cardiorespiratory fitness.[6,7] Lower intensity exercise appears to be more appealing for most Americans, promoting better long-term compliance. (See Figure 8.1.)

It is the behavioral aspects of the exercise prescription that need more attention. Only a minority of Americans are exercising appropriately according to the F.I.T. model (11–28 percent, depending on the definition, as discussed in Chapter 1.) A less technical, informal approach to exercise might be more attractive to the American public. The message that might appeal to the society at large is simply to become more active by watching less television, walking more, using stairs, and adopting other physically active leisure-time pursuits.[8–13] This type of activity may confer substantial health benefits, even though $\dot{V}O_{2max}$ is only moderately affected.

Thus, as a public guide, the exclusive emphasis on the F.I.T. model and the importance of increasing $\dot{V}O_{2max}$ may be untenable. The public health goal is to increase the percentage of the population who are physically active. To attract the greatest number of people to physical activity, recommendations for physical activity should include the widest range of intensity and duration that is consistent with known health and fitness benefits.

This public health theme will be the focus of this chapter. The ACSM F.I.T. model will be described fully, with an emphasis on strategies that have the potential to include a majority of Americans as regular exercisers.

The Individualized Approach

People vary widely in their health and fitness status, motivation, goals, occupation, age, needs, desires, and education.[3, 14] Thus, to give an *exercise prescription* that best meets a person's needs in a safe and effective manner requires a clear understanding of that person.

In Section 2, emphasis was placed on obtaining medical, health, and physical fitness information for each participant to be given an exercise prescription. This cannot be emphasized enough. An exercise prescription must never be written before this information is available. In addition, it is a good idea to sit down with the person and get to know him, discussing interests, felt needs, future goals, reasons for starting an exercise program, and feelings about the results of the physical fitness tests. (See Physical Fitness Activity 8.1.) (See Figure 8.2.)

Once these preliminary requirements have been met, then the participant can be educated about the principles of exercise, and given adequate leadership and direction through the use of an exercise prescription.

The focus in the 1990s is to utilize a comprehensive physical fitness approach. During the boom years of the

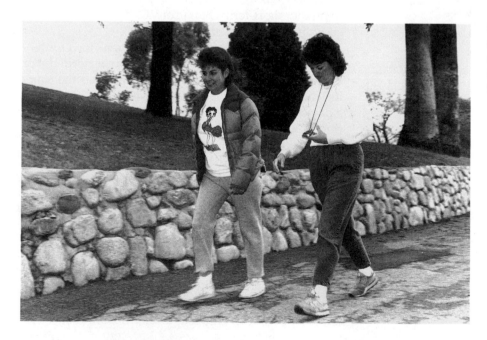

Figure 8.1 Lower intensity exercise, such as brisk walking, is more appealing to many Americans than more vigorous exercise such as running.

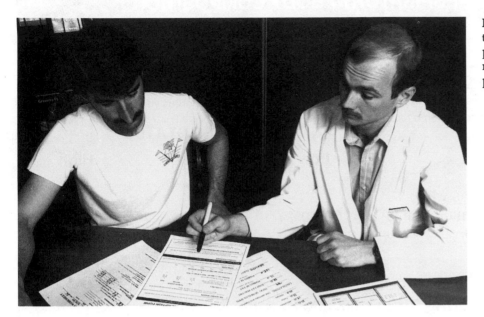

Figure 8.2 A clear understanding of the individual to be given the exercise prescription can be gained by reviewing medical, health, and physical fitness test information.

aerobic movement in the 1970s and 1980s, cardiorespiratory conditioning was often the only type of exercise for many, leaving out exercises for flexibility and muscular strength and endurance. This was the reverse of what happened during the 1950s and 1960s when muscular strength was preeminent, to the detriment of exercises for the heart and lungs. The comprehensive approach that now is emerging gives attention to both cardiorespiratory and musculoskeletal fitness. On the other hand, cardiorespiratory training is still the foundation of any exercise prescription, because most of the health benefits related to physical activity are associated with dynamic, whole-body, continuous, sustained activity.[15, 16]

Figure 8.3 summarizes the comprehensive approach to physical fitness, emphasizing a five-step approach. Each step, in the order given, is considered important for the development of "total fitness." The rest of this chapter will focus on describing these five steps.

Before discussing this conditioning format, an important point needs to be made. In order to realize the full benefits of regular exercise and physical activity, the development of physical fitness must be seen as one of several important components contributing to wellness and health. Other components include adequate rest, a proper diet, management of stress, wholesome social and family influences, sufficient sunshine, pure air and water, sanitation, and a nurturing sense of

spirituality. All these factors work together to promote health, happiness, and "good feelings."

Cardiorespiratory Endurance/ Body Composition

Warm-Up

As shown in Figure 8.3, the purpose of the *warm-up* is to slowly elevate the pulse to an aerobic level. The suggested routine is five minutes of slow aerobic-type exercises to gradually ease into the aerobic session.

There is quite a strong debate at present over the constituents of a true warm-up. Many fitness leaders advocate *flexibility exercises* during the warm-up ("joint-readiness exercises") to prepare for the aerobic session.[17–19] Others advocate at least 5–10 minutes of slow aerobic activity to elevate body temperature before even thinking of any flexibility exercises.[20–27]

Holding *static flexibility* positions before the muscle becomes warm can be potentially injurious.[20, 23] A good plan for athletes is to start slowly, then exercise intensely, and finally finish with a gentle cool-down with range-of-motion exercises. Larsen, a track coach at UCLA, has his runners first jog for one and one-half to two miles, going out at a very easy pace, wearing sweats, to work up heat in their joints and muscles.[21] Then he has them engage in static flexibility exercises,

THE EXERCISE PRESCRIPTION FORM

STAGE ONE - CARDIORESPIRATORY / BODY COMPOSITION

1. **WARM-UP** _____

Purpose: To slowly elevate the pulse to an aerobic level by engaging in 5 min of slow aerobic activity.

2. **THE AEROBIC SESSION**

Purpose: To improve the cardiorespiratory system of the body by exercising vigorously for at least 20-30 min, 3 times/wk, on a regular basis.

FITNESS STATUS

F.I.T. GUIDELINES	**Low**	**Average**	**High**
F Frequency (sessions/wk)	3	3-4	≥5
I Intensity (% heart rate reserve)	50-60%	60-75%	75-85%
T Time (min/session)	10-20	20-30	30-60

MODE SELECTION (your personal) _____

▶ TRAINING HR = [(Max HR - RHR) x 50-85%] + RHR

_____ = _____ − _____ × _____ + _____

▶ DAYS OF WEEK AND TIME OF EXERCISE SESSIONS

Sun_____   Mon_____   Tue_____   Wed_____   Thu_____   Fri_____   Sat_____

3. **WARM-DOWN** _____

Purpose: to slowly decrease the heart rate by engaging in slow aerobic activity for at least 5 min

STAGE TWO - MUSCULOSKELETAL FITNESS

1. **FLEXIBILITY EXERCISES** _____

_____

Purpose: to stretch the major muscles and joints, especially those involved in the aerobic session, using static stretching techniques.

2. **MUSCULAR STRENGTH AND ENDURANCE EXERCISES** _____

_____

Purpose: to build muscular endurance and strength, especially in the muscles not developed in the aerobic session, using appropriate weight training and calisthenic exercises.

* Note: fill in the blanks

Figure 8.3   This exercise prescription form can be used to organize the exercise prescription process.

believing that stretching after the muscles are warm is safer, and that they can be stretched further. States Larsen:[21]

> "I realize many runners stretch and then jog, but most highly competitive runners jog first before stretching. I really don't know why it's that way, but most seem to prefer that procedure."

International-class gymnasts have long prepared for performances by running lightly (or engaging in other slow-aerobic exercise) to raise body temperature, inducing a light perspiration, and then engaging in flexibility exercises.[22]

The physiological benefits of the warm-up are listed in Box 8.1.[23,24,26,28] In general, a thorough warm-up (meaning an elevation in body temperature) before hard aerobic exercise will enhance the activity of enzymes in the working muscles, reduce the viscosity of muscle, improve the mechanical efficiency and power of the moving muscles, facilitate the transmission speed of nervous impulses augmenting coordination, increase muscle blood flow and thus improve delivery of necessary fuel substrates, increase the level of free fatty acids in the blood, help prevent injuries to the muscles and various supporting connective tissues, and allow the heart muscle to adequately prepare itself for aerobic exercise (possibly preventing abnormal EKG changes).

For these reasons, researchers advise that the warm-up consist of the specific exercise that will be engaged in during the aerobic session, but in slow motion, allowing for a gradual increase in body temperature.[23,26,27] This not only warms the body, but also provides a slight rehearsal of the event that is to take place. Flexibility exercises should not be engaged in until the body is warm. Muscle, tendon, and ligament elasticity depends on blood saturation. Cold connective

tissues, which have a low blood saturation, can be more susceptible to damage.

For athletes, the best plan is to stretch just after the warm-up and just after the warm-down. Recreational exercisers can concentrate on flexibility exercises after the aerobic session is over. Stretching at this time has the special advantage of allowing one to stretch warm muscles that have been contracting forcibly during aerobic exercise. It makes sense that muscles that have been continually contracting and shortening should be lengthened after the session is over. This is safer, helps ease the after-effects of the aerobic exercise, and allows one to stretch further because of decreased muscle viscosity.

For example, a runner would start his exercise session by walking for a minute or so, then jogging easily for two to four more minutes, and then finally building up speed to elevate the pulse to the training level intensity. After warming-down with jogging/walking for several minutes (reversing the warm-up), static-flexibility exercises can be performed for at least five minutes, emphasizing the posterior leg, lower back, and upper-front chest areas (muscles that are shortened during running). (See Figure 8.4.) The same would be true for swimmers or cyclers, except that flexibility exercises would be directed more toward shoulder and thigh areas respectively.

The Aerobic Session

To be most effective, an exercise prescription must give specific written instructions for the frequency, intensity, and time of exercise. These are known as the F.I.T. criteria of cardiorespiratory endurance training. Figure 8.3 outlines the basic guidelines for aerobic exercise prescription. Many articles have been written on exer-

---

Box 8.1   Beneficial Effects of Warm-Up Before Strenuous Exercise

1. Increases breakdown of oxyhemoglobin, allowing greater delivery of oxygen to the working muscle,

2. increases the release of oxygen from myoglobin,

3. decreases the activation energy for vital cellular metabolic chemical reactions,

4. decreases muscle viscosity, improving mechanical efficiency and power,

5. increases speed of nervous impulses; sensitivity of nerve receptors is also augmented,

6. increases blood flow to the muscles,

7. decreases number of injuries to muscles, tendons, ligaments, and other connective tissues,

8. improves the cardiovascular response to sudden, strenuous exercise (especially heart muscle blood flow), and

9. leads to earlier sweating which reduces risk of high body temperature during exercise.

Source: adapted from: Shellock FG. Physiological Benefits of Warm-up. Physician Sportsmed 11:134-139, 1983. Used with permission from The Physician and Sportsmedicine, a McGraw-Hill publication.

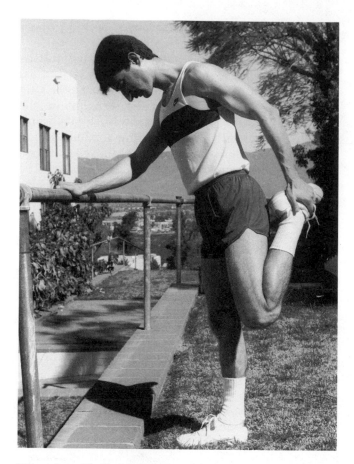

Figure 8.4 Flexibility exercises are best conducted when the body is warm from aerobic activity.

cise prescription.[3, 14, 15, 29–43] A discussion of the major criteria follows.

Frequency

Frequency of exercise refers to the number of exercise sessions per week in the exercise program. In order both to improve cardiorespiratory endurance and keep body fat at optimal levels, most reviewers have concluded that it is necessary to exercise at least three times weekly with no more than two days between workouts.[31, 40, 41] Some studies have shown some cardiorespiratory improvements with an exercise frequency of less than three days per week, but such improvements are at most minimal to modest, and result in little or no body fat loss.[14, 32, 36, 41]

When a person is initiating an aerobic exercise program, conditioning every other day is recommended.[14] This is especially true for running programs with those who are unfit and have been previously sedentary. For such people, the musculoskeletal system is unable to adapt quickly to hard daily exercise, and it will lead to muscle soreness, fatigue, and injury.

In one study,[32] the injury rate related to the foot, ankle, and knee joints increased dramatically when beginning joggers initially trained more than three days per week. The rate of injuries for the five-day per week beginner jogger group was three times that of the three-day per week group. If those starting a running program want to exercise more frequently than three days per week, jogging days should be mixed with days of walking, bicycling, or swimming, which are easier on the musculoskeletal system.[14]

The following advice has been given in the ACSM position statement on "The Recommended Quantity and Quality of Exercise for Developing and Maintaining Fitness in Healthy Adults":[40]

> "For the non-athlete, there is not enough information available at this time to speculate on the value of added improvement found in programs that are conducted more than 5 days per week. Participation of less than two days per week does not show an adequate change in $\dot{V}O_{2max}$."

This statement brings up the principle of the *"The Law of Diminishing Returns."* There appears to be a certain amount of training that most humans will respond quickly and fruitfully to. But every step beyond that level brings less return for the time and effort invested. With three to five days per week of aerobic training come many benefits—increasing the frequency beyond this means putting in more time for smaller gains. This is why most researchers agree with Dr. Kenneth H. Cooper when he contends that people exercising more than five times a week, 30 minutes per session, are doing it for something other than health or fitness (e.g., for competition, ego, special outdoor activities.[44]

Participants who desire to increase their frequency of training can gradually do so, depending on age, initial fitness status, and other personal factors.[14] (See section on rate of progression.)

Intensity

As described previously, the *maximum heart rate* represents the maximum attainable heart rate at the point of exhaustion from all-out exertion.[45] During a treadmill test, the EKG heart rate recorder measures the maximum heart rate when the person reaches total exhaustion. If the oxygen uptake is measured at this same point, the $\dot{V}O_{2max}$ can be determined ($ml \cdot kg^{-1} \cdot min^{-1}$).

For healthy adults to develop and maintain cardiorespiratory fitness and proper body composition, the

American College of Sports Medicine and others have emphasized that the *intensity of exercise* needs to be between 50–85 percent of *"heart rate reserve,"* which is approximately the same as 50–85 percent of maximum oxygen uptake capacity ($\dot{V}O_{2max}$).[3, 14, 30, 40] However, as described in the beginning section of this chapter, some researchers are reporting that cardiorespiratory endurance improvement can be measured at intensities as low as 42 percent $\dot{V}O_{2max}$.[6, 7]

In light of this research, reviewers are urging ACSM to lower their intensity range, and in order to enhance compliance, to urge the American public to exercise at the lower end of the range.[2] The question is whether improvement in $\dot{V}O_{2max}$ is more important than such factors as avoidance of chronic disease, decrease in anxiety and depression, avoidance of injury, and improvement in musculoskeletal fitness, which are related to lower exercise intensity levels. It probably is not.

For athletes, the greatest improvements in aerobic power occur when intensity is high (90–100% $\dot{V}O_{2max}$).[41] When exercise duration exceeds 35 minutes, training intensity is reduced to 70–80% $\dot{V}O_{2max}$ and training effects are no higher than those from training at higher intensities for shorter durations. Athletes need to balance this information with the consistent finding that high intensity exercise increases the risk of injury.

Calculating Exercise Intensity

Exercise intensity can be assessed using the results of the graded exercise test.[3] Based on the length of time the participant stays on the treadmill, $\dot{V}O_{2max}$ can be estimated. (See Chapter 4.) This $\dot{V}O_{2max}$ can be expressed in *METS* (3.5 ml · kg^{-1} · min^{-1} = 1 MET). If the subject desires to exercise at 70 percent of $\dot{V}O_{2max}$, then the MET value is simply multiplied by 70 percent. For example, if a participant has a $\dot{V}O_{2max}$ of 10 METS, then 70 percent times 10 METS is 7 METS. Tables 8.1 and 8.2 can then be consulted to determine the types of activities that represent the 7-MET level.[46]

However, using a set MET level for exercise can have some disadvantages. Various environmental factors such as wind, hills, sand, snow, heat, cold, humidity, altitude, pollution, and bulky or restrictive clothing, can increase or decrease the amount of actual work being accomplished during a given activity.[3] Also, as the person improves in fitness, different MET levels will be needed to ensure an adequate training stimulus. For these reasons, the training heart rate, or rating of perceived exertion (RPE) are often used instead as an indicator of exercise intensity. The heart rate and RPE are indicators of exercise intensity that adjust for environmental factors and realistically predict improvement in fitness.

As indicated, exercise intensity can also be prescribed in terms of heart rate. There are several methods of determining the *training heart rate.* The first method used by researchers is to plot the slope of the line between a person's exercise heart rates and the exercise workload in METS or $\dot{V}O_2$.[3] From this relationship, the exercise heart rate pertaining to a given percent of $\dot{V}O_{2max}$ can be obtained.

A second method for determining the exercise heart rate for training is to calculate a given percentage of the maximum heart rate (MHR).[3] To equate this method with the other methods, the following formula has been developed to make the appropriate 15 percent adjustment:

Training Heart Rate = (MHR × 70 percent) × 1.15

For example, if the MHR is 200: (200 × 70%) × 1.15 = 161.

Some exercise programs instruct participants to multiply their MHR by 50–85 percent, without the 15-percent upward adjustment. This will lead to an underestimation of the heart rate needed to improve cardiorespiratory endurance.

The third method for determining training heart rate was developed by Dr. M. Karvonen of Scandinavia.[47, 48] The *Karvonen Formula* attempts to calculate the training heart rate using a percentage of the "heart rate reserve," which is the difference between the maximum and resting heart rates. (See Figure 8.5.)

Training Heart Rate =
[(MHR – RHR) × 50–85 percent] + RHR

(MHR = maximum heart rate; RHR =
resting heart rate).

The intensity range of 50–85 percent of "heart rate reserve" is approximately equal to 50–85 percent of $\dot{V}O_{2max}$. Table 8.3 shows the relationship between these two factors and the percentage of maximum heart rate.

There are two methods of determining maximum heart rate. The most accurate way is to directly measure the maximum heart rate with an EKG recorder during graded exercise testing. The other way is to estimate MHR by using the simple formula:

MHR = 220 – AGE (low estimate) or 210 –
(0.5 × AGE) (high estimate).[3]

The problem with estimations of maximum heart rate is that they are based on population averages, with a standard deviation of plus or minus 10–12 bpm. If

Table 8.1 MET Values for Various Physical Activities

Physical Activity	MET Range	Physical Activity	MET Range
Archery	3–4	Running	
Backpacking	5–11	12 min per mile	8.7
Badminton	4–9	11 min per mile	9.4
Basketball		10 min per mile	10.2
Non-game	3–9	9 min per mile	11.2
Gameplay	7–12	8 min per mile	12.5
Bed Exercise (cardiac)	1–2	7 min per mile	14.1
Bicycling		6 min per mile	16.3
Pleasure	3–8	Sailing	2–5
10 mph	7.0	Scubadiving	5–10
Bowling	2–4	Skating, ice and roller	5–8
Canoeing, Rowing, Kayaking	3–8	Skiing, snow	
Calisthenics	3–8	Downhill	5–8
Dancing		Cross country	6–12
Social and square	3–7	Skiing, water	5–7
Aerobic	6–9	Sledding, tobogganing	4–8
Fencing	6–10	Snowshoeing	7–14
Fishing		Squash	8–12
Bank, boat, or ice	2–4	Soccer	5–12
Stream, wading	5–6	Stairclimbing	4–8
Football (touch)	6–10	Swimming	4–8
Golf		Table tennis	3–5
Power cart	2–3	Tennis	4–9
Walking, with bag or cart	4–7	Volleyball	3–6
Handball	8–12	Walking	
Hiking, cross country	3–7	1.7 mph	2.3
Horseback riding	3–8	2.0 mph	2.4
Horseshoe pitching	2–3	2.5 mph	2.9
Hunting, walking		3.0 mph	3.3
Small game	3–7	3.4 mph	3.6
Big game	3–14		
Mountain climbing	5–10		
Music playing	2–3		
Paddleball, racquetball	8–12		
Rope jumping	8–12		

Source: American College of Sports Medicine. Guidelines for Graded Exercise Testing and Exercise Prescription. Philadelphia: Lea & Febiger, 1986. Used with permission from the American College of Sports Medicine.

estimations are used, the accuracy of the Karvonen formula is lessened. When the training heart rate is based on an estimated maximum heart rate, it should not be used as a precise measure, and should be readjusted if the exercise participant complains that perceived exertion (using the Borg scale) is "very hard" or higher.

To determine the resting heart rate, it is best to take one's pulse while in a sitting position upon waking in the morning.[14] This should be done three mornings in a row, and then the values are averaged. After waking, one should allow the heart to calm down, which might mean sitting quietly for a few minutes or emptying the bladder.

Resting heart rates taken prior to graded exercise testing are often elevated because of pretest apprehension. In such situations, it is best to estimate the resting heart rate based on the health and fitness history of the person. (See Appendix B, Table 38 for resting heart rate norms.) Some people are in the habit of taking their RHRs on a periodic, regular basis, and if they are validated with careful questioning, these reported values can be used.

Based on the results of the graded exercise test and/or exercise history, and the exercise goals of the person, the intensity percentile used in the Karvonen formula can be varied, as summarized in Table 8.4.

To summarize with an example, the exercise train-

Table 8.2 Occupation Activities and MET Values

METS	Occupational Activities
1.5-2	Desk work, driving auto, electric calculating machine operation, light housework—polishing furniture or washing clothes.
2-3	Auto repair, radio and TV repair, janitorial work, riding lawn mower, light woodworking.
3-4	Brick laying, plastering, wheelbarrow (100 lb load), machine assembly, welding, cleaning windows, mopping floors, vacuuming.
4-5	Painting, masonry, paperhanging, light carpentry, raking leaves.
5-6	Digging garden, shoveling light earth.
6-7	Shoveling 10 times/min (10 lb), splitting wood, snow shoveling.
7-8	Digging ditches, carrying 36 kg or 80 lb, sawing hardwood.
8-9	Shoveling 10 times/min (14 lb).
10+	Shoveling 10 times/min (16 lb).

Source: Fox SM, et al. Physical Activity and Cardiovascular Health. Mod Concepts Cardiovasc Dis 41:25-30, 1972. Used with permission of The American Heart Association, Inc.

Note: Since 1 MET = 1 $kcal \cdot kg^{-1} \cdot hour^{1}$, multiply the MET value by the body weight of the person in kg, and divide by 60 min per hour to obtain the energy expenditure in $kcal \cdot min^{-1}$. Example for a 65 kg person playing golf while carrying his clubs: 5 METS = 5 $kcal \cdot kg^{-1} \cdot hour^{1} \cdot$ (5 $kcal \cdot kg^{-1} \cdot hour^{-1} \times 65$ kg)/60 $min \cdot hr^{-1}$ = 5.4 $kcal \cdot min^{-1}$.

ing heart rate for a 30-year-old male of average cardiorespiratory fitness and a resting heart rate of 70 bpm would be calculated as follows:

(MHR − RHR) × Intensity percentage + RHR = training heart rate

(190 − 70) × 70% + 70 = 154 bpm

So this 30-year-old person of average fitness status would need to exercise at an intensity of 154 bpm, for 15–30 minutes, three to four days a week, to develop and maintain a healthy level of cardiorespiratory fitness and proper body composition. Figure 8.6 summarizes the training heart rate zone for people of varying ages.

Assessment of Training Heart Rate

Training heart rate can be assessed by three methods:[3, 14]

- The metabolic method (the use of METS or kcal · min⁻¹) (Tables 8.1, 8.2),

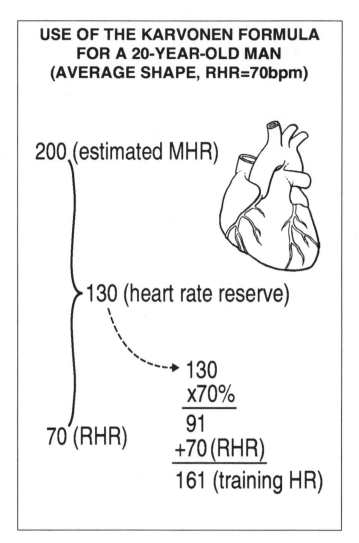

USE OF THE KARVONEN FORMULA FOR A 20-YEAR-OLD MAN (AVERAGE SHAPE, RHR=70bpm)

200 (estimated MHR)

130 (heart rate reserve)

$$\begin{array}{r} 130 \\ \times 70\% \\ \hline 91 \\ +70 \text{ (RHR)} \\ \hline 161 \text{ (training HR)} \end{array}$$

70 (RHR)

Figure 8.5 The Karvonen formula calculates the training heart rate using a percentage of the "heart rate reserve," which is the difference between the maximum and resting heart rates.

Table 8.3 Relation Between Percent Maximum Heart Rate, Percent $\dot{V}O_{2max}$, Heart Rate Reserve,* and RPE

Percent Maximum Heart Rate	Percent $\dot{V}O_{2max}$ or Percent Heart Rate Reserve	Rating of Perceived Exertion
54-67	30-49	10–11 Light
68-84	50-75	12–13 Moderate/ Somewhat hard
85-90	76-85	14–16
>90	>85	>16

*Resting heart rate of 70 used in calculations.

Table 8.4 Criteria for Choosing Intensity Percentile for Karvonen Formula

Criteria	Intensity Range
Low fitness status and/or desiring lower intensity, longer duration program	50%-65%
Average fitness status	70%-75%
Excellent fitness status and/or an an athlete desiring to improve fitness for competition	80%-90%

- Measurement of training heart rate by taking pulse for 10 sec, and
- The use of the Borg rating of perceived exertion scale.

To measure his training heart rate during exercise, the participant should stop every five minutes or so during the initial days of the exercise program and count his pulse. He should locate it quickly, within one to two seconds.[31]

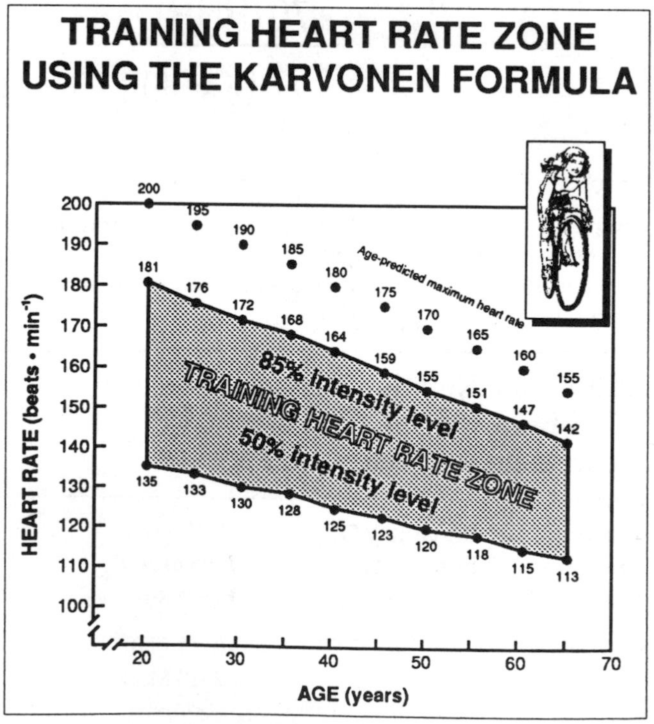

Figure 8.6 Maximal heart rates and the training heart rate zone for people of varying ages using the Karvonen formula. The resting heart rate is assumed to be 70 bpm.

The pulse is best counted using the carotid pulse; when properly done this method is safe and accurate[49] (although this is still being debated by some researchers).[50] When palpating the carotid pulse, two fingers of one hand should be placed lightly on one side of the neck adjacent to the larynx or voice box area. (See Figure 8.7.)

Beginners should compare resting heart rates taken by both carotid and radial palpations (the latter taken on the thumb side of the bottom of the wrist). If the carotid pulse rate is consistently lower than the radial count, it is advisable to use the radial count because some people's heart rates slow down when their carotid pulse is palpated, especially when excessive pressure is applied. However, during exercise the radial pulse is more difficult to locate because it is smaller and lies among the tendons of the hand and finger flexors. So if possible, it is best to learn to take the carotid pulse properly (as lightly as possible).

To take your pulse during an exercise bout, count for 10 seconds, and then multiply by six.[14] Table 8.5 gives 10-second pulse count values for varying age groups. These training heart rate values have been figured using the Karvonen formula, assuming average fitness status and resting heart rates of 70 bpm.

Various heart rate monitors have been developed to aid the exerciser in counting the pulse.[51] The best ones use chest-strap transmitters that wirelessly signal the heart rate to a monitor on the wrist. These types of heart rate monitors have been found to agree within one or two heart beats per minute with EKG recordings. (See Appendix C for a listing of companies that sell these monitors.) (See Figure 8.8.)

Although monitoring exercise heart rates with the 10-second carotid pulse count has been popular and generally satisfactory, errors do occur, arising from pulse counting mistakes, difficulty in finding the palpation site, and from taking too long.[52] Heart rate monitors are also expensive (about $250). In addition, some participants do not like to worry about taking their heart rates, or feel that it is unnecessary.

Borg has therefore developed a psychophysical scale for *ratings of perceived exertion* (RPE), which have been shown to have a high correlation with heart rates and other metabolic parameters.[53–57] Two types of scales are most common, the original RPE scale, and the revised ratio scale. (See Table 8.6.)

Borg's original RPE scale was convenient for indirectly tracking heart rate and oxygen consumption, which increase linearly with increased workload. This scale did not account for variables such as lactic acid and excessive ventilation, which rise in a non-linear fashion.

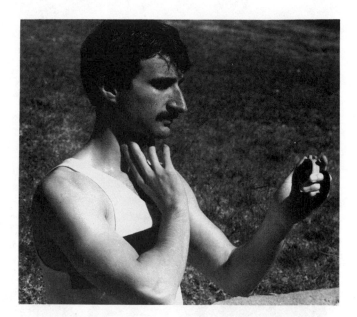

Figure 8.7 To measure the training heart rate during exercise, the participant should stop periodically and count his pulse using the carotid pulse.

Table 8.5 10-Second Pulse Count Values for Varying Ages Based on the Karvonen Formula for Average Fitness Status and RHR of 70 BPM

Age Range	10 Second Pulse Count
20-24	27
25-29	26
30-34	25-26
35-39	25
40-44	25
45-49	24-25
50-54	24
55-59	23-24
60-64	23
65-69	22-23

Consequently, the new, revised category scale with ratio properties was developed. The ratio scale uses verbal expressions, which are simple to understand and more accurately describe sensations such as aches and pain. Both scales have been used to rate effort signals from the entire body during exercise.

There is widespread consensus that perception of effort during aerobic exercise is determined by a combination of sensory inputs from local factors (sensations of strain and/or discomfort in the exercising muscles and joints) and central factors (sensations related to rapid heart beat and breathing rates).[55–57] The RPE scale is often used during graded exercise testing to indicate perceived exertion. (See Figure 8.9.)

Available evidence suggests that RPE independently or in combination with pulse rate can be effectively used for prescribing exercise intensity.[55] Indeed, an RPE of "somewhat hard or strong" may be more effective than heart rate in estimating the percentage of $\dot{V}O_{2max}$ necessary to elicit a training effect.

Trained and untrained men and women have been found to perceive the exercise intensity at the lactate threshold (intensity at which lactate begins to accumulate in the blood) as "somewhat hard or strong" (13 to 14 on the original RPE Borg scale, 4 on the newer, 10-point scale).[56] In other words, despite gender or state

Table 8.6

The original RPE scale is here contrasted with the newer revised ratio scale.

RPE (original scale)		New Rating Scale	
6		0	Nothing at all
7	Very, very light	0.5	Very, very weak
8		1	Very weak
9	Very light	2	Weak
10		3	Moderate
11	Fairly light	4	Somewhat strong
12		5	Strong
13	Somewhat hard	6	
14		7	Very strong
15	Hard	8	
16		9	
17	Very hard	10	Very, very strong
18			Maximal
19	Very, very hard		

Source: Borg GAV. Med Sci Sports Exerc 14:377-387, 1982. Noble B., Borg GAV, Jacobs I., Ceci R., Kaiser P. Med Sci Sports Exerc 15:523-528, 1983.

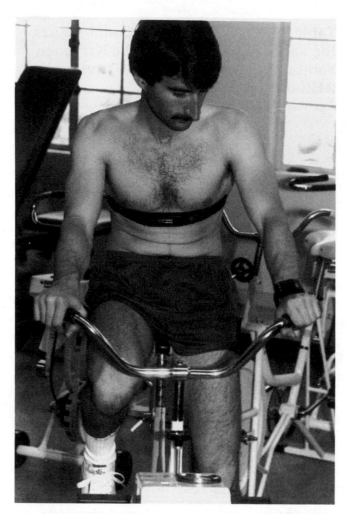

Figure 8.8 Heart rates can be accurately monitored using chest-strap transmitters that wirelessly signal the heart rate to a monitor on the wrist.

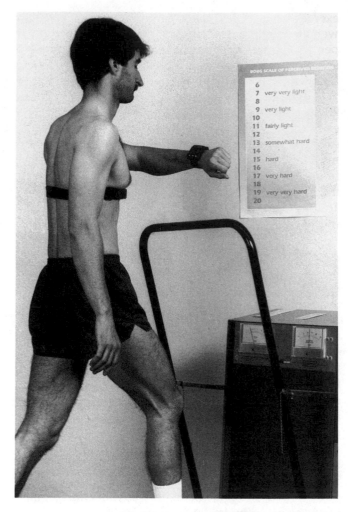

Figure 8.9 The RPE scale is commonly used during graded exercise testing to indicate progress toward maximal exertion.

of cardiorespiratory fitness, exercising at what exercisers characterized as the "somewhat hard" level correlates with exercising at the lactate threshold, a point that is recommended as the ideal exercise intensity.

When exercising at the "somewhat hard" level, one can think, talk intermittently with a partner, look around and enjoy the scenery, and engage in prolonged endurance activity. When exercising at a "very hard" level, the pulse is too high, and it is difficult to talk or exercise for prolonged periods of time. When exercising below "somewhat hard," the exercise stimulus is not adequate to develop cardiorespiratory endurance. The level of training intensity that can be tolerated depends on several factors, such as age, experience, fitness status, health, and motivation.[3, 14] Long distance runners are capable of running 26.2 mile marathons at 80–90 per-

cent $\dot{V}O_{2max}$, while most beginners can not tolerate this level for more than 5–15 minutes. For this reason, beginners should choose a lower intensity level, near 50–60 percent of heart rate reserve. The intensity percentage can gradually be increased during ensuing weeks of training.

Time

Time of exercise refers to the duration of time in minutes that the proper intensity level is maintained. Beginners should start with 10–20 minutes of aerobic activity, those in average shape should go for 20–30 minutes, and highly fit people can exercise for 30–60 minutes.[3, 14]

The most important factor in cardiorespiratory endurance improvement is persisting in the aerobic exercise bout until 200–400 kcal (or 4 kcal/kg of body weight) is expended (at an intensity level above 50 percent aerobic capacity or 50 percent heart rate reserve).[3, 30] This is thus a function of both time and intensity.

Dr. Michael Pollock conducted a study with men 20–35 years of age for 20 weeks[32] in three groups who exercised for different lengths of time. The intensity of exercise was standardized at 85–90 percent of maximum, and the men all participated three days per week. Improvement in $\dot{V}O_{2max}$ was then correlated with varying exercise durations. $\dot{V}O_{2max}$ improved 8.5 percent, 16.1 percent, and 16.8 percent with the 15-, 30-, and 45-minute duration groups, respectively.

Notice that there was little difference between the 30-minute and 45-minute groups. This study and others like it prompted Dr. Kenneth H. Cooper, as stated earlier, to say that exercise sessions lasting longer than 30 minutes are "for something other than fitness."[44] Research shows that injuries increase above this level, and overall coronary risk shows little further reduction.

It appears that the body responds fruitfully to four to five days per week of aerobic exercise with sessions lasting 20–30 minutes. Most of the psychological, cardiorespiratory, and heart disease benefits from physical activity appear to be positively affected within this exercise range.

The proper balance between exercise risks and benefits is hotly debated, and will be discussed in Section 4. In general, as with all lifestyle habits that promote health, moderation is the key. Too much of any good thing becomes a definite evil.

Mode of Exercise

If frequency, intensity, and duration of training are similar, and a minimum of 200–400 kcal are expended during the session, the training result appears to be independent of the *mode* of aerobic activity.[3, 14, 40] Activities should be selected on the basis of individual functional capacity, interests, time availability, equipment and facilities, and personal goals and objectives.[3] Any activity that uses large muscle groups, that can be maintained continuously, and is rhythmical and cardiorespiratory in nature, can be used. Common examples include running/jogging, walking/hiking, swimming, skating, bicycling, rowing, cross-country skiing, rope skipping, and various endurance sports. Table 8.7 lists some of the better modes for developing cardiorespiratory endurance.

One of the trends of the 1980s and 1990s is the movement toward participation in a variety of aerobic activities for enjoyment rather than intense concentration on one sport.[15] Multi-sports participation carries several benefits, including decreased risk of overuse injury, reduced boredom, increased compliance, and increased overall fitness.

Rating the Cardiorespiratory Exercises

Dr. Kenneth H. Cooper has rated the various cardiorespiratory exercises.[44] Using physical fitness criteria, the top five physical activities, listed in descending order of exercise value, are estimated by Dr. Cooper to be as follows:[44]

- **Cross-country skiing:** Involves both upper and lower body muscles, and therefore gives the greatest aerobic benefit. Additional overload factors include the high altitude, cold weather, and heavier clothing.

- **Swimming:** This exercise also involves both the upper and lower body muscles, providing more of a total conditioning effect than many other sports. Swimmers also tend to have fewer injury problems because of less pressure on the bones and joints. For this reason swimmers can put in more exercise time than runners.

- **Jogging/running:** The level of skill required and the amount of equipment is minimal. In addition, running is the most convenient activity—there's always an available road or path for running. But a significant proportion of runners, especially those who do not warm-up properly and who are overzealous about going long distances, are injured, especially in the knees, feet, and ankles. It is very important to progress gradually in a running program, realizing that more than 15 miles a week is not needed for health and fitness.

- **Outdoor cycling:** This exercise causes less trauma to the joints and muscles than running, because the weight is borne on the bicycle seat. But high speeds with the bicycle are needed for a training effect, and bicycle safety on the roads becomes a problem.

- **Brisk walking:** The great advantage of walking is that it can be done anywhere by anyone, regardless of age or sex. The major disadvantage is that more time is required to gain the same aerobic benefit from walking as from running. When walking is conducted in hilly terrain, or with a backpack, the benefits rise sharply.

Table 8.7 Activities that Rate High in Cardiorespiratory Benefits and Their Approximate Energy Requirements

Summarized are some of the better cardiovascular-respiratory exercises and the number of Kcal expended per hour of the exercise. An important concept is to select several of these activities that are enjoyable, and to use them in such a way that scheduled exercise sessions are looked forward to, not dreaded.

Caloric consumption is based on a 150 lb. person. There is a 10% increase in caloric consumption for each 15 lbs. over this weight and a 10% decrease for each 15 lbs. under.

Activity	Kcal Per Hour	Activity	Kcal Per Hour
Badminton, competitive singles	480	Skating, ice or roller, rapid	700
Basketball	360–660	Skiing, downhill, vigorous	600
Bicycling		Skiing, cross-country	
10 mph	420	2.5 mph	560
11 mph	480	4 mph	600
12 mph	600	5 mph	700
13 mph	660	8 mph	1,020
Calisthenics, heavy	600	Swimming, 25–50 yards per min.	360–750
Handball, competitive	660	Walking	
Rope skipping, vigorous	800	Level road, 4 mph (fast)	420
Rowing machine	840	Upstairs	600–1,080
Running		Uphill, 3.5 mph	480–900
5 mph	600	Gardening, much lifting, stooping, digging	500
6 mph	750	Mowing, pushing hand mower	450
7 mph	870	Sawing hardwood	600
8 mph	1,020	Shoveling, heavy	660
9 mph	1,130	Wood chopping	560
10 mph	1,285		

Source: Wynder EL. The Book of Health: The American Health Foundation. New York: Franklin Watts, Inc., 1981. Used with permission.

Dr. Cooper has developed an "aerobics point" system to help participants choose their amounts and kinds of exercises.[44] (The reader is referred to Cooper's excellent series of books for a description.) A point system is not really needed, however; the system described within this chapter, using frequency, time, and intensity, is simpler and more practical.

Brisk Walking

As mentioned earlier, moderate-intensity activities of longer duration are being promoted more and more by fitness leaders, because these types of activities are more acceptable to the masses, increasing the likeli-hood of a permanent change in lifestyle.[15] Also, the musculoskeletal risk is less, and studies show that health benefits are still realized, especially when total energy expenditure averages at least 1000 kcal per week.[2-11]

Brisk walking for exercise is now one of the fastest growing activities in the United States. (See Chapter 1.) Several recent studies are demonstrating that from a public health viewpoint, brisk walking is probably the best overall exercise for the majority of American adults.[10,11,58-61] Walking has been found to have a higher compliance rate than other physical activities because it can easily be incorporated into a busy time schedule, does not require any special skills, equipment, or facility, is companionable, and is much less apt to cause injuries.[10]

When you run, the forces between the ground and your feet are normally 2.5–3.0 times your body weight, whereas when you walk, they are never more than 1.25 times your body weight. In addition, there is less foot pronation during walking.[11]

We need to provide an opportunity for the 80 percent of Americans who do not exercise appropriately to become involved. Two factors are critical in adherence—convenience and enjoyability—and brisk walking fits the bill for many.

Several studies have shown that brisk walking can be used to improve aerobic capacity.[58–61] In most walking studies, a walking pace equal to 60 percent $\dot{V}O_{2max}$ has been found to increase the $\dot{V}O_{2max}$ of previously sedentary adults 10 to 20 percent within 5 to 20 weeks.[58, 60, 61] In one study of people ages 30–69, more than 90 percent of the women and 67 percent of the men were able to reach the training zone by walking.[59] With visual feedback from heart rate monitors, all participants with high $\dot{V}O_{2max}$ values were able to maintain appropriate training heart rates if the walking pace was appropriately adjusted.[59] The researchers concluded that fast walking offers an adequate aerobic training stimulus for nearly all adults. The $\dot{V}O_{2max}$ of competitive race walkers averages 63 ml · kg^{-1} · min^{-1}, which is an excellent cardiorespiratory fitness level.[11]

While walking burns fewer calories than running, its energy cost can be increased by carrying weights. Many recent studies have verified that hand/wrist weights increase the energy expenditure of walking significantly more than ankle weights.[62–68] The use of 3-pound hand/wrist weights increases the oxygen cost of walking by 1 MET, with an associated 7–13 beat per minute increase in exercise heart rate.[65, 67] The hand/wrist weights also tend to improve upper body muscle endurance.

The Rockport Company has been active in the promotion and development of walking programs, equipment, and fitness tests. Brochures and a newsletter are available by writing: The Rockport Company, 72 Howe Street, Marlboro, Massachusetts 01752.

Aerobic Dance

Aerobic dance traces its origins to Jacki Sorenson, the wife of a naval pilot, who began conducting exercise classes at a U.S. Navy base in Puerto Rico in 1969.[69] The original aerobic dance programs consisted of an eclectic combination of dance forms, including ballet, modern jazz, disco, and folk, as well as calisthenic-type exercises.

More recent innovations include water aerobics (done in a swimming pool), non-impact or low-impact aerobics (one foot on the ground at all times), specific dance aerobics, and "assisted" aerobics with weights on the wrists and/or ankles.

Several studies have now shown that when aerobic dancers follow the F.I.T. criteria, aerobic dancing is similar to other aerobic activities in improving the cardiorespiratory system.[69–75] Aerobic dancing also builds the endurance of upper body muscles, enhancing musculoskeletal fitness.

One cause of concern for the aerobic dance movement has been the alarming number of reported injuries.[69] This will be discussed in greater detail in Chapter 15. *Low-impact aerobics* has been growing in popularity to help reduce the number of injuries.[76] At least one foot is touching the floor throughout the aerobic portion. Movements are not ballistic, but focus on large upper body movements, combined with leg kicks and high-powered steps and lunges. However, to achieve appropriate intensity, low-impact aerobics must be performed at a high rate.[76] Ankle and wrist weights are often used to increase the intensity of exercise.

Aerobic dance in the water uses many of the same upper body movements practiced on the aerobic dance floor, but without the associated stress on the legs and feet.[77] These *"aquasize"* programs are especially beneficial for the obese, elderly, and those with physical disabilities.

The International Dance-Exercise Association (*IDEA*) Foundation has published a manual and provides certification standards designed to foster a high degree of professionalism within the dance-exercise industry. The manual provides the basic information an instructor needs to conduct classes.[73]

Racquet Sports

Many people just do not like the structure and monotony of the continuous aerobic exercises like running, swimming, and cycling. A large number have found *racquet sports* like racquetball, squash, and tennis to be more attractive. The competitive and social aspects of these sports make them enjoyable for many, and help promote long-lasting compliance.

When played at appropriate intensity levels, racquet sports provide an adequate cardiorespiratory stimulus.[78–81] (See Figure 8.10.) Racquetball participants of intermediate ability have expended an average of 600 kcal per hour, playing at 51 percent $\dot{V}O_{2max}$.[80] Players of intermediate ability average 61 percent of their heart rate reserve during singles matches, but only 33 percent playing doubles.[81]

Such competitive activities, however, are not recommended by the American College of Sports Medi-

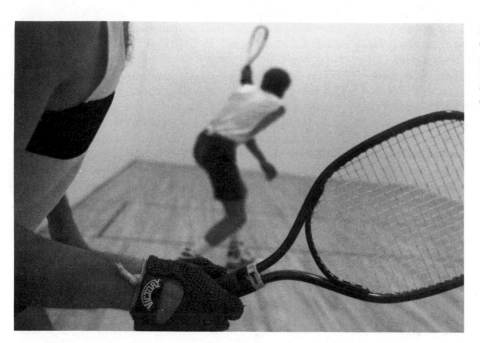

Figure 8.10 Racquetball participants of intermediate ability have been found to expend an average of 600 kcal per hour of play, which provides an adequate stimulus for cardiorespiratory improvement.

cine for previously sedentary or high-risk people until they have prepared themselves with an initial 6–10-week conditioning program.[3]

Other Modes of Activity

Some people find vigorous work activities more satisfying. Tables 8.2 and 8.7 show that various occupational activities like wood chopping, heavy shoveling and gardening, using a hand mower for mowing grass, or sawing hardwood can lead to an energy expenditure of close to 300 kcal in 30 minutes (the recommended amount). In addition, the upper body is given a good workout along with the heart and lungs (and a direct, purposeful task is accomplished).

Some have wondered if *circuit weight training programs,* which involve 8–12 repetitions with various weight machines at 7–14 stations while moving quickly from one station to the next, develop cardiorespiratory endurance. Most studies have concluded that there is little or no cardiorespiratory improvement (at most a 5 percent in $\dot{V}O_{2max}$) with such regimens.[82–86] Circuit weight lifting tends to elevate the heart rate substantially, with average heart rates of 150 (80 percent of maximum heart rate) reported.[84] However, actual oxygen uptake is relatively low—about 40 percent of $\dot{V}O_{2max}$. The heavy muscle exertion increases the heart rate through sympathetic nervous system stimulation, but because the involved muscle mass is small, the blood flow and oxygen uptake is low.

Such weight lifting circuits, however, should not be confused with circuit training systems like the *Parcourse,* which emphasize running between stations which each call for various calisthenics or weight lifting maneuvers. Outdoor circuit training systems of this sort have been shown to burn 400 kcal in 30 min, and contribute to high cardiorespiratory endurance improvement.[87]

For some, the convenience of indoor aerobic exercise equipment is important, and there is a wide variety of such equipment available today. (See Appendix C for a list of equipment, including company addresses.) However, expensive indoor equipment is not needed for a good aerobic workout. Such forms of indoor, home exercise as rope skipping, stationary running, or aerobic calisthenics to music have all been shown to be beneficial to the cardiorespiratory system.[44, 88, 89]

Some experts predict that more and more people will choose home exercise because it is the most convenient and practical way to obtain needed exercise. Because of this, there is a big push by equipment suppliers for Americans to purchase expensive indoor exercise equipment. Potential buyers should consider carefully before making the investment.

There are certainly good reasons for preferring home to outdoor exercise—including unpleasant weather, environmental pollution, darkness, and safety concerns. Home exercise equipment can help make exercising enjoyable and effective. The concern is that such devices will quickly lose their appeal and end up cluttering the garage.

Popular equipment includes stationary bicycles, rowing machines, motorized treadmills, and simulated cross-country skiing machines. (See Appendix C.) The rowing machine and cross-country skiing equipment are especially valuable, because they give the entire body a workout along with the cardiorespiratory system.[90–93]

Rate of Progression

Appropriate progression in an exercise conditioning program depends on a person's fitness status, health status, age, needs or goals, family support, and many other factors.[3] The American College of Sports Medicine defines three progression stages for the aerobic phase of the exercise prescription:

- **Initial Conditioning Stage:** This stage typically lasts 4–6 weeks, but should depend on the adaptation of the participant to the program. ACSM suggests that exercise intensity be 1 MET lower than the estimated 50–80 percent $\dot{V}O_{2max}$, to help avoid muscle soreness, injury, discomfort, and discouragement. It is always best to be very conservative when starting an exercise program, and then gradually progress. Participants can start at 12 minutes, and slowly work up to 20 minutes of exercise during this stage.

- **Improvement Conditioning Stage:** This stage usually lasts 12–20 weeks, and the rate of progression is more rapid. The exercise intensity is increased to 50–80 percent of $\dot{V}O_{2max}$, and the duration of exercise can be increased every two to three weeks. The degree and frequency of progression during this stage depend largely on the age of the participant. For each decade of life after age 30, it takes approximately one week longer for the body to adapt to a higher conditioning stimulus.[3] During this stage, participants can build from 20 minutes up to 30 minutes per session. All should strive to burn 300 kcal per session (usually accomplished in 30 minutes), and 1000 kcal per week (at least three sessions per week).

- **Maintenance Conditioning Stage:** Once the desired level of fitness is reached, the person enters the maintenance stage of the exercise program. This stage usually begins 6 months after the start of training and continues on a regular, long-term basis (lifetime commitment). Here particularly, it is important to select aerobic exercises you find enjoyable.[3]

Systems of Cardiorespiratory Training

There are several systems of cardiorespiratory training.[29, 94]

- **Continuous Training:** This involves continuous exercise like jogging, swimming, walking, or cycling, at "somewhat hard to hard" intensities without rest intervals. The prescribed exercise intensity is maintained consistently throughout the exercise session.

- **Interval Training:** *Interval training* involves a repeated series of exercise work bouts interspersed with rest periods. Higher intensities can be used during the exercise to overload the cardiorespiratory system because the exercise is discontinuous. A miler training for competition, for example, could use an interval regimen where he runs very fast for one lap (440 yards), then walks one lap, repeating this cycle 5–20 times. In time, the "rest" interval of walking can gradually be increased in intensity, until the miler can run at a high intensity for four full laps.

  Interval training is necessary for athletes who wish to compete.[94] A good endurance base (at least 1–2 months of regular aerobic training) and a 10-minute warm-up are prerequisites to interval training. In addition, the first interval training sessions should be moderate, with gradual transitions to higher intensity levels. Interval sessions should not number more than one or two per week. Above all, never run hard anaerobic workouts on consecutive days.

- **Fartlek Training:** *Fartlek training* is like interval training, but it is a free form of training done out on trails or roads. People who abhor track running can do Fartlek training on roads, golf courses, or trails. The exercise-rest cycle is not systematic or precisely timed and measured, but is based on the feelings of the participant.

- **Circuit Training:** As noted previously, *circuit training* involves 10–20 stations of varying calisthenic and weight lifting exercises interspersed with running. The Parcourse is a good example.

The Question of Supervision

- **Unsupervised Exercise Programs:** Asymptomatic participants with $\dot{V}O_{2max}$ values of 8 METS or more can usually exercise safely in an unsupervised conditioning program.[3] Participant safety and compliance can be improved by individualizing the exercise prescription. Some people find it more enjoyable to exercise alone at home; some like the group support of a community exercise class.

- **Supervised Exercise Programs:** Exercise should be supervised for asymptomatic people with $\dot{V}O_{2max}$ values of less than 8 METS, participants with known heart disease risk factors, and for heart disease patients.[3] These programs should be under the combined guidance of a physician and an exercise program director or exercise specialist (ACSM certified). Direct supervision of each session by a physician is not required, but the attendance of qualified personnel is mandatory. Several types of supervised exercise programs exist, including inpatient (in-hospital programs for heart disease patients), outpatient (continuation of inpatient after hospital discharge), home, and community (for people at 5 METS capacity or above).

Warm-Down

The purpose of the *warm-down* (cool-down) is to slowly decrease the pulse rate that has been elevated during the aerobic phase. This is effectively and safely done by keeping the feet and legs moving, by walking, light jogging, slow swimming, or bicycling. In other words, the warm-down is the warm-up in reverse.

There are at least three important physiological reasons for it:[95, 96]

- By moving during recovery for about 5 minutes (more or less, depending on fitness status, state of fatigue, and environmental factors), muscle and blood lactic acid levels decrease more rapidly than if one completely rests. In other words, moving during the warm-down promotes faster recovery from fatigue.

- Mild activity following heavy aerobic exercise keeps the leg muscle "pumps" going and thus prevents the blood from pooling in the legs. The leg muscles promote venous return by the "milking" action of the contraction and relaxation cycle. Preventing the pooling of the blood reduces the possibility of delayed muscular stiffness, and also reduces any tendency toward fainting and dizziness.

- Following very hard aerobic exercise, there is an increase of catecholamines in the blood. Among high-risk people, this can adversely affect the heart, causing cardiac irregularities.[44, 96] The majority of severe cardiac irregularities that can be

dangerous appear to occur following exercise, not during it. Although such exercise-related irregularities of the heart are relatively rare, a careful warm-down is only prudent.

Musculoskeletal Conditioning

Flexibility Exercises

The major reason for performing flexibility exercises after the aerobic phase is to more safely and effectively stretch the warm muscle groups and joints that were involved in the aerobic exercise.[23, 26] Appendix D contains pictures and descriptions of eight common flexibility exercises.

One study of 238 athletes participating in a wide variety of sports showed that nearly all the athletes pursued a stretching program of some kind, but their practices varied greatly.[97] Only 39 percent of the athletes stretched daily, 37 percent stretched before activity, and 33 percent stretched both before and after exercise. In the author's study of 2310 Los Angeles Marathon runners, 26 percent reported that they usually didn't stretch, with 10 percent stretching after running, 24 percent before, and 40 percent both before and after running. (See Figure 8.11.)

It is commonly accepted that flexibility is an important factor in reducing the potential for injury and in improving performance, and serves as an important component of overall physical fitness.

The literature, however, contains conflicting reports about the relationship between injury and flexibility.[97-99] Although neglect of stretching is cause for concern, there is little evidence to support the concept that stretching helps prevent injury. In one study of 181 soccer players, no correlation was found between past injuries and existing muscle tightness.[98] In another study, gymnasts with low back pain had greater toe-touching ability than those without symptoms.[99]

Four types of stretching techniques have been developed by athletes, dancers, and physical therapists.[26, 100-105] *Ballistic* methods, commonly referred to as "bouncing" stretches, use the momentum of the moving body segment to produce the stretch. Slow movements often used by dancers are a second method, in which muscle stretching occurs as the movement progresses gradually from one body position to another and then smoothly returns to the starting point. However, the two other techniques—*static stretching* and

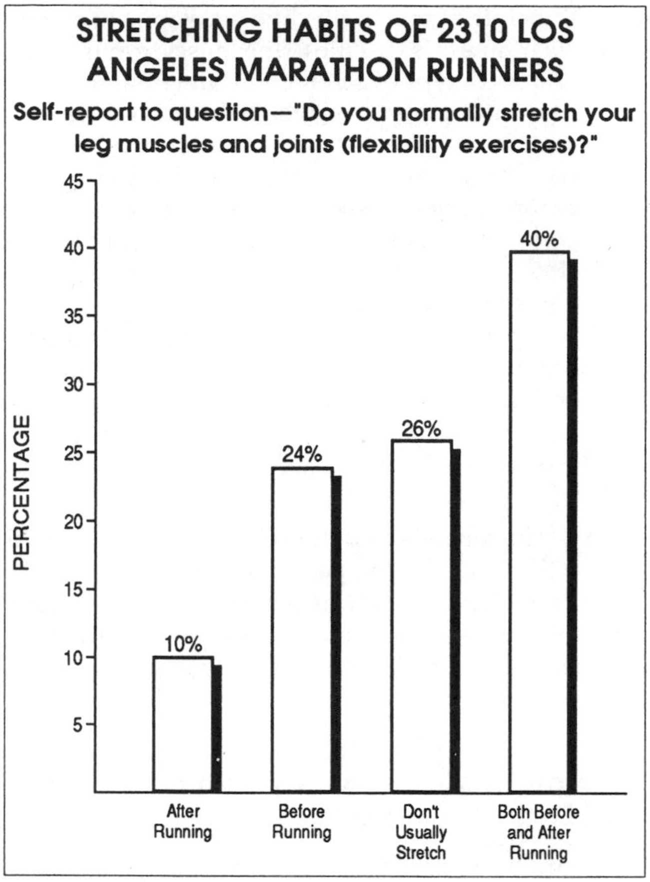

STRETCHING HABITS OF 2310 LOS ANGELES MARATHON RUNNERS

Self-report to question—"Do you normally stretch your leg muscles and joints (flexibility exercises)?"

Figure 8.11 Stretching habits in marathon runners vary widely. *Source:* Nieman DC, Johansen LM, Lee JW. Training Habits in Los Angeles Marathon Runners. (Unpublished data.)

proprioceptive neuromuscular faciliation—are considered best for developing flexibility.

Static Stretching

Static stretching involves slowly applying stretch to the muscle, and then holding it in a lengthened position for a period of 10–30 seconds.[104] During this easy, held stretch, one relaxes, focusing attention on the muscles being stretched. The feeling of slight tension in the stretching muscle should slowly subside. Then one stretches a bit further, until the mild tension is again felt (never any pain), and held for 30–60 seconds. The tension should again slowly subside. One should be breathing easily, and feel relaxed.

Each major joint and muscle group of the body should be stretched. Appendix D contains pictures of eight common static stretching exercises.

Proprioceptive Neuromuscular Facilitation

Studies have shown that proprioceptive neuromuscular facilitation (PNF) flexibility techniques are more effective than conventional stretching methods for increasing joint range of motion.[100-103] Muscle relaxation using PNF is first induced by a contraction of the muscle to be stretched, followed by a static stretching of the same muscle group. There are two ways to do PNF:

- **Contract-relax:** An isometric contraction of the muscle group being stretched precedes the slow, static stretching (relaxation) of the same muscle group. Theoretically, the isometric contraction of the muscles to be stretched induces a reflex relaxation.

- **Contract-relax with agonist contraction:** This is the same as the contract-relax technique, except that at the same time the muscle is stretched, the opposing muscle group is submaximally contracted. This is supposed to facilitate even more relaxation in the stretched muscles.

PNF is usually done with a partner. The following steps are recommended:

- First stretch the muscle group by moving the joint to the end of its range of motion.

- Next, have a partner provide resistance as the same muscle group is statically contracted (for example, in a sit-and-reach stretch, after the person stretching has extended his reach forward, the partner will push on his back as he strives to lean back).

- Finally, have the partner apply pressure to aid in a slow, static stretch of the muscle group, while the person stretching contracts the opposing muscle group (for example, in the sit-and-reach, the partner pushes down on the person's back while he tries to relax the hamstrings and contract his quadriceps).

PNF appears to produce the largest gains in flexibility.[100] However, it is associated with more pain and muscle stiffness, requires a partner, and takes more time. For these reasons, the static stretching method is often the most practical one. Risk of injury and pain is low with static stretching, and it requires little time and assistance.

Muscular Strength and Endurance Exercises

The fifth and final stage of the comprehensive or "total" fitness workout involves the development of muscular strength and endurance. The American College of Sports Medicine recommends that this stage include a minimum of one set of eight to twelve repetitions of eight to ten different exercises that condition all of the major muscle groups at least twice per week.[40] Dr. Kenneth H. Cooper, who suggests that this stage last a minimum of 10 minutes, advises that muscular strength and endurance exercises follow the aerobic session.[44] Such exercise before the aerobic session can create an oxygen debt, leading to fatigue before the start of the important cardiorespiratory endurance stage. In addition, the aerobic phase warms up the muscles, allowing weight training to take place more safely. It is also common to alternate days of aerobic training with musculoskeletal training.

The American College of Sports Medicine[3] warns that strength exercise increases systemic blood pressure. This increases the work of the heart, and its requirement for oxygen. Heavy lifts can cause a reduction in venous return, and result in decreased blood flow to the heart and brain (*Valsalva's maneuver*).

Therefore, maximal muscular tensions should be discouraged for those at risk for cardiovascular disease. High risk patients should use dynamic exercises utilizing low-resistance. Exhalation on effort should be encouraged. Warm-up and warm-down should surround the weight lifting session, with care to maintain correct body position and utilize proper weight lifting techniques.

Principles of Weight Training

There are three major principles of weight training:[95, 106–109]

- **Overload principle:** Strength and endurance development is based on what is known as the overload principle. This states that the strength, endurance, and size of a muscle will increase only when the muscle performs for a given period of time at its maximal strength and endurance capacity (against workloads that are above those normally encountered). Muscle endurance and strength will only improve when brought to a state of fatigue.
- **Progressive resistance principle:** The resistance (pounds of weight) against which the muscle works should be increased periodically as gains in strength and endurance are made, until the desired state is achieved.

- **Principle of specificity:** The development of muscular fitness is specific to the muscle group that is exercised, type of contraction, and training intensity. In other words, weight-resistance training appears to be motor-skill specific. Thus, weight-training programs should exercise the muscle groups actually used in the sport or activity the person is training for, and should simulate as closely as possible the movement patterns involved in that activity.

Research has shown that training should be conducted at high speeds, because gains in strength and endurance are specific to the speed trained at, with maximal gains for activities at velocities equal to or slower, but not faster than the training velocity.

The movement pattern involved in the sports skill for which the person is training should be simulated as closely as possible during the training sessions. The maximal number of contractions should be 8–15, with three sets of each exercise used.

Systems of Muscular Strength and Endurance Training

There are three classifications of muscle contractions: *isometric, isotonic (concentric),* and *isotonic (eccentric).*

Isometric

In isometrics, the muscle group contracts against a fixed, immovable resistance. (See Figure 8.12.) For example, the hands could be placed under a desk while sitting in a chair with arms at a 90 degree angle. The biceps are then contracted, but there is no movement as the hands attempt to push up on the heavy desk.

Maximum gains in strength appear to come from 5–10, six-second isometric contractions at 100 percent of maximal strength, repeated at three different points in the full range of motion. Isometric exercises are easy to perform, can be done nearly anywhere, and require little time or expense. But it is important to do each exercise at several different angles for each joint, because strength gain is specific to the angle at which the isometric exercise is performed.

Isotonic

Traditionally, isotonic training has involved the use of weights in the form of barbells, dumbbells, and pulleys, or heavy calisthenics such as push-ups, sit-ups, leg squats, etc. Appendix D summarizes some of the

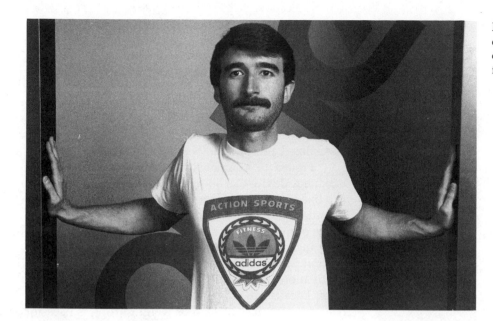

Figure 8.12 In isometric muscle contractions, the muscle group contracts without shortening against a fixed, immovable resistance.

some of the more common calisthenics used to develop muscular endurance and strength.

Isotonic muscular contractions take two forms: concentric, or muscle contraction with shortening, and eccentric, or muscular contraction with lengthening. For example, when a heavy weight is lowered, there is eccentric muscle contraction resisting the downward movement of the weight. Running downhill involves eccentric muscle contraction.

A muscle can maximally produce 40 percent more tension eccentrically than concentrically. However, training with eccentric contractions produces no greater increases in strength than isotonic programs. The major problem with eccentric contraction is its association with muscle soreness. Thus will be discussed in more detail in Chapter 15. (See Figure 8.13.)

Isotonic muscle movement usually centers around *sets* and *repetitions*. A repetition is defined as one particular weight lifting or calisthenic movement, with a set defined as a certain number of these repetitions. *One repetition maximum* (1-RM) is defined as the maximal load a muscle or muscle group can lift just once. Six-repetitions maximum (6-RM), for example, is the greatest amount of weight that can be lifted six times.

The best weight lifting system for increasing both muscular strength and endurance is the 3-set, 6–8 repetitions maximum system.[106–109] In this system, a weight is chosen that can only be lifted 6–8 times, and then the sequence is repeated two more times with three minutes rest in between. Weight lifting systems that use more repetitions do not increase muscular strength as

much, but do tend to improve muscular endurance a bit more. There are many other types of muscle training programs. These are summarized in Table 8.8.[106]

The isotonic weight-training program should be planned for every other day. Chronic fatigue can develop from daily training. Some athletes will focus on the upper body one day, and then the lower body the next, allowing 48 hours for exercised muscle groups to recover.

When beginning a weight-training program, it is important to start easy. A 1-set, 10 RM program with 8–10 different exercises, 2–3 times per week is good for beginners. This can help avoid the muscle soreness that will lead to noncompliance.

Bodybuilding is a unique activity in which competitors work to develop the mass, definition, and symmetry of their muscles, rather than the strength, skill, or endurance required for traditional athletic events.[108] In one study of 31 competitive bodybuilders (15 female, 16 male) who were free of steroids, the average was four to six 90-minute weight-training workouts each week. Particular muscle groups were generally exercised twice a week, using several different exercises for each muscle group. Each exercise was performed to the point of muscle failure, using a resistance that achieved this effect with from 8 to 15 repetitions. Exercises were repeated for 5 to 8 sets.

There was no regular aerobic training except during the weeks prior to competition, when 12 of the women and 3 of the men cycled to increase caloric expenditure. Women bodybuilders averaged 14.4 percent body fat,

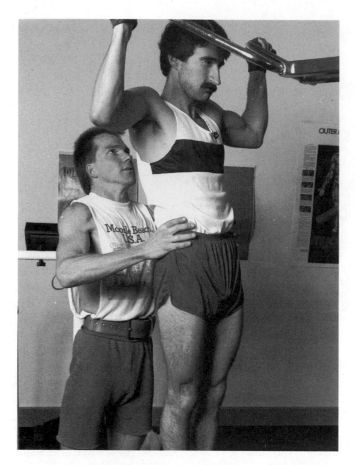

Figure 8.13 Eccentric muscle contractions involve muscle lengthening as it develops tension. For example, if at the top of a pull-up, a partner pulls you down as you attempt to resist the downward action, muscle eccentric contraction will take place. Eccentric muscle contraction is associated with muscle soreness.

and men 7.2 percent. Women were capable of bench pressing 111 pounds (92 percent of body weight), and men 322 pounds (193 percent body weight). Flexibility was excellent. $\dot{V}O_{2max}$ averaged 39.5 ml $\cdot$ kg^{-1} $\cdot$ min^{-1} for the women and 46.1 ml $\cdot$ kg^{-1} $\cdot$ min^{-1} for the men.

Table 8.9 summarizes some of the more common weight lifting exercises, with a description of technique, overall benefits, and the specific muscle groups improved. Consult Appendix E for identification of the involved muscles.

Isokinetic

This type of muscular training is relatively new. In all joint motion, the muscles controlling the movement have points at which strength is greater, and points where it is less. For example, the greatest tension or strength of the elbow flexors (biceps, brachialis) is at 120°, with the least tension and strength at 30°. In true isokinetic exercise, the resistance adjusts so that it is exactly matched to the force applied by the muscle throughout the full range of joint motion. This means that the muscle can apply maximal tension during the entire lift. This is accomplished by controlling the speed of the movement (iso = same, kinetic = motion) with specialized equipment. (See Figure 8.19.)

Figure 8.20 demonstrates use of the *Cybex II*, an isokinetic device that allows the exercising limb to work at a fixed speed with a variable resistance that is totally accommodating to the individual throughout the entire range of motion.[107]

In comparing the different systems, there are several advantages and disadvantages with each.[107] Motivation is generally superior with isotonic exercises, because they are self-testing in nature. Also, if heavy calisthenics instead of weight lifting is used for isotonic training, no special equipment is needed. (See Appendix D.) Isometrics can also be performed without equipment and done anywhere. But gains in strength are joint-angle specific (within 20°), and care must be taken to exercise at several angles. As for isokinetics, studies show that muscular strength and endurance development is somewhat better with such programs, but the specialized, expensive equipment makes this type of training impractical for most.

It should be noted that Nautilus, Hydra-fitness, and similar equipment are not isokinetic in concept (fixed speed, accommodating resistance), but actually isotonic equipment that attempts imperfectly to vary the resistance using cam devices, etc., working around the weak points of each lift.

The Problem of Compliance

As outlined in Chapter 1, only 28 percent of the U.S. adult population are considered physically active. Although exercise is generally regarded as health-promoting in developed nations, available estimates from North America, Europe, and Australia indicate that 30–60 percent of their populations can be defined as sedentary. In the United States, 60 percent have been found to be either sedentary or irregularly active.

At the worksite, considered one of the most promising places for adults to obtain regular exercise, only 20 percent of eligible workers will join exercise programs, and up to 50 percent of them will drop out of the program over the first 6–12 months.[110] In supervised exercise programs, a dropout or noncompliance rate near 50 percent is typical over a 3–12 month period.

Table 8.8 Systems of Resistance Training

1. Single Set System	Each weight lifting exercise is performed for one set, 8-12 RM. Although improvement is not as good as with a multiple set system, this system may be appropriate for those with little time to dedicate to weight training.
2. Multiple Set System	A minimum of three sets, 4-6 RM, are performed.
3. Light-to-Heavy System	As the name implies, the light-to-heavy system entails progressing from light to heavy resistances. A set of 3-5 repetitions are performed with a relatively light weight. Five pounds are then added to the bar and another set, 3-5 reps are performed. This is continued until only one repetition can be executed.
4. Heavy-to-Light System	This is a reversal of the light-to-heavy system. The research suggests that this produces better strength gains than the light-to-heavy system.
5. The Triangle Program	This consists of the light-to-heavy system followed immediately by the heavy-to-light system. It is used by many power lifters.
6. Super Set System	This is used by bodybuilders. Two types are used. In one, multiple sets of two exercises for the same body part but opposing muscle groups (biceps vs triceps, for example) are performed without any rest in-between. The second type of super setting uses one set of several exercises in rapid succession for the same muscle group or body part. Both types of super setting involve many sets of 8-10 reps, with little or no rest between sets and/or exercises.
7. Circuit Program	Circuit programs consist of a series of resistance-training exercises performed one after the other with minimal rest (15-30 seconds) between exercises. Approximately 10-15 reps of each exercise are performed per circuit, at a resistance of 40-60% RM. Cardiorespiratory endurance can increase about 5% with such programs.
8. Split Routine System	Many body builders use a split routine system. Body builders like to perform many sets and many types of exercises for each body part to cause hypertrophy. This is a time-consuming process, and not all parts of the body can be exercised in a single session. A typical split routine system may entail the training of arms, legs and abdomen on Monday, Wednesday, and Friday, and chest, shoulders, and back on Tuesday, Thursday, and Sunday.

Source: Fleck SJ, Kraemer WJ. Designing Resistance Training Programs. Champaign, IL: Human Kinetics Publishers, 1987.

Large numbers of participants leave exercise programs within the first few weeks.[111-112]

Even in well-structured programs for cardiac patients, 30–70 percent of them will drop out, the majority within the first 3 months.[111] This is remarkable in light of the perceived benefits of exercise, especially for these patients who stand to benefit the most.

As discussed in Chapter 7, exercise patterns must be maintained to realize benefits.[113] The chronic adaptations to exercise are lost within 4–8 weeks following termination of regular exercise. Former college varsity athletes have been found to be just as likely as nonathletes to have coronary disease unless they continued regular exercise habits after college sports participation.[114]

National goals call for participation in regular aerobic exercise by 90 percent of the youth and 60 percent of adults by 1990.[115] To achieve these goals, much work needs to be done in creating an environment to help Americans motivate themselves to engage in regular exercise.

Past promotional efforts to increase physical activity have been frustrated by a poor understanding of the factors that motivate participation in exercise.[111, 112, 116] Table 8.10 summarizes current understanding of some of these factors, with much more research needed to refine this listing. Based on available evidence, blue collar workers, low socioeconomic and low education groups, middle age groups, and people with high risk for coronary heart disease, particularly smokers, are relatively inactive in leisure time, and are unlikely to participate in supervised exercise programs.

It is now clear that promotions designed to increase leisure physical activity and exercise that do not address behavioral skills and environments which enable and reinforce participation cannot expect to be successful.[111-112] Campaigns that focus solely on knowledge and information alone will have little influence

Table 8.9 Common Weight Lifting Exercises and Description

1. Bench Press (see Figure 8.14):	Lie down on the bench with shoulders just in back of the bar. Space the hands evenly on the bar. Let the bar down to the chest, and then forcefully push the bar back up to a straight arm position. Breathe in as the bar is lowered, and exhale as you raise the bar.
	Overall benefit: Builds up the front of the chest and back of upper arms.
	Muscle involved: Forearm extensors (triceps), arm flexors (pectoralis major, anterior deltoid).
2. Lat Pull (see Figure 8.15)	Kneel directly below the handle with your hands grasping it, arms straight. Forcefully pull the bar down behind the head.
	Overall benefit: Develops the "lats," which helps give the back the "V-shaped look."
	Muscle involved: Forearm flexors (biceps brachii, brachialis); arm extensors and adductors (latissimus dorsi, posterior deltoid, pectoralis major, teres major).
3. Two Arm Curl (see Figure 8.16)	Grasp the bar with palms up and away from body. Standing straight, forcefully raise hands to chest. Try not to arch the lower back or let the elbows drive backwards during the lift.
	Overall benefit: Develops the biceps, a muscle important for carrying objects when arms are bent at a 90-degree angle.
	Muscle involved: Forearm flexors (biceps brachii, brachialis).
4. Military Press (see Figure 8.17)	Grasp the bar with hands shoulder-width apart, arms down, and palms toward body. Raise the bar to shoulder height, and then press hands straight up above body.
	Overall benefit: Develops the shoulder area, and firms back of arm.
	Muscle involved: Arm abductors (deltoid, supraspinatus), forearm extensor (triceps).
5. Leg Squats (see Figure 8.18)	A partner places the bar on the shoulders behind the head. Squat down so that the legs are at a 90-degree angle (to a bench), and then stand back up.
	Overall benefit: Develops the front of the thigh, giving better strength for climbing stairs and hills, bicycling, and kicking in various sports. The buttock muscles are also firmed.
	Muscles Involved: knee extensors (quadriceps--rectus femoris and vastus lateralis, medialis, and intermedius), thigh extensors (gluteus maximus, adductor magnus, posterior part).

unless combined with an emphasis on behavioral skills and environmental reinforcement.

Physical activity and exercise require a unique commitment: they are more complex, time-consuming, and strenuous than most other health-related behaviors, and they are only weakly associated with other health habits. Successful exercise programs must provide accessible and convenient facilities, support and reinforce behavior change, and remove barriers. Social support from care providers, family, friends, and peers is also important.

The most common reason for dropping out of or not starting an exercise program is lack of time.[110, 117, 118–120] Another is the perception of the sedentary that they are getting enough exercise already. A national Gallup Poll in 1984 found that among those who did not exercise, 39 percent reported they had no time for such activity, and 20 percent felt that they received enough exercise in their daily routine without doing anything extra.[119]

Dr. Roy Shephard of Toronto points out that although people report lack of time as the number one

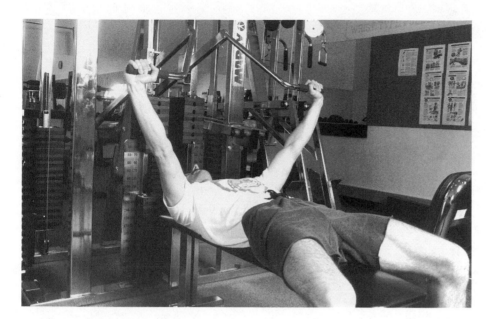

Figure 8.14   Bench Press

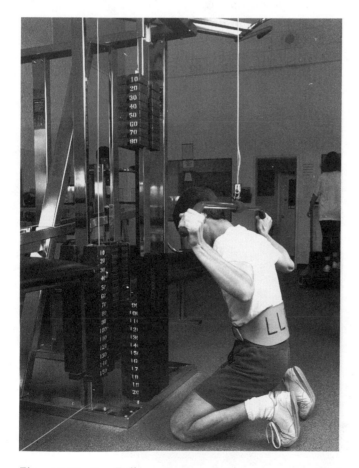

Figure 8.15   Lap Pull

obstacle to exercise, it is really a poor excuse.[110, 118] The average American has 15–18 hours of leisure per week, and has the TV on for 7 hours a day at home. The obstacle to exercise is not so much lack of time as lack of desire. The 1984 Gallup Poll on American attitudes towards exercise showed that 77 percent of those who do exercise find time in their normal schedules without alterations.[119] Shephard concludes that correcting the misconception about lack of time would do more to increase exercise participation than anything else (including more information, better leadership, or more facilities and equipment).[110]

The most frequently pursued aerobic activities of Americans (walking, swimming, cycling, jogging) tend to require little organization or equipment, and no partner.[110, 118] In other words, Americans who are already active have chosen convenient activities. In trying to urge more Americans to exercise, focus must be placed on simple programs, preferably those that can be pursued at home or as a family unit. Expensive, formal, vigorous exercise classes appeal to a limited clientele, and have high dropout rates.

Informal Physical Activity

There is growing opinion that Americans need not only to increase formal exercise patterns, but more importantly, their informal patterns of physical activity. Dr. Per Olaf Astrand of Sweden believes that optimal func-

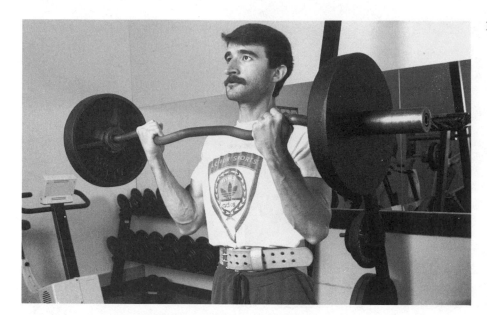

Figure 8.16   Two Arm Curl

tion and health demands more than formalized aerobic activity.[1] He believes that at least 60 minutes per day need to be spent in informal, moderate physical activity. This can take several forms:

▪ Transportation exercise: e.g., taking the stairs instead of the elevator, walking or cycling to work, walking as much as possible during the day. (See Figure 8.21.)

▪ Home exercise: e.g., active gardening with hand tools, sawing, chopping, and splitting wood, cutting the lawn with a hand mower instead of a power mower, etc.

▪ Active leisure-time hobbies: e.g., weekend excursions to the mountains, beach, or lake for hiking and swimming; evening walks with the family; half-court basketball games; touch football with friends and family, etc.

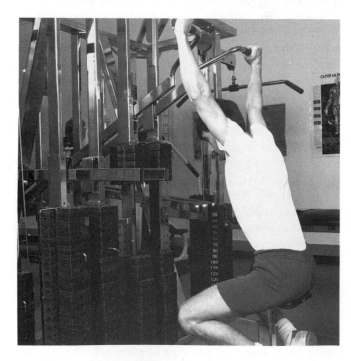

Figure 8.17   Military Press

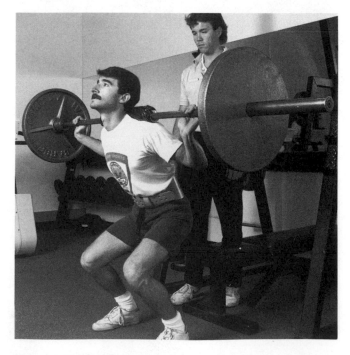

Figure 8.18   Leg Squats

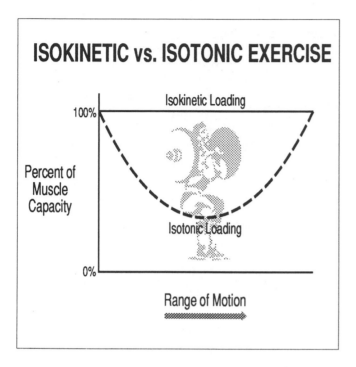

ISOKINETIC vs. ISOTONIC EXERCISE

Isokinetic Loading

Percent of Muscle Capacity

100%

Isotonic Loading

0%

Range of Motion

Figure 8.19 During isotonic muscle contraction, the amount of weight that can be utilized must be adjusted to the weakest point of the lift. Thus the muscle is not operating at 100 percent capacity during all parts of the lift. With isokinetic exercise, the specialized equipment allows the muscle to contract maximally throughout the entire range of motion.

Developing an "exercise mentality," consciously building exercise into regular daily functions, can be an easy way of clearing the motivation hurdle for many. Some like the feeling of "accomplishing something useful" while exercising. In this age of urbanization, mechanization, and technology, this approach to building in physical activity can fill a great need.

Relating exercise to regular daily activities has several advantages:[8, 9]

- Informal physical activity is more convenient, and can be integrated into the regular routine without special scheduling.

- Such activities are purposeful, and can seem to be a good use of time. When a person can accomplish two things at once (e.g., exercise while commuting to work, or doing home chores), there is greater potential for satisfaction.

- They can be more fun (e.g., active leisure time pursuits with family and friends in the out-of-doors).

- When done frequently enough, and at the proper intensity, cardiorespiratory endurance can be enhanced, and health status improved.

This latter point needs more clarification. Several studies have found that cardiovascular disease risk can be lowered with moderate, normal lifestyle activities. In one study of 2,161 women and 1,870 men in four north-

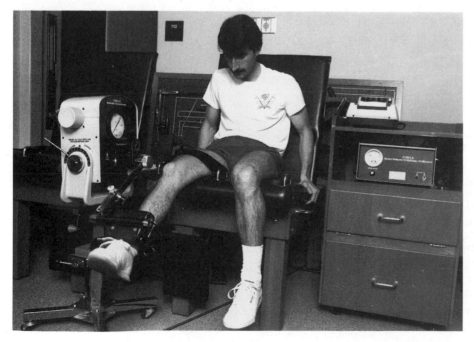

Figure 8.20 The Cybex II allows isokinetic exercise, keeping all movement at a specific speed while varying the resistance to allow maximal effort throughout the range of motion.

Table 8.10 Summary of Variables that May Determine the Probability of Exercise

Determinant	Changes in probability	
	Supervisd Program	Spontaneous Program
Personal Characteristics		
Past program participation	+ +	
Past activity outside of programs	+	
School athletics, 1 sport	+	0
School athletics, >1 sport		+
Blue-collar occupation	- -	-
Smoking	- -	
Overweight	- -	
High risk for coronary heart disease	+ +	
Type A behavior	-	
Health and exercise knowledge	-	0
Attitudes	0	+
Enjoyment of activity	+	
Perceived health	+ +	
Mood disturbance	- -	- -
Education	+	+ +
Age	00	-
Expect personal health benefit	+	
Self-efficacy for exercise		+
Intention to adhere	0	0
Perceived physical competence	00	
Self-motivation	+ +	0
Evaluating costs and benefits	+	
Behavioral skills	+ +	
Environmental Characteristics		
Spouse support	+ +	+
Perceived available time	+ +	+
Access to facilities	+ +	0
Disruptions in routine	- -	
Social reinforcement (staff, exercise partner)	+	
Family influences		+ +
Peer influence		+ +
Physical influences		+
Cost		0
Medical screening	-	
Climate	-	
Incentives	+	
Activity Characteristics		
Activity intensity	00	-
Perceived discomfort	- -	-

Key: + + repeatedly documented increased probability
      + weak or mixed documentation of increased probability
      00 repeatedly documented that there is no change probability
      0 weak or mixed documentation of no change in probability
      - weak or mixed documentation of decreased probability
      - - repeatedly documented decreased probability blank spaces indicate no data

Source Dishman R, Sallis J. Orenstein D. The Determinants of Physical Activity and Exercise. Public Health Reports 100:158–171, 1985.

ern California communities, body mass index scores were significantly lower for people reporting lifestyle exercise (informal exercise).[8] Diastolic blood pressures were significantly lower for the lifestyle exercise group, among younger women and men. Men ages 35–49 who engaged in moderate lifestyle exercise had more favor-

able blood lipid and lipoprotein profiles. In sum, low to moderate levels of physical activity can reduce risk of cardiovascular disease, even though they do not produce substantial changes in cardiorespiratory function.

A team of researchers in Finland measured the training effects of on–the–job stairclimbing for both

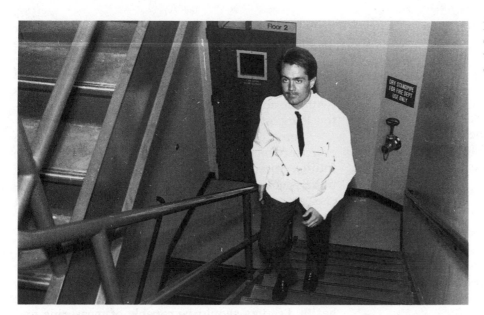

Figure 8.21 Taking the stairs instead of the elevator can be integrated into the daily routine, promoting cardiorespiratory fitness.

male and female employees.[5,6] Participants averaged 30 flights of stairs per workday over a 10–week period. The average number of continuous flights used during climbing was 7.0. $\dot{V}O_{2max}$ improved 15.1% in the stairclimbing group, demonstrating that stairclimbing is a suitable on–the–job physical activity program.

In other words, we need to get away from the image that one must jog around a track, or swim back and forth to get the best exercise. This turns off many potential participants. Fun and excitement should be included as often as possible.

In addition, the pleasure provides more than just motivation for the exercise. Research results have demonstrated that although active people tend to expect and believe that they receive personal health benefits from exercise, the positive feelings gained from the activity seem more important than the actual health benefits.[117] By far, the number one reason given by active people for remaining active is that they "feel better."[117,120]

Sports Medicine Insight
How to Implement Successful Exercise Programs

The Problem

During the 1980s, fitness and health clubs became popular. The National Club Association estimates that there are now between 16,000 and 18,000 member–owned clubs in the country, including yacht clubs, tennis clubs, swim clubs, country clubs, university clubs, and dining clubs.[121] Of these, close to half offer some sort of recreational or fitness service.

Investor–owned clubs fall into three categories: fitness or health clubs, full–service racquet and athletic clubs, and resorts and spas. There are more than 2000 YMCAs, with 10 million members, representing 3–5 percent of the facilities in the industry.

As the fitness club industry has grown, problems have become apparent.[121–124] Fitness and health clubs have few internal standards and little external regulation, and there are no professional standards for the industry. Membership attrition is very high, ranging from 30 to 50 percent of members who join.

There is a growing consensus among club operators that the "revolving door" syndrome is not good for the industry. It is creating consumer cynicism toward fitness that could threaten the industry's long-range potential for growth. Consumer surveys show that the average dissatisfied customer will tell at least nine other people about his or her displeasure.

More than half the states in the country are considering or have passed legislation to regulate the activities of commercial health clubs. The image of the health club industry is badly tainted because of high-pressure sales tactics, insistence on long-term member contracts and up-front fees, misrepresented pre-opening membership sales, and abrupt club closings and bankruptcies leaving prepaid members holding the bag. The major problem is that clubs are taking money in advance for services to be rendered later.[123]

Principles for Successful Programs

Successful formal exercise programs, particularly in a club setting, tend to follow common guidelines.[123-129] The following exercise program principles and motivational strategies can enhance participant interest, enthusiasm, and long-term compliance:

- Provide qualified, enthusiastic exercise leaders.
- Encourage group participation.
- Emphasize variety and enjoyment in the physical activity program. Also, play music during exercise sessions when appropriate.
- Minimize musculoskeletal injuries with a moderate exercise prescription and a slow rate of progression.
- Incorporate effective behavioral and programmatic techniques into the physical conditioning regimen (personal goal setting, contracting).
- Employ periodic testing to assess participants' response to the program.
- Recruit spouse support.
- Provide progress charts to document exercise achievements.
- Recognize participant accomplishments through a system of rewards.
- Downplay exercise performance while awarding individualized achievement of goals.
- Facilitate participation through a system of incentives, such as released time from work with pay, compensation per amount of exercise, and awards for reaching goals.
- Think simple and do what you can to minimize concerns and maximize convenience—in terms of time, travel, and disruptions of family relationships.

The Important Considerations

The challenge for each fitness program is to maximize convenience, to overcome the major obstacle of "lack of time." The best, most successful worksite fitness programs have onsite facilities for just this reason.

Onsite facilities can be inexpensive. Showers and lockers can often be provided with simple refurbishing of unused storage rooms. Showers and locker room facilities can encourage workers to engage in "transpor-

tation exercise," getting to and from work by jogging or cycling. With professional leadership, much can be done (e.g. calisthenics to music, simple testing, walking, jogging) without sophisticated equipment. Use of local community pools, health clubs, and running tracks (with subsidized membership fees) can provide effective low-cost facilities.

Some companies provide incentives for home exercise (which some feel will be the biggest trend of the future). Specific incentives include helping with the purchase of stationary bicycles and other indoor exercise equipment, and monetary rewards for meeting set exercise and fitness goals.

Professional leadership is perhaps the key element behind successful worksite wellness programs. Program directors and exercise leaders should have rigorous academic preparation in exercise physiology, health education, physical education, and/or public health. Leaders should be capable of measuring and interpreting individual fitness characteristics, prescribing safe and effective exercise programs, and motivating participants to join and adhere to an exercise program. A health professional can best assess the needs, set priority objectives, organize personnel, equipment, and facilities, and implement and carry on periodic evaluation research.

The optimal combination appears to be two to three professionals per 1,000 employees. The American College of Sports Medicine administers an extensive certification program for leaders of preventive and rehabilitative exercise programs. It has published a complete list of competency requirements for exercise leaders and technicians. (See Chapter 3.)

To succeed, fitness programs must be attractive, effective, visible, accessible, and convenient.[129,130] Clubs and centers should offer the widest possible range of exercise programs (with as many modes as possible), and should offer services at times that are optimally convenient. Fitness activities should be complemented by nutrition education, smoking cessation, and stress management programs. Screening and testing should precede the exercise programs for each participant, with periodic reevaluation for monitoring of progress and success.

Documented improvement is a strong motivator for continued participation. Long-term adherence to exercise should be promoted through the use of appropriate award systems. Spouses and family members should be involved in the program as well, to provide social support networks. The support of "significant others" may provide the key to long-term adherence to a healthful lifestyle.

Competition can add a potent motivation factor to an exercise program.[128] Typically it takes the form of contests between groups to see who can lose the most weight, record the greatest increases in exercise, stop smoking in the greatest numbers, etc. Such competitions are highly visible, they reduce attrition, influence behavior change, and are cost-effective. They work because they stress motivation and capitalize on existing social networks, providing ongoing support for behavior modification.

A substantial number of dropouts report lack of interest and boredom. One way to offset this is by making workouts interesting, educational, and/or competitive.

Cooperative goal setting events are gaining popularity. One, often conducted at school sites, plays on the around-the-world-in-80-days theme (200–300 people run 1–3 miles a day for 80 days, equalling the distance around the world). Another uses a coast-to-coast concept, with a huge map of the United States hung in the fitness center, reflecting with markers individual progress biking, swimming, walking, or running across the U.S. Different equipment can be mandated for certain sections of the country (rowing machines or swimming for lakes and rivers, cross country ski simulators for snowy areas, etc.).

Administration of Exercise Programs

The American College of Sports Medicine has published general administrative guidelines for exercise programs.[3] Successful programs have well-defined organizational relationships with clearly identified, specific personnel responsibilities and sources of authority.

Ultimate accountability for the program should reside with a governing body/advisory committee composed of appropriate professionals. The governing committee should draw up income and expenditure accounting procedures (with a member with accounting experience facilitating the process). Budget development should be based on many factors, including goals, analysis, and personnel needs.

Marketing precedes public relations,[131] and involves assessing the current and future target population, looking at age, income, marital status, gender, occupation, and education. The interest and demand level should also be assessed, looking at sensitivity to prices, whether the demand is stable, volatile, growing, declining, or maturing. The competition should be looked at, including their location, quality and type of service, and pricing.

Public relations are important. The function of public relations is to influence opinion through communication with the community and participants. Public relations can utilize community service organizations, newsletters, radio, TV, workshops, seminars, news releases, demonstration projects, brochures, flyers, and most importantly, word-of-mouth.

The program must be promoted. Promoting service is different from promoting goods. Persuasion is needed to overcome the various barriers that stand between your service and the customer. These include: distance, time, and knowledge of the services and the values of the service.

Program evaluation should be periodic and ongoing. The manager should evaluate program effectiveness in terms of cost, staff productivity, public image and, most importantly, service to the participants and community. Sources for evaluation include the program staff, the participants in the programs, and nonparticipating members of the community.

Summarizing the Process and Necessary Staff Components

The elements of an effective process for developing programs for worksites, schools, communities, and commercial clubs include:[132]

1. **Needs Assessment:** Use of market research techniques to evaluate the needs and interests of a target audience.

2. **Establishing Objectives:** Development of long and short-term objectives that have been identified through prior needs assessment.

3. **Program Development:** Development of product/services that address market needs and meet program objectives.

4. **Program Positioning and Promotion:** Packaging and promoting programs.

5. **Staffing:** Personnel to develop, implement and produce programs. Developing advisory or management committees.

6. **Facility Program and Design:** Space requirements for office, classes, and exercise programs.

7. **Types of Programs:** Specific form of programs offered.

Important program staff qualities include:

- B.S. or M.S. in physical education, health education, or recreation.
- Knowledge of the physiology of exercise.
- Experience and knowledge in exercise testing and exercise prescription.
- Knowledge and experience in health education and motivational techniques.
- Good writing and verbal communication skills.
- Excellent people skills.
- Experience in facility planning and equipment selection.
- Prior internship or prior staff position in a corporate, hospital, or community program.
- Certification through ACSM or YMCA.
- Experience in program design.
- Ability to integrate and relate other health promotion topics (e.g., stress management, weight control, nutrition, etc.) within total program design.

Summary

1. A comprehensive approach to exercise prescription should be used to provide all of the elements of physical fitness:

   Warm-Up—in slow aerobic activity for several minutes to gradually elevate the pulse for hard aerobic activity. This will prepare the body by elevating the pulse, warming the body, and increasing blood flow. Flexibility exercises should not be done before the muscles and joints are warm.

   Frequency—start with three days per week and gradually build up to five or more days. Less than three days per week of aerobic activity does not build adequate fitness or help keep body fat under control. More than five days per week brings less fitness returns for the time and effort invested.

   Intensity—should be between 50–85 percent of maximal capacity, depending on fitness status. The Karvonen formula is helpful for determining the training heart rate. The heart rate should be periodically counted (10-second pulse count) during exercise.

   Time—the duration of an aerobic workout should be 20–60 minutes, depending on fitness status, intensity of exercise, and age. Time and intensity are interrelated and can be adjusted as

long as 4 kcal/kg of body weight is expended. Informal exercise for one hour a day is advised to complement the formal exercise program.

   Mode—if frequency, intensity, and duration of training are similar, and a minimum of 4 kcal/kg are expended during the session, the training result is independent of the mode of exercise. Aerobic activities that are enjoyable should be utilized. A variety of exercises will enhance compliance.

   Warm-Down—the purpose is to slowly decrease the pulse rate that has been elevated during the aerobic phase by engaging in slow aerobics. This will enhance recovery by reducing the muscle and blood lactic acid levels, and promoting venous return to the heart.

   Flexibility—engage in flexibility exercises after the aerobic session to stretch warm muscle groups that have been especially involved in the aerobic activities. Static stretching is advised, with each specific position held for two sets of about 15–30 seconds each.

   Conditioning exercises for muscular endurance and strength—strength, size, and endurance of muscle tissue is enhanced when the muscle performs for a period of time at its maximal strength and endurance capacity against workloads above those normally encountered. The resistance should be gradually increased until the desired state is achieved. Isometric, isotonic, and isokinetic muscle training systems have been developed.

2. Adherence to exercise programs is a major problem. Based on available evidence, blue collar workers, low socioeconomic and low education groups, middle age groups, and those at high risk for coronary heart disease, particularly smokers, are relatively inactive during their leisure time and are unlikely to participate in supervised exercise programs.

3. To improve compliance, it is now clear that physical activity promotions must address behavioral skills and utilize environments that enable and reinforce participation.

4. A less technical, informal approach to exercise may be more attractive to the American public. The message that may appeal to the society at large is simply to become more active by watching less television, walking more, using stairs, and adopting other physically active

leisure-time pursuits. This type of activity can confer substantial health benefits, even though $\dot{V}O_{2max}$ is only moderately affected.

5. As the fitness club industry has grown, problems have become apparent. Exercise program principles and motivational strategies were reviewed that may enhance participant interest, enthusiasm, and long-term compliance.

References

1. Astrand PO. Optimal Function and Health. Bibl Cardio 36:11–18, 1976.

2. Simons-Morton BG, Parcel GS, O'Hara NM, Blair SN, Pate RR. Health-Related Physical Fitness in Childhood: Status and Recommendations. Annu Rev Public Health 9:403–425, 1988.

3. American College of Sports Medicine. Guidelines for Exercise Testing and Prescription (4th Ed). Philadelphia: Lea & Febiger, 1991.

4. Ilmarinen J, Ilmarinen R, Koskela A, Korhonen O, et al. Training Effects of Stair-Climbing During Office Hours on Female Employees. Ergonomics 22(5):507–516, 1979.

5. Ilmarinen J, Rutenfranz J, Knauth P, Ahrens M, et al. The Effect of an On the Job Training Program—Stairclimbing—On The Physical Working Capacity of Employees. Eur J Appl Physiol 38:25–40, 1978.

6. Gaesser GA, Rich RG. Effects of High- and Low-Intensity Exercise Training on Aerobic Capacity and Blood Lipids. Med Sci Sports Exerc 16:269–274, 1984.

7. Gossard D, Haskell WL, Taylor CB, Mueller JK, Rogers F, et al. Effects of Low- and High-Intensity Home Based Exercise Training on Functional Capacity in Healthy Middle-Aged Men. Am J Cardiol 57:446–449, 1986.

8. Sallis JF, Haskell WL, Fortmann SP, Wood PD, Vranizan KM. Moderate-Intensity Physical Activity and Cardiovascular Risk Factors: The Stanford Five-City Project. Prev Med 15:561–568, 1986.

9. Sallis JF, Haskell WL, Fortmann SP, et al. Predictors of Adoption and Maintenance of Physical Activity in a Community Sample. Prev Med 15:311–341, 1986.

10. Kriska AM, Bayles C, Cauley JA, et al. A Randomized Exercise Trial in Older Women: Increased Activity Over Two Years and the Factors Associated With Compliance. Med Sci Sports Exerc 18:557–562, 1986.

11. A Round Table. Walking for Fitness. Physician Sportsmed 14(10): 145–159, 1986.

12. Wankel LM. Personal and Situational Factors Affecting Exercise Involvement: The Importance of Enjoyment. Res Quart Exerc Sport 56:275–282, 1985.

13. Dishman RK. Exercise Adherence Research: Future Directions. Am J Health Promotion 3(1):52–56, 1988.

14. Pollock ML, Wilmore JH, Fox SM. Exercise In Health and Disease. Philadelphia: W.B. Saunders, Co., 1984.

15. Porcari JP, Ebbeling CB, Ward A, Freedson PS, Rippe JM. Walking for Exercise Testing and Training. Sportsmed 8:189–200, 1989.

16. Haskell WL, Montoye HJ, Orenstein D. Physical Activity and Exercise To Achieve Health-Related Physical Fitness Components. Public Health Rep 110:202–212, 1985.

17. Sharkey BJ. Physiology of Fitness. Champaign, Illinois: Human Kinetics Publishers, 1979.

18. Cooper KH. The Aerobics Way. New York: M. Evans and Co., Inc., 1977.

19. Getchell B. Physical Fitness: A Way of Life. New York: John Wiley and Sons, 1983.

20. Shyne K, Dominquez RH. To Stretch or Not to Stretch? Physician Sportsmed 10:137–140, 1982.

21. Larsen B. The Warmup. Runner's World, Annual, 1983, p. 45.

22. Maddux GT. Men's Gymnastics. Pacific Palisades, CA: Goodyear Publishing Co., Inc., 1970.

23. Shellock FG. Physiological Benefits of Warm-up. Physician Sportsmed 11:134–139, 1983.

24. Hetzler RK, Knowlton RG, Kaminsky LA, Kamimori GH. Effect of Warm-up on Plasma Free Fatty Acid Responses and Substrate Utilization During Submaximal Exercise. Res Quart Exerc Sport 57:223–228, 1986.

25. Wiktorsson-Möller M, Oberg B, Ekstrand J, Gillquist J. Effects of Warming Up, Massage, and Stretching on Range of Motion and Muscle Strength in the Lower Extremity. Am J Sports Med 11:249–252, 1983.

26. Shellock FG, Prentice WE. Warming-Up and Stretching for Improved Physical Performance and Prevention of Sports-Related Injuries. Sports Med 2:267–278, 1985.

27. Moffatt RJ. Strength and Flexibility Considerations for Exercise Prescription. IN: Blair SN, Painter P, Pate RR, Smith LK, Taylor CB (eds). Resource Manual for Guidelines for Exercising Testing and Prescription. Philadelphia: Lea & Febiger, 1988.

28. Moneta-Chivalbinska J, Hänninen O. Effect of Active Warming-Up on Thermoregulatory, Circulatory, and Metabolic Responses to Incremental Exercise in Endurance-Trained Athletes. Int J Med 10:25–29, 1989.

29. Heyward VH. Designs for Fitness. Minneapolis: Burgess Publishing Co., 1984.

30. Haskell WL, et al. Physical Activity and Exercise to Achieve Health-Related Physical Fitness Components. Public Health Rep 100:202–212, 1985.

31. Gibson SB, Gerberich SG, Leon AS. Writing the Exercise Prescription: An Individualized Approach. Physician Sportsmed 11:87–110, 1983.

32. Pollock ML. How Much Exercise Is Enough? Physician Sportsmed 6: 1978.

33. Birrer RB. Exercise Prescription. Postgrad Med 77:219–230, 1985.

34. Gutin B. Basic Principles of Training and Fitness. Contemporary OB/GYN: The Active Woman. May, 1985, pp: 33–46.

35. Gettman LR, et al. Physiological Responses of Men to 1,3, and 5 Day Per Week Training Programs. Res Quart Exerc Sport 47:638–646, 1976.

36. Pollock ML, Ward A, Ayres JJ. Cardiorespiratory Fitness: Response to Differing Intensities and Durations of Training. Arch Physical Med Rehabil 58:467–473, 1977.

37. Wilmore JH. Individual Exercise Prescription. Am J Cardiol 33:757–759, 1974.

38. Cooper KH. Guidelines in the Management of the Exercising Patient. JAMA 211:1663–16567, 1970.

39. Wilmore JH, Haskell WL. Use of the Heart Rate-Energy Expenditure Relationship in the Individualized Prescription of Exercise. Am J Clin Nutr 24:1186–1192, 1971.

40. American College of Sports Medicine. Position Statement on the Recommended Quantity and Quality of Exercise for Developing and Maintaining Fitness In Healthy Adults. Med Sci Sports Exerc 10:vii–x, 1978.

41. Wenger HA, Bell GJ. The Interactions of Intensity, Frequency and Duration of Exercise Training in Altering Cardiorespiratory Fitness. Sports Med 3:346–356, 1986.

42. Getchell LH. Exercise Prescription for the Healthy Adult. J Cardiopulmonary Rehabil 6:46–51, 1986.

43. Vaccaro P, Mahon A. Cardiorespiratory Responses to Endurance Training in Children. Sports Med 4:352–363, 1987.

44. Cooper KH. The Aerobics Program for Total Well-Being. New York: M.Evans and Company, Inc., 1982.

45. Wilmore JH. The Physiological Basis of the Conditioning Process. Boston: Allyn and Bacon, Inc., 1982.

46. Fox SM, et al. Physical Activity and Cardiovascular Health. Mod Concepts Cardiovasc Dis 41:25–30, 1972.

47. Karvonen M, Kentala E, Mustala O. The Effects of Training On Heart Rate. A Longitudinal Study. Ann Med Exper Biol Fenn 35:307–315, 1957.

48. Davis JA, Convertino VA. A Comparison of Heart Rate Methods for Predicting Endurance Training Intensity. Med Sci Sports Exerc 7:295–298, 1975.

49. Couldry W, Corbin CB, Wilcox A. Carotid vs Radial Pulse Counts. Physician Sportsmed 10:67–72, 1982.

50. Boone T, Frentz KL, Boyd NR. Carotid Palpation At Two Exercise Intensities. Med Sci Sports Exerc 17:705–709, 1985.

51. Allen D. Heart-Rate Monitors: The Ideal Exercise Speedometer. Fitness Management Nov/Dec 1988, pp 34–37.

52. Smutok MA, et al. Exercise Intensity: Subjective Regulation by Perceived Exertion. Arch Phys Med Rehabil 61:569–574, 1980.

53. Borg G. Perceived Exertion as Indicator of Somatic Stress. Scand J Rehabil Med 2:92–98, 1970.

54. Noble BJ, Borg GAV, Jacobs I., Ceci R., Kaiser P. A Category-Ratio Perceived Exertion Scale: Relationship to Blood and Muscle Lactates and Heart Rate. Med Sci Sports Exerc 15:523–528, 1983.

55. Carton RL, Rhodes EC. A Critical Review of the Literature on Ratings Scales for Perceived Exertion. Sports Med 2:198–222, 1985.

56. Demello JJ, Cureton KJ, Boineau RE, et al. Ratings of Perceived Exertion at the Lactate Threshold in Trained and Untrained Men and Women. Med Sci Sports Exerc 19:354–362, 1987.

57. Birk TJ, Birk CA. Use of Ratings of Perceived Exertion for Exercise Prescription. Sports Med 4:1–8, 1987.

58. Pollock ML, et al. Effects of Walking on Body Composition and Cardiovascular Function of Middle-aged Men. J Appl Physiol 30:126–130, 1971.

59. Porcari J, McCarron R, Kline G, et al. Is Fast Walking an Adequate Aerobic Training Stimulus for 30- to 69-Year-Old Men and Women. Physician Sportsmed 15(2):119–129, 1987.

60. Jette M, Sidney K, Campbell J. Effects of a Twelve-Week Walking Program on Maximal and Submaximal Work Output Indices in Sedentary Middle-Aged Men and Women. J Sports Med 28:59–66, 1988.

61. Nieman DC, Haig JL, De Guia ED, Dizon GP, Register UD. Reducing Diet and Exercise Training Effects on Resting Metabolic Rates in Mildly Obese Women. J Sports Med 28:79–88, 1988.

62. Zarandonz JE, Nelson AG, Conlee RK, Fisher AG. Physiological Responses to Hand-Carried Weights. Physician Sportsmed 14(10):113–120, 1986.

63. Miller JF, Stamford BA. Intensity and Energy Cost of Weighted Walking vs. Running for Men and Women. J Appl Physiol 62:1497–1501, 1987.

64. Auble TE, Schwartz L, Robertson RJ. Aerobic Requirements for Moving Handweights Through Various Ranges of Motion While Walking. Physician Sportsmed 15(6):133–140, 1987.

65. Graves JE, Pollock ML, Montain SJ, et al. The Effect of Hand-Held Weights on the Physiological Responses to Walking Exercise. Med Sci Sports Exerc 19:260–265, 1987.

66. Claremont AD, Hall SJ. Effects of Extremity Loading Upon Energy Expenditure and Running Mechanics. Med Sci Sports Exerc 20:167–171, 1988.

67. Graves JE, Martin AD, Miltenberger LA, Pollock ML. Physiological Responses to Walking With Hand Weights, Wrist Weights, and Ankle Weights. Med Sci Sports Exerc 20:265–271, 1988.

68. Makalous SL, Arujo J, Thomas TR. Energy Expenditure During Walking With Hand Weights. Physician Sportsmed 16(4):139–148, 1988.

69. Garrick JG, Requa RK. Aerobic Dance: A Review. Sports Med 6:169–179, 1988.

70. Watterson VV. The Effects of Aerobic Dance On Cardiovascular Fitness. Physician Sportsmed 10:138–145, 1984.

71. Milburn S, Butts NK. A Comparison of the Training Responses to Aerobic Dance and Jogging In College Females. Med Sci Sports Exerc 15:510–513, 1983.

72. Cearly ML, et al. The Effects of Two- and Three-Day-Per-Week Aerobic Dance Programs on Maximal Oxygen Uptake. Res Quart Exerc Sport 55:172–174, 1984.

73. Gelder NV, Marks S. Aerobic Dance-Exercise Instructor Manual. San Diego: International Dance-Exercise Association (IDEA) Foundation, 1987.

74. Nelson DJ, Pels AE, Geenen DL, White TP. Cardiac Frequency and Caloric Cost of Aerobic Dancing in Young Women. Res Quart Exerc Sport 59:229–233, 1988.

75. Williford HN, Blessing DL, Barksdale JM, Smith FH. The Effects of Aerobic Dance Training on Serum Lipids, Lipoproteins and Cardiopulmonary Function. J Sports Med 28:151–157, 1988.

76. Williford HN. Is Low-Impact Aerobic Dance An Effective Cardiovascular Workout? Physician Sportsmed 17(3º)95–109, 1989.

77. Koszuto LE. From Sweats to Swimsuits: Is Water Exercise the Wave of the Future? Physician Sportsmed 17(4):203–206, 1989.

78. Morgans LF, Scovil JA, Bass KM. Heart Rate Responses During Singles and Doubles Competition. Physician Sportsmed 12:64–72, 1984.

79. Friedman DB, Ramo BW, Gray GJ. Tennis and Cardiovascular Fitness in Middle-Aged Men. Physician Sportsmed 12:87–92, 1984.

80. Montpetit RR, Beauchamp L, Léger L. Energy Requirements of Squash and Racquetball. Physician Sportsmed 15(8):106–112, 1987.

81. Morgans LF, Jordan DL, Baeyens DA, Franciosa JA. Heart Rate Responses During Singles and Doubles Tennis Competition. Physician Sportsmed 15(7):67–74, 1987.

82. Hurley BF, et al. Effects of High-Intensity Strength Training On Cardiovascular Function. Med Sci Sports Exerc 16:483–488, 1984.

83. Gettman LR, Ayres JJ, Pollock ML, Jackson A. The Effect of Circuit Weight Training on Strength, Cardiorespiratory Function, and Body Composition of Adult Men. Med Sci Sports Exerc 10:171–176, 1978.

84. Ballor DL, Becque MD, Katch VL. Metabolic Responses During Hydraulic Resistance Exercise. Med Sci Sports Exerc 19:363–367, 1987.

85. Harris KA, Holly RG. Physiological Response to Circuit Weight Training in Borderline Hypertensive Subjects. Med Sci Sports Exerc 19:246–252, 1987.

86. Dudley GA, Fleck SJ. Strength and Endurance Training: Are They Mutually Exclusive? Sports Med 4:79–85, 1987.

87. Sleamaker RH. Caloric Cost of Performing the Perrier Parcourse Fitness Circuit. Med Sci Sports Exerc 16:283–286, 1984.

88. Quirk JE, Sinning WE. Anaerobic and Aerobic Responses of Males and Females to Rope Skipping. Med Sci Sports Exerc 14:26–29, 1982.

89. Town GP, Sol N, Sinning WE. The Effect of Rope Skipping Rate On Energy Expenditure of Males and Females. Med Sci Sports Exerc 12:295–298, 1980.

90. Eisenman PA, Johnson SC, Bainbridge CN, Zupan MF. Applied Physiology of Cross-Country Skiing. Sports Med 8:67–79, 1989.

91. Mahler DA, Andrea BE, Ward JL. Comparison of Exercise Performance on Rowing and Cycle Ergometers. Res Quart Exerc Sport 58:41–46, 1987.

92. Rosiello RA, Mahler DA, Ward JL. Cardiovascular Responses to Rowing. Med Sci Sports Exerc 19:239–245, 1987.

93. Hagerman FC, Lawrence RA, Mansfield MC. A Comparison of Energy Expenditure During Rowing and Cycling Ergometry. Med Sci Sports Exerc 20:479–488, 1988.

94. Daws R. All In Good Time. Runner's World, August 1987, pp 32–39.

95. Fox EL, Mathews DK. The Physiological Basis of Physical Education and Athletics. New York: Saunders College Publishing, 1981.

96. Dimsdale JE, Hartley LH, Guiney T, et al. Postexercise Peril: Plasma Catecholamines and Exercise. JAMA 251:630–632, 1984.

97. Levine M, Lombardo J, McNeeley J, Anderson T. An Analysis of Individual Stretching Programs of Intercollegiate Athletes. Physician Sportsmed 15(3):130–137, 1987.

98. Ekstrand J, Gillquist J. The Frequency of Muscle Tightness and Injuries in Soccer Players. Am J Sports Med 10:75–78, 1982.

99. Kirby RL, Simms FC, Symingtom VJ, Garner JB. Flexibility and Musculoskeletal Symptomatology in Female Gymnasts and Age-Matched Controls. Am J Sports Med 9:160–164, 1981.

100. Etnyre BR, Lee JA. Chronic and Acute Flexibility of Men and Women Using Three Different Stretching Techniques. Res Quart Exerc Sport 59:222–228, 1988.

101. Etnyre BR, Abraham LD. Antagonist Muscle Activity During Stretching: A Paradox Re-Assessed. Med Sci Sports Exerc 20:285–289, 1988.

102. Cornelius WL, Craft-Hamm K. Proprioceptive Neuromuscular Facilitation Flexibility Techniques: Acute Effects on Arterial Blood Pressure. Physician Sportsmed 16(4):152–161, 1988.

103. Moore MA, Hutton RS. Electromyographic Investigation of Muscle Stretching Techniques. Med Sci Sports Exerc 12:322–329, 1980.

104. Anderson B. Stretching. Bolinas, CA: Shelter Publications, 1980.

105. Zebas CJ, Rivera ML, Retention of Flexibility In Selected Joints After Cessation of a Stretching Exercise Program. IN: Dotson CO, Humphrey JH (eds): Exercise Physiology: Selected Research. New York: AMS Press, Inc., 1985.

106. Fleck SJ, Kraemer WJ. Designing Resistance Training Programs. Champaign, IL: Human Kinetics Publishers, 1987.

107. Davies GJ. A Compendium of Isokinetics in Clinical Usage. S & S Publishers, 1707 Jennifer Court, Onalaska, Wisconsin 54650. 1987.

108. Elliot DL, Goldberg L, Kuehl KS, Catlin DH. Characteristics of Anabolic- Androgenic Steroid-Free Competitive Male and Female Bodybuilders. Physician Sportsmed 15(6):169–180, 1987.

109. Anderson T, Kearney JT. Effects of Three Resistance Training Programs on Muscular Strength and Absolute and Relative Endurance. Res Quart Exerc Sport 53:1–7, 1982.

110. Shephard RJ. Motivation: The Key to Fitness Compliance. Physician Sportsmed 13:88–101, 1985.

111. Dishman RK. Exercise Adherence Research: Future Directions. Am J Health Promotion 3(1):52–56, 1988.

112. Sallis JF, Hovell MF, Hofstetter CR, et al. A Multivariate Study of Determinants of Vigorous Exercise in a Community Sample. Prev Med 18:20–34, 1989.

113. Serfass RC, Gerberich SG. Exercise for Optimal Health: Strategies and Motivational Considerations. Prev Med 13:79–99, 1984.

114. Paffenbarger RS, Wing AL, Hyde RT. Physical Activity as an Index of Heart Attack Risk in College Alumni. Am J Epidemiol 108:161–175, 1978.

115. Department of Health and Human Services, Office of Disease Prevention and Health Promotion: Prevention '82. DHHS Publication No. (PHS) 82–50157. U.S. Government Printing Office, Washington, D.C., 1982.

116. Sonstroem RJ. Psychological Models. IN: Dishman RK (ed). Exercise Adherence. Champaign, Illinois: Human Kinetics Books, 1988.

117. Dishman RK. Public Health Rep 100:158–171, 1985.

118. Shephard RJ. Factors Influencing the Exercise Behavior of Patients. Sports Med 2:348–366, 1985.

119. Public Attitudes and Behavior Related to Exercise: conducted for American Health Magazine by The Gallup Organization, Inc., 53 Bank Street, Princeton, New Jersey 08542. February, 1985.

120. Gettman LR, Pollock ML, Ward A. Adherence to Unsupervised Exercise. Physician Sportsmed 11:56–64, 1983.

121. Anonymous. An Industry In Transition. Athletic Business (April):40–46, 1987.

122. Anonymous. Update. Club Industry, November 1986.

123. Anonymous. More State Regulation? Athletic Business (April):20–24, 1987.

124. Anonymous. Designing Clubs That Encourage Use. Athletic Business, November 1986, pp 34–39.

125. Franklin BA. Program Factors That Influence Exercise Adherence: Practical Adherence Skills for the Clinical Staff. In: Dishman RK (ed). Exercise Adherence. Champaign, Illinois: Human Kinetics Books, 1988.

126. Wankel LM. Personal and Situational Factors Affecting Exercise Involvement: The Importance of Enjoyment. Res Quart Exerc Sport 56:275–282, 1985.

127. Fielding JE, Piserchia PV. Frequency of Worksite Health Promotion Activities. Am J Public Health 79:16–20, 1989.

128. Brownell KD, Felix MRJ. Competitions to Facilitate Health Promotion: Review and Conceptual Analysis. Am J Health Promotion 2(1):28–36, 1987.

129. Pate RR, Blair SN. Physical Fitness Programming for Health Promotion at the Worksite. Prev Med 12:632–643, 1983.

130. Hargadine HK. Health Promotion Programs: Limited Funds No Stumbling Block. Occup Health Safety 54:69–74, 1985.

131. Singer JL, Monteson PA. But Will It Work? Athletic Business, June, 1985, pp. 100–106.

132. Pfeiffer GJ. Management Aspects of Fitness Program Development. Am J Health Promotion 1(2):10–18, 1986.

Physical Fitness Activity 8.1— Writing the Exercise Prescription

In this physical fitness activity, you will be writing an exercise prescription for someone needing your guidance (choose a fellow student, family member, or friend). There are several steps that should be followed. In order they are:

1. Have the client you are writing the exercise prescription for fill out the medical/health questionnaire. (See Appendix A.) Review this questionnaire with the client to gain a complete picture of his background, present health status, and future goals. Next classify him according to the American College of Sports Medicine criteria listed in Chapter 3 (apparently healthy, individual at higher risk, or patient with disease). Make an appropriate judgment as to the need for further testing with physician supervision. (Review Chapter 3.)

2. Review physical fitness testing results. It is preferable to have test results indicating the cardiorespiratory, body composition, and musculoskeletal status of the client you are counseling. Make sure the client understands the test results and their ranking within the norm tables.

3. Now that you have a better understanding of the medical, health, and physical fitness status of the client, start the exercise prescription process by reviewing the preferred mode of exercise. Using Table 8.7, have the person mark at least two cardiorespiratory endurance activities that he has either enjoyed in the past, or feels he can utilize in his present circumstances. Review the summary of variables that may determine the probability of exercise (Table 8.10), and challenge the client to think through perceived available time, access to facilities and equipment, social reinforcement, family and peer influences, cost, climate, and other environmental characteristics.

4. Using the form in Figure 8.3, go step-by-step through each stage of the exercise prescription, explaining the basic concepts involved. It is a good idea to have the client fill in the blanks to facilitate acceptance of the information. Important concepts to keep in mind with each stage of the exercise prescription include the following:

Cardiorespiratory—Warm-Up: Emphasize the importance of elevating body temperature through slow aerobic activity, preferably the aerobic activity that will be utilized in the workout session. Explain that flexibility exercises are best done when the body is warm after the aerobic session.

Cardiorespiratory/Body Composition—Aerobic Session: Circle the appropriate F.I.T. criteria based on the fitness status of the client. Help the client determine his training heart rate using the Karvonen formula, and fill in the appropriate blanks. Explain how to measure the training heart rate, and fill in the blank for the 10-sec pulse count. Review the concept of rating of perceived exertion, explaining that an RPE of "somewhat hard" appears appropriate for most people. Caution against overexertion. Fill in the mode selected by the client. Discuss the concept of informal exercise, and the importance of using the stairs when possible, walking during work breaks, etc. Finally, have the client mark the appropriate blanks indicating the time and days of the week the exercise sessions will be planned for.

Cardiorespiratory—Warm-Down: Explain that this is basically the warm-up in reverse to help the body through the transition from hard aerobic exercise to rest.

Musculoskeletal—Flexibility: Using the exercises pictured in Appendix D, review the principles of flexibility calisthenics, and the particular importance of stretching the muscles utilized in the aerobic session.

Musculoskeletal—Muscular Strength and Endurance: First find out whether or not your client has access to a weight training facility. If so, discuss the principles of weight training, and the basic lifts as summarized in Table 8.9. If not, review the calisthenics pictured in Appendix D.

Before starting the exercise prescription process with your clients, a few concepts about counseling are helpful for providing better service. It is important to understand that no one person can motivate another. One can only create a climate that will facilitate others to motivate themselves. In other words, motivation comes from within. People tend to be motivated by challenge, growth, achievement, promotion, and recognition. Emphasis should be placed on providing a proper environment for self-growth by challenging clients, giving responsibility, encouraging, and giving full range to individual strength. The good exercise counselor develops warm personal relationships with each participant, and regards each as worthy of his/her genuine concern and attention.

Traits of a good counselor include:

- **Empathy**—ability to climb into the world of the client and communicate back feelings of understanding.

- **Respect**—a deep and genuine appreciation for the worth of the client, separate and apart from his behavior. The strength and ability of the client to overcome and adjust is appreciated.

- **Warmth**—communication of concern and appropriate affection.

- **Genuineness**—being freely and deeply one's self. One is congruent, and not just playing a role.

- **Concreteness**—essential ideas and elements are ferreted out.

- **Self-Disclosure**—revelations about self for the benefit of the client at the appropriate time.

- **Potency and Self-Actualization**—one is dynamic, in command, conveys feelings of trust and warmth, is competent, inner directed, creative, sensitive, not judgmental, productive, serene, satisfied—and this comes across to the client in a helpful way.

Chapter 9

Nutrition and Physical Performance

"Aside from the limits imposed by heredity and the physical improvements associated with training, no factor plays a bigger role in exercise performance than does nutrition." [1]

Introduction: Ten Cardinal Sports Medicine Principles

Paul Anderson, who once raised the greatest weight ever lifted by a human, 6,270 pounds, had a special drink he used while in training. Using his bare hands, he would squeeze the blood from two pounds of raw hamburger into a glass of tomato juice, and then drink the mixture. [2]

Milo of Crotona, legendary wrestler of the ancient Greeks who was never once brought to his knees over five Olympiads (532–516 B.C.), ate gargantuan amounts of meat. [3] Swimmer Jim Montgomery, winner of four gold medals in the 1976 Olympics, normally ate a breakfast consisting of eight eggs, a pound of bacon, a loaf of bread, and a quart of orange juice. Don Kardong, Olympic marathon runner, proudly boasts of his huge intake of ice cream, soda pop, cookies, pastries, and beer. [4] Seoul Olympic marathoner Cathy O'Brien skips breakfast, consumes only 1,300 Calories a day, and has a weakness for Pepsi and whole milk. [5]

On the other hand, there are many fine athletes who are very meticulous about their diets. Nancy Ditz, America's top ranked female marathoner, emphasizes carbohydrates, averaging 65 percent to 75 percent of her daily energy intake. [5] Dave Scott, world record holder in the Ironman Triathlon, eats a diet high in complex carbohydrates—74 percent of total Calories, consisting of brown rice, tofu, low-fat dairy products, and up to 20 pieces of fruit and vegetables per day . [6] Olympic marathoner Margaret Groos also emphasizes a high carbohydrate diet (over 60 percent of total energy intake), emphasizing such foods as English muffins, rice cakes, fruit, pasta, high-carbohydrate drinks, and low-fat dairy products. [5]

These examples point out the obvious: among our top athletes, dietary practices cover a wide range. Questions that naturally arise are: (1) Could athletes or fitness enthusiasts improve their ability to train and perform by optimizing their diet? (2) What is the optimal diet for people who exercise regularly and/or compete? (3) Can regular exercise protect one from the effects of a bad diet (e.g., high blood cholesterol, high blood pressure, heart disease, etc.)? (4) Are the nutritional stresses imposed by hard training greater than can be met by ordinary foods, without protein, vitamin, or mineral supplementation?

In this chapter, these and other questions will be answered through a discussion of ten cardinal sports nutrition principles. This listing represents a summary of the most recent and important research in this area.

These principles apply to both the basic fitness exerciser and even more importantly to the competitive endurance athlete.

Before reviewing these principles, it is important to realize that the ability to exercise hard and perform well depends on much more than diet. In fact, most sports nutrition experts feel that proper nutrition ranks third behind *talent* and *training* as factors affecting athletic accomplishment.[1]

However, researchers have also shown that athletes can *maximize* this talent and training by putting into practice the ten sports nutrition principles listed in this chapter. You cannot eat your way to Olympic gold, but a prudent diet can definitely improve your chances. On the other hand, don't expect to run your fastest 10-K right after improving your diet, unless you also improve the quality of your training program. What you can expect is that a good diet will help you feel better from day to day, allowing you to train harder.

PRINCIPLE 1 The Prudent Diet is the Cornerstone

The *prudent diet* will be defined here as the diet adhering to the 1988 *Surgeon General's Report on Nutrition and Health*.[7] (See Table 9.1.) As noted in the Surgeon General's report, our nutritional problems today are no longer related to deficiency, but to excess. As the incidence of diseases of nutritional deficiency has diminished (e.g., scurvy from lack of vitamin C, or pellagra from a lack of niacin), it has been replaced by an increased incidence of diseases of dietary excess and imbalance.

Eight of the top ten causes of illness and death in the United States (in particular, heart disease and cancer) have been associated with diet and excessive alcohol intake. While many food factors are involved, "chief among them is the disproportionate consumption of foods high in fats, often at the expense of foods high in complex carbohydrates and fiber that may be more conducive to health," states the Surgeon General.

The same basic diet that enhances health (the prudent diet) is also advocated for fitness enthusiasts (those exercising 3 to 5 days per week, 15 to 30 minutes per session). (See Table 9.2.) For the competitive endurance athlete (who trains more than one hour a day), several adaptations *beyond* the prudent diet are beneficial. (See especially sports nutrition principles #2–5.) Heavy training imposes special nutritional stresses because of the high intensity of effort expended over a relatively short time period, demanding extra energy, carbohydrate, water, and iron.

As time spent in endurance activity increases, the quantity of fat in the diet should decrease and be replaced by carbohydrate. This is best accomplished by consuming less visible fat (margarine, oil, salad dressing, mayonnaise, etc.), fewer high-fat dairy products (most cheeses, whole milk, butter, cream cheese, etc.), less high-fat meat (fried meats, bacon, corned beef, ground beef, ham, sausages, processed meats, etc.), and more grain products (pasta, bagels, breads, brown rice, cereals, etc.), tubers (potatoes, yams), legumes (kidney beans, pinto beans, etc.), dried fruits (raisins, dates, etc.), fresh fruits, and fresh vegetables.

Dietary Practices of Athletes

Despite the considerable number of publications on nutrition for athletes, very few formal studies of the dietary intake and eating behaviors of athletes have been published.[8]

Table 9.3 summarizes some of the cross sectional studies that have evaluated dietary intakes by athletes.[8, 22]

Examination of Table 9.3 reveals that there is a wide range of energy intake among athletes.[8, 9, 22] In general, however, athletes tend to be high energy consumers, with the size of the participant and the energy demands of the sport having much to do with the amount of Calories each consumes. Very large athletes training intensively for several hours each day (e.g., football players in the early fall) have the highest caloric requirements. Smaller athletes who transport their body mass over long distances on a regular basis (e.g., cross-country skiers and distance runners) also have high caloric requirements.[8]

Athletes who purposely keep their body weights below natural weight for competition (e.g., wrestlers, gymnasts, and ballet dancers) tend to have reported caloric intakes that appear to fall way below calculated energy expenditure. Several researchers have reported that athletes in sports that emphasize leanness are exceptionally preoccupied with weight, tend to use unhealthy methods for weight-control, tend toward eating disorders, and demonstrate poor nutrition knowledge.[16, 17, 19–21, 23–26]

The desire of the highly competitive wrestler to alter body weight without medical supervision has caused much concern among sports medicine professionals.[19] A high percentage induce dehydration, utilizing sauna baths, fluid restriction, and rubber or plastic suits. Some also resort to laxatives, diuretics, and vomiting. Such practices may endanger health, adversely affect performance, and can affect a younger person's growth potential.

Table 9.1 Surgeon General Recommendations for Most People

Fats and cholesterol	Reduce consumption of fat (especially saturated fat) and cholesterol. Choose foods relatively low in these substances, such as vegetables, fruits, whole grain foods, fish, poultry, lean meats, and low-fat dairy products. Use food preparation methods that add little or no fat.
Energy and weight control	Achieve and maintain a desirable body weight. To do so, choose a dietary pattern in which energy intake is consistent with energy expenditure. To reduce energy intake, limit consumption of foods relatively high in calories, fats and sugars, and minimize alcohol consumption. Increase energy expenditure through regular and sustained physical activity.
Complex carbohydrates and fiber	Increase consumption of whole grain foods and cereal products, vegetables (including dried beans and peas), and fruits.
Sodium	Reduce intake of sodium by choosing foods relatively low in sodium and limiting the amount of salt added in food preparation and at the table.
Alcohol	To reduce the risk for chronic disease, take alcohol only in moderation (no more than two drinks a day), if at all. Avoid drinking any alcohol before or while driving, operating machinery, taking medications, or engaging in any other activity requiring judgment. Avoid drinking alcohol while pregnant.
Other Issues for Some People	
Fluoride	Community water systems should contain fluoride at optimal levels for prevention of tooth decay. If such water is not available, use other appropriate sources of fluoride.
Sugars	Those who are particularly vulnerable to dental caries (cavities), especially children, should limit their consumption and frequency of use of foods high in sugars.
Calcium	Adolescent girls and adult women should increase consumption of foods high in calcium, including low-fat dairy products.
Iron	Children, adolescents, and women of childbearing age should be sure to consume foods that are good sources of iron, such as lean meats, fish, certain beans, and iron-enriched cereals and whole grain products. This issue is of special concern for low-income families.

Source: U.S. Department of Health and Human Services. The Surgeon General's Report on Nutrition and Health. DHHS (PHS) Publication No. 88-50211. U.S. Government Printing Office: Washington, DC, 1988.

As long as wrestling competition is organized by weight categories, the popular practice of competing at the lowest possible weight will probably continue.[25] Some sort of control, such as limiting the amount of weight that can be lost or establishing a minimum body fat percentage level, may be necessary.

As can be seen from Table 9.3, protein in athletes' diets accounts on the average for about 13–17 percent of energy intake, but the proportions among different athletes can vary from 10–36 percent.[8,9] Protein intakes tend to be lower among endurance athletes, and higher among some groups of power and strength athletes, who often consume more than 20 percent of their energy as protein.[22] Relative to body weight, protein intakes usually exceed 1.5 g/kg/day, and intakes exceed-ing 2.0 g/kg/day are common. Although the Recommended Dietary Allowance (RDA) is only 0.8 g/kg/day, athletes do not appear to be much different than the non-athletic population, who tend to consume nearly double the RDA.

Table 9.3 also shows that fat accounts for about 36 percent of athletes' energy intakes. This is close to the 37 percent reported in national diet surveys.[27] Again the proportions for athletes vary, and range from about 20 percent to more than 50 percent.[8,9] Power and strength athletes tend to have higher fat intakes than endurance athletes, and these higher fat intakes are often associated with their higher protein intakes.[23]

Carbohydrate provides about 46 percent of the energy consumed by athletes, nearly the same as it does

Table 9.2 The Sports Nutrition Continuum

Percent of Total Caloric Intake*

	Average American	Prudent Diet	Heavy Endurance Athlete
Carbohydrate	48%	55%	70%
Fat	37%	30%	15%
Protein	15%	15%	15%

*Note: Often nutritionists like to discuss the *percentage of total Calories* represented by protein, carbohydrate, and fat. This is useful information and is based on the following:

> 1 gram carbohydrate = 4 Calories
> 1 gram protein = 4 Calories
> 1 gram fat = 9 Calories

For example, Grape Nuts has 110 Calories per serving, with 23 grams from carbohydrate, 3 grams from protein, and none from fat. To figure what percentage of the Calories is provided by protein or carbohydrate or fat, the gram amount of each should be multiplied by the Calories/gram factor listed above, and then divided by the total energy (110 Calories). For example:

> Percent Calories as carbohydrate = (23g×4)/110 = 83.6 percent
>
> Percent Calories as protein = (3g×4)/110 = 10.9 percent
>
> Percent Calories as fat = (0g × 9)/110 = 0.0 percent

for the average American.[27] (See Table 9.2.) The range of percentages is wide, and intakes of from 22–72 percent have been reported.[8,9] Triathletes are unique in that they tend to have higher carbohydrate intakes than other athletes.[10,11]

A growing number of studies are reporting a full analysis of the diets of athletes and their estimated intakes of vitamins and minerals.[8–23,28,31] In nearly all of these studies, the regular diets of most athletes contain vitamins and minerals in excess of the RDA, because they eat more food. However, despite the adequacy of minerals and vitamins in their diets, athletes make widespread use of dietary supplements. (This will be discussed further in the section on vitamins and minerals in this chapter.)

Athletes in sports which emphasize leanness, however, (including wrestling), have been found to consume insufficient quantities of vitamins and minerals, largely because of inadequate energy intake.[16,17,19–21] Close to half of all gymnasts, wrestlers, and ballet dancers, for example, have been reported to consume less than two-thirds the RDA for various important minerals and vitamins.[16,17,19,21]

The author conducted the largest dietary study ever done on endurance athletes.[28] Three-day food records were collected from 347 participants in the Los Angeles Marathon (291 males, 56 females). Their overall intake of vitamins and minerals was adequate, and substantially higher than that of the general population, and came closer to meeting current prudent dietary recommendations. (See Figure 9.1.) However, both caloric intake and percent energy consumed as carbohy-

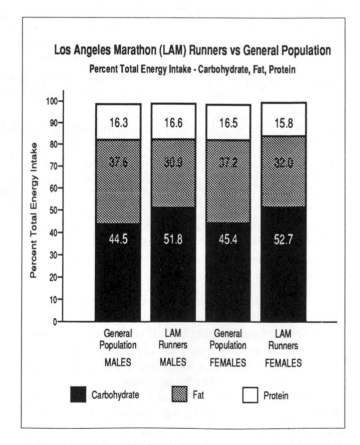

Figure 9.1 The diets of Los Angeles Marathon runners (N = 347) in this study tended to contain less fat and more carbohydrate than the diets of the general population. However, the percentage of total energy intake obtained from carbohydrate was lower than what is recommended for endurance runners.[28]

Table 9.3 Dietary Intakes by Athletes Reported in the Literature

Sport	Daily Calories	Protein Grams/%	Fat Grams/%	Carbohydrate Grams/%
Aerobic:				
Males				
cross country skier	3492-5500	153/13	215/38	600/49
triathlete	3623-6400	130/13	124/28	560/59
Females				
cross country skier	2414-3963	114/14	146/41	333/42
swimmers	2030-4000	99/15	111/38	309/47
triathlete	1500-3500	80/13	85/31	351/56
Aerobic-Anaerobic:				
Males				
soccer	3000-5000	140/15	175/40	460/45
football	2000-11000	196/16	212/40	539/44
basketball	2000-9000	180/15	212/41	503/44
wrestler	1100-6700	95/14	100/34	400/52
Females				
basketball	1900-3900	108/14	145/40	379/46
volleyball	1100-3200	103/16	95/34	314/50
Power				
Males				
track/field	3500-4700	175/17	330/36	470/47
body builders	3575	200/23	157/40	320/36
Skill				
Males				
gymnast	600-4300	77/15	92/40	231/45
ballet dancers	1740-4100	122/17	140/42	300/38
Females				
gymnast	1360-1923	69/15	76/37	225/48
ballet dancers	900-2900	70/15	69/34	230/50

Note: for diets of runners, see Table 9.4. *Source:* See references 8-22.

drate were lower than the amounts recommended for endurance exercise. (See Table 9.2.)

The basic results of the Los Angeles Marathon study are shown in Table 9.4 (under Nieman), and compared with results from other dietary studies on runners. The composition of runners' diets in general, when expressed as a percentage of total energy intake, is surprisingly consistent across the wide range of training distances reported. Both energy and carbohydrate intake are lower than recommended for marathon runners, but slightly higher than those of the general population. (See Table 9.2.) Generally, energy consumption increased with an increase in distance trained,

when expressed as kcal/kg. In other words, people who tend to train more, consume more Calories per kilogram of body weight. In all studies that measured nutrient consumption, the vitamin and mineral intake was at least 67 percent of the RDA (the minimum cut-off point).

Some researchers[3] have suggested that when people start an exercise program, they may also tend to start eating better.[38] Data from the author's study on the Los Angeles marathoners support this view—the majority of the runners reported their present dietary habits were much improved compared to those in pre-running years.[28] (See Figures 9.2 A and B.) The average

Table 9.4 Summary of Dietary Studies on Long Distance Runners

Reference	N	wt (kg)	km/wk	kcal	carb (%)	fat (%)	prot (%)	alco (%)	(RDA (met)	kcal/kg
Males										
Blair (29)	34	71.0	65	2959	40	41	14	6	—	41.7
Clement (30)	35	—	77	3020	49	34	16	—	—	—
Peters (31)	15	68.9	91	3292	49	31	15	5	yes	47.8
Short (22)	9	—	—	4121	49	36	14	—	yes	—
Weight (32)	30	70.2	≥70	2468	60	21	19	—	yes	35.2
Nieman (28)										
total gp	281	73.1	46	2552	52	31	17	3	yes	34.9
low km/wk gp	82	74.2	18	2447	51	31	17	3	yes	33.0
mid km/wk gp	106	73.4	42	2624	52	31	16	3	yes	35.7
high km/wk gp	93	71.7	76	2560	54	29	17	2	yes	35.7
Females										
Blair (29)	27	54.0	55	2386	39	42	16	5	—	44.2
Clement (30)	17	—	70	2026	50	39	15	—	—	—
Dale (33)	37	51.6	73	2217	46	39	15	—	yes	43.0
Deuster (34)	51	51.7	113	2397	55	32	13	—	yes	46.4
Drinkwater (35)	14	57.9	40	1965	52	36	13	—	—	33.9
Moore (36)	45	55.5	50	1765	40	42	17	4	—	31.8
Nelson (37)	17	55.4	64	2250	51	34	15	—	—	40.6
Nieman (28)										
total gp	53	55.6	40	1882	53	32	16	1	yes	33.8
low km/wk gp	20	57.2	16	1774	53	32	15	1	yes	31.0
mid km/wk gp	19	53.9	42	1760	54	30	16	1	yes	32.6
high km/wk gp	14	55.3	70	2193	53	30	17	2	yes	39.7

Note: N = number of people in study; km/wk = average kilometers per week of training; RDA met = at least 67% of the RDA met for the protein, vitamins and minerals that were analyzed; — = data not available; kcal/kg = caloric intake per kilogram of body weight. *Source:* reference 28.

Los Angeles marathoner had been running for 7.5 years, and reported that compared to pre-running years, present dietary habits included a higher consumption of fruit, vegetables, whole grains, poultry and fish, and a lower consumption of red meats, eggs, sugar, salt, and fats.

A longitudinal, randomized, controlled study is needed to see if these perceptions are real. Diets among educated people have tended to improve during the last 10 years,[27] and runners, who are more educated than the average American, may simply be joining this trend.

Nutrition Knowledge of Athletes and Coaches

Surveys conducted on the nutrition knowledge of athletes and coaches have shown, in general, that both are lacking in adequate nutrition knowledge.[39–41] In one study, only 11 percent of coaches had formally studied nutrition as a separate course, yet 73 percent saw themselves as adequately prepared in this regard. Eighty-six percent of the coaches dispensed nutrition knowledge regularly, yet they received low grades (less than 55 percent) when given a standard nutrition test.

Two-thirds of athletes studied were not familiar with the Dietary Goals. In another study of 70 female varsity athletes, scores on a nutritional knowledge test averaged 34 percent, which was no better than the average score of non-athletic female university students.[41]

There are now several excellent books written for the lay-person, some especially for coaches and athletes. (See Box 9.1.) Athletes respond well to dietary counseling, and in particular have learned the importance of emphasizing carbohydrate intake while moderating dietary fat and cholesterol.[18]

In general, athletes of all descriptions do not eat much differently than the general population does, including consuming more fat and less carbohydrate

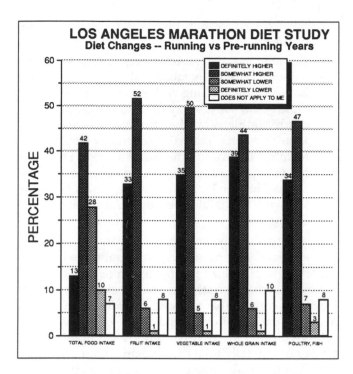

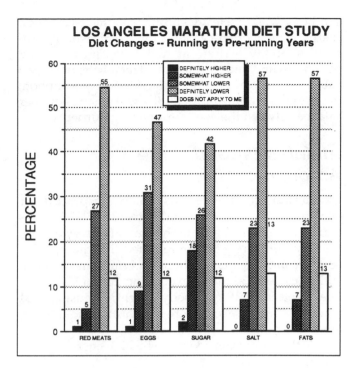

Figures 9.2 A and B Los Angeles Marathon runners (N = 347) who had been training an average of 7.5 years used a five-point Likert scale to estimate the kind of changes in their diets compared to pre-running years. More than 75 percent of the runners reported somewhat or definitely higher intakes of fruits, vegetables, whole grains, poultry and fish, and lower intakes of red meat, eggs, sugar, salt, and fats. *Source:* reference 28.

Box 9.1   Sports Nutrition Books for Coaches, Athletes, and the Lay Public

- **Eating for Endurance** by Ellen Coleman, M.P.H., R.D. Palo Alto, CA: Bull Publishing Co., 1988.

- **Food For Sport** by Nathan Smith, M.D. and Bonnie Worthington-Roberts, Ph.D. Palo Alto, CA: Bull Publishing Co., rev. ed., 1989.

- **Food Power: A Coach's Guide to Improving Performance** by the National Dairy Council, Rosemont, Illinois 60018-4233. 1984.

- **Nutrition for Sports and Dance** by the American Heart Association. Alameda County Chapter, 11200 Golf Links Road, Oakland, California 94605. 1984.

- **Nutrition for Sport Success** by The American Alliance for Health, Physical Education, Recreation and Dance, 1900 Association Drive, Reston, Virginia 22091. 1984.

- **Sports Nutrition: A Guide for the Professional Working with Active People** by the Sports and Cardiovascular Nutritionists (SCAN). The American Dietetic Association, 430 North Michigan Avenue, Chicago, Illinois, 60611. 1986.

than is recommended for both health and athletic effectiveness. The vast proportion of athletes obtain adequate levels of vitamins and minerals in their diets. So what is the bottom line? It is that athletes need to be educated to improve the carbohydrate content of their diets.[42] (This is the basis of sports nutrition principle #3.)

PRINCIPLE 2 Increase Total Energy Intake

If body weight is normal, and exercise is engaged in regularly, energy consumption will need to be higher than that of the average sedentary American to maintain body weight. Heavy endurance athletes are high energy consumers because of their high working capacities, ability to train at high intensities for long periods of time, and elevated basal metabolic rates. (See Table 9.5.) In planning additional food consumption, the guidelines of the prudent diet will ensure a proper balance between the energy-providing nutrients.

Athletes Expend Large Amounts of Energy

As physical activity increases, Calories expended per kilogram of body weight steadily increase.[28, 38] Athletes are capable of amazingly high levels of energy output. A study from Great Britain reported that during a 24-hour cycling time trial in a human performance lab, one athlete cycled 430 miles, expending 20,166 Calories.[43] The athlete lost 1.19 kg of body weight, because only 54 percent of energy needs were met through liquids and food.

Athletes are considered to be high energy expenders for three major reasons:

▪ **High Working Capacities:** As discussed in Chapter 7, one of the best indicators of fitness is the maximum amount of oxygen one can consume during maximal exercise ($\dot{V}O_{2max}$). Male athletes commonly have maximum oxygen uptakes exceeding 4.5 liters/min and some can achieve more than 6.0 liters/min. Female athletes, because of their smaller size, have $\dot{V}O_{2max}$ values about 30 percent lower. For every liter of oxygen consumed, approximately five Calories are expended, which for athletes with high maximal oxygen uptakes means high rates of energy expenditure.

▪ **Ability to Work at High Percent of Maximal Capacity:** During competition and training, athletes often exercise at levels ranging from 70–90 percent of $\dot{V}O_{2max}$. With high $\dot{V}O_{2max}$ capacities to begin with, exercising at high percentages of $\dot{V}O_{2max}$

results in exceedingly high levels of energy expenditure.[8]

▪ **Elevated Basal Metabolic Rates:** Researchers have shown that basal metabolic rates stay elevated for hours following long and intense exercise.[44] (See Figure 9.3.) The twenty-four hour energy expenditure of athletes can therefore be 10 percent higher than that for a normally sedentary person performing the same amount of work. (This only holds for vigorous exercise, however; as we will see in Chapter 11, mild exercise, e.g., a two-mile jog, has a negligible effect on basal metabolic rate during recovery.)

Athletes are not only high energy expenders, they also have a unique pattern of energy utilization, which has important implications for the design of athletic diets. Although endurance athletes tend to expend amounts of energy comparable to those of workers in heavy-labor occupations, they expend a large quantity of their Calories during short time periods—as much as 40 percent of the daily total in less than 2 hours. This has special nutritional implications because of athletes':

▪ high utilization of glycogen (higher carbohydrate needs)

▪ high sweat rates (higher water needs plus possible mineral imbalances)

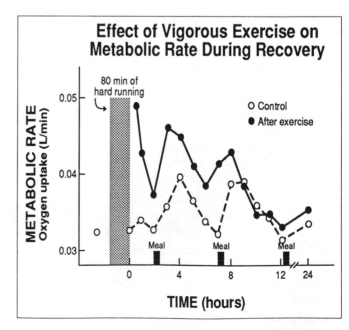

Figure 9.3 Following 80 min of intense running, metabolic rate can stay elevated for more than 8 hours, increasing total energy expenditure substantially. *Source:* reference 44.

Table 9.5 The Relationship Between Caloric Intake and Exercise

	Caloric Intake	
	Males	Females
Average sedentary American	2550	1600
Fitness enthusiast	2700	1800
Heavy endurance athlete	3500	2400

- musculoskeletal trauma (may effect protein and iron needs), and
- gastrointestinal disturbances (may effect iron balance).

Energy and ATP Production

Muscular contraction for any sport or physical activity is produced by movement within the muscle powered by energy released from the separation of high energy phosphate bonds from adenosine triphosphate (ATP).[45-47] (See Chapter 7.)

Although ATP is the immediate energy source for muscular contraction,[45] the amount of ATP present in a muscle is so small that it must be constantly replenished or it will be depleted after several seconds of high intensity exercise. ATP is replenished by two separate systems, the anaerobic (which produces ATP in the absence of oxygen from the small ATP-PC stores and the lactate system), and the aerobic or the oxygen system. (See Figure 9.4.)

The three sources from which ATP is supplied are:

- **ATP-PC Stores:** The body stores a small amount of ATP and CP (creatine phosphate). The muscles can depend on these stores for most of the ATP for up to 10 seconds for such events as sprinting and weight lifting before they are depleted.

- **Lactate Path:** ATP is produced at a high rate from carbohydrate (glycogen) stores within the muscle (see Chapter 7), but lactic acid is also produced. Because of the lactic acid by-product, which accumulates to cause muscle fatigue, ATP production from the lactate system can empower intense exercise for only 1–3 minutes (for such sporting events as 400–800-meter runs, 100-meter swimming events, and boxing).

- **Oxygen System:** This system, which can utilize fatty acids, produces ATP at a slower rate than the other two energy systems, but it represents an enormous potential source of energy—the body supply of fats and carbohydrates for exercise are more than enough for five continuous days of exercise. Oxygen is required, however, which is why the oxygen utilization capacity of the athlete depending on this energy source becomes critically important. The oxygen system is the main provider of ATP in events lasting more than 3 minutes, and in such events as the 26.2-mile marathon, becomes by far the main provider of ATP.

The aerobic and anaerobic systems work in tandem. When the exercise rate is pushed beyond the capability of the ventilation-circulation system to provide oxygen in sufficient amounts, the muscle cells rely more and more on the lactate system to provide ATP. When this reliance becomes too great, glycogen stores may be depleted, and the accumulation of lactic acid may cause debilitating fatigue.

Figure 9.5 summarizes the anaerobic-aerobic continuum. In sports where both systems are utilized (such as in boxing), the training schedule should be designed to develop the capacities of both systems. (See Chapter 8.)

As can be seen in Table 9.6, the body has relatively limited supplies of carbohydrate (1,880 Calories). These are generally distributed in the forms of blood glucose (80 Calories), and liver (350 Calories) and muscle (1,450 Calories) glycogen. On the other hand, fat stores total 142,844 Calories.

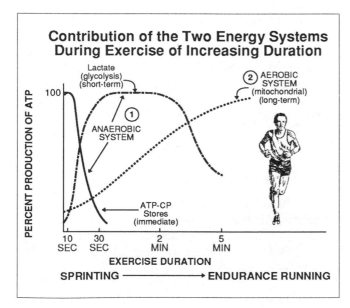

Factors That Determine Type of Fuel Used for ATP Production

Fat and carbohydrate are the primary fuels for endurance exercise; protein is a minor fuel source.

There are three factors that determine which primary fuel, fat or carbohydrate, will be utilized for ATP production:[1, 46, 47]

Figure 9.4 The anaerobic energy system provides ATP to the working myofilaments from ATP-PC stores and the lactate or glycolysis path. The aerobic system supplies ATP from the mitochondria, which require oxygen to burn carbohydrates and fats.

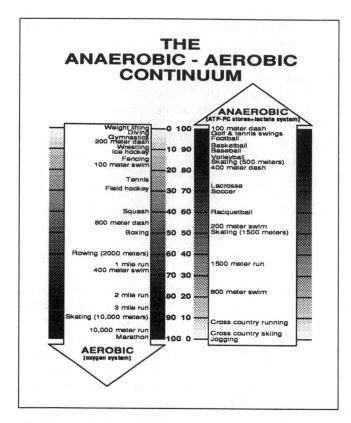

THE ANAEROBIC - AEROBIC CONTINUUM

ANAEROBIC
(ATP-PC stores+lactate system)

Anaerobic %		Aerobic %	
Weight lifting	0	100	100 meter dash
Diving			Golf & tennis swings
Gymnastics			Football
200 meter dash			
Wrestling	10	90	Basketball
Ice hockey			Baseball
Fencing			Volleyball
100 meter swim			Skating (500 meters)
	20	80	400 meter dash
Tennis			
Field hockey	30	70	Lacrosse
			Soccer
Squash	40	60	Racquetball
800 meter dash			
Boxing	50	50	200 meter swim
			Skating (1500 meters)
Rowing (2000 meters)	60	40	
1 mile run			1500 meter run
400 meter swim			
	70	30	
2 mile run	80	20	800 meter swim
3 mile run			
Skating (10,000 meters)	90	10	
10,000 meter run			Cross country running
Marathon	100	0	Cross country skiing
			Jogging

AEROBIC
(oxygen system)

Figure 9.5 While the 100-meter dash is considered a pure anaerobic event, and the marathon a pure aerobic event, most other activities use ATP from both systems. Athletes should train both systems in accordance with the demands of their sport.

1. **Instensity and Duration of Exercise:** The high-intensity, low-duration events (for example, sprinting), depend primarily on carbohydrate, utilizing the anaerobic (without oxygen) system. Carbohydrate is the only fuel that can be used anaerobically.

   As the intensity decreases and the duration increases (e.g., hiking), fat becomes the major preferred fuel source. Carbohydrate is still utilized, especially during the beginning portion of the exercise. Table 9.7 summarizes the utilization of metabolic fuels by muscles at different intensities of exercise.[8, 45–47]

   During prolonged exercise, the usage of carbohydrate is at first high. As the exercise continues, more and more fat is used to supply ATP for the working muscle. (See Figure 9.6.)

2. **Fitness Status:** With an improvement in aerobic fitness status, at any given workload there is an increase in the utilization of fat to produce ATP,

Table 9.6   Substrate Stores of a "Normal Man"

Fuel	Weight (Kg)	Energy (Kcal)
Circulating Fuels		
Glucose	0.020	80
Free fatty acids	0.0004	4
Triglycerides	0.004	40
Total		124
Tissue Stores		
Fat		
adipose	15.0	140,000
intramuscular	0.3	2,800
Protein (muscle)	10.0	41,000
Glycogen		
liver	0.085	350
muscle	0.350	1,450
Total		185,600

Source: see references 8, 46, 47.

preserving the limited carbohydrate stores, and decreasing lactate levels.[1, 48, 49] This greater utilization of fat stores (which are relatively unlimited) enables the athlete to perform longer before muscle glycogen stores are depleted.

3. **Previous Diet:** Early in the 20th Century it was discovered that where the pre-event diet was high in carbohydrate, relatively more carbohydrate was used at any given workload for ATP production. With a high-fat diet, relatively more fat is used.[1] The influence of diet will be discussed fully under sports nutrition principle #3.

PRINCIPLE 3 Keep the Carbohydrate Intake High (55–70 Percent)

Use of a high-carbohydrate diet is probably the most important nutritional principle for both the fitness enthusiast and the endurance athlete.[50–57] (See Table 9.2.) Body carbohydrate stores (glycogen) are extremely important because they are the primary fuel source for the working muscles. When muscle glycogen levels drop too low, the ability to exercise falls, and one feels more stale and tired and is more prone to injury. Athletes in heavy training may need more than 8 grams of carbohydrate per kilogram of body weight in their diet per day, which translates to approximately 70 percent of their total energy intake.

Table 9.7 How Intensity Affects Which Fuel the Muscle Uses

Exercise Intensity	Fuel Used by Muscle
Less than 30% $\dot{V}O_{2max}$	Mainly muscle fat stores
40–60% $\dot{V}O_{2max}$	Fat and CHO used evenly
75% $\dot{V}O_{2max}$	Mainly CHO
+80% $\dot{V}O_{2max}$	Nearly 100% CHO

Source: Adapted from references 8, 45–47.

The Importance of Carbohydrate During Heavy Training

The story of carbohydrate (CHO) in endurance performance began in 1939, when Scandinavian researchers demonstrated the effect of exercise intensity on the fuel used by the muscle during exercise.[58,59] They found that as the intensity of the exercise increased, the relative contribution of CHO as muscular fuel increased.

The development of the biopsy needle in 1962 allowed researchers to extend these findings by measuring the actual amounts of glycogen in the muscle. (See Figure 9.7.) A series of experiments by other Scandinavian investigators during the late 1960s demonstrated that the ability to exercise at 70–80 percent of $\dot{V}O_{2max}$ was related to the preexercise level of muscle glycogen.[60,61]

Several basic principles are now clear regarding the relationship between exercise and dietary carbohydrate, and muscle glycogen synthesis:[1,8,50–57]

- Body glycogen stores play an important role in hard exercise (70–85 percent of $\dot{V}O_{2max}$) that is either prolonged and continuous (e.g., running, swimming, cycling), or of an extended intermittent, mixed anaerobic-aerobic nature (e.g., soccer, basketball, ice hockey, repeated running intervals). The higher the intensity of exercise, the more dependent the working muscle is on glycogen. (See Figure 9.8.) For example, 2 hours of cycling at 30 percent of $\dot{V}O_{2max}$ will only reduce muscle glycogen by about 20 percent, whereas performing at 75 percent of $\dot{V}O_{2max}$ results in almost complete muscle glycogen depletion.[1]

- Because of limited CHO body stores (see Table 9.6), the body adapts in various ways to maximize its use of these stores. Endurance training leads to higher stored levels of muscle glycogen, nearly double those of untrained people.[62] Endurance training also leads to a greater utilization of fat at any given workload, sparing the glycogen. In other words, aerobically fit people consume more fat at any given workload, sparing the glycogen. (See Figure 9.8.) Triglyceride stores within the muscle also increase, by as much as 75–100 percent.[62]

- Exhaustion during prolonged, hard exercise is tied to low muscle glycogen levels. CHO stores are thus the *limiting* factor in exercise bouts lasting longer than 60 minutes.[1,50,63] (See Figure 9.9.) Fatigue in shorter events is due to other factors, especially the buildup of metabolic by-products such as lactic acid and hydrogen ions within the muscle cells.

- When muscle glycogen is low, a high work output cannot be maintained. Marathoners use the term "hitting the wall" to describe the fatigue and pain that is associated with reaching low glycogen levels. There is an apparent obligatory requirement of muscle glycogen breakdown for intense exercise. The breakdown of fat cannot sustain metabolic rates during exercise at levels much above 50–65 percent of $\dot{V}O_{2max}$. In other words, when muscle glycogen levels are low, the exerciser

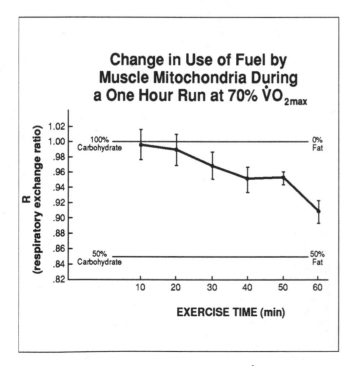

Change in Use of Fuel by Muscle Mitochondria During a One Hour Run at 70% $\dot{V}O_{2max}$

Figure 9.6 During a one-hour run at 70% $\dot{V}O_{2max}$, the muscles gradually use more and more fat to produce ATP. *Source:* Nieman DC, Carlson KA, Brandstater ME, et al. Running Endurance in 27-h Fasted Humans. J Appl Physiol 63:2502–2509, 1987.

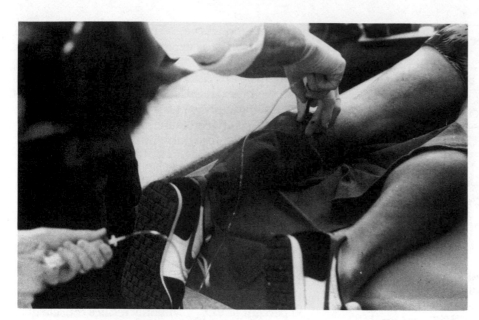

Figure 9.7 The needle biopsy allows researchers to obtain a small sample of muscle tissue to measure the amount of glycogen. A small incision is made in the muscle (after anesthetizing the area), the biopsy needle is inserted, suction pressure is applied, and a small piece of muscle is cut with a sliding knife device in the needle.

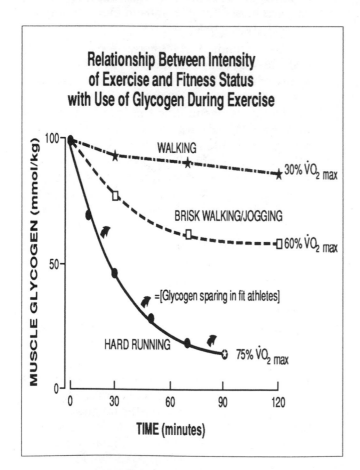

Figure 9.8 With increasing intensity of exercise, more and more glycogen is utilized by the muscle. As the arrows depict, with aerobic training fit athletes tend to use less glycogen during any given workload, sparing the glycogen.

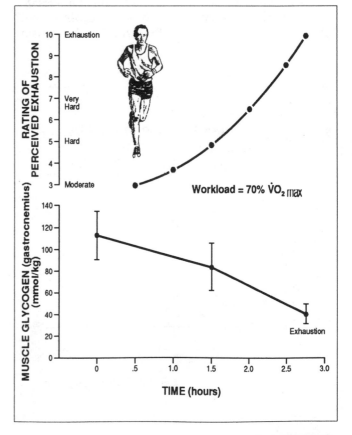

Figure 9.9 Nine experienced marathoners ran for nearly 3 hours on a treadmill at 70 percent $\dot{V}O_{2max}$. As the muscle glycogen levels fell, the rating of perceived exertion climbed strongly. Exhaustion was associated with low glycogen levels in the muscles of the runners. *Source:* see reference 63.

will not be able to exercise at intensities above 50–65 percent of $\dot{V}O_{2max}$—which for many runners means a painful shuffle or jog.

CHO produces five percent more energy per liter of oxygen consumed than fats, which places fewer demands upon the heart and lung systems. In addition, CHO is needed for the oxidation of fat. Thus when muscles are depleted of glycogen, the muscle cells are unable to support fat metabolism.[1, 46]

■ During the first hour of hard exercise, nearly all of the CHO and fat (triglycerides) come from within the muscle, which is an amazing depot of fuel.[62] (See Figure 9.10.) As the exercise continues beyond one hour, more and more demands are placed upon adipose tissue fat fuel sources and blood glucose as muscle glycogen levels begin to be depleted. The longer the exercise period, the greater the need for glucose from the liver to keep pace with the increasing glucose demands of the glycogen-depleted working muscle.[1]

■ During strenuous training, muscle glycogen stores undergo rapid day-to-day fluctuation. Sedentary people on normal mixed diets have glycogen stores of only 70–110 mmol per kilogram wet muscle.[54] Athletes on mixed diets, after 24 hours of rest, have glycogen levels of 130–135 mmol/kg wet muscle, and after 48 hours of rest with a high carbohydrate diet, they have 140–230 mmol/kg.[1]

As Figure 9.11 shows, glycogen levels of athletes can be reduced 50 percent after a 2-hour

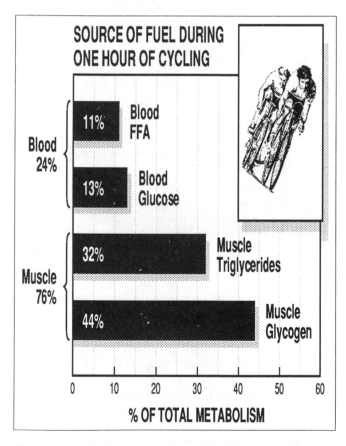

Figure 9.10 During the first hour of cycling, about three-fourths of the fuel comes from within the muscle itself (primarily muscle glycogen). Blood borne fuels become a more important factor as exercise continues beyond one hour, and muscle glycogen stores begin to be depleted.

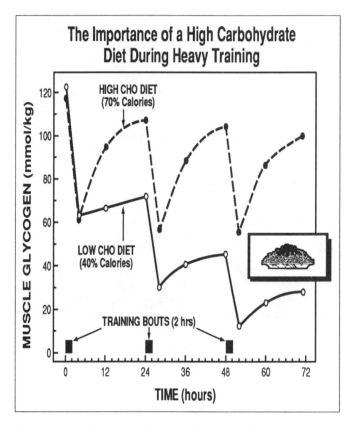

Figure 9.11 Daily, two-hour workouts deplete muscle glycogen stores by about 50 percent. A low-carbohydrate diet (40 percent of Calories) does not adequately restore this depleted glycogen, and there will be a progressive reduction in muscle glycogen as the daily workouts continue. A high-carbohydrate diet (70 percent of Calories) helps to keep muscle glycogen stores near normal despite heavy training, preventing chronic fatigue. *Source:* Costill DL, Miller JM. Nutrition for Endurance Sports: Carbohydrate and Fluid Balance. Int J Sports Med 1:2–14, 1980. Used with permission from Georg Thieme Verlag, Publishers, Stuttgart 1, West Germany.

workout. If the carbohydrate content of the diet is low (about 40 percent of total Calories), little muscle glycogen is restored during the following day, and with a 2-hour work-out the next day, there will be increasing fatigue because of initially low glycogen levels. If this cycle continues, chronic fatigue will be felt.[1, 64-66] On the other hand, a high carbohydrate diet (about 70 percent of total caloric intake) can help counter this glycogen depletion.

Practical Implications for Athletes

In general, glycogen synthesis increases in proportion to the amount of consumed CHO. Six hundred and twenty-five grams of dietary CHO leads to near maximal replenishment of muscle glycogen following a strenuous training bout.[67] More than 8 grams of CHO are needed per kilogram of body weight each day for the endurance athlete who is training for more than 60–90 minutes.[65] Athletes in heavy training should consume a diet of at least 70 percent CHO (525 grams per 3000 Calories), which will result in a synthesis of 70–80 mmol glycogen per kilogram wet muscle within 24 hours, enabling the athlete to continue heavy training.

This is more carbohydrate than most athletes would ordinarily choose, however, and they need to be educated to include in this large amount.[52] Athletes commonly underestimate their carbohydrate needs, and are thus susceptible to feeling "stale" from glycogen depletion.

When muscle glycogen stores are depleted, a sense of tiredness, fatigue, mistakes, and injuries increase.[8, 64]

Table 9.8 is a sample listing of high-carbohydrate foods, in descending order of amount of the carbohydrate they contain (in grams per cup). Notice that foods high in simple sugars lead the list, followed by dried fruits, cereals, potatoes, rice, legumes, and fruit juices. Although high-sugar foods such as honey, jams, and syrups provide high amounts of carbohydrate (and although glycogen synthesis appears to be unaffected by the form of carbohydrate consumed),[67, 68] too much simple sugar in the diet invites shortages of necessary vitamins and minerals.

Table 9.9 outlines a sample menu for an athlete who is training more than 60–90 minutes a day aerobically. Notice that grain products and fruits predominate in this high-carbohydrate diet. The use of fatty meats and dairy products, nuts, olives, and oils should be limited to ensure that sufficient carbohydrate is consumed to replete muscle glycogen stores.

PRINCIPLE 4 Drink Large Amounts of Water During Training and the Event

Probably the second most important dietary principle for those who exercise is to drink large quantities of water. As little as a 2 percent drop in body weight caused by water loss (primarily from sweat) can reduce exercise capacity. In other words, if a runner weighs 150 pounds and loses 3.0 pounds during an exercise bout, his performance ability is reduced—and what is more, he enters the zone of impending exhaustion.

Thirst lags behind actual body needs. So before, during, and after the exercise bout, one should drink plenty of fluids, beyond the demands of thirst. A plan recommended by some sports medicine experts is to drink two cups of water immediately before the exercise bout, one cup every 15 minutes during the exercise session, and then two more cups after the session. (Whether or not to include carbohydrates and electrolytes in the exercise drink is important, and will be discussed below.)

The Importance of Water for Temperature Regulation During Exercise

About 80 percent of the energy released during exercise is heat.[8] If this were retained by the body, body heat would potentially increase up to 1°C every 5 minutes,[69] resulting in lethal heat injury (hyperthermia) within 20 minutes.

During steady state exercise at 75 percent of capacity, average heat loss from the body may range from 900–1500 kcal/hour. An addition of up to 100–150 kcal/hour may be gained from the sun.

The body's chief avenue of heat loss is sweat evaporation—during exercise in the heat, more than 80 percent of the total heat loss is produced by sweat evaporation.[70] For every liter of sweat evaporated on the skin, close to 600 kcal are given off, preventing an increase in body temperature of a full 10°C.

Circulatory adjustments increase skin blood flow so that heat can be carried off through convection and radiation. Figure 9.12 shows the avenues of heat loss from the exercising human body, sweat evaporation being by far the most important.[69-82]

The sweat glands draw fluid from stores between and within the body cells, and then from the plasma

Table 9.8 High-Carbohydrate Foods—One Cup Portions

Food	Grams of Carbohydrate/Cup	Calories/Cup	% Kcal CHO
Honey	272	1040	100
Pancake syrup	238	960	100
Jams/preserves	224	880	100
Molasses	176	720	100
Dates (chopped)	131	489	100
Raisins	115	434	100
Prunes	101	385	100
Grape Nuts	94	407	92
Whole wheat flour	85	400	85
Dried apricots (uncooked)	80	310	100
Sweet potato (boiled, mashed)	80	344	93
Sweetened applesauce	51	194	100
Brown rice	50	232	86
Prune juice	45	181	100
Kidney beans	42	230	73
Rolled wheat (cooked)	41	180	91
Macaroni (cooked)	39	190	82
Lentils (cooked)	39	210	74
Grape juice	38	155	98

Source: USDA Handbook No. 8 (revised)

volume of the blood in the skin.[71] (See Figure 9.13.) The efficiency of sweat evaporation is greatly affected by humidity.[72, 73] If the humidity is so high that the sweat rolls off the skin without evaporation, no heat is given off and body temperature rises. This can result in heat injury, including heat exhaustion and heat stroke. (See Chapter 15.) In heat stroke, the brain shuts off the sweat glands to protect blood fluid levels, resulting in dry, hot, and red skin and a deadly rise in body temperature.

Exercise in hot and humid weather can be dangerous. During the 1986 Pittsburgh Marathon, the temperature reached 87°F and the humidity 60 percent; one-half of the 2,879 runners were treated for heat injuries.[83] (The American College of Sports Medicine has established guidelines for race directors to follow to avoid this type of disaster.) (See Chapter 15.)

Sweat losses of 1.5 liters per hour are common in endurance sports. Under extremely hot conditions, sweat rates (of fit participants) have been measured at over 2.5 liters per hour.[8, 74] During the 1984 Los Angeles Olympic games, U.S. runner Alberto Salazar lost 12 pounds (8.1 percent of body weight) during the marathon, despite drinking nearly 2 liters of water during the race. Alberto's sweat rate was 3.7 liters per hour, one of the highest ever measured.[75]

Loss of body water from sweating beyond 2 percent of body weight will significantly impair endurance capacity, through elevation of body temperature and decreased cardiac output. When sweat output exceeds water intake, both intracellular and extracellular water levels fall, and plasma volume decreases, resulting in an increase in body temperature, a decrease in the ability of the heart to pump blood, and a decrease in endurance performance.[76, 77] During just 30 minutes of cycling in the heat, plasma volume can fall an average of 13 percent.[78]

Table 9.10 outlines the adverse effects of dehydration.[79] Those most vulnerable to dehydration during exercise are the obese, unfit, unacclimatized, overclothed, or ill, exercising on hot, humid, sunny days.[84] Early warning signals include clumsiness, stumbling, excessive sweat, cessation of sweating, headache, nausea, or dizziness.

People who are accustomed to exercising in the heat go through physiological changes which have been termed the "acclimatization process."[85–87] Acclimatization (using a gradual progression for safety) can occur within as few as 5–10 days of training in the heat. The acclimatized person has a higher plasma volume (400 to 700 ml increase), and sweat glands that produce more sweat earlier in the exercise session with less loss of sodium. During exercise, the acclimatized person's body temperature and heart rate do not rise as strongly as those of unacclimatized people.

Fluid replacement during exercise dramatically reduces the adverse effects of dehydration.[42, 82, 88-91] Fluid consumption during exercise can slow the rise in core temperature, maintain plasma volume and cardiac output, improve endurance, and lessen the risk of heat injury.

In one study,[82] a physically active middle-aged male performed treadmill simulations of 10-mile races

---

Table 9.9 Sample Menu of 3,500 Kcal, High-Carbohydrate (79 Percent Total Kcal)

The foods listed below represent a one-day sample of the type of diet recommended for the average male runner training for long endurance events. This type of diet is also recommended for "carbohydrate loading" during the three-day period before a long endurance race. This sample diet meets the recommended dietary allowance (RDA) for all nutrients and follows the guidelines of the "prudent diet." Most of the calories come during breakfast and lunch, with a lighter supper, to allow a better night's rest.

Portion	Food	Kilocalories
Breakfast		
1 cup	Grape Nuts	404
2 cup	2% lowfat milk	242
1 whole	banana	105
.5 cup	seedless raisins	247
2 cup	orange juice	224
1 piece	whole wheat bread	84
2 tsp	honey	43
Lunch		
2 piece	whole wheat bread	168
1 tbs	peanut butter	96
2 whole	apple	162
2 cup	cooked brown rice	464
2 cup	mixed vegetables	105
1 tsp	seasonings	5
1 cup	low fat yogurt	231
2 whole	bagels	330
Supper		
.5 whole	fresh tomato	12
.5 cup	loose leaf lettuce	5
2 oz.	cooked chicken	108
2 piece	whole wheat bread	168
1 tbs	low-cal dressing	35
2 cup	canned pineapple juice	278

Meal	Kilocalories	Total CHO	% CHO
Breakfast	1349	290	86%
Lunch	1561	292	75%
Supper	606	108	71%
Totals	3516	690	79%

Nutrients	Protein	Iron	Zinc	Calcium	Vit C	Vit A	Vit B1
Day Totals	116 g	25 mg	18 mg	1579 mg	425 mg	15009 IU	4.2 mg
% RDA	207%	250%	120%	197%	708%	300%	280%

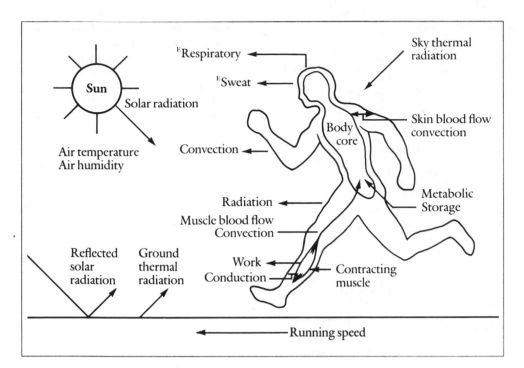

Figure 9.12 As the muscles contract during exercise, heat is produced, causing the core body temperature to rise. A small amount of heat is also gained by the body from the environment. The primary route for this heat to exit is sweat evaporation. Other routes include convection, radiation, conduction, and respiration. *Source:* Gisolfi CV, Wenger CB. Temperature Regulation During Exercise: Old Concept, New Ideas. Exercise and Sports Sciences Reviews, Volume 12, 1984. Edited by Terjung RL. Lexington: Collamore Press.

Table 9.10 Adverse Effects of Dehydration

% Body Wt Loss	Symptoms
.5	Thirst
2.0	Stronger thirst, vague discomfort, loss of appetite
3.0	Increasing hemoconcentration, dry mouth, reduction in urine
4.0	Increased effort for exercise, flushed skin, impatience, apathy
5.0	Difficulty in concentrating
6.0	Impairment in exercise temperature regulation, increased HR
8.0	Dizziness, labored breathing in exercise, mental confusion
10.0	Spastic muscles, inability to balance with eyes closed, general incapacity, delirium and wakefulness, swollen tongue
11.0	Circulatory insufficiency, marked hemoconcentration and decreased blood volume, failing renal function

Source: Greenleaf JE, Fink WJ. Fluid Intake and Athletic Performance. IN: Nutrition and Athletic Performance (Haskell W, ed). Palo Alto: Bull Publishing Co., 1982. Used with permission of Bull Publishing Co.

Sources of Fluid for Sweat Production

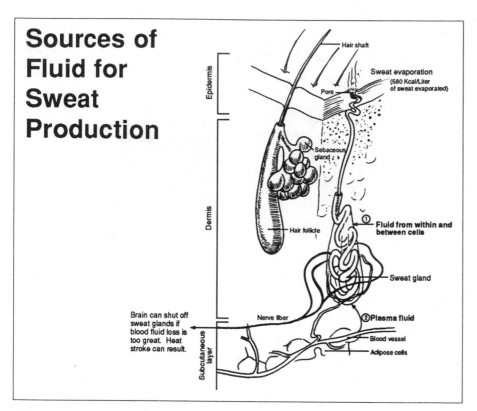

Figure 9.13 The sweat glands draw fluids from between and within cells and from the blood to produce sweat during exercise. If blood volume levels fall too low, the brain will shut off sweat gland activity. Continued exercise can result in heat stroke.

on two separate days in a heated chamber (95°F). (See Figure 9.14.) In the first trial, cold fluids were force-fed in 400-ml volumes at 20-minute intervals before and during the run. In the second trial, the exercise was repeated in the same fashion, but without fluids. Beyond four miles the benefits of fluid intake were manifested by substantially lower heart rate and temperature responses (both core and skin). In the no-fluid trial, premature exhaustion occurred at 6.8 miles with exertional hyperthermia (40.5°C, core temperature).

How much water should one drink during exercise to avoid dehydration? It is common to lose 2–4 percent of body weight during vigorous workouts.[92, 93] Marathoners can lose 6–8 percent of their body weight in water during the 26.2-mile event, with plasma volume decreasing 13–18 percent. A 4-percent drop in body weight for a 150-pound person means a loss of six pounds, or three quarts of water. It is not uncommon for such a man, if he were running in a hot environment, to lose half a pound per mile after the first hour. That would amount to a cup of water every mile, or every 6–8 minutes.

For most athletes, it is hard to drink this much water, mainly because such intake is beyond the demands of thirst. Exercise tends to blunt thirst (which does not generally reflect dehydration in any event), so

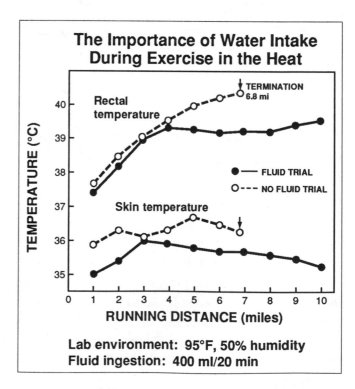

The Importance of Water Intake During Exercise in the Heat

Lab environment: 95°F, 50% humidity
Fluid ingestion: 400 ml/20 min

Figure 9.14 Use of cold fluids during exercise in the heat can prolong endurance time while keeping core body temperature at lower levels. *Source:* see reference 82.

a systematic plan should be followed for fluid consumption during exercise.[42] (When athletes drink only what they desire during exercise, their plasma volume tends to fall 8–10 percent, leading to impaired performance.)[94] Most sports nutrition experts recommend 200–400 ml of water every 20 minutes of exercise, or 500 ml every 30 minutes. The majority of 400 ml of water will be out of the stomach within 15 minutes, being absorbed in the small intestine.

When exercise intensity climbs above 75 percent $\dot{V}O_{2max}$, however, gastric emptying decreases[95] as compared with that for more moderate exercise.

The water should be 40–50°F, or refrigerator cold when drunk during exercise. The coldness does not interfere with gastric emptying (or cause cramps), and helps stabilize the core temperature of the body.[96] In one study conducted by the author, ten marathoners were able to maintain plasma volume at normal levels despite running for three hours in a laboratory (70°F, 50-percent humidity) at 70 percent of $\dot{V}O_{2max}$ by forcing down 500 ml of cold water every 30 minutes.[88]

Can body temperature be controlled and dehydration prevented by wetting the head and skin during exercise? Although this may be psychologically pleasing, researchers have shown that skin wetting does not reduce sweat rates or reduce core body temperature.[70, 75] In these studies, however, only 50 ml of water were sprayed on the skin every 10 minutes. The possibility exists that greater amounts of cold water may be beneficial. More research is needed in this area.

Should Electrolytes and Carbohydrates be Used During Exercise?

There are a wide variety of sports drinks available containing varying levels of electrolyte and carbohydrate. (See Table 9.11.) There are three purposes promoted for using these drinks: (1) to avoid dehydration; (2) to counter the loss of electrolytes; (3) to oppose the loss of body carbohydrate stores.[97, 98]

Should electrolytes (sodium, potassium, and chloride) be added to the exercise drink? The electrolyte content of sweat is relatively very low. Although sodium, chloride, potassium, magnesium, calcium, zinc, and some vitamins are excreted with the sweat, most studies have shown that such losses are rarely significant for properly nourished and acclimatized people.[8] In particular, athletes are very unlikely to develop sodium chloride deficiency, even with high sweat rates, because training develops adaptive mechanisms that

conserve salt. The salt content of a trained athlete's sweat is one third that of an untrained person.

There are exceptions to this in extreme endurance events. Low levels of sodium (hyponatremia) have been measured in ultramarathoners and Ironman triathletes.[99–101] If large quantities of plain water are consumed during exercise exceeding 4 hours duration, low blood sodium levels become a concern. Therefore, athletes engaging in events lasting longer than 4 hours are urged to drink fluids containing electrolytes.

However, except for such extreme endurance events, the addition of electrolytes in fluid replacement beverages is generally not justified. One exception can be the addition of small amounts of sodium to water, which has been found to speed gastric emptying and fluid absorption from the intestine.[97] But even here, recent evidence suggests that differences in gastric emptying rates among beverages are not particularly important unless they exceed 10 percent concentration (more than 10 grams of CHO per 100 ml water).[102–107]

However, the addition of limited carbohydrate to replacement fluids can be helpful. Although the results of earlier studies suggested that solutions with more than 2.5 percent glucose slow the rate of passage of the fluid through the stomach, recent gastric emptying studies conducted during 2–4 hours of exercise show that 4–10 percent CHO solutions, regardless of CHO type, can be emptied from the stomach at rates similar to water.

Beverages containing simple sugars or glucose polymers (4–6 glucose units) with or without small amounts of electrolytes minimize disturbances in temperature regulation and cardiovascular function as well as ordinary water, maintain blood glucose levels better than water, and enhance athletic performance more than water. Most reviewers now conclude that sports drinks that contain 4–10 percent CHO of any type (glucose polymer, glucose, or sucrose) in volumes of 200–400 ml consumed every 15–20 minutes are preferable to plain water.[97, 98] Some research suggests that fructose can cause gastrointestinal distress and may compromise performance,[89] so this type of sugar should be avoided.

Figure 9.15 summarizes this information. The importance of CHO in the drink solution lies in its ability to elevate blood glucose levels. Several studies have shown that even when muscle glycogen levels are low, ingestion of CHO solutions during the later stages of long endurance exercise (at least 30 minutes before fatigue) can counter the drop in blood glucose levels and prolong exercise by as much as 20–30 percent.[97, 108–112] Apparently the elevated blood glucose levels from

Table 9.11 A Comparison of Sports Drinks (Per Cup or 8 Fluid Ounces)

Sports Drink	Type of Carbohydrate	Recommended Concentration	Sodium	Other Electrolytes	Calories
Body fuel 100	Glucose polymer	0.3%	28 mg	none	5
Body fuel 450	Glucose polymer Fructose	4%	80 mg	K–20 mg	40
Carbo plus	Glucose polymer	16%	5 mg	K–100 mg Mg-100 mg	170
Exceed	Glucose polymer Sucrose	7.2%	66 mg	K–56 mg Mg–6 mg	68
Gatorade	Sucrose/glucose	6%	110 mg	K–25 mg	50
Gookinaid ERG	Glucose	5.7%	70 mg	K-100 mg	45
Max	Glucose polymers	7.5%	15 mg	none	70
R.P.M.	Fructose	7.6%	0 mg	K–70 mg	70

Source: Adapted from Applegate L. Choosing a Sport Drink. Runner's World, July 1986, pp 18–19. K = potassium, Mg = magnesium.

the CHO ingestion during exercise can support exercise even at 60–70 percent $\dot{V}O_{2max}$ levels.

In one study of cyclers, feeding them 3 g/kg of glucose polymers (50–percent solution) after 135 minutes of exercise (30 minutes before estimated fatigue) allowed the athletes to cycle 21 percent longer, restoring normal blood glucose levels.[112] As discussed earlier, during long endurance exercise, there appears to be a gradual shift from intramuscular glycogen toward blood-borne glucose as muscle glycogen is depleted.

However, plasma glucose concentrations can drop late in exercise (hypoglycemia), leading to fatigue.[113] This is because the liver is incapable of keeping up with the glucose demands of intense endurance exercise. This can be reversed to an extent by ingesting glucose polymers in large quantities (about 800 Calories' worth).

The researchers concluded that there appears to be no benefit to ingesting glucose polymers throughout exercise.[112] This is especially true for athletes who carbohydrate load before-hand.[114] What appears to be critical is to ingest about 200 grams of CHO (800 Calories) about 30 minutes before the estimated onset of fatigue to restore blood glucose levels. If the CHO is taken at the time of fatigue, blood glucose levels do not rise sufficiently to allow continued exercising. Interestingly, the stomachs of the athletes appeared capable of emptying a 50 percent CHO drink quickly enough to support continued exercise.

So in summary, one of the most important measures for an endurance athlete is to develop the habit of drinking plenty of water just before, during, and after exercise. The water should be cold, and drunk in 200–400 ml quantities every 20 minutes (more than thirst calls

for). During prolonged exercise, CHO in concentrations of 4–10 percent helps prevent the exercise-induced drop in blood glucose levels, allowing exercise to continue even though muscle glycogen levels are low. There is some evidence to suggest that there is no practical benefit in consuming carbohydrate throughout the exercise session, so long as it is taken in large quantities 30 minutes before fatigue begins.

There is little need for electrolytes in the fluids except for extreme endurance events such as ultramarathons. Most people will easily obtain all needed electrolytes in the food they eat following the exercise. The one exception would be the usefulness of including a small amount of sodium in the fluid replacement drink, to help the stomach empty the solution faster and allow quicker absorption of water in the small intestine.

PRINCIPLE 5 Keep a Close Watch on Possible Iron Deficiency

An alarming number of athletes, especially elite male and female endurance athletes, test positive for mild iron deficiency, best measured by evaluating serum ferritin levels. On the other hand, very few athletes reach a state of anemia, which is measured when the hemoglobin falls below 12 md/dl for females and 13 md/dl for males. In general, fitness enthusiasts do not usually need to be concerned with iron deficiency, because moderate amounts of exercise have not been shown to cause any iron deficiency.

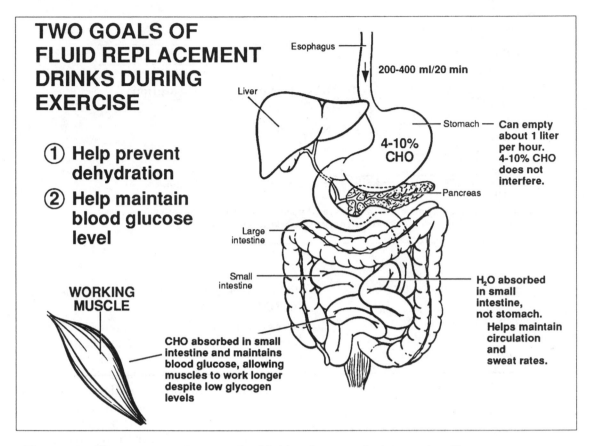

TWO GOALS OF FLUID REPLACEMENT DRINKS DURING EXERCISE

① **Help prevent dehydration**

② **Help maintain blood glucose level**

WORKING MUSCLE

CHO absorbed in small intestine and maintains blood glucose, allowing muscles to work longer despite low glycogen levels

Esophagus

200-400 ml/20 min

Liver

Stomach — **Can empty about 1 liter per hour. 4-10% CHO does not interfere.**

4-10% CHO

Pancreas

Large intestine

Small intestine

H₂O absorbed in small intestine, not stomach.

Helps maintain circulation and sweat rates.

Figure 9.15   There are two primary goals of fluid replacement during exercise: (1) to prevent dehydration; (2) to help maintain blood glucose levels.

The Problem of Iron Deficiency

Several reports in the literature suggest that endurance athletes, especially runners, may be prone to iron deficiency.[42, 115-125] Using serum ferritin levels as a criteria (less than 12 ng/ml), between 10 and 80 percent of male and female athletes, depending on the study, have mild iron deficiency. Serum ferritin falls in about half of those tested within four weeks, when exercise is increased to high levels.[122]

While most of these reports have been on runners, one study of swimmers found that 11 percent of males and 57 percent of females had low serum ferritin levels.[123] In nearly all studies, however, it is extremely rare to find that hemoglobin is low (an indication of anemia). And iron deficiency has not been a problem for fitness enthusiasts who exercise moderately (20–40 minutes per session, 3–5 sessions per week).[126]

Iron deficiency is commonly divided into three stages,[127-129] which form a continuum, each shading gradually into the other. (See Table 9.12.)

The first stage is mild iron depletion, which is characterized by decreased or absent bone marrow iron stores, and measured sensitively, by a drop in plasma ferritin. There is usually 1000 mg of iron in the bone marrow of male adults, and 300 mg in the marrow of female adults. At this stage other indices of iron deficiency are normal. Serum ferritin levels below 20 ng/ml are suboptimal, and levels below 12 ng/ml are associated with very low bone marrow iron stores.

Stage 2 follows the exhaustion of bone marrow iron stores, and is characterized as a diminishing iron supply to the developing red cell. Iron-deficient erythropoiesis (formation of red blood cells) occurs and is measured by increased total iron binding capacity and reduced serum iron and percent saturation (<16 percent is abnormal). The red blood cell protoporphyrin (a derivative of hemoglobin which has an atom of iron deleted) increases above 70 mcg/dl.

Stage 3 is iron deficient anemia, characterized by a drop in hemoglobin. Hemoglobin levels below 12 g/dl for females, and 13 g/dl for males are considered anemic.[128-131] The range of normal hemoglobin levels is 13–16 g/dl for men and 12–16 g/dl for women. The bone marrow produces an increasing number of smaller and less brightly red colored red blood cells. This is

Table 9.12 Stages of Iron Deficiency

Stage	Blood Indices						Bone Marrow FE	Iron Absorption
	SF	FE	TIBC	SAT	HGB	RBC		
Iron deficient mild	D	N	N	N	N	N	0	I
Iron deficient erythropoiesis	D	D	I	D	N	N	0	I
Iron deficient anemia	D	D	I	D	D	D*	0	I

N = Normal; D = decrease; I = increase, 0 = none; SF = serum ferritin; FE = serum iron; TIBC = total iron binding capacity; SAT = transferrin saturation; HGB = hemoglobin.

*Red blood cells in ron deficient anemia become small (microcytic) and less red (hypochromic). The amount of RBC protoporphyrin, a derivative of hemoglobin with one atom of iron deleted, increase. *Source:* See references 128, 129.

measured when the mean corpuscular volume (MCV) falls below 80 fl.

Anemia is generally acknowledged to be the most common single nutritional deficiency in both developing and developed countries. However, it is not particularly associated with athletes. In the United States, 5 percent of female and 1.5 percent of male adults are anemic.[129] In one study of 85 female marathon runners, only 2 percent were anemic.[124]

Menstruating females are particularly at risk for iron deficiency.[132] The combination of growth, menstruation, and strenuous training can put the young female athlete at a high level of risk.[133] Some researchers conjecture that the relatively high incidence of amenorrhea among runners and dancers may be partially explained by low iron body stores, as the body seeks to prevent any further iron loss. (See Chapter 15.)

Iron deficiency, with or without anemia, is particularly undesirable for athletes. An essential constituent of hemoglobin, myoglobin, and several iron-containing respiratory enzymes, iron plays a vital role in energy production.[131] Relatively small decreases in hemoglobin (1–2 g/dl) have been shown to impair physical performance.[134,135] There is a very close association between the hemoglobin content of the blood and $\dot{V}O_{2max}$. (More recently, iron deficiency without anemia has been examined, and has also been shown to reduce physical work capacity,[127,136,137] although not all researchers agree on this.)[124,138]

Several factors explain why runners in particular (especially females) are at high risk for iron deficiency.[42,118,127,131,139–144]

- **Inadequate Dietary Iron:** The average Western diet supplies only 5–6 mg per 1,000 Calories.[128] The best studies measuring the diets of female athletes have shown them consuming less than the RDA of 18 mg.[28,105]

- **Increased Hemolysis:** Several studies provide evidence to suggest that exercise causes an accelerated destruction of red blood cells.[123,127,141,142,145] Some authors have suggested that the breakdown of red blood cells inside the capillaries (measured by a decrease in blood haptoglobin), together with kidney excretion of hemoglobin may be contributing to the low hemoglobin concentrations reported among athletes. Some researchers have attributed this to the mechanical trauma imposed on the capillaries of the feet from running.[142,145] Other factors may include elevated body temperatures, increased blood flow, acidosis, and the effects of catecholamines.

- **Decreased Iron Absorption:** Mean absorption of dietary iron is about 5–10 percent when body iron stores are adequate and about 15–20 percent when stores are low.[128,132] However, the tendency of iron absorption to increase as iron stores are depleted has not been clearly demonstrated with iron-deficient athletes—who show half the absorption rates of controls with depleted iron stores.[117] Runners may have an absorption disturbance, because of a faster clearance of food through the gastrointestinal tract.[139]

- **Increased Iron Loss in Sweat, Feces, and Urine:** Athletes' iron losses in sweat can be substantial, averaging about 0.25 mg per liter of sweat.[143,144] This is important, because normally only a small portion of dietary iron is absorbed, about 1–2 mg per day.[128] Running (especially when racing) has been found to induce gastrointestinal bleeding, which can be measured in the feces.[146,147] One study showed that of 24 runners, 21 had an increase of fecal hemoglobin after racing (10K–42.2K).[117] Seven runners lost over 2 mg of iron during the one day of their race. Hemoglobin can also be found in the urine of athletes, especially after hard exercise.[127] Intense running may cause slight damage to the hollow gut and bladder, due to the trauma of the sides rubbing each other.

Practical Implications for Athletes

Treatment of iron deficiency should first involve a checkup with a physician to ensure that there is no underlying illness or medical disorder.[127]

It is very difficult to help a person recover from iron deficiency with diet alone.[124, 148] Oral iron therapy must often be considered, consisting of 30–75 mg of elemental iron given as a ferrous salt administered 3 times daily, on an empty stomach. In addition, ascorbic acid can help enhance absorption.[149] However, for many athletes, the most effective therapy is to reduce iron losses by reducing the amount of exercise to more moderate levels.

Despite the prevalence of iron deficiency among runners, iron supplements should not be given routinely to athletes without medical supervision. In addition to the possibility of inducing deficiencies of other trace minerals, such as copper and zinc, a high iron intake can produce an iron overload in some people.[150, 151] Therefore, athletes should be encouraged to increase iron intake by eating foods high in iron. High iron foods include, fortified breakfast cereals, dried fruit, legumes, molasses, lean meats, and nuts.[11] (See Table 9.13.)

Animal tissue has an average of 40 percent heme iron and 60 percent nonheme iron, while plant products are composed of 100 percent nonheme iron.[128] Nonheme iron absorption is enhanced by consuming vitamin C during the meal, and absorption from plant sources is also increased if meat is eaten at the same time. Vegetarian athletes, who may be at special risk for iron deficiency, should be sure to include vitamin C foods with each meal.[140, 152]

PRINCIPLE 6 Vitamin and Mineral Supplements are Not Needed

As we shall see in this section, most studies show that the intake of major vitamins and minerals by people who exercise is above recommended levels. People who

Table 9.13 Iron in One Cup Portions of Plant Foods

Food	Iron Per Cup of Food (Mg)
Pumpkin seeds	20.7
Raisin bran cereal	16.4
Wheat germ	10.3
Sunflower seeds	9.8
Cashews	8.2
Wheat chex cereal	7.3
Dried apricots	6.1
Grape Nuts cereal	4.9
Great north beans (cooked)	4.9
Soybeans (cooked)	4.9
Almonds	4.8
Peanut butter	4.6
Red kidney beans (cooked)	4.6
Lentils (cooked)	4.2
Prunes	4.0
Blackeye cowpeas (cooked)	3.6
Lima beans (cooked)	3.5
Raisins	3.0
Fish, bass, broiled	2.9
Turkey	2.5
Ham, extra lean	2.1
Lobster	1.9
Tuna	1.5

Source: USDA Handbook No. 8 (revised)

Note: Although meats have lower concentrations of iron, their iron is more easily absorbed than iron from plant foods. Vitamin 3, however, greatly improves the availability of iron from plant foods.

exercise are at an advantage because they tend to eat more than sedentary people, thereby providing their bodies with more vitamins and minerals. The American Dietetic Association, in their publication "Nutrition for Physical Fitness and Athletic Performance for Adults," has stated that heavy endurance exercise ". . . may increase the need for some vitamins and minerals, but this can easily be met by consuming a balanced diet in accordance with the extra caloric requirement."[42] Although a nutritional deficiency can impair physical performance and cause several other detrimental effects, there is no conclusive evidence of performance enhancement with intakes in excess of the recommended dietary intake levels.

Reasons Not to Use Supplements

There is considerable misinformation and exaggeration regarding the relationship between vitamins and minerals, and exercise.[153] Coaches' magazines, popular fitness journals, and training table practices of sports superstars send the message that high levels of vitamins and minerals are needed as an energy boost, to maximize performance, to compensate for less-than-optimal diets, to meet the unusual nutrient demands induced by heavy exercise, and to help alleviate the stress of competition. Advocates of supplementation have exaggerated the needs for all 13 recognized vitamins, and have even created some new ones, such as pangamic acid or vitamin B-15. (See Table 9.14 for the United States Recommended Dietary Allowance guidelines used as a criteria on food labels.)

The relationship between vitamins, minerals, and exercise can be looked at in two ways: (1) Do vitamin and mineral supplements improve performance? (2) Does exercise impose requirements for vitamins and minerals greater than the amounts obtainable from the diet? (See Figure 9.16.)

As discussed in this chapter previously, most studies that have examined the mineral and vitamin contents of athletic diets have found that athletes exceed 67 percent the RDA for all vitamins and minerals measured, except for iron for females.[154] Figure 9.17 (A and B) shows that male and female Los Angeles marathon runners met or exceeded 100 percent of the RDA for all major nutrients except for vitamin B-6 and iron in women.[28]

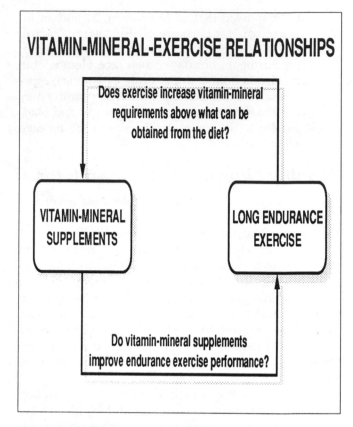

Figure 9.16 The relationship between vitamins, minerals, and exercise can be looked at in two ways.

Table 9.14 U.S. Recommended Dietary Allowances (U.S. RDAs)

Nutrient	Adults and Children Over 4 Years	Infants and Children Under 4 Years	Pregnant or Lactating Women
Protein	65 mg	25-28 g	65 g
Vitamin A	5000 IU	2500 IU	8000 IU
Vitamin C	60 mg	40 mg	60 mg
Thiamin	1.5 mg	0.7 mg	1.7 mg
Riboflavin	1.7 mg	0.8 mg	2.0 mg
Niacin	20 mg	9.0 mg	20 mg
Calcium	1.0 g	0.8 g	1.3 g
Iron	18 mg	10 mg	18 mg
Vitamin D	400 IU	400 IU	400 IU
Vitamin E	30 IU	10 IU	30 IU
Vitamin B-6	2.0 mg	0.7 mg	2.5 mg
Folacin	0.4 mg	0.2 mg	0.8 mg
Vitamin B-12	6.0 mcg	3 mcg	8 mcg
Phosphorus	1.0 g	0.8 g	1.3 g
Iodine	150 mcg	70 mcg	150 mcg
Magnesium	400 mg	200 mg	450 mg
Zinc	15 mg	8 mg	15 mg
Copper	2.0 mg	1 mg	2 mg
Biotin	0.3 mg	0.15 mg	0.3 mg
Pantothenic Acid	10 mg	5 mg	10 mg

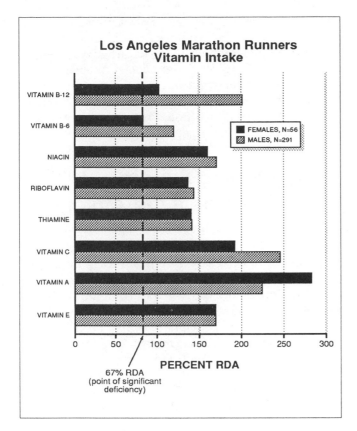

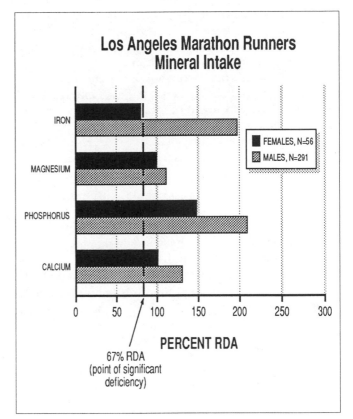

Figure 9.17 A and B   In this study of 291 male and 56 female Los Angeles marathon runners, three-day food records revealed that vitamin and mineral intake was adequate except for a slight deficiency of vitamin B-6 and iron for women.

Despite what appear to be adequate diets for athletes (mainly because of their high caloric intakes), many feel the need to supplement their diets with vitamins and minerals. Research evidence shows that between 53 and 80 percent of athletes use vitamin/ mineral supplements on a regular basis.[155–159] (This compares with 52 percent of the American public as measured in the 1985 Nationwide Food Consumption Survey, Continuing Survey of Food Intakes by Individuals.)[160]

The American Medical Association, the American Dietetic Association, the American Institute of Nutrition, the American Society for Clinical Nutrition, and the National Council Against Health Fraud have submitted formal statements to the effect that there are no demonstrated benefits of self supplementation beyond the Recommended Dietary Allowances except in special cases.[161, 162]

There are several reasons for advising against vitamin and mineral supplementation by athletes.

▪ Extensive reviews of the literature have failed to find any convincing support for the role of supple-

mentation in enhancing performance, hastening recovery, or decreasing the rate of injury in healthy, well-nourished adults undergoing athletic training.[8, 56, 153, 154, 164] After over 40 years of research, there is no conclusive evidence to suggest that vitamin supplementation improves the performance of adequately nourished people.[153, 165–168]

Although heavy endurance exercise is associated with an increased need for many nutrients, including iron, zinc, copper, magnesium, chromium, vitamin B-6, riboflavin, and ascorbic acid,[169–180] these demands are usually met when the athlete matches energy expenditure through increased consumption of the conventional food supply.

This approach is supported in a recent technical support paper from the American Dietetic Association (ADA).[42] The ADA took the position that extended physical activity may increase the need for some vitamins and minerals, but that these could easily be met by consuming a balanced diet in proportion to the extra caloric requirement.

Other reviews of the sports nutrition literature have also consistently concluded that except in special cases, vitamin and mineral supplementation by athletes is unwarranted.[8, 153]

Many studies have shown clearly that the capacity to perform exercise is obviously hindered by the development of vitamin deficiency states, and that performance is returned to normal when the deficiency is corrected.[153,154,181,182] However, vitamin/mineral deficiencies are probably rare among athletes.[9–12, 28]

■ There are problems associated with high intakes of vitamins and minerals. Considerable evidence has now been gathered to show that dietary excess of one nutrient may have a detrimental effect on another.[150, 151, 183–191] High intakes of specific nutrients especially fat soluble vitamins like A, D, E, and K, can be toxic in themselves and indirectly dangerous because they block the action of other nutrients. Excessive intake of water soluble vitamins can also cause problems. Too much niacin can in time lead to liver toxicity, too much vitamin C to red blood cell hemolysis and impaired white blood cell activity, and too much vitamin B-6, to peripheral nervous system toxicity.

A deficiency of one nutrient can be caused by an excess of another. Excessive zinc decreases copper and iron absorption and vice-versa; excessive vitamin C decreases copper absorption; high levels of folic acid decrease zinc absorption; excess fructose decreases copper absorption; large amounts of calcium, phytates, and fiber in the diet cause the formation of insoluble iron, zinc, or copper complexes, making these minerals unavailable for absorption; high sugar intakes decrease chromium levels in the body; excess manganese decreases iron absorption.

In other words, too much of a good thing becomes a definite evil. Water and sunshine are both necessary for life, but excesses of either can kill you.

Some coaches and other leaders still feel that giving supplements is beneficial, even if there is no proven physiological benefit, because the athlete thinks the supplement will help and thus performs better (placebo effect). It would be better to help the athlete believe in something that really works, such as a nutritious, varied diet, high in carbohydrate and liquids—providing him with both physiological and psychological support.

For the athlete who is poorly nourished (often to "make weight"), the best solution is education

to provide a better diet. Supplements can reinforce unhealthy eating habits, as evidenced by some athletes who tend to excuse their poor eating habits with supplements. Dietary imbalances can only who tend to get worse in this situation. Thus every effort must be made to convince athletes that their best nutritional resource for optimum performance is proper eating habits.

PRINCIPLE 7 Extra Protein Does Not Benefit the Athlete

Many people who exercise, especially weight lifters, feel that consumption of high protein foods and protein supplements is necessary to build muscle mass. The average sedentary person has been advised to consume 0.8 grams of dietary protein per kilogram of body weight. As we shall see in this section, recent research is showing that highly active people may need up to 50 percent more than this, because 5–15 percent of the energy needs of long endurance exercise or weight lifters comes from protein. Does this mean that athletes should use protein supplements—or should they concentrate on high protein foods in their diets?

Changes in Protein Metabolism During Exercise

The importance of protein for athletics has been debated for many years. In 1842, the great German chemist and physiologist, Justus von Liebig, reported that the primary fuel for muscular contraction was derived from muscle protein, and he suggested that large quantities of meat be eaten to replenish the supply.[152,192] A number of studies during the late 1800s that measured urinary urea excretion, however, failed to confirm his results, and the concept became established that changes in protein metabolism during exercise are nonexistent or minimal at best[193,194] (and the idea persists today in some textbooks).

However, recent studies using newer technology and improved techniques have concluded that protein is a much more important fuel source during exercise than was previously thought.[192–199]

Four basic changes in protein metabolism take place with exercise.[194, 195] (See Figure 9.18.)

■ **Depression of Protein Synthesis:** During exercise (endurance exercise or heavy weight lifting) normal protein synthesis is depressed by 17–70 percent, depending on the intensity and duration of

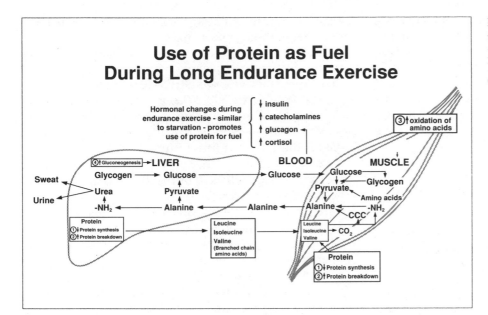

Figure 9.18 This figure summarizes the various pathways by which protein can be used as fuel by the working muscles (see text for an explanation).

the exercise. This depression leaves amino acids available as fuel for the working muscle. Later, during recovery, muscle protein synthesis increases, augmenting incorporation of amino acids into muscle protein (hypertrophy).[199, 200]

The average 70-kg man has 12 kg of protein in his body, nearly half in the actin and myosin myofilaments found in muscle.[201] The body depot of protein is highly labile, with some 200–500 g (50 g nitrogen) of new protein being synthesized every day, and only 10 g N/day excreted. Five tons of protein are thus synthesized in one's lifetime, while total dietary protein intake is only one ton, indicating the extensive reutilization of body amino acids. For young adults, muscle accounts for 25–30 percent of total body protein turnover.

The fact that exercise temporarily interrupts this protein turnover and synthesis is very important, making amino acids immediately available for fuel. (Following exercise, protein synthesis is accelerated, leading to hypertrophy—temporary unless maintained).

▪ **Increased Muscle Breakdown:** There is not a clear consensus, but more and more studies are supporting the concept that exercise leads to a breakdown of the muscle protein.[195, 202–204] Many researchers have reported that hard exercise leads to significant muscle cell damage that can be measured when muscle enzymes leak into the plasma.[193, 205] (See Chapter 15.)

With the combination of reduced muscle protein synthesis and increased muscle protein break-

down, more amino acids are available in the body for fuel during exercise and the repair and buildup of muscle cells after exercise.[194]

▪ **Increase in Amino Acid Oxidation:** During rest, 10–20 percent of ATP regeneration comes from protein. Many studies have now shown that exercise increases the rate of amino acid oxidation.[194, 195, 198, 204] During cycling exercise, for example, it has been reported[198] that there is a 240-percent increase in leucine oxidation, with a 21-percent decrease in leucine synthesis.

▪ **Increase in Gluconeogenesis:** Sixteen of the amino acids that are in the human body can be changed into glucose by the liver. This gluconeogenic process is extremely important during exercise, because it can contribute to the supply of glucose to prevent hypoglycemia during long endurance exercise.[195] During exercise, there is a steady stream of alanine passing from the muscle to the liver,[193–195] where it is converted into glucose, which then enters the blood and feeds the working muscle. (See Figure 9.18.) This appears to be most important during prolonged exercise. After three hours of exercise, about 60 percent of glucose used by the working muscle comes from the liver, which is producing glucose from alanine, lactate, glycerol, and other metabolic by-products.[113]

The increase in liver gluconeogenesis during long endurance exercise, and the use of protein for fuel is probably hormonally controlled.[195] Exercise causes several changes in blood hormone levels, including a decrease in insulin and increases in catecholamines (epinephrine and norepinephrine), glucagon, and cortisol. These hormonal changes are amazingly similar to what happens during starvation (which tends to increase the use of protein for fuel).[207] From the evidence available, it seems likely that endurance exercise and heavy weight lifting cause a transient increase in the use of protein that is somewhat analogous to the changes caused by starvation.

Practical Implications for Athletes

The practical advice in light of this information is still conjectural.[8, 42, 193–195, 208–210] It does appear certain that the contribution of protein as an energy source during endurance training is about 5–15 percent (instead of next to nothing as previously thought). The actual amount of protein utilized during such exercise depends on the intensity, duration, and fitness status, with long, hard exercise by trained athletes leading to the greatest protein utilization.[194, 211]

Various reviewers have suggested that the current protein RDA is insufficient for both strength and endurance athletes,[8, 194, 210] for whom the actual requirement may be 50 to 100 percent higher than the RDA.[194] In light of this information, the American Dietetic Association has advised that endurance athletes take in 1 g/kg daily.[42] For athletes in unusually heavy training, more than 1.5 g/kg may be needed.[193] A good rule for endurance athletes to be sure that protein intake is adequate is to keep caloric intake of protein at 12 to 15 percent of the diet. Regardless of exercise level, this should provide sufficient protein, because caloric intake generally rises with energy expenditure.[194]

Most endurance athletes are already getting this much protein, and would not need to supplement their diets with protein powder or concern themselves with eating high protein foods. In the study by the author of 347 Los Angeles Marathon runners, the average male and female runner consumed 1.4 and 1.3 g/kg, respectively.[28] Table 9.9 demonstrates that even on a high-carbohydrate diet with relatively little meat and few dairy products, protein intake is still 116 grams, or 13 percent of total caloric intake. What is amazing is that the sedentary public consumes more than one gram of protein per kilogram per day, about 16 percent of total caloric intake.[27] The general public needs to worry more about exercise supplementation than protein supplementation! (See Table 9.15.)

Contrary to popular opinion, weight lifters need less protein than endurance athletes.[210] Muscle mass increase can only come from specific heavy resistance

exercise training.[8] Eating large quantities of protein does not increase muscle mass.

Protein is needed to form increased lean body weight, but more than enough is provided by a normal diet. Young men who weight 75–80 kg can increase their lean body mass by 500–1,000 g/week. If 20 percent of this lean body mass increase is pure protein, this will require up to 14–28 grams of extra protein in the diet per day. If these weight lifters burn 500–1,000 Calories in their exercise per day, they need 13–25 grams more than the normal need reflected by the RDA. So the total extra need may range from 25–50 grams of protein per day during active muscle-building training. This extra 25–50 grams of protein, plus the RDA, is only 80–105 grams (about 1.1 g/kg), which is easily obtained in the diet. There is absolutely no need to consume protein powders or to emphasize high-protein foods.

Too much protein in the form of supplements can overload the liver and kidneys, generally impairing health.

PRINCIPLE 8 Rest and Eat Carbohydrate Before Long Endurance Events

The preparation during the last few days and hours before the endurance event can mean the difference between success and failure. In this section, we will discuss the concept of "carbohydrate loading" (or "glycogen loading"). As we shall see, the best scheme for endurance athletes preparing for any exercise event lasting longer than 60–90 minutes is to taper off the exercise gradually during the week before the event, while consuming more than 70 percent carbohydrate during the three days before the event. If the exercise event lasts less than 90 minutes, "carbohydrate loading" is unnecessary.

The "pre-event meal" is another important consideration. The meal three to five hours before the event should be 500–800 Calories of light, low-fiber, starch. There are various pros and cons concerning the use of different sugar solutions.

How to "Carbohydrate Load" Before the Big Event

As discussed earlier, the human body can maintain limited stores of CHO. Exercise training at 60–80 percent $\dot{V}O_{2max}$ leads to muscle glycogen depletion after 100–120 minutes.[1, 53] Exercise at 80–95 percent $\dot{V}O_{2max}$

Table 9.15   Protein Needs, Intake, and Exercise Requirements

	Protein Intake (Grams/Day)	
	Males	Females
Recommended intake level for sedentary Americans (0.8 g/kg)	56	44
Average sedentary American (actual intake)	95	65
Average fitness enthusiast (1 g/kg)	70	55
Recommended level for bodybuilder (1.1 g/kg)	90	70
Recommended level for heavy endurance athlete (1.5 g/kg)	105	80

Source: see references 42, 194, 210.

can lead to muscle glycogen depletion even sooner.

Various researchers have therefore tried to manipulate muscle glycogen stores using a combination of the high-CHO diet and varying levels of exercise and rest to increase glycogen levels above normal in the belief that exercise time to exhaustion could be prolonged.

The original Scandinavian researchers set up a regimen now known as the "classical" method of "muscle glycogen supercompensation."[1, 50–55, 58–60] According to this plan, athletes first deplete their muscles of glycogen by eating a low-carbohydrate diet for 3 days (e.g., Sunday, Monday, and Tuesday) while engaging in intense, prolonged exercise sessions for at least two of these days. Next, athletes would "supercompensate" their muscles with glycogen, by resting for three days before competition while eating a very high (90-percent) carbohydrate diet.

This regimen has been found to create muscle glycogen levels as high as 220 mmol/kg wet muscle (with total body CHO stores of more than 1,000 grams).[212] Unfortunately, this program causes several undesirable side effects during the depletion phase, including marked physical and mental fatigue, elevation of fat metabolic by-products in the blood (ketosis), low blood sugar levels (hypoglycemia), muscle cell damage, electrocardiographic abnormalities, depression, and irritability.[8, 213] In addition, during the high carbohydrate phase, the athlete often feels heavy and stiff in the legs.

Because of these side effects, researchers have modified the depletion phase.[214–216] Instead of three days of a low-carbohydrate diet and hard exercise, the modified scheme utilizes a slow tapering of exercise over a six-day period, without any intensive exercise

the day before competition. During the week, the diet should provide more than 8 g CHO/kg (about 70 percent CHO).[42] (See Table 9.9 for a sample menu.)

Recent research is showing that it takes 4 to 5 days of a high carbohydrate diet to saturate the body with glycogen.[212] This modified regimen has been found to create muscle glycogen levels of approximately 200 mmol/kg, nearly the same as the old classical method, without the side effects. (See Figure 9.19.)

With the muscles "loaded" or "supercompensated" with glycogen, runners are able to maintain their racing pace for longer periods of time. (See Figure 9.20.) The overall race time is lower, though the fastest running pace per mile does not improve. In other words, runners can maintain speed longer, and thus reduce the total time.[1, 50, 217, 218]

The Pre-Event Meal

The meal before competition can make a difference both physiologically and psychologically.[42] Most sports nutrition experts advise 1–2 glasses of water, followed within 20–30 minutes by a light (500–800 kcal) meal of rapidly digestible, low-fiber starch (e.g., cream of wheat hot cereal, white bread, bagels, pasta, refined cereals). The food should be consumed 3–5 hours before the event, so that the stomach will be empty at the time of competition to avoid uncomfortable feelings of fullness or cramping.[42] The use of proteins, fats, known gas-forming foods, high-fiber foods, and foods known to act as laxatives is not recommended.[1, 52]

The so-called "liquid meals" (Ensure, Nutriment, Sustagen, and SustaCal) are becoming increasingly popular. They are low in fiber, but may be too high in fat

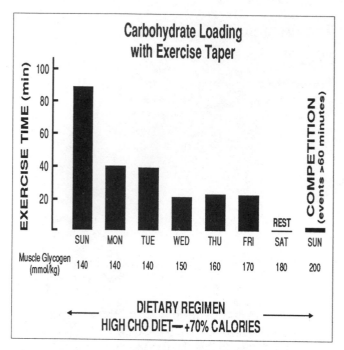

Figure 9.19 The best scheme for increasing muscle glycogen stores before endurance competition is to consume a high carbohydrate diet while tapering the exercise to complete rest. *Source:* adapted from reference 214.

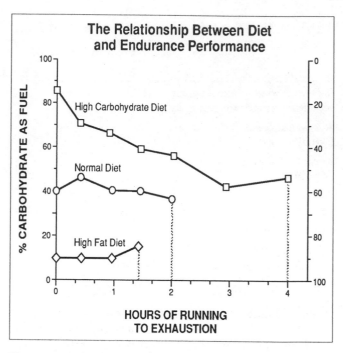

Figure 9.20 Following at least three days of a high-carbohydrate diet, runners are able to maintain their pace two to three times longer than with high-fat, low-carbohydrate diets. *Source:* see references 58,59

and protein for optimal competitive performance.

Many athletes feel that drinking soda-pop 30–60 minutes before hard exertion will enhance performance.[42] Earlier studies examining intakes of glucose or sucrose 30–60 minutes before exercise reported that blood glucose rose sharply, causing an increase in blood insulin concentrations, which then stimulated the muscles to utilize blood glucose. This resulted in rebound low blood sugar levels, and later, debilitating muscle glycogen depletion.[219, 220]

More recent studies, however, have not been able to confirm these earlier findings.[221-223] The use of 75-gram glucose solutions (about 300 Calories) 30–45 minutes before endurance performance has not been associated with low blood glucose levels, increased glycogen depletion, or decreased performance. In fact, researchers reported that a glucose meal 30–60 minutes before exercise increased the amount of carbohydrate available to the working muscle, enhancing endurance performance.[221]

In one study of ten well-trained cyclists, researchers found that the best possible pre-event eating schedule was a 200-gram carbohydrate meal (800 Calories) four hours before the event, and a 45-gram CHO snack immediately before high-intensity endurance exercise.[224]

Authorities are not in agreement, and the best advice would appear to be to eat a 500–800 Calorie CHO meal 3–5 hours before exercise, in combination with a 150–200 Calorie CHO meal 5 minutes before exercise.

Does it help to drink unusually large quantities of water just before long endurance exercise? In one study, athletes who drank about two liters of water just before cycling for 45 minutes experienced a shortened delay in onset of sweating and a lower increase in body temperature.[225] Although such a practice may help in preventing dehydration, the practical problem of having to stop to urinate more frequently may be counterproductive.

Some athletes feel that fasting before long endurance exercise will make them feel lighter and more energetic. In a study conducted by the author, a one-day fast by male marathon runners resulted in a 45-percent decrease in endurance performance.[63] Fasting caused significant increases in oxygen uptake, heart rate, rating of perceived exertion, ventilation, and psychological fatigue. In general, the metabolic data appeared to suggest that the responses at the start of the runners who had fasted were like those of the runners who had eaten after 90 minutes of exercise. (See Figure 9.21.)

Immediately after the event, the recovery of glycogen stores has been found to be improved by consum-

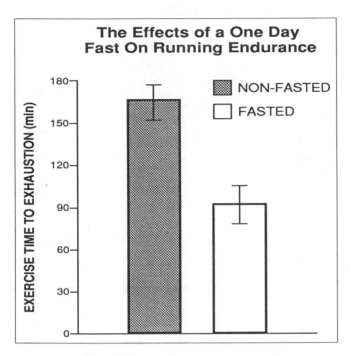

The Effects of a One Day Fast On Running Endurance

NON-FASTED
FASTED

EXERCISE TIME TO EXHAUSTION (min)

Figure 9.21 Fasting for one day before long endurance running led to a 45 percent reduction in exercise time to exhaustion. *Source:* see reference 63.

ing 500–800 Calories of CHO solutions.[226–228] In other words, CHO is important both immediately before and immediately after exercise.

PRINCIPLE 9 Use of Ergogenic Aids is Unethical

Ergogenic aids are defined as substances that increase one's ability to exercise harder. Although there are many worthless ergogenic aids (e.g., bee pollen, B-15 or pangamic acid, alcohol, wheat germ oil, lecithin, kelp, brewer's yeast, phosphates, etc.), others confer impressive benefits (caffeine, sodium bicarbonate, blood doping, steroids, etc.). These may enhance performance, but the ethical issues of equitable competition and fair play claim a higher priority.

For thousands of years, warriors and athletes have used a wide variety of substances in the attempt to enhance physical performance.[230] The ancient Greek athletes believed in the value of meat;[152] ancient Muslim warriors used hashish; during World War II some German soldiers experimented with anabolic-androgen steroid hormones to increase their aggressiveness in combat; American soldiers were given the stimulant amphetamine to improve their endurance and atten-

tiveness; amphetamines became popular among bicycle racers in the 1960s, leading to several deaths; strychnine was used by some of the early prize fighters; and many athletes today use everything from anabolic-androgen steroids to caffeine to doses of blood to improve endurance performance.[230]

Why is the use of drugs and ergogenic aids so pervasive today? This is best answered in a statement made in 1972 by The Medical Commission of the International Olympic Committee:[231]

> The merciless rigor of modern competitive sports, especially at the international level, the glory of victory, and the growing social and economical reward of sporting success (in no way any longer related to reality) increasingly forces athletes to improve their performance by any means available.

Categories of Ergogenic Aids

The term "ergogenic" means "tending to increase work." Thus ergogenic aids are any substances or methods that tend to increase performance capacity.[229]

These aids fall into five categories:

- Nutritional aids:
  Carbohydrates, proteins, vitamins, minerals, iron, water, electrolytes, and miscellaneous substances (e.g., bee pollen, B-15),
- Pharmacological aids:
  Amphetamines, caffeine, anabolic steroids, alcohol, $NaHCO_3$,
- Physiological aids:
  Oxygen, blood doping,
- Psychological aids:
  Hypnosis, covert rehearsal strategies, stress management, and
- Mechanical aids:
  Biomechanical aids, physical warm-up.

Miscellaneous Nutritional Aids

A number of nutritional substances are advocated to improve performance. Included are the various vitamins and minerals, and extracts from various foods. (See principle #6 on vitamin and mineral supplements.)

Miscellaneous nutritional aids also include bee pollen, wheat germ oil, brewer's yeast, amino acids, ginseng, spirulina, royal jelly, DNA and RNA, L-carnitine, phosphate, various vitamin and mineral preparations, and kelp.[42, 232–241] Many of these substances have been studied under double blind placebo conditions, and have been found to be worthless.

Bee pollen, for example, has been tested extensively at Louisiana State University.[239] When compared with placebo capsules, bee pollen was "absolutely not a significant aid in metabolism, workout training, or performance." This was confirmed in another study of 20 swimmers.[240]

Pangamic acid (B-15) is another example of a substance thought to hold special ergogenic value.[241] The active ingredient, N,N-Dimethylglycine (DMG), is thought to supply methyl groups to the muscle cell that aid in liberating muscle energy to form phosphocreatine. Athletes use B-15 in the belief that it will act to keep muscle tissue operating at peak efficiency through heavy exercise. Most of the studies used to back up these claims come from Russia. The best U.S. study utilizing a double blind procedure on 16 male athletes over a 3-week period showed no performance advantage.[241]

L-carnitine first received media attention in 1982 when the Italian national soccer team credited its World Cup victory to the "miracle drug."[235] L-carnitine is an amine responsible for transporting fatty acids into the mitochondria for oxidation. Some have urged that L-carnitine supplements may increase the amount of fatty acid oxidation during exercise, sparing the glycogen. However, L-carnitine supplements have never been shown in reputable, double-blind, controlled studies to improve the athletic performance of a healthy person.[233–235] It appears that the increased demand for fatty acid oxidation resulting from exercise is adequately supported by levels of carnitine normally found in the body.[233]

The Placebo Effect

Despite such evidence, many athletes are convinced that various nutritional substances do lead to improved performance. If these substances have no value, why do athletes continue to use and believe in them?

The Food and Drug Administration has concluded that "people are often helped, not by the food or drug being touted, but by a profound belief it will help."[239] In other words, the placebo effect is powerful enough to actually produce a benefit. A review of the literature shows that an average of 35 percent of the members of any group will respond favorably to placebos (with a variation of zero to 100 percent).[242]

The challenge of the health professional working with an athlete is to use this placebo effect to advantage by instilling a "profound belief" in food substances that have proven worth (e.g., carbohydrate, water, and nutritious foods). This can be summarized as follows:

1 (placebo effect) + 0 (substance of no worth) = 1
1 (placebo effect) + 1 (substance of worth) = 2

Use of Caffeine to Improve Performance in Long Endurance Events

Despite the widespread use of caffeinated beverages by Americans, a growing number of studies are providing evidence that this drug is not as benign as once thought.[243] One in three Americans consumes approximately 200 mg caffeine (equivalent to 1–2 cups of coffee) per day. Caffeine is an alkaloid present in more than 60 plant species. Peak plasma levels after ingestion occur within 15 to 45 minutes, with a plasma half-life ranging from 2.5 to 7.5 hours. The metabolism by the liver, storage, and clearance rate of caffeine may vary greatly between acute and chronic users.

Caffeine stimulates the central nervous system, increases secretion of gastric acid and pepsin, increases urinary volume and sodium excretion, increases LDL-C and total cholesterol levels in the blood, and especially in nonusers, increases blood pressure and ventilation, and causes an increase in cellular calcium levels that could contribute to the onset of arrhythmias. Most chronic consumers of caffeine develop a tolerance to it.[243]

Over the past 15 years, researchers have been divided in their opinion as to whether caffeine enhances performance.[244–256] Caffeine tends to elevate free fatty acids in the blood. When exercising muscles are presented with elevated levels of free fatty acids at the beginning of exercise, the muscles will increase their utilization of fat, sparing the muscle glycogen, resulting in improved endurance.

With cyclers who are not carbohydrate loaded and other athletes not accustomed to the use of caffeinated beverages who have taken caffeine in 4–5 mg/kg doses one hour before exercise (about 2–4 cups of coffee), time to exhaustion has been prolonged by 7–19 percent.[244–247, 249–251] With runners, however, or athletes habituated to the use of caffeine, caffeine has been found to have little effect.[245, 248, 254, 255]

The American College of Sports Medicine does not recommend the use of caffeine for enhancement of performance.[50] The International Olympic Committee has banned caffeine urine testing at levels greater than 15 micrograms per ml.[257]

Caffeine increases the urine output, contributing to dehydration. In addition, the use of caffeine, at least for cyclers, violates the principle of all athletic competition: equitable competition and fair play for all. Caffeine does not predictably enhance performance, may increase the incidence of premature ventricular contractions in those susceptible, and regular, heavy consumption may raise blood cholesterol and increase the risk of heart attack. Thus, the use of caffeine cannot be recommended for athletes.[246]

"Soda Loading" for Anaerobic Exercise

During high intensity exercise, the requirement for oxygen exceeds the capacity of the aerobic supply system to supply it, increasing glycolysis and therefore lactic acid levels. The buildup of lactic acid finally inhibits the energy supplying chemical reactions, with resulting fatigue. Exercise of one- to four-minutes' duration is limited by lactic acid buildup.[258]

Several recent studies have shown that sodium bicarbonate (as found in Alka Seltzer) augments the body's buffer reserve, counteracts the buildup of lactic acid, and improves anaerobic exercise performance.[256-265] The use of sodium bicarbonate in doses of 0.3 g/kg (spread out over a 2–3 hour period and given with water) has been shown to improve 400-meter running times by an average of 1.5 seconds, and 800–meter running times by 2.9 seconds.[259, 264] For the 800-meter, this translates to a 19-meter advantage, often the difference between first and last place. The practical implications are that in any event demanding hard exercise over a 1–4 minute period, performance can be enhanced because the usual limiting factor, lactic acid, is partially controlled and buffered.

As with all ergogenic aids, however, there are some adverse effects. As many as half of those using soda may suffer from "urgent diarrhea" one hour after the soda loading is completed. The effects of repeated ingestion are unknown, and caution is advised.

And once again, as with caffeine, there is the ethical issue of equitable competition and fair play. Soda loading should be banned because of the unfair advantage it offers. Bicarbonate rises sharply in the urine after sodium bicarbonate is used, and can be measured to detect "soda loaders."

Blood Doping for Endurance

Just as Roman gladiators drank the blood of foes to gain strength, modern Olympians have infused the blood of friends as well as their own to gain endurance.[266] Increased performance after blood transfusion was first demonstrated 40 years ago, but the technique did not attract attention until the early 1970s, when it was dubbed "blood doping" by the media. Although earlier studies on blood doping reported mixed results, recent studies have shown that this practice has strong ergogenic value.[267-275]

Blood doping involves removing 900 ml of blood (about 2 units) from an athlete, freeze storing it at –80°C for six to eight weeks, and then reinfusing the blood back into the athlete one to seven days before the competition. (See Figure 9.22.) This increases the hemoglobin ten percent, leading to a 5–10 percent increase in $\dot{V}O_{2max}$.

Training with a lower amount of red blood cells and blood triggers a physiologic response similar to that which occurs when runners train at high altitudes.[276] In general, a runner's performance will drop by 10–20 percent immediately after giving 900 ml of blood, but it will gradually return to normal over the next 6–8 weeks.

Cardiorespiratory endurance performance is improved following the reinfusion, because the oxygen carrying capacity of the blood is greater, cardiac output is increased, and lactate levels are reduced.[270] Treadmill time to exhaustion is increased, 10-kilometer (6.2 miles) times drops 69 seconds,[274] 5-mile time performances drop an average of 49 seconds (10 seconds faster per mile), and 3-mile time performances drop 23.7 seconds.[267]

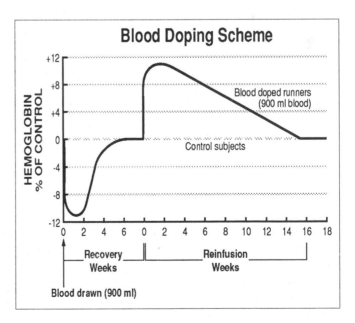

Figure 9.22 Blood doping usually involves removing 900 ml of one's own blood, storing it for 6–8 weeks as the body builds back to its normal amount, and then, shortly before competition, reinfusing the 900 ml blood to increase blood volume and hemoglobin levels to higher than normal levels. *Source:* see reference 267.

After blood doping, the hemoglobin level rises about 10 percent (e.g., from 15 to 16.5 g/dl). Because the normal range of hemoglobin is 14–18 g/dl, detecting blood doping has proven to be very difficult. Blood doping was forbidden by the International Olympic Committee after the 1984 Olympics, despite the fact that no methods had been devised for unequivocal detection.

Data now suggest that blood doping can be detected to some extent, by taking two blood samples with a minimum interval of 1–2 weeks. Changes are then noted in hemoglobin, combined with increases in serum iron and bilirubin, and a decrease in serum erythropoietin. With these measures, blood doping can be detected in 50 percent of blood doped athletes during the first 2 weeks.[277] Other detection techniques are being developed.

Anabolic-Androgenic Steroids for Muscular Strength and Size

Anabolic-Androgenic Steroids

The use of anabolic-androgenic steroids by athletes worldwide has become symbolic of what athletes are willing to go through to achieve excellence and success in competition.[278–287] The use of steroids by Ben Johnson, which led to his loss of the 1988 Olympic 100-meter dash gold medal, has been widely reviewed and decried by the media.

Sports Illustrated has highlighted the case histories of athletes who have developed mental and physical problems because of anabolic-androgenic steroids (see Chaikin T with Rick Telander. The Nightmare of Steroids. *Sports Illustrated*, 1988). The February 20, 1989 issue of *Sports Illustrated* carried the tragic story of Benji Ramirez, a high school football player who died from steroid usage.

Obtaining accurate statistics on steroid use by athletes has proven very difficult. Conservative estimates put the black market cost at $100 million per year.[284] The reason given most often for using steroids was improved athletic performance.

Steroid abuse is particularly common among athletes in strength sports. In one survey of 250 weight lifters, almost half admitted using steroids at some time.[279] In another study of elite power lifters, 33 percent admitted to having used steroids.[281]

Results from a nationwide study of high school seniors showed that 6.6 percent of all male students currently used or had used anabolic steroids.[280] Over two-thirds of the students initiated use when they were 16 years of age or younger.

Approximately 21 percent of users reported that a health professional was their primary source. The primary motivation for steroid usage among the high school seniors was strength and appearance.

The most common side effects reported were heightened sex drive, acne, and increased body hair.

The problems of anabolic-androgenic steroids can be considered from three different perspectives: pharmacological—the possibility that these substances may provide a real physiological advantage for the athletes; psychological—the importance of winning and the placebo effect of drugs; and ethical—the concept of violation of fair play.[278]

Anabolic steroids are synthetic androgens that have greater anabolic activity (building up of the body) relative to androgenic (masculinization) activity than testosterone. (See Box 9.2.) Testosterone is the principal circulating androgen in humans, concentrated 20 times as much in men as in women. Anabolic-androgenic steroids are derivatives of testosterone.[283] The esterified steroids are usually given intramuscularly, whereas the

---

Box 9.2 Anabolic-Androgenic Steroids Banned by the U.S. Olympic Committee

Bolasterone

Boldenone

Clostebol

Dehydrochlormethyl testosterone

Fluoxymesterone

Mesterolone

Metenolone

Methandienone

Methyltestosterone

Nandrolone

Norethandrolone

Oxandrolone

Oxymesterone

Oxymetholone

Stanozolol

Testosterone and related compounds

Source: The Physician Sportsmed 16(2):160, 1988.

alkylated steroids are given orally. The effects of steroids depend on the type used, the size and frequency of the doses, the overall length of treatment, and the route of administration.

Anabolic steroids have been used by athletes for decades in the belief that they increase body mass, muscle tissue, strength, and aggressiveness. More recently, testosterone has been used because it is more difficult to detect in drug screening programs. Although study results have been mixed, an intensive exercise program coupled with a high-protein diet and anabolic steroids may increase muscular strength and size for some people.[230, 278, 279]

Reasons given by athletes for using steroids include: decreasing body fat, increasing muscle mass and strength, improving appearance, increasing red blood cell count, and increasing training tolerance (greater intensity, better recovery).[283] Athletes often take doses 10–40 times greater than clinical therapeutic doses.

The side-effects are legion.[283–286] Use of these substances can affect the reproductive system, leading to temporary infertility, atrophy of the testicles, decreased production of sperm, and reduced levels of several reproductive hormones. Steroids also produce liver abnormalities, decrease HDL-C and increase LDL-C, and increase the incidence of acne. Among women, androgenic hormones produce masculinizing effects (e.g., clitoris enlargement and increased hair growth).

While most of the effects of anabolic steroid use among adults may be reversible, several studies suggest that they may have more serious biophysical consequences for adolescents, particularly with regard to premature skeletal maturation, spermatogenesis, and an elevated risk of injury.[280]

The use of steroids may also expose athletes to a risk of injury to ligaments and tendons, and these injuries may take longer to heal. There is also some evidence of anabolic steroid association with cancer, death, edema, fetal damage, heart disease, prostate enlargement, sterility, swelling of feet or lower legs, and yellowing of the eyes or skin.[284]

However, the most worrisome of the problems associated with anabolic steroids may be their potential to induce severe adverse psychiatric effects.[286] In one recent study[287] researchers found manic symptoms in 13 of 41 bodybuilders and football players who had used steroids. Of those 13, at least five had experienced full-scale psychotic episodes while using steroids.

It has been known for years that anabolic steroids increase aggressiveness. Athletes using steroids have exhibited increased levels of anger and hostility and overall mood disturbance.

Human Growth Hormone

In contrast to the abuse of anabolic steroids, the abuse of human growth hormone is a relatively new phenomenon. This hormone is now used by some athletes for body growth and strength, and has the advantage of being undetectable by drug testing procedures. Its use is probably limited by its great expense, however.

Growth hormone is a potent regulator of somatic growth, promoting protein storage as well as fat mobilization and oxidation. In one well designed study, growth hormone supplements in large doses decreased body fat while increasing the fat-free weight of a group in weight training.[288]

The side-effects have not yet been researched extensively, but may include acromegaly (characterized by elongation and enlargement of bones of the extremities and certain head bones, especially the frontal bone and jaws).

Use of Alcohol for Sports Performance

Endurance athletes are being advised by various magazines to drink alcoholic beverages to gain certain benefits. Beer has been presented as a "soup to replace lost electrolytes," and it is claimed that beer and wine will "relax muscles and improve emotional state."[289] Runners are urged to "have a beer with your pasta" to carbohydrate load before a race,[290] and to drink wine or beer to recover from a race, to remove aches and pains.[291]

Some athletes believe that drinking wine or beer during long endurance events will enhance performance. For example, during the 1979 Great Hawaiian Footrace, a 500-km road run held over 20 days, athletes averaged seven cans of beer per day.[292]

The combination of ethanol with exercise is not new. The ancient Greek games were accompanied by great revelry and the drinking of prodigious amounts of wine.[289] Spiridon Loues, winner of the first Olympic marathon in 1896, drank several cups of white-resin wine during the race, supposedly to power him to victory. At the turn of the century, it was standard practice for runners to quaff champagne or brandy immediately before a race.[293]

Claims that wine and beer provide substantial carbohydrate and electrolytes are false. According to the Nutrient Data Research Group of the USDA, one 12-oz. can of beer, or 3.5-oz. glass of wine provides only about 50 Calories of carbohydrate, enough to run about a half mile. Since these amounts also contain a half ounce of ethanol, to obtain enough carbohydrate to run just 2.5 miles would require enough ethanol to raise the blood alcohol level to 0.10, which would violate the drinking and drunk driving laws of most states. In other words, to get enough carbohydrate from beer or wine to get anywhere, one would be too drunk to be a legal driver.

The amounts of minerals and vitamins in beer and wine are too low to be of value; all the electrolyte levels are very low. (See Table 9.16.)

When a half-ounce of ethyl alcohol (the average amount in a standard drink) enters the stomach, about 20 percent of it is absorbed into the blood stream through the stomach walls. The rest is absorbed into the blood from the small intestine. Five to 10 percent is eliminated unchanged in the urine, perspiration, and breath. The remainder is metabolized in the liver. It is unavailable to the working muscle for energy.[294] (The enhanced alcohol elimination during exercise is probably due to increased liver enzyme activity induced by an increase in body temperature.)

Ethanol has various acute and chronic metabolic and physiological effects. Lactate levels are increased, urine output increases, the central nervous system is sedated, myocardial contraction is depressed, the blood vessels dilate, and blood glucose levels decrease.[295]

Because of these metabolic properties, performance is not helped, and in most cases, is hurt.[296] Even small to moderate doses of alcohol have a deleterious effect on a wide variety of psychomotor skills. Tests of endurance exercise have shown alcohol (in moderate doses equivalent to 3 to 5 cans of beer) to be detrimental to submaximal performance, especially affecting the function of the heart muscle during recovery from exercise. In cold environments, alcohol leads to impairment of thermoregulation and hypoglycemia.[298]

The American College of Sports Medicine[296] and the American Dietetic Association[42] have both concluded that alcohol has no real ergogenic properties, and in most instances appears to be detrimental to optimal performance.

PRINCIPLE 10 Nutrition for the Active Individual is Important for More than Performance

Research has shown that athletes have no guarantee of protection from heart disease unless they continue prudent habits of exercise and diet after their days of competition are over. (See Chapter 10.) Even during heavy training, a high saturated fat diet can raise serum cholesterol to alarming levels. Regular endurance exercise will not fully negate bad nutritional habits. Fitness enthusiasts and endurance athletes are well advised to consider not only performance, but also general health, in making their dietary choices.

Dietary Fats, Performance, and Health

As discussed earlier, as a person becomes trained aerobically, the muscles utilize more fat for fuel at any given workload, sparing the precious glycogen. This has encouraged various researchers to consider whether dietary manipulations can mimic the training effect by providing the muscles with more fats, thus sparing glycogen.

Research has centered around the following dietary manipulations:

- High-fat diets for 3–5 days before exercise,
- High-fat diets immediately before exercise (following normal carbohydrate diets),
- Fat supplements during exercise, and
- High-fat diets for one month prior to the exercise event.

Early researchers concluded that the consumption of a low-carbohydrate, high-fat diet for 3–7 days significantly decreased carbohydrate stores in the muscles, reducing endurance time dramatically.[1, 299] Such a fat-rich diet (with fat accounting for 70 percent of total Calories) tends to increase the relative contribution of fat (supplied mainly by plasma free fatty acids). Although this leads to decreased CHO utilization, performance is impaired because of low muscle glycogen levels.[299, 300]

Very few studies have examined the impact of a fatty meal 1–5 hours before exercise after several days of a normal diet.[301-304] Potentially, oil supplements 1–5 hours before prolonged exercise could cause the muscles to utilize more free fatty acids for fuel, sparing the muscle glycogen, but researchers have been unable to confirm this.[303, 304] In one study, 400 Calories of fat given one hour before prolonged bicycling failed to improve exercise time to exhaustion.[303]

In an evaluation of the impact of a month-long high-fat diet on cycling time to exhaustion, five highly trained bicyclists were given a normal training diet for one week.[305] Then for 3–4 weeks they were given a diet containing the same amount of Calories, but providing less than 20 grams of CHO daily. At the end of the period their endurance performance time on a bicycle

Table 9.16 Alcoholic Beverages—Nutrients—Percent USRDA

Type of Alcoholic Beverage	Quantity	Kcals	Vitamin A	Thiamin	Riboflavin	Vitamin C	Calcium	Iron	Magnesium
80 Proof Gin, Rum, Vodka, Whiskey (100% Kcal-OH)	1.25 oz	80	0	0	0	0	0	0	0
Wine-Red (89% Kcal-OH)	4 oz	85	0	0	2	0	1	3	4
Wine-White (96% Kcal-OH)	4 oz	79	0	0	0	0	1	2	3
Beer-Regular (61% Kcal-OH)	12 oz	146	0	1	5	0	2	1	5
Beer-Light (79% Kcal-OH)	12 oz	100	0	2	6	0	2	1	4
Bloody Mary (80% Kcal-OH)	5 oz	116	5	3	2	34	1	3	3
Daquiri (85% Kcal-OH)	2 oz	111	0	1	0	2	0	0	0
Manhattan (95% Kcal-OH)	2 oz	128	0	0	0	0	0	0	0
Martini (99% Kcal-OH)	2.5 oz	156	0	0	0	0	0	0	0
Screwdriver (54% Kcal-OH)	7 oz	174	1	9	2	111	2	1	4

Note: Notice that the two drinks, Bloody Mary and Screwdriver, are high in vitamin C because they contain tomato juice and orange juice, respectively.

ergometer was unchanged. Muscle glycogen use dropped four-fold, with lipid oxidation providing the difference. It was concluded that muscle metabolic adaptations to high-fat diets permit performance comparable to what would be achieved after a high-carbohydrate diet.

Because even lean people have much greater fat stores than glycogen stores, this could provide an advantage.[306] However, there is the factor of health to consider, and the potential adverse effects of high-fat diets.[307]

An experiment with three highly trained cyclers training 300 miles per week provided three consecutive diets for 28 days each. On high saturated-fat diets, the athletes' serum cholesterol levels rose to 250 mg/dl, and on the low saturated-fat diet, they fell to 160 mg/dl. So despite heavy exercise, the diets caused dramatic changes in serum cholesterol.[308]

These studies appear to show that even athletes who are exercising hard can derive health benefits from prudent diet choices. Although long-term adaptation to a high-fat diet may provide performance ability comparable to that of high-carbohydrate diets, the health risk makes it a bad choice.

Sports Medicine Insight
A Practical Nutrition Scheme
for a Marathon

For the highly active endurance athlete, maximizing muscle glycogen stores for the "big event" is vital. This sports medicine insight deals with the necessary preparation and race-day activities for a marathon-type event (more than 2 hours).

1. **Train long and hard to help the muscles adapt.** During the months of training for the marathon-type event, train at a hard pace for a minimum of 90–120 minutes several times per month, to train the muscles both to store more glycogen and to utilize fat more efficiently (sparing the glycogen stores). Remember, nutrition is not as important as talent and training. The minimum amount of training for a marathon (26.2 miles) is 50 miles per week for 3 months before the event. The best athletes in the world work up to a schedule of 80–120 miles per week, but this takes many months of gradual training progression.

2. **During the months of training, emphasize a high-carbohydrate diet with plenty of rest and water.** Adequate recovery from hard training means consuming a high carbohydrate diet (at least 60 to 70 percent of total Calories). The carbohydrate should be primarily starch, not sugar, to ensure adequate vitamin and mineral intake. A wide variety of healthful foods should be used to obtain all nutrients without supplementation. A conscious effort must be made to drink more water than desired.

3. **During the week before the event, rest and eat primarily carbohydrate-rich foods.** The exercise should gradually taper to total rest the day before the event. During the three days just before the event, eat a very high carbohydrate diet (close to 70–80 percent of total Calories).

4. **Three to four hours before the event, consume a high-carbohydrate meal.** About 20–30 min before eating the meal, consume 2–4 glasses of water to ensure that your body is adequately hydrated to provide digestive juices for the meal. The meal should be consumed 3–4 hours before the event to allow the stomach time to empty all its contents. If the event is early in the day, get up early. The meal should be light (500–800 Calories) and high in carbohydrate, but low in dietary fiber. Refined hot cereal, fruit juices, bagels, white bread and jam, white rice, or pasta (without any fats added) are good choices. Just before the event (5 minutes before), consuming 150–200 Calories of a diluted CHO solution can help maintain blood glucose levels.

5. **During the event, emphasize water, adding CHO toward the end.** Drink 200–400 ml of cold water every 15–20 minutes during the event. Plain water is preferable during the first portion of the race, especially if you have had a high CHO pre-event meal. Approximately 30 minutes before you estimate that you will feel fatigued, drink a glucose polymer solution that has 3 grams of glucose polymer per kilogram of body weight in a 50 percent solution. (For example, if you weigh 70 kg, prepare a drink that has 210 grams of glucose polymer mixed in 420 grams of water.) Prepare this drink ahead of time, and have a friend hand it to you at the appropriate spot in the race. This will restore blood glucose levels, allowing you to continue exercising vigorously. There appears to be little benefit to consuming CHO drinks earlier in the race.

6. **After the event, consume a high carbohydrate diet to replenish muscle glycogen stores.** Recovery from the marathon-type event is hastened by consuming a high CHO diet.

Summary

Principle #1—The prudent diet is the cornerstone. The same diet that enhances health (the prudent diet) is the one that also maximizes performance for most athletes. For some athletes in heavy training, however (defined as more than two hours a day of aerobic or intermittent anaerobic-aerobic activity), several adaptations beyond the prudent diet are beneficial. Heavy training imposes special nutritional stresses because of the high intensity of effort over a relatively short time period, demanding extra energy, carbohydrate, water, and iron.

Principle #2—Increase total energy intake. Athletes are high energy consumers because of their high working capacities, high intensity training levels, elevated basal metabolic rates, and higher-than-normal lean body masses. Many athletes need more than 50 kcal per kilogram of body weight. Most of this extra energy should come in the form of carbohydrate from grains, dried fruits, breads, and pasta.

Principle #3—Keep the carbohydrate intake high (55–70 percent) during training. A high-carbohydrate diet is probably the most important nutritional factor for athletes. Body carbohydrate stores (glycogen) are extremely labile because they are the chief fuel source for the working muscle. When muscle glycogen levels drop too low, exercise performance is impaired, and the athlete feels stale and tired and is more prone to injury. Athletes in heavy training need up to 625 grams of carbohydrate in their diet per day, which for some athletes means receiving close to 70 percent of total Calories as carbohydrate. The high levels of carbohydrate are usually more than athletes want, so they must be trained to eat high-carbohydrate diets.

Principle #4—Drink large amounts of water during training and the event. Probably the second most important diet principle for athletes is to drink large quantities of water. As little as a 2 percent drop in body weight from water loss has been associated with impaired performance. Athletes tend to sweat earlier and more than nonathletes, so they tend to lose more body water with exercise. The thirst desire of an athlete lags behind actual body needs, so athletes should be encouraged to force fluids beyond what is desired. No electrolytes are needed except in ultramarathon events— they are easily obtained with normal meals after the event. Carbohydrate added to the drink taken during exercise can help maintain blood glucose levels. Research suggests that 3 g CHO/kg should be taken in a 50 percent solution 30 minutes before fatigue.

Principle #5—Keep a close watch on possible iron deficiency. An alarming number of athletes, especially runners, have Stage 1 iron deficiency, best measured by evaluating serum ferritin levels. Because performance is impaired with even mild iron deficiency, athletes should have periodic serum ferritin evaluations. To help prevent iron deficiency, runners (especially menstruating females) should consume high-iron foods. Under the supervision of a physician, some runners may benefit from moderate iron supplementation.

Principle #6—Vitamin and mineral supplements are not needed. Most studies show that athletes are above RDA levels for all nutrients (except iron for females). Athletes are at an advantage because their high caloric intakes provide more than adequate quantities of vitamins and minerals. The sedentary are actually at greater risk because of their low caloric intakes. Athletes should not use vitamins or mineral supple-

ments in amounts above the RDA; many studies are showing the potential for nutrient imbalances in the body.

Principle #7—Extra protein does not benefit the athlete. Although 5–15 percent of the energy needed in long endurance exercise or weight lifting come from protein, athletes obtain more than enough protein in their normal diets. There is absolutely no need for protein supplements.

Principle #8—Rest and eat carbohydrate before long endurance events. The best scheme for preparing for any exercise event lasting longer than 60–90 minutes is to taper the exercise gradually, while consuming more than 70 percent carbohydrate during the seven days before the event. (Depletion of muscle glycogen during the initial phase of "glycogen loading" is no longer recommended. The pre-event meal should be 500–800 Calories, of light, low-fiber starch, three to five hours before the event.

Principle #9—Use of ergogenic aids is unethical. Although there are many worthless ergogenic aids (e.g., bee pollen, B15, alcohol), many provide impressive performance benefits (caffeine, sodium bicarbonate, phosphorus, blood doping). These enhance performance, but the ethical issue of equitable competition and fair play claim a higher priority.

Principle #10—Nutrition for the athlete is important for more than performance. Research has evaluated the effects of fat in the diet before and during exercise, and performance is not enhanced. Adapting to a high-fat diet for one month has been found to aid endurance in some studies, but such adaptation may be harmful to health in the long term. Athletes have no guarantee of protection from heart disease unless they continue prudent habits of exercise and diet after their days of competition are over. Even during heavy training, a high saturated fat diet can raise serum cholesterol to alarming levels—exercise is not powerful enough to fully negate bad nutritional habits. Athletes can maximize both performance and health through wise dietary choices.

References

1. Costill DL. Carbohydrates for Exercise: Dietary Demands for Optimal Performance. Int J Sports Med 9:1–18, 1988.

2. Mirkin G. The Sportsmedicine Book. Boston: Little, Brown, and Co., 1978.

3. Ryan AJ. Anabolic Steroids Are Fool's Gold. Fed Proc 40:2682, 1981.

4. Freeman P. Muscle Meals. California Living, March 4, 1984.

5. Higdon H. What's Diet Got To Do With It? Runner's World, October, 1988.

6. Pritikin N. The Brave Soldiers in the Ironman Army Travel on Their Stomachs. Runner's World, February, 1984, p 127.

7. U.S. Department of Health and Human Services. The Surgeon General's Report on Nutrition and Health. DHHS (PHS) Publication No. 88–50211. U.S. Government Printing Office: Washington, DC, 1988.

8. Brotherhood JR. Nutrition and Sports Performance. Sports Med 1:350–389, 1984.

9. Barr S.I.: Women, nutrition and exercise: A review of athletes' intakes and a discussion of energy balance in active women. Prog Food Nutr Sci 11:307, 1987.

10. Knoo C-S, Rawson NE, Robinson ML, Stevenson RJ. Nutrient Intake and Eating Habits of Triathletes. Ann Sports Med 3:144–150, 1987.

11. Burke LM, Diet GD, Read RSD. Diet Patterns of Elite Australian Male Triathletes. Physician Sportsmed 15(2):140–155, 1987.

12. Ellsworth NM, Hewitt BF, Haskell WL. Nutrient Intake of Elite Male and Female Nordic Skiers. Physician Sportsmed 13(2):78–92, 1985.

13. Hickson JF, Duke MA, Risser WL, et al. Nutritional Intake From Food Sources of High School Football Athletes. J Am Diet Assoc 87:1656–1659, 1988.

14. Nowak RK, Knudsen KS, Schultz LO. Body Composition and Nutrient Intakes of College Men and Women Basketball Players. J Am Diet Assoc 88:575–578, 1988.

15. Perron M, Endres J. Knowledge, Attitudes, and Dietary Practices of Female Athletes. J Am Diet Assoc 85:573–576, 1985.

16. Benson J, Gillien DM, Bourdet K, Loosli AR. Inadequate Nutrition and Chronic Calorie Restriction in Adolescent Ballerinas. Physician Sportsmed 13(10):79–89, 1985.

17. Loosli AR, Benson J, Gillien DM, Bourdet K. Nutrition Habits and Knowledge in Competitive Adolescent Female Gymnasts. Physician Sportsmed 14(8):118–130, 1986.

18. Welch PK, Zager KA, Endres J, Poon SW. Nutrition Education, Body Composition, and Dietary Intake of Female College Athletes. Physician Sportsmed 15(1):63–74, 1987.

19. Steen SN, McKinney S. Nutrition Assessment of College Wrestlers. Physician Sportsmed 11(14):100–116, 1986.

20. Cohen JL, et al. A Nutritional and Hematologic Assessment of Elite Ballet Dancers. Physician Sportsmed 13(5):43–54, 1985.

21. Moffatt RJ. Dietary Status of Elite High School Gymnasts. J Am Diet Assoc 84:1361, 1984.

22. Short SH, Short WR. Four-Year Study of University Athletes' Dietary Intake. J Am Diet Assoc 82:632–645, 1983.

23. Faber M, Bénad AJS, van Eck M. Dietary Intake, Anthropometric Measurements, and Blood Lipid Values in Weight Training Athletes (Body Builders). Int J Sports Med 7:342–346, 1986.

24. Borgen JS, Corbin CB. Eating Disorders Among Female Athletes. Physician Sportsmed 15(2):89–95, 1987.

25. Yarrows SA. Weight Loss Through Dehydration in Amateur Wrestling. J Am Diet Assoc 88:491–493, 1988.

26. Rosen LW, Hough DO. Pathogenic Weight-Control Behaviors of Female College Gymnasts. Physician Sportsmed 16(9):141–146, 1988.

27. U.S. Department of Agriculture, Human Nutrition Information Service. 1985. Nationwide Food Consumption Survey, Continuing Survey of Food Intakes by Individuals: Women 19–50 Years and Their Children 1–5 Years, 1 Day, 1985. U.S. Dept. of Agric., Rpt. No 85–1. Men 19–50 Years, 1 Day, 1985. U.S. Dept. of Agric., Rpt. No 85–3.

28. Nieman DC, Butler JV, Pollett LM, Dietrich SJ, Lutz RD. Nutrient Intake of Marathon Runners. J Am Diet Assoc 89:1273–1278, 1989.

29. Blair SN, Ellsworth NM, Haskell WL, Stern MP, Farquahr JN, and Wood PD. Comparison of Nutrient Intake in Middle-Aged Men and Women Runners and Controls. Med Sci Sports Exerc 13:310–315, 1981.

30. Clement DB, Asmundson RC. Nutritional Intake and Hematological Parameters in Endurance Runners. Physician Sportsmed 10(3):37, 1982.

31. Peters AJ, Dressendorfer RH, Rimer J, Keen CL. Diets of Endurance Runners Competing in a 20-day Road Race. Physician Sportsmed 14(7):63, 1986.

32. Weight LM, Noakes TD, Graves J, Jacobs P, Berman PA. Vitamin and Mineral Status of Trained Athletes Including the Effects of Supplementation. Am J Clin Nutr 47:186, 1988.

33. Dale E, Goldberg DL. Implications of Nutrition in Athletes' Menstrual Cycle Irregularities. Can J Appl Sports Sci 7:74, 1982.

34. Deuster PA, Kyle SB, Moser PB, Vigersky RA, Singh A, and Schoomaker EB. Nutritional Survey of Highly Trained Women Runners. Am J Clin Nutr 45:954, 1986.

35. Drinkwater BL, Nilson K, Chestnut CH, Bremner WJ, Shainholtz S, Southworth MB: Bone Mineral Content of Amenorrheic and Eumenorrheic Athletes. N Engl J Med 311:277, 1984.

36. Moore CE, Hartung GH, Mitchell RE, Kappus CM, Hinderlitter J. The Relationship of Exercise and Diet on High-Density Lipoprotein Cholesterol Levels in Women. Metabolism 32:189, 1983.

37. Nelson ME, Fisher EC, Catsos PD, Meredith CN, Turksoy RN, Evans WJ: Diet and Bone Status in Amenorrheic Runners. Am J Clin Nutr 43:910, 1986.

38. Blair SN, Jacobs DR, Powell KE. Relationships Between Exercise or Physical Activity and Other Health Behaviors. Public Health Rep 100:172–179, 1985.

39. Bedgood BL, Tuck MB. Nutrition Knowledge of High School Athletic Coaches in Texas. J Am Diet Assoc 83:672–677, 1983. See also: J Am Diet Assoc 84:1198, 1984.

40. Parr RB, et al. Nutrition Knowledge and Practice of Coaches, Trainers, and Athletes. Physician Sportsmed 12:127, 1984.

41. Barr SI. Nutrition Knowledge of Female Varsity Athletes and University Students. J Am Diet Assoc 87:1660–1664, 1987.

42. Nutrition for Physical Fitness and Athletic Performance for Adults: Technical Support Paper. J Am Diet Assoc 87:934, 1987.

43. White JA. Ergogenic Demands of a 24-Hour Cycling Event. Br J Sports Med 18:165, 1984.

44. Hermansen L. Post Exercise Elevation of Resting Oxygen Uptake: Possible Mechanisms and Physiological Significance. IN: Physiological Chemistry of Training (Marconnet and Poortmans, Eds). Basel: Karger, 1984.

45. Chasiotis D. Role of Cyclic AMP and Inorganic Phosphate in the Regulation of Muscle Glycogenolysis During Exercise. Med Sci Sports Exerc 20:545–550, 1988.

46. Gollnick PD. Metabolism of Substrates: Energy Substrate Metabolism During Exercise and As Modified By Training. Fed Proc 44:353–357, 1985.

47. Fox El, Mathews DK. The Physiological Basis of Physical Education and Athletics. Philadelphia: Saunders College, 1981.

48. Koivisto VC, et al. Influence of Physical Training on the Fuel-Hormone Response to Prolonged Low Intensity Exercise. Metabolism 31:192–196, 1982.

49. Holloszy JO. Muscle Metabolism During Exercise. Arch Phys Med Rehabil 63:231–233, 1982.

50. Sherman WM, Costill DL. The Marathon: Dietary Manipulation to Optimize Performance. Am J Sports Med 12:44–51, 1984.

51. Evans WJ, Hughes VA. Dietary Carbohydrates and Endurance Exercise. Am J Clin Nutr 41:1146–1154, 1985.

52. Costill DL. Carbohydrate Nutrition Before, During, and After Exercise. Federation Proceedings 44:364–368, 1985.

53. Burke LM, Read RSD. Sports Nutrition: Approaching the Nineties. Sports Med 8:80–100, 1989.

54. Coyle EF. Effectiveness of Carbohydrate Feeding in Delaying Fatigue During Prolonged Exercise. Sports Med 1:446, 1984.

55. Sherman WM. Carbohydrates, Muscle Glycogen, and Muscle Glycogen Super-Compensation. In: Ergogenic Aids in Sports (William MH, ed). Champaign: Human Kinetics Publishers, 1983.

56. Williams MH. Nutritional Aspects of Human Physical and Athletic Performance (2nd edition). Springfield, Illinois: Charles C. Thomas, Publisher, 1985.

57. Conlee RK. Muscle Glycogen and Exercise Endurance: A Twenty-Year Perspective. IN: Pandolf KB (ed). Exercise and Sports Sci Rev New York: Macmillan Publishing Company, 1987.

58. Christensen EH, Hansen O. Hypoglykamie, Arbeitsfahigkeit and Ermudung. Scand Archd Physiol 81:172–179, 1939.

59. Christensen EH, Hansen O. Respiratorischer Quotient and O2 Aufnahme. Scand Arch Physiol 81:180–189, 1939.

60. Bergstrom J, Hermansen L, Hultman E, et al. Diet, Muscle Glycogen and Physical Performance. Acta Physiol Scand 71:140–150, 1967.

61. Bergstrom J, Hultman E. A Study of the Glycogen Metabolism During Exercise in Man. Scan J Clin Lab Invest 19:218–228, 1967.

62. Fox EL. Sports Physiology. New York: Saunders College Publishing, 1984.

63. Nieman DC, Carlson KA, Brandstater ME, Naegele RT, Blankenship JW. Running Endurance in 27-h-Fasted Humans. J Appl Physiol 63:2502–2509, 1987.

64. Costill DL, Flynn MG, Kirwan JP, et al. Effects of Repeated Days of Intensified Training on Muscle Glycogen and Swimming Performance. Med Sci Sports Exerc 20:249–254, 1988.

65. Kirwan JP, Costill DL, Mitchell JB, et al. Carbohydrate Balance in Competitive Runners During Successive Days of Intense Training. J Appl Physiol 65:2601–2606, 1988.

66. Costill DL, Miller JM. Nutrition for Endurance Sports: Carbohydrate and Fluid Balance. Int J Sports Med 1:2–14, 1980.

67. Costill DL, Sherman WM, Fink WJ, et al. The Role of Dietary Carbohydrate in Muscle Glycogen Resynthesis After Strenuous Running. Am J Clin Nutr 34:1831–1836, 1982.

68. Brewer J, Williams C, Patton A. The Influence of High Carbohydrate Diets on Endurance Running Performance. Eur J Appl Physiol 57:698–706, 1988.

69. Haymes EM. Physiological Responses of Females Athletes to Heat Stress: A Review. Physician Sportsmed 12:45–59, 1984.

70. Bassett DR, Nagle FJ, Mookerjee S, et al. Thermoregulatory Responses to Skin Wetting During Prolonged Treadmill Running. Med Sci Sports Exerc 19:28–32, 1987.

71. Nose H, Mack GW, Shi X, Nadel ER. Shift in Body Fluid Compartments After Dehydration in Humans. J Appl Physiol 65:318–324, 1988.

72. Gisolfi CV, Wenger CB. Temperature Regulation During Exercise: Old Concepts, New Ideas. Exerc and Sport

Sciences Rev (Terjung RL, ed). Lexington: Collamore Press, 1984.

73. Hanson PG. Heat Injury in Runners. Physician Sportsmed 7:91–96, 1979.

74. Hecker AL, Wheeler KB. Impact of Hydration and Energy Intake On Performance. Athletic Training 19:260–266, 1984.

75. Armstrong LE, Hubbard RW, Jones BH, Daniels JT. Preparing Alberto Salazar for the Heat of the 1984 Olympic Marathon. Physician Sportsmed 14(3):73–81, 1986.

76. Sinclair JD, et al. Circulatory Effects of Fluid Loss and Fluid Intake During Exercise. J Sports Sciences 1:175–183, 1983.

77. Sawka MN, et al. Influence of Hydration Level and Body Fluids on Exercise Performance In the Heat. JAMA 252:1165–1169, 1984.

78. Fortney SM, Vroman NB, Beckett WS, et al. Effect of Exercise Hemoconcentration and Hyperosmolality on Exercise Responses. J Appl Physiol 65:519–524, 1988.

79. Greenleaf JE, Fink WJ. Fluid Intake and Athletic Performance. IN: Nutrition and Athletic Performance (Haskell W, ed). Palo Alto: Bull Publishing Co., 1982.

80 Nash HL. Treating Thermal Injury: Disagreement Heats Up. Physician Sportsmed 13:134–144, 1985.

81. Gisolfi CV, et al. Symposium On the Thermal Effects of Exercise In the Heat. Med Sci Sports Exerc 11:29–71, 1979.

82. Herbert WG. Water and Electrolytes. IN: Ergogenic Aids In Sport (Williams MH, ed). Champaign, Illinois: Human Kinetics Publishers, 1983.

83. Perlmutter EM. The Pittsburgh Marathon: 'Playing Weather Roulette.' Physician Sportsmed 14(8):132–138, 1986.

84. ACSM Position Statement. Prevention of Thermal Injuries During Distance Running. Physician Sportsmed 12:43–51, 1984.

85. Hopper MK, Coggan AR, Coyle EF. Exercise Stroke Volume Relative to Plasma-Volume Expansion. J Appl Physiol 64:404–408, 1988.

86. Buono MJ, Sjoholm NT. Effect of Physical Training on Peripheral Sweat Production. J Appl Physiol 65:811–814, 1988.

87. Kirby CR, Convertino VA. Plasma Aldosterone and Sweat Sodium Concentrations After Exercise and Heat Acclimation. J Appl Physiol 61:967–970, 1986.

88. Nieman DC, Berk LS, Simpson-Westerberg M, Arabatzis K, Youngberg WS, Tan SA, Lee JW, Eby WC. The Effects of Long Endurance Running on Immune System Parameters and Lymphocyte Function in Experienced Marathoners. Int J Sports Med 10:317–323, 1989.

89. Murray R, Paul GL, Seifert JG, et al. The Effects of Glucose, Fructose, and Sucrose Ingestion During Exercise. Med Sci Sports Exerc 21:275–282, 1989.

90. Murray R, Eddy DE, Murray TW, et al. The Effect of Fluid and Carbohydrate Feedings During Intermittent Cycling Exercise. Med Sci Sports Exerc 19:597–604, 1987.

91. Pitts GL, Johnson RE, Consolzio FC. Work in the Heat As Affected By Intake of Water, Salt, and Glucose. Am J Physiol 142:253–259, 1944.

92. Nadel ER. Recent Advances in Temperature Regulation During Exercise In Humans. Fed Proc 44:2286–2292, 1985.

93. Hughson RL, Staudt LA, Mackie JM. Monitoring Road Racing In the Heat. Physician Sportsmed 11:94–105, 1983.

94. Wells CL, Stern JR, Kohrt WM, et al. Fluid Shifts With Successive Running and Bicycling Performance. Med Sci Sports Exerc 19:137–142, 1987.

95. Neufer PD, Young AJ, Sawka MN. Gastric Emptying during Walking and Running: Effects of Varied Exercise Intensity. Eur J Appl Physiol 59:440–445, 1989.

96. McArthur KE, Feldman M. Gastric Acid Secretion, Gastrin Release, and Gastric Emptying in Humans As Affected by Liquid Meal Temperature. Am J Clin Nutr 49:51–54, 1989.

97. Lamb DR, Brodowicz GR. Optimal Use of Fluids of Varying Formulations to Minimize Exercise-Induced Disturbances in Homeostasis. Sports Med 3:247–274, 1986.

98 Ryan AJ, Bleiler TL, Carter JE, Gisolfi CV. Gastric Emptying During Prolonged Cycling Exercise in the Heat. Med Sci Sports Exerc 21:51–58, 1989.

99. Frizzell RT, Lang GH, Lowance DC, Lathan SR. Hyponatremia and Ultramarathon Running. JAMA 255:772–774, 1986.

100. Hiller WDB, O'Toole ML, Massimino F, et al. Plasma Electrolyte and Glucose Changes During the Hawaiian Ironman Triathalon. Med Sci Sports Exerc 17:219, 1985.

101. Noakes TD, Goodwin N, Rayner BL, et al. Water Intoxication: A Possible Complication During Endurance Exercise. Med Sci Sports Exerc 17:370–375, 1985.

102. Mitchell JB, Costill DL, Howard JA, et al. Gastric Emptying: Influence of Prolonged Exercise and Carbohydrate Concentration. Med Sci Sports Exerc 21:269–274, 1989.

103. Neufer PD, Costill DL, Fink WJ, et al. Effects of Exercise and Carbohydrate Composition on Gastric Emptying. Med Sci Sports Exerc 18:658–662, 1986.

104. Murray R, Eddy DE, Murray TW, et al. The Effect of Fluid and Carbohydrate Feedings During Intermittent Cycling Exercise. Med Sci Sports Exerc 19:597–604, 1987.

105. Murray R. The Effects of Consuming Carbohydrate-Electrolyte Beverages on Gastric Emptying and Fluid Absorption During and Following Exercise. Sports Med 4:322–351, 1987.

106. Mitchell JB, Costill DL, Houmard JA, et al. Effects of Carbohydrate Ingestion on Gastric Emptying and Exer-

cise Performance. Med Sci Sports Exerc 20:110–115, 1988.

107. Davis JM, Lamb DR, Pate RR, Slentz CA, Burgess WA, Bartoli WP. Carbohydrate-Electrolyte Drinks: Effects On Endurance Cycling in the Heat. Am J Clin Nutr 48:1023–1030, 1988.

108. Coggan AR, Coyle EF. Reversal of Fatigue During Prolonged Exercise by Carbohydrate Infusion or Ingestion. J Appl Physiol 63:2388–2395, 1987.

109. Coyle EF, Coggan AR, Hemmert MK, Ivy JL. Muscle Glycogen Utilization During Prolonged Strenuous Exercise When Fed Carbohydrate. J Appl Physiol 61:165–172, 1986.

110. Hargreaves M, Briggs CA. Effect of Carbohydrate Ingestion on Exercise Metabolism. J Appl Physiol 65:1553–1555, 1988.

111. Coggan AR, Coyle EF. Effect of Carbohydrate Feedings During High-Intensity Exercise. J Appl Physiol 65:1703–1709, 1988.

112. Coggan AR, Coyle EF. Metabolism and Performance Following Carbohydrate Ingestion Late In Exercise. Med Sci Sports Exerc 21:59–65, 1989.

113. Winder WW. Role of Cyclic AMP in Regulation of Hepatic Glucose Production During Exercise. Med Sci Sports Exerc 20:551–560, 1988.

114. Flynn MG, Costill DL, Hawley JA, et al. Influence of Selected Carbohydrate Drinks on Cycling Performance and Glycogen Use. Med Sci Sports Exerc 19:37–40, 1987.

115. Clement DB, Asmundson RC. Nutritional Intake and Hematological Parameters in Endurance Runners. Physician Sportsmed 10:37–43, 1982.

116. Hunding A, Jordal R, Pauley PE. Runner's Anemia and Iron Deficiency. Acta Med Scand 209:315–318, 1981.

117. Ehn L, Carlmark B, Hoglund S. Iron Status In Athletes Involved In Intense Physical Activity. Med Sci Sports Exerc 12:61–64, 1980.

118. Carlson DL, Mawdsley RH. Sports Anemia: A Review of the Literature. Am J Sports Med 14:109–112, 1986.

119. Manore MM, Besenfelder PD, Wells CL, et al. Nutrient Intakes and Iron Status in Female Long-Distance Runners During Training. J Am Diet Assoc 89:257–259, 1989.

120. Durstine JL, Pate RR, Sparling PB, et al. Lipid, Lipoprotein, and Iron Status of Elite Women Distance Runners. Int J Sports Med 8 (suppl):119–123, 1987.

121. Risser WL, Lee EJ, Poindexter HBW, et al. Iron Deficiency in Female Athletes: Its Prevalence and Impact on Performance. Med Sci Sports Exerc 20:116–121, 1988.

122. Magazanik A, Weinstein Y, Dlin RA, et al. Iron Deficiency Caused by 7 Weeks of Intensive Physical Exercise. Eur J Appl Physiol 57:198–202, 1988.

123. Selby GB, Eichner ER. Endurance Swimming, Intravascular Hemolysis, Anemia, and Iron Depletion. Am J Med 81:791–794, 1986.

124. Matter M, Stittfall T, Graves J, et al. The Effect of Iron and Folate Therapy on Maximal Exercise Performance in Female Marathon Runners with Iron and Folate Deficiency. Clin Sci 72:415–422, 1987.

125. Wishnitzer R, Berrebi A, Hurwitz N, Vorst E, Eliraz A. Decreased Cellularity and Hemosiderin of the Bone Marrow in Healthy and Overtrained Competitive Distance Runners. Physician Sportsmed 14(7):86–100, 1986.

126. Blum SM, Sherman AR, Boileau RA. The Effects of Fitness-Type Exercise on Iron Status in Adult Women. Am J Clin Nutr 43:456–463, 1986.

127. Clement DB, Sawchuk LL. Iron Status and Sports Performance. Sports Med 1:65–74, 1984.

128. Herbert V. Recommended Dietary Intakes (RDI) of Iron in Humans. Am J Clin Nutr 45:679–686, 1987.

129. Expert Scientific Working Group. Summary of a Report on Assessment of the Iron Nutritional Status of the United States Population. Am J Clin Nutr 42:1318–1330, 1985.

130. Pate RR. Sports Anemia: A Review of the Current Literature. Physician Sportsmed 11:115–131, 1983.

131. Puhl JL, Van Handel PJ, Williams LL, et al. Iron Status and Training. IN: Butts NK, Gushiken TT, Zarins B (eds): The Elite Athlete. New York: Spectrum Publications, 1985.

132. Finch CA, Cook JD. Iron Deficiency. Am J Clin Nutr 39:471–477, 1984.

133. Nelson RA. Nutrition and Physical Performance. Physician Sportsmed 10:55–63, 1982.

134. Perkkio MV, et al. Work Peformance in Iron Deficiency of Increasing Severity. J Appl Physiol 58:1477–1480, 1985.

135. Woodson RD. Hemoglobin Concentration and Exercise Capacity. Am Rev Respir Dis 129:(Suppl)S72–S75, 1984.

136. Schoene RB, et al. Iron Repletion Decreases Maximal Exercise Lactate Concentrations in Female Athletes With Minimal Iron-Deficiency Anemia. J Lab Clin Med 102:306–312, 1983.

137. Rowland TW, Deisroth MB, Green GM, Kelleher JF. The Effect of Iron Therapy on the Exercise Capacity of Nonanemic Iron-deficient Adolescent Runners. Am J Dis Child 142:165–169, 1988.

138. Newhouse IJ, Clement DB, Taunton JE, McKenzie DC. The Effects of Prelatent/Latent Iron Deficiency on Physical Work Capacity. Med Sci Sports Exerc 21:263–168, 1989.

139. Lampe JW, Slavin JL, Apple FS. Poor Iron Status of Women Runners Training for a Marathon. Int J Sports Med 7:111–114, 1986.

140. Snyder AC, Dvorak LL, Roepke JB. Influence of Dietary Iron Source on Measures of Iron Status Among Female Runners. Med Sci Sports Exerc 21:7–10, 1989.

141. O'Toole ML, Hiller WDB, Roalstad MS, Douglas PS. Hemolysis During Triathlon Races: Its Relation to Race Distance. Med Sci Sports Exerc 20:272–275, 1988.

142. Miller BJ, Pate RR, Burgess W. Foot Impact Force and Intravascular Hemolysis During Distance Running. Int J Sports Med 9:56–60, 1988.

143. Brune M, Magnusson B, Persson H, Hallberg L. Iron Losses in Sweat. Am J Clin Nutr 43:438–443, 1986.

144. Lamanca JJ, Haymes EM, Daly JA et al. Sweat Iron Loss of Male and Female Runners During Exercise. Int J Sports Med 9:52–55, 1988.

145. Falsetti HL, et al. Hematological Variations After Endurance Running With Hard- and Soft-Soled Running Shoes. Physician Sportsmed 11:118–124, 1983.

146. Stewart JG, et al. Gastrointestinal Blood Loss and Anemia in Runners. Ann Int Med 100:843–845, 1984.

147. McMahon LF, et al. Occult Gastrointestinal Blood Loss in Marathon Runners. Ann Int Med 100:846–847, 1984. See also: Br Med J 287:1427, 1983.

148. Haymes EM, Lamanca JJ. Iron Loss in Runners During Exercise: Implications and Recommendations. Sports Med 7:277–285, 1989.

149. Hallberg L, Brune M, Rossander L. Iron Absorption in Man: Ascorbic Acid and Dose-Dependent Inhibition by Phytate. Am J Clin Nutr 49:140–144, 1989.

150. Simmer K, Iles CA, James C, et al. Are Iron-Folate Supplements Harmful? Am J Clin Nutr 45:122–125, 1987.

151. Yadrick MK, Kenney MA, Winterfeldt EA. Iron, Copper, and Zinc Status: Response to Supplementation with Zinc or Zinc and Iron in Adult Females. Am J Clin Nutr 49:145–150, 1989.

152. Nieman DC. Vegetarian Dietary Practices and Endurance Performance. Am J Clin Nutr 48:754–761, 1988.

153. Belko AZ. Vitamins and Exercise—An Update. Med Sci Sports Exerc 19:S191–S196, 1987.

154. Van der Beek EJ. Vitamins and Endurance Training: Food for Running or Faddish Claims? Sports Med 2:175–197, 1985.

155. Grandjean AC. Vitamins, Diet, and the Athlete. Clin Sports Med 2:105, 1983.

156. Khoo C-S, Rawson NE, Robinson ML, Stevenson RJ: Nutrient intake and eating habits of triathletes. Ann Sports Med 3:144, 1987.

157. Clark N, Nelson, M, Evans W: Nutrition education for elite female runners. Physician Sportsmed 16(2):124, 1988.

158. Deuster, PA, Kyle SB, Moser PB, Vigersky RA, Singh A, Schoomaker EB: Nutritional Survey of Highly Trained Women Runners. Am J Clin Nutr 45:954, 1986.

159. Nieman DC, Gates JR, Butler JV, Pollett LM, Dietrich SJ, and Lutz RD. Supplementation Patterns in Marathon Runners. J Am Diet Assoc 89:1615–1619, 1989.

160. U.S. Department of Agriculture, Human Nutrition Information Service. 1985. Nationwide Food Consumption Survey, Continuing Survey of Food Intakes by Individuals: Women 19–50 Years and Their Children 1–5 Years, 1 Day, 1985. U.S. Dept. of Agric., Rpt. No 85–1. Men 19–50 Years, 1 Day, 1985. U.S. Dept. of Agric., Rpt. No 85–3.

161. Council on Scientific Affairs: Vitamin Preparations as Dietary Supplements and as Therapeutic Agents. JAMA 257:1929, 1987.

162. Callaway, CW, McNutt K, Rivlin RS: Statement on Vitamin and Mineral Supplements. Am J Clin Nutr 46:1075, 1987.

163. Barnett DW, Conlee RK. The Effects of a Commercial Dietary Supplement On Human Performance. Am J Clin Nutr 40:586–590, 1984.

164. Haskell WH, Scala J, Whittam J. Nutrition and Athletic Performance. Palo Alto, CA: Bull Publishing Co., 1982.

165. Keys A, et al. Vitamin Supplementation of U.S. Army Rations In Relation to Fatigue and the Ability to Do Muscular Work. J Nutrition 23:259–269, 1942. See also: Am J Physiol 144:5, 1945.

166. Barnett DW, Conlee RK: The effects of a commercial dietary supplement on human performance. Am J Clin Nutr 40:586, 1984.

167. Weight LM, Noakes TD, Graves J, Jacobs P, Berman PA: Vitamin and Mineral Status of Trained Athletes Including the Effects of Supplementation. Am J Clin Nutr 47:186, 1988.

168. Read MH, McGuffin SL: The Effect of B-complex Supplementation on Endurance Performance. J Sports Med 23:178, 1983.

169. Haymes EM: Nutritional Concerns: Need for Iron. Med Sci Sports Exerc 19:S197, 1987.

170. McDonald R, Keen CL: Iron, Zinc and Magnesium Nutrition and Athletic performance. Sports Med 5:171, 1988.

171. Keen CL, Lowney P, Gershwin E, et al. Dietary Magnesium Intake Influences Exercise Capacity and Hematologic Parameters in Rats. Metabolism 36:788–793, 1987.

172. Campbell WW, Anderson RA. Effects of Aerobic Exercise and Training on the Trace Minerals Chromium, Zinc and Copper. Sports Med 4:9–18, 1987.

173. Deuster PA, Dolev E, Kyle SB, et al. Magnesium Homeostasis During High-Intensity Anaerobic Exercise in Men. J Appl Physiol 62:545–550, 1987.

174. Manore MM, Leklem JE, Walter MC. Vitamin B-6 Metabolism as Affected by Exercise in Trained and Untrained Women Fed Diets Differing in Carbohydrate and Vitamin B-6 Content. Am J Clin Nutr 46:995–1004, 1987.

175. Stendig-Lindberg G, Shaprio Y, Epstein Y, et al. Changes in Serum Magnesium Concentration After Strenuous Exercise. J Am Coll Nutr 6:35–40, 1987.

176. Belko AZ, Roe DA, et al. Effects of Exercise on Riboflavin Requirements of Young Women. Am J Clin Nutr 37:509–517, 1983.

177. Belko AZ, Roe DA, et al. Effects of Aerobic Exercise and Weight Loss On Riboflavin Requirements of Moderately Obese, Marginally Deficient Young Women. Am J Clin Nutr 40:553–561, 1984.

178. Belko AZ, Roe DA, et al. Effects of Exercise On Riboflavin Requirements: Biological Validation In Weight Reducing Women. Am J Clin Nutr 41:270–277, 1985.

179. Leklem JE, Shultz TD. Increased Plasma Pyridoxal 5'-phosphate and Vitamin B6 in Male Adolescents After a 4500 Meter Run. Am J Clin Nutr 38:541–548, 1983.

180. Anderson RA, Bryden NA, Polansky MM, Deuster PA. Exercise Effects on Chromium Excretion of Trained and Untrained Men Consuming a Constant Diet. J Appl Physiol 64:249–252, 1988.

181. van der Beck EJ, van Dokkum W, Schrijver J, et al. Thiamin, Riboflavin, and Vitamins B-6 and C: Impact of Combined Restricted Intake on Functional Performance in Man. Am J Clin Nutr 48:1451–1462, 1989.

182. Powers HJ, Bates CJ, Lamb WH, et al. Effects of a Multivitamin and Iron Supplement on Running Performance in Gambian Children. Hum Nutr: Clin Nutr 39C:427, 1985.

183. Fischer PWF, et al. Effect of Zinc Supplementation On Copper Status In Adult Man. Am J Clin Nutr 40:743–746, 1984.

184. Finley EB, Cerklewski FL. Influence of Ascorbic Acid Supplementation On Copper Status In Young Adult Men. Am J Clin Nutr 37:553–556, 1983.

185. Greger JL, Baier MJ. Effect of Dietary Aluminum On Mineral Metabolism of Adult Males. Am J Clin Nutr 38:411–419, 1983.

186. Alexander M, et al. Relation of Riboflavin Nutriture In Healthy Elderly to Intake of Calcium and Vitamin Supplements: Evidence Against Riboflavin Supplementation. Am J Clin Nutr 39:540–546, 1984.

187. Solomons NW, et al. Studies On the Bioavailability of Zinc In Humans: Intestinal Interaction of Tin and Zinc. Am J Clin Nutr 37:566–571, 1983.

188. Milne DB, et al. Effect of Oral Folic Acid Supplements On Zinc, Copper, and Iron Absorption and Excretion. Am J Clin Nutr 39:535–539, 1984.

189. O'Dell BL. Bioavailability of Trace Elements. Nutr Rev 42:301–308, 1984.

190. Institute of Food Technologists' Expert Panel on Food Safety and Nutrition. Food Nutrient Interactions. Food Tech, October, 1984, pp. 59–63.

191. Dawson-Hughes B, Seligson FH, Hughes VA. Effects of Calcium Carbonate and Hydroxyapatite on Zinc and Iron Retention in Postmenopausal Women. Am J Clin Nutr 44:83–88, 1986.

192. Goodman MN, Ruderman NB. Influence of Muscle Use On Amino Acid Metabolism. Exerc Sports Sci Rev 10:1–25, 1982.

193. Lemon PWR. The Importance of Protein for Athletes. Sports Med 1:474–488, 1984.

194. Lemon PWR. Protein and Exercise: Update 1987. Med Sci Sports Exerc 19:S179–S190, 1987.

195. Dohm GL. Protein Metabolism During Endurance Exercise. Fed Proc 44:348–352, 1985.

196. Lemon PWR, Nagle FJ. Effects of Exercise On Protein and Amino Acid Metabolism. Med Sci Sports Exerc 13:141–149, 1981.

197. Bier DM, Young VR. Exercise and Blood Pressure: Nutritional Considerations. Ann Intern Med 98:864–869, 1983.

198. Evans WJ. Protein Metabolism and Endurance Exercise. Physician Sportsmed 11:63–71, 1983.

199. Young VR, Torun B. Physical Activity: Impact on Protein and Amino Acid Metabolism and Implications for Nutritional Requirements. Prog Clin Biol Res 77:57–85, 1981.

200. Hickson JF, Wolinsky I, Rodriguez GP, et al. Failure of Weight Training to Affect Urinary Indices of Protein Metabolism in Men. Med Sci Sports Exerc 18:563–567, 1986.

201. Stein TP. Nutrition and Protein Turnover: A Review. J Parenter Enter Nutr 6:444–454, 1982.

202. Dohm GL, Tapscott EB, Kasperek GJ. Protein Degradation During Endurance Exercise and Recovery. Med Sci Sports Exerc 19:S166–S171, 1987.

203. Hickson JF, et al. Exercise and Protein Intake Effects On Urinary 3-Methylhistidine Excretion. Am J Clin Nutr 41:246, 1985.

204. Pivarnik JM, Hickson JF, Wolinsky I. Urinary 3-methylhistidine Excretion Increases with Repeated Weight Training Exercise. Med Sci Sports Exerc 21:283–287, 1989

205. Hagerman FC, et al. Muscle Damage in Marathon Runners. Physician Sportsmed 12:39–48, 1984.

206. Ji LL, Miller RH, Nagel FJ, et al. Amino Acid Metabolism During Exercise in Trained Rats: The Potential Role of Carnitine in the Metabolic Fate of Branched-Chain Amino Acids. Metabolism 36:748–752, 1987.

207. Nair KS, Woolf PD, Welle SL, Matthews DE. Leucine, Glucose, and Energy Metabolism After 3 Days of Fasting in Healthy Human Subjects. Am J Clin Nutr 46:557–562, 1987.

208. Wolfe RR. Does Exercise Stimulate Protein Breakdown in Humans?: Isotopic Approaches to the Problem. Med Sci Sports Exerc 19:S172–S178, 1987.

209. Butterfield GE. Whole-Body Protein Utilization in Humans. Med Sci Sports Exerc 19:S157–S165, 1987.

210. Tarnopolsky MA, MacDougall JD, Atkinson SA. Influence of Protein Intake and Training Status on Nitrogen Balance and Lean Body Mass. J Appl Physiol 64:187–193, 1988.

211. Lemon PWR. Effect of Intensity on Protein Utilization During Prolonged Exercise. Med Sci Sports Exerc 16:151, 1984.

212. Acheson KJ, Schutz Y, Bessard T, et al. Glycogen Storage Capacity and De Novo Lipogenesis During Massive Carbohydrate Overfeeding in Man. Am J Clin Nutr 48:240–247, 1988.

213. Goss FL, Karam C. The Effects of Glycogen Supercompensation On the Electrocardiographic Response During Exercise. Res Quart Exerc Sport 58:68–71, 1987.

214. Sherman WM, Costill DL, Fink WJ, et al. The Effect of Exercise Diet Manipulation On Muscle Glycogen and Its Subsequent Utilization During Performance. Int J Sports Med 2:114–118, 1981.

215. Blom PCS, Costill DL, Vollestad NK. Exhaustive Running: Inappropriate as a Stimulus of Muscle Glycogen Supercompensation. Med Sci Sports Exerc 19:398–403, 1987.

216. Roberts KM, Nobel EG, Hayden DB, Taylor AW. Simple and Complex Carbohydrate-Rich Diets and Muscle Glycogen Content of Marathon Runners. Eur J Appl Physiol 57:70–74, 1988.

217. Pernow B, Saltin B. Availability of Substrates and Capacity for Prolonged Heavy Exercise. J Appl Physiol 31:416–422, 1971.

218. Karlsson J, Saltin B. Diet, Muscle Glycogen, and Endurance Performance. J Appl Physiol 31:203–206, 1971.

219. Foster C, Costill DL, Fink WJ. Effects of Preexercise Feedings On Endurance Performance. Med Sci Sports Exerc 11:1–5, 1979.

220. Keller K, Schwarzkopf R. Preexercise Snacks May Decrease Exercise Performance. Physician Sportsmed 12:89–91, 1984.

221. Gleeson M, Maugham RJ, Greenhaff PL. Comparison of the Effects of Pre-Exercise Feeding of Glucose, Glycerol, and Placebo On Endurance and Fuel Homeostatsis in Man. Eur J Appl Physiol 55:645–653, 1986.

222. Fielding RA, Costill DL, Fink WJ, et al. Effects of Preexercise Carbohydrate Feedings On Muscle Glycogen Use During Exercise in Well-Trained Runners. Eur J Appl Physiol 56:225–229, 1987.

223. Hargreaves M, Costill DL, Fink WJ, et al. Effect of Pre-Exercise Carbohydrate Feedings on Endurance Cycling Performance. Med Sci Sports Exerc 19:33–36, 1987.

224. Neufer PD, Costill DL, Flynn MG, et al. Improvements in Exercise Performance: Effects of Carbohydrate Feedings and Diet. J Appl Physiol 62:983–988, 1987.

225. Grucza R, Szczypaczewska M, Koziowski S. Thermoregulation in Hyperhydrated Men During Physical Exercise. Eur J Appl Physiol 56:603–607, 1987.

226. Ivy JL, Katz AL, Cutler CL, et al. Muscle Glycogen Synthesis After Exercise: Effect of Time of Carbohydrate Ingestion. J Appl Physiol 64:1480–1485, 1988.

227. Ivy JL, Lee MC, Brozinick JT, Reed MJ. Muscle Glycogen Storage After Different Amounts of Carbohydrate Ingestion. J Appl Physiol 65:2018–2023, 1988.

228. Brewer J, Williams C, Patton A. The Influence of High Carbohydrate Diets on Endurance Running Performance. Eur J Appl Physiol 57:698–706, 1988.

229. Williams MH. Ergogenic Aids in Sports. Champaign, Illinois: Human Kinetics Publishers, 1983.

230. Strauss RH. Drugs and Performance in Sports. Philadelphia: W.B. Saunders Company, 1987.

231. Percy EC. Ergogenic Aids In Athletics. Med Sci Sports Exerc 10:298–303, 1978.

232. Aronson V. Protein and Miscellaneous Ergogenic Aids. Physician Sportsmed 14(5):199–202, 1986.

233. Oyono-Enguelle S, Freund H, Ott C, et al. Prolonged Submaximal Exercise and L-Carnitine in Humans. Eur J Appl Physiol 58:53–61, 1988.

234. Greig C, Finch M, Jones DA, et al. The Effect of Oral Supplementation With L-Carnitine on Maximum and Submaximum Exercise Capacity. Eur J Appl Physiol 56:457–460, 1987.

235. Marconi C, Sassi G, Carpinelli A, et al. Effects of L-carnitine Loading on the Aerobic and Anaerobic Performance of Endurance Athletes. Eur J Appl Physiol 54:131–135, 1985. DiPalma JR: L-carnitine: Its Therapeutic Potential. Am Fam Physician 34(6):127–130, 1986.

236. Duffy DJ, Conlee RK. Effects of Phosphate Loading on Leg Power and High Intensity Treadmill Exercise. Med Sci Sports Exerc 18:674–677, 1986.

237. Ahlberg A, Weatherwax RS, Deady M, et al. Effect of Phosphate Loading on Cycle Ergometer Performance. Med Sci Sports Exerc 18:S11, 1986.

238. Bredle DL, Stager JM, Brechue WF, Farber MO. Phosphate Supplementation, Cardiovascular Function, and Exercise Performance in Humans. J Appl Physiol 65:1821–1826, 1988.

239. Larkin T. Bee Pollen As A Health Food. FDA Consumer, April 1984, p. 21.

240. Mirkin G. Bee Pollen: Living Up to Its Hype? Physician Sportsmed 13:159–160, 1985. See also: Br J Sports Med 16:142, 1982.

241. Gray ME, Titlow LW. B-15: Myth or Miracle? Physician Sportsmed 10:107–112, 1982.

242. Fennema O. The Placebo Effect of Foods. Food Tech, December 1984, pp. 57–67.

243. Leonard TK, Watson RR, Mohs ME. The Effects of Caffeine on Various Body Systems: A Review. J Am Diet Assoc 87:1048–1053, 1987.

244. Butts NK, Crowell D. Effect of Caffeine Ingestion on Cardiorespiratory Endurance in Men and Women. Res Quart Exerc Sport 56:301–305, 1985.

245. Fisher SM, McMurray RG, Berry M, et al. Influence of Caffeine on Exercise Performance in Habitual Caffeine Users. Int J Sports Med 7:276–280, 1986.

246. Eichner ER. The Caffeine Controversy: Effects on Endurance and Cholesterol. Physician Sportsmed 14(12):124–132.

247. Weir J, Noakes TD, Myburgh K, et al. A High Carbohydrate Diet Negates the Metabolic Effects of Caffeine During Exercise. Med Sci Sports Exerc 19:100–105, 1987.

248. Sasaki H, Takaoka I, Ishiko T. Effects of Sucrose or Caffeine Ingestion on Running Performance and Biochemical Responses to Endurance Running. Int J Sports Med 8:203–207, 1987.

249. McNaughton L. Effects of Two Levels of Caffeine Ingestion on Blood Lactate and Free Fatty Acid Responses During Incremental Exercise. Res Quart Exerc Sport 58:255–259, 1987.

250. Costill DL, Dalsky GP, Fink WJ. Effects of Caffeine Ingestion On Metabolism and Exercise Performance. Med Sci Sports Exerc 10:155–158, 1978.

251. Ivy JL, Costill DL, Fink WJ, Lower RW. Influence of Caffeine and Carbohydrate Feedings On Endurance Performance. Med Sci Sports Exerc 11:6–11, 1979.

252. MacIntosh BR, Gardiner PF. Muscle Fatigue: Reversal by Caffeine. Med Sci Sports Exerc 16:145, 1984.

253. Messier G, et al. Effect of Caffeine Ingestion Before Exercise In Rats On A Glycogen Loading Diet. Med Sci Sports Exerc 15:127, 1983.

254. Casal DC, Leon AS. Failure of Caffeine to Affect Substrate Utilization During Prolonged Running. Med Sci Sports Exerc 17:174–179, 1985.

255. Knapil JJ, et al. Influence of Caffeine On Serum Substrate Changes During Running In Trained and Untrained Individual. Biochem Exerc 13:514–519, 1983.

256. Powers SK, Dodd S. Caffeine and Endurance Performance. Sports Med 2:165–174, 1985.

257. Lombardo JA. Stimulants and Athletic Performance (Part 1 or 2): Amphetamines and Caffeine. Physician Sportsmed 11(14):128–140, 1986.

258. Gledhill N. Bicarbonate Ingestion and Anaerobic Performance. Sports Med 1:177–180, 1984.

259. Wilkes D, Gledhill N, Smyth R. Effect of Acute Induced Metabolic Alkalosis on 800-m Racing Time. Med Sci Sports Exerc 15:277–280, 1983.

260. Costill Dl, et al. Acid-Base Balance During Repeated Bouts of Exercise: Influence of HCO3-. Int J Sports Med 5:228–231, 1983.

261. Rupp JC, et al. Effect of Sodium Bicarbonate Ingestion On Blood and Muscle pH and Exercise Performance. Med Sci Sports Exerc 15:115, 1983.

262. Robertson RJ, Falkel JE, Drash AL, et al. Effect of Blood pH on Peripheral and Central Signals of Perceived Exertion. Med Sci Sports Exerc 18:114–122, 1986.

263. Bouissou P, Defer G, Guezennec CY, Estrade PY, Serrurier B. Metabolic and Blood Catecholamine Responses to Exercise During Alkalosis. Med Sci Sports Exerc 20:228–232, 1988.

264. Goldfinch J, Naughton LM, Davies P. Induced Metabolic Alkalosis and Its Effects on 400-m Racing Time. Eur J Appl Physiol 57:45–48, 1988.

265. Horswill CA, Costill DL, Fink WJ, et al. Influence of Sodium Bicarbonate on Sprint Performance: Relationship to Dosage. Med Sci Sports Exerc 20:566–569, 1988.

266. Eichner ER. Blood Doping: Results and Consequences From the Laboratory and the Field. Phys Sportsmed 15(1):121–129, 1987.

267. Gledhill N. The Ergogenic Effect of Blood Doping. Physician Sportsmed 11:87–90, 1983.

268. Legwold G. Blood Doping and the Letter of the Law. Physician Sportsmed 13:37–38, 1985.

269. Klein HG. Blood Transfusion and Athletics. N Eng J Med 312:854–856, 1985.

270. Spriet LL, Gledhill N, Froese AB, Wilkes DL. Effect of Graded Erythrocythemia on Cardiovascular and Metabolic Responses to Exercise. J Appl Physiol 61:1942–1948, 1986.

271. Sawka MN, Dennis RC, Gonzalez RR, et al. Influence of Polycythemia on Blood Volume and Thermoregulation During Exercise-Heat Stress. J Appl Physiol 62:912–918, 1987.

272. Duda M. Blood Doping Improves Endurance and Heat Tolerance, Studies Say. Physician Sportsmed 15(8):123–127, 1987.

273. Sawka MN, Young AJ, Muza SR, et al. Erythrocyte Reinfusion and Maximal Aerobic Power. JAMA 257:1496–1499, 1987.

274. Brien AJ, Simon TL. The Effects of Red Blood Cell Infusion on 10-km Race Time. JAMA 257:2761–2765, 1987.

275. Berglund B, Hemmingson P. Effect of Reinfusion of Autologous Blood on Exercise Performance in Cross-Country Skiers. Int J Sports Med 8:231–233, 1987.

276. Giel D. Should Runners Donate Blood? Physician Sportsmed 16(7):30–32, 1988.

277. Berglund B. Development of Techniques for the Detection of Blood Doping in Sport. Sports Med 5:127–135, 1988.

278. Council on Scientific Affairs. Drug Abuse in Athletes: Anabolic Steroids and Human Growth Hormone. JAMA 259:1703–1705, 1988.

279. American College of Sports Medicine. Position Statement on Anabolic-Androgenic Steroids. Sports Med Bull 19:8–12, 1984.

280. Buckley WE, Yesalis CE, Friedl KE, et al. Estimated Prevalence of Anabolic Steroid Use Among Male High School Seniors. JAMA 260:3441–3445, 1988.

281. Yesalis CE, Herrick RT, Buckley WE, Friedle KE, et al. Self-Reported Use of Anabolic-Androgenic Steroids by Elite Power Lifters. Physician Sportsmed 16(12):91–100, 1988.

282. Chaikin T with Rick Telander. The Nightmare of Steroids. Sports Illustrated, 1988.

283. Alen M, Rahkila P. Anabolic-Androgenic Steroid Effects on Endocrinology and Lipid Metabolism in Athletes. Sports Med 6:327–332, 1988.

284. Miller RW. Athletes and Steroids: Playing a Deadly Game. FDA Consumer, November: 17–21, 1987.

285. Lenders JWM, Demacker PNM, Vos JA, et al. Deleterious Effects of Anabolic Steroids on Serum Lipoproteins, Blood Pressure, and Liver Function in Amateur Body Builders. Int J Sports Med 9:19–23, 1988.

286. Lubell A. Does Steroid Abuse Cause—or Excuse—Violence? Physician Sportsmed 17(2):176–185, 1989.

287. Pope HG, Katz DL. Affective and Psychotic Symptoms Associated with Anabolic Steroid Use. Am J Psychiatry 145:487–490, 1988

288. Crist DM, Peake GT, Egan PA, Waters DL. Body Composition Response to Exogenous GH During Training in Highly Conditioned Adults. J Appl Physiol 65:579–584, 1988.

289. Benyo R, Herbert MR. Wine: It's Not Just Vintage Folklore. Runner's World. January 1982, pp. 32–39.

290. Hartbarger JN. Carbohydrates. Runner's World. March 1982, p. 37.

291. Costill D, Higdon H. The Drink's On Us. The Runner. June 1980, pp. 62–71.

292. Dressendorfer RH, et al. High Density Lipoprotein Cholesterol in Marathon Runners During A 20-Day Road Race. JAMA 247:1715–1717, 1982.

293. Whorton JC. Crusaders for Fitness. Princeton: Princeton University Press, 1982.

294. Schurch PM, et al. The Influence of Moderate Prolonged Exercise and a Low Carbohydrate Diet on Ethanol Elimination and On Metabolism. Eur J Physiol 48:407–414, 1982.

295. Katzung BG. Basic and Clinical Pharmacology. Los Altos: Lange Medical Publications, 1982.

296. American College of Sports Medicine Position Statement: The Use Of Alcohol In Sports. Med Sci Sports Exerc 14:ix–xi, 1982.

297. Sinyor D, et al. The Role of a Physical Fitness Program In the Treatment of Alcoholism. J Stud Alcohol 43:380–386, 1982.

298. Graham TE. Alcohol Ingestion and Sex Differences on the Thermal Responses to Mild Exercise in a Cold Environment. Hum Biol 55:463–476, 1983.

299. Hultman E, Bergstrom J. Muscle Glycogen Synthesis In Relation to Diet Studied In Normal Subjects. *Acta Med Scand* 182:109–111, 1967.

300. Jansson E, Kaijser L. Effect of Diet On The Utilization of Blood-Borne and Intramuscular Substrates During Exercise In Man. Acta Physiol Scand 115:19–30, 1982.

301. Falecka-Wieczorek I, Kaciuba-Uscilko H. Metabolic and Hormonal Responses to Prolonged Physical Exercise in Dogs After A Single Fat-Enriched Meal. Eur J Appl Physiol 53:273–276, 1984.

302. Costill DL, et al. Effects of Elevated Plasma FFA and Insulin On Muscle Glycogen Usage During Exercise. J Appl Physiol 43:695–699, 1977.

303. Satabin P, Portero P, Defer G, et al. Metabolic and Hormonal Responses to Lipid and Carbohydrate Diets During Exercise in Man. Med Sci Sports Exerc 19:218–223, 1987.

304. Ivy JL, Costill DL, et al. Contribution of Medium and Long Chain Triglyceride Intake to Energy Metabolism During Exercise. Int J Sports Med 1:15–29, 1980.

305. Phinney SD, et al. The Human Metabolic Response to Chronic Ketosis Without Caloric Restriction: Preservation of Submaximal Exercise Capability With Reduced Carbohydrate Oxidation. Metabolism 32:769–776, 1983.

306. Miller WC, Bryce GR, Conlee RK. Adaptations to a High-Fat Diet That Increase Exercise Endurance In Male Rats. J Appl Physiol 56:78–83, 1984.

307. Lukaski HC, et al. Influence of Type and Amount of Dietary Lipid On Plasma Lipid Concentrations In Endurance Athletes. Am J Clin Nutr 39:35–44, 1984.

308. Thompson PD, et al. The Effects of High-Carbohydrate and High-Fat Diets on the Serum Lipid and Lipoprotein Concentrations of Endurance Athletes. Metabolism 33:1003–1010, 1984.

Physical Fitness Activity 9.1—What Is the Carbohydrate Quality of Your Diet?

Starch and most types of dietary fiber are complex carbohydrates. Chemically they are chains of many sugar molecules, such as table sugar (sucrose), honey, corn syrup and such, which are simple carbohydrates.

During digestion, starch and sugars are broken down into simple sugar molecules before being absorbed into the body and used for energy. The links between the sugar molecules in dietary fiber cannot be broken by human digestive enzymes. Thus, fiber passes down the intestinal tract and forms bulk for the stool.

Take the following quiz to check your diet for starch and fiber.

	Seldom or never	1–2/wk	3–4/wk	Almost daily

How often do you eat:

1. Several servings of breads, cereals, pasta, or rice? _____ _____ _____ _____

2. Starch vegetables like potatoes, corn, peas, or dishes made with dry beans or peas? _____ _____ _____ _____

3. Whole-grain breads or cereals? _____ _____ _____ _____

4. Several servings of vegetables? _____ _____ _____ _____

5. Whole fruit with skins and/or seeds (apples, pears, berries, etc.)? _____ _____ _____ _____

The best answer to all of the above is *almost daily*. Breads, cereals, and other grain products and starch vegetables provide starch. Whole-grain products, and fruits and vegetables, especially those with edible skins and seeds, are good sources of fiber.

Note: if you would like a full, computerized analysis of your diet, an excellent computer software program for nutritional analysis can be obtained from:

Wellsource Inc.
P.O. Box 569
15431 SE 82 Dr., Ste. E
Clackamas, OR 97015
(503) 656-7446
Ask for "Nutrition Profile Plus."

Part 4

Benefits and Precautions in Physical Activity

Chapter 10

Physical Activity and Heart Disease

Epidemiological studies have left no doubt as to the existence of a strong inverse relationship between physical exercise and coronary heart disease risk. The questions we need to address are not whether exercise is a real element for cardiovascular disease health, but what kind of exercise is needed, and how much, i.e., with what frequency, intensity, timing, and duration.—Dr. Ralph Paffenbarger[1]

Definitions and Statistics of Heart Disease

Heart disease is the leading killer in the United States and developed countries worldwide. (See Table 10.1.) In this chapter, each of the three major risk factors for heart disease—cigarette smoking, high blood pressure, and high blood cholesterol levels—will be reviewed, with special attention given to their relationship to physical activity. In addition, the importance of physical activity in preventing heart disease will be highlighted.

Heart Disease

Heart disease (also termed *cardiovascular disease*) is not a single illness, but a general name for more than 20 different diseases of the heart and its vessels.[2] *Arteriosclerosis* is a generic term that includes practically any arterial disease that leads to thickening and hardening of the arteries. *Atherosclerosis* is a specific form of arteriosclerosis. Its most distinctive feature is the accumulation of lipid in the inner layer *(intima)* of large elastic arteries like the aorta, and medium-sized muscular arteries like the coronary, femoral, and carotid arteries. (See Figure 10.1.)

Atherosclerosis is the underlying factor in 85 percent of all cardiovascular deaths. The atherosclerotic plaques range from small yellows streaks to advanced lesions with ulceration, *thrombosis* (formation or existence of a blood clot within the blood vessel system), hemorrhage, and calcification.

There is not yet complete agreement among researchers as to the origin of atherosclerosis. Various theories have included the "lipid theory" and the "injury theory."[3–5]

The arterial wall can be injured by a variety of factors, including high blood pressure *(hypertension)*, high blood cholesterol levels *(hypercholesterolemia)*, cigarette smoking, toxins and viruses, and blood flow turbulence disturbance.[5] Such an injury appears to cause smooth muscle cells from the *media* (middle layer of muscle in the artery wall) to migrate into the intima. This migration is enhanced by the release of chemicals and growth factors from blood platelets and white blood cells that adhere to the injured site.[5] These smooth muscle cells and monocytes accumulate cholesterol (primarily from low-density lipoproteins), and make collagen, elastic fibers, and carbohydrate-containing proteins, all of which lead to the formation of an atherosclerotic plaque.[4]

Table 10.1   Estimated Total Deaths and Percent of Total Deaths for the Ten Leading Causes of Death: United States, 1987

Rank	Cause of Death	Number	Percent
1	Heart diseases	759,400	35.7
	Coronary heart disease	511,700	24.1
	Other heart disease	247,700	11.6
2	Cancers	476,700	22.4
3	Strokes	148,700	7.0
4	Unintentional injuries	92,500	4.4
5	Chronic obstructive lung diseases	78,000	3.7
6	Pneumonia and influenza	68,600	3.2
7	Diabetes mellitus	37,800	1.8
8	Suicide	29,600	1.4
9	Chronic liver disease and cirrhosis	26,000	1.2
10	Atherosclerosis	23,100	1.1

Source; National Center for Health Statistics, Monthly Vital Statistics Report, vol. 37, no. 1, April 25, 1988.

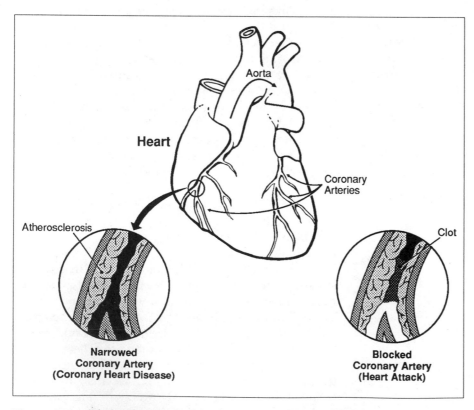

Figure 10.1 Atherosclerosis can form in the coronary arteries of the heart, resulting in a progressive narrowing of the lumen. If a clot forms, blood flow through the coronary artery can be blocked, resulting in a heart attack.

This entire process can begin in infancy, with clinical manifestations in early adulthood. The end result of the atherosclerotic process is a progressive narrowing of the blood vessel *lumen* (opening).

Coronary Heart Disease

Coronary heart disease (CHD) (also referred to as *coronary artery disease* (CAD)) is the major form of heart disease.[2] Nearly one of every three deaths is the result of CHD, making it the single leading cause of death in the United States.

The heart muscle, like every other organ of the body, needs its own blood supply. The heart is not nourished by the blood that is being pumped to the lungs and body. The heart's blood is supplied through the *coronary arteries* (three major branches). The narrowing, hardening, and blocking of these arteries by atherosclerosis leads to CHD. A blood clot may form in a narrowed coronary artery and block the flow of blood to the part of the heart muscle supplied by that artery. This is referred to as a *myocardial infarction* or *heart attack*. (See Figure 10.1.)

When part of the heart muscle does not get enough blood (oxygen and nutrients), it begins to die. When CHD closes the coronary artery by about two-thirds, it causes chest pain called *angina pectoris*, which usually occurs during emotional excitement or physical exertion. (The treadmill EKG test for victims of angina pectoris can cause a depression of the ST segment.) (See Chapter 4.)

The first indications of a heart attack may be any of several warning signals, including those listed in Box 10.1.

Stroke

Stroke is a form of cardiovascular disease that affects the blood vessels that supply oxygen and nutrients to the brain.[2] The blood flow of most stroke victims is blocked from atherosclerosis and/or a clot that forms inside the cerebral artery (*cerebral thrombosis*). Stroke can also be caused by a wandering clot (*embolus*) that breaks loose from another atherosclerotic site elsewhere in the body. A *hemorrhage* can also cause stroke when a defective artery in the brain bursts, often from an *aneurysm* (arterial weak point that balloons).

Important risk factors for stroke include high blood pressure, gender, family history, abdominal obesity, and race.[2, 6] Warning signals of stroke include unexplained dizziness, sudden temporary weakness or numbness on one side of the face, arm, leg, or body generally, temporary loss of speech, and/or temporary dimness or loss of vision in one eye.[2]

Hypertension

As discussed in Chapter 4, blood pressure is the force of blood against the walls of the arteries and veins, created by the heart as it pumps to every part of the body. High blood pressure or *hypertension* is a condition in which the blood pressure is chronically elevated above optimal levels.

The diagnosis of adult hypertension is confirmed when the average of two or more diastolic measurements on at least two subsequent visits is 90 mm Hg or higher, or when the average of multiple systolic measurements on two or more subsequent visits is consistently greater than 140 mm Hg. (See Chapter 4.)

An estimated 60 million Americans over the age of six have high blood pressure (systolic BP $\geq$140 mm Hg and/or diastolic BP $\geq$90 mm Hg).[7] For adults, 33 percent of white males, 38 percent of black males, 25 percent of white females, and 39 percent of black females have high blood pressure. In 90 percent of the cases, high blood pressure has no identifiable specific cause. Contributing factors include age, race, heredity, sex, obe-

---

Box 10.1 Warning Signals of a Heart Attack

- An uncomfortable pressure, fullness, squeezing or pain in the center of the chest behind the breastbone.

- The sensation may spread to the shoulders, neck, or arms. If it lasts for two minutes or more, it may be a heart attack.

- There may also be severe pain, dizziness, fainting, sweating, nausea, or shortness of breath, but not always.

Note: If any of these signals are experienced, seek help immediately, or go as quickly as possible to an emergency room. Each year 300,000 Americans die from heart attack before reaching the hospital. *Source:* 1989 Heart Facts, The American Heart Association.

sity, sodium sensitivity, alcohol consumption, use of oral contraceptives, and lack of exercise.

High blood pressure adds to the workload of the heart and arteries, and contributes to heart failure and atherosclerosis. When the heart is forced to work harder than normal for a long period of time, it tends to enlarge. A heart that is very much enlarged has a difficult time keeping up with the demands on it. Arteries and arterioles eventually become hardened, less elastic, and scarred. A person may have high blood pressure for years and never know it because usually there are no symptoms.[2]

Trends and Statistics

Table 10.2 gives the American Heart Association's estimated statistics for heart disease.[2] Heart disease is the leading killer of Americans, and ranks second behind unintentional injuries and ahead of a cancer in years of potential life lost prior to age 65.[2, 8]

From 1920–1950, there was a sharp rise in deaths from heart disease, primarily from acute myocardial infarction among men.[9] The causes are unknown, but during this time Americans moved off farms into cities, began driving cars, and increased their consumption of saturated fats and cigarettes. In 1953, awareness of the growing epidemic grew with the publication of a study of American soldiers killed in action in Korea.[10] Of 300 autopsies on soldiers, whose average age was 22 years old, 77.3 percent of the hearts showed some gross evidence of coronary arteriosclerosis. Of all cases, 12.3 percent had plagues causing luminal narrowing of over 50 percent.

Since the mid-1960s, the trend has reversed—the sharp rise of the earlier period has been reversed by an equally sharp fall in deaths from coronary disease.[11–16] From 1964 to 1985, CHD death rates dropped by more than 42 percent, resulting in 350,000 fewer deaths.[11] This fall, impressive for white men and even steeper for women and blacks, began in California and spread east.[9, 15] The lowest mortality now is in the Rocky Mountain states and the highest in the southeastern states. Death rates for CHD have also fallen in Canada, Australia, New Zealand, and Finland, whereas Eastern Europe and the Soviet Union have seen marked upturns.[16]

The death rate attributable to stroke has been declining for more than 50 years in the United States.[17] Between 1973 and 1985 alone, stroke death rates fell 50 percent. (See Figure 10.2.) Increasing control of hypertension (through lifestyle adjustments and modification) is probably the major cause. In the 1960s, only about 15–20 percent of hypertensive patients had their blood pressures under control, compared with 50–70 percent in the 1980s.[17] Figure 10.2 summarizes the dramatic decreases in stroke and coronary heart disease between 1973 and 1985.

Much has been written regarding the causes of this dramatic turnaround.[9, 18–23] Dr. Goldman of Harvard has calculated that approximately 60 percent of the decline in CHD is related to changes in lifestyle, specifically to reductions in serum cholesterol levels and ciga-

Table 10.2 American Heart Association Statistics On Heart Disease

Prevalence	65,980,000	Cardiovascular disease
	60,130,000	Hypertension (adults)
	4,940,000	Coronary heart disease
	2,180,000	Rheumatic disease
	2,020,000	Stroke
Cardiovascular Disease Deaths	978,500	1986 (47% of all deaths) 20% are under age 65.
Heart Attack Deaths	524,100	1986 (#1 cause of death)
	4,940,000	Alive today have history of heart attack or angina pectoris.
	300,000	Per year die before reaching hospital
	1,500,000	Projected heart attacks in 1989. 36% will die.
Stroke	147,800	1986 (2,020,000 victims alive today)
CAB Surgery	284,000	Coronary bypass operations, 1986.

Source: 1989 Heart Facts, American Heart Association.

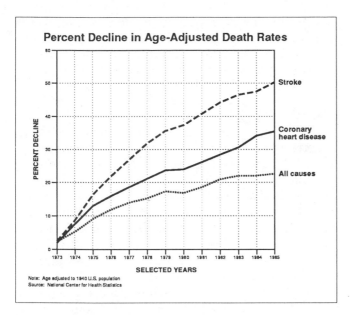

Figure 10.2 Since 1973, death rates for coronary heart disease and stroke fell 3 and 4 percent per year, respectively. *Source:* see reference 14.

Table 10.3 Improvement in American Diet (ages 19–50), 1977–1985

Food group	Comparison of Food Intake Between 1977 and 1985	
	Males	Females
beef	–35%	–45%
pork	– 7%	–22%
whole milk	–25%	–35%
eggs	–26%	–28%
fish	+50%	+18%
low-fat milk	+53%	+60%

Source: See references 24 and 25.

rette smoking.[21] In comparison, about 40 percent of the decline can be directly attributed to specific medical interventions (e.g., coronary care units, medical treatment of hypertension and heart disease).

The Intersociety Commission for Heart Disease Resources has noted many of the coincident changes in lifestyle, including a decrease in per capita consumption of milk, butter, eggs, and animal fats, and a decrease in cigarette smoking.[19] In one study using dietary information and coronary heart disease mortality data between 1909 and 1980, dietary substitutions towards less saturated fatty acids were found to be associated with less CHD.[24]

The lifestyle changes preceded the reductions in CHD mortality rates by 10 to 20 years. Decreases in egg, dairy product, whole-milk, and butter consumption began around 1950. These trends have continued, as shown by a comparison of 1977 and 1985 intake data (the latter from the 1985 Nationwide Food Consumption Survey.[25] See Table 10.3.)

Risk Factors for Heart Disease

Extensive clinical and statistical studies have identified several risk factors for heart attack and stroke.[2,26] These are outlined in Box 10.2. (Though associated with heart disease, they are not necessarily causal.)

Box 10.2   Risk Factors of Heart Disease

- male sex
- family history of premature CHD (definite myocardial infarction or sudden death before age 55 of a parent or sibling)
- cigarette smoking (currently smokes more than 10 cigarettes per day)
- hypertension (systolic BP >140 mm Hg and/or diastolic BP >90 mm Hg)
- high total cholesterol (≥240 mg/dl) and/or low density lipoprotein cholesterol (LDL-C) (≥160 mg/dl)
- low HDL-C (<35 mg/dl confirmed by repeated measurements)
- history of definite stroke or occlusive peripheral vascular disease
- severe obesity (≥30% overweight)

Source: National Cholesterol Education Program. See reference 26.

The risk factors listed in Box 10.2 do not explain all heart disease, but do appear to account for the majority of cardiovascular disease in this country.[19] Many other factors are probably important, but not enough is known to include them at this time. For example, blue collar workers and people with less education have higher CHD death rates than white collar workers and those with more education .[27, 28] Also, those with poor social relationships have been found to be at increased risk for cardiovascular disease.[29]

In Chapter 13, the relationship of Type A Behavior and stress to cardiovascular disease will be reviewed. In general, although Type A Behavior has not consistently been found to predict increased risk of CHD, high stress levels do appear to be an important risk factor.[27-35] For example, people who have occupations involving low decision latitude and high psychological work load have increased serum cholesterol and systolic blood pressure levels and increased death rates from CHD.[34, 35]

People with a family history of premature CHD are at a risk two to five times that of those with no family CHD history, particularly if first-degree relatives are involved.[19,36-39] One study in Utah showed that one-half of all heart attacks before age 55 among men and before age 60 among women are clustered in only 5 percent of families.[36]

The role of genetic factors in atherosclerosis is difficult to evaluate precisely, however, because various coronary risk factors tend to cluster within families.[19] For example, in one study of women who had died before age 55 with CHD, 62 percent had first-degree relatives with early coronary disease compared with 12 percent of women who did not die before age 55 with CHD.[38] However, smoking, hypertension, hyperlipidemia, and diabetes were all two to three times more common among the women who had died from CHD.

The danger of heart attack increases with the number of risk factors. Often people who are stricken with heart disease have several risk factors, each of which is only marginally abnormal. One researcher has concluded that a combined lowering of Americans' average serum cholesterol from 210 mg/dl to 190 mg/dl, and diastolic blood pressure to an average of 80 mm Hg, would reduce cardiovascular disease deaths by 70 percent.[20] A similar type of estimate predicted that if Americans ate the American Heart Association diet, had a serum cholesterol of 200 mg/dl (rather than 240 mg/dl), a systolic blood pressure of 120 mm Hg (rather than 140 mm Hg), and did not smoke, they would add 11.8 years to their life expectancy due to decreased CHD deaths.[23]

It has long been agreed that clotting factors are important in the development of atherosclerosis. High levels of fibrinogen (a globulin in the blood association with blood clotting) correlated positively in the Framingham Study with risk of cardiovascular disease.[42] The impact of fibrinogen value on risk of cardiovascular disease was comparable to that of the major risk factors, such as blood pressure, cigarette smoking, and diabetes.

Table 10.4 shows the effect of age, race, and gender on death rates for coronary heart disease.[11] Nothing can be done about any of these. On the other hand, age may be less important than lifestyle, which of course can be altered.[43] The decline in CHD death rates has occurred at all ages during a period when the percentage of the population over 65 has increased dramatically.

Cigarette Smoking

Cigarette smoking is the most important of the known modifiable risk factors for CHD in the United States.[44] A brief background of this major health problem points up its importance.[44-55]

Trends and Background Information

Deaths from cigarette smoking in the U.S. are estimated to exceed 350,000 annually.[45] An additional 10 million Americans suffer increased rates of various debilitating and chronic diseases caused by smoking, including bronchitis, emphysema, peptic ulcer disease, and arte-

---

Table 10.4 Death Rate for Coronary Heart Disease by Age, Race, and Gender, United States, 1985. Death Rate per 100,000 Population

Age (years)	White Men	Black Men	White Women	Black Women
Under 45	8.2	13.2	1.7	4.3
45-64	294.5	317.8	85.1	161.1
65-74	1,132.6	990.6	506.0	645.9
75 and over	3,071.8	2,205.0	2,010.2	1,717.5

Source: National Center for Health Statistics. See reference 11.

riosclerosis. Tobacco contributes to 30 percent of all cancer deaths yearly, including 85 percent of all lung cancer deaths. Those who smoke two or more packs a day have lung cancer mortality rates 15–25 times greater than nonsmokers.

Using national data, the National Cancer Institute has determined that as many as one-third of heavy smokers (more than 25 cigarettes per day) age 35 will die before age 85 of diseases caused by their smoking.[52] Cigarette smoking causes more premature deaths than the combined total from acquired immunodeficiency syndrome, cocaine, heroin, alcohol, fire, automobile accidents, homicide, and suicide. A tobacco-free society would add 15 years to the lives of the 350,000 people who are victims of tobacco-related deaths.[53]

Evidence also is mounting for the adverse health effects of *passive smoking*.[45, 56–60] New studies strongly indicate an increased risk for cancer, and heart disease, and exacerbation of respiratory disorders from passive smoking. The 1986 Surgeon General's Report on the health consequences of involuntary smoking drew three major conclusions:[57] (1) Involuntary smoking is a cause of disease, including lung cancer; (2) The children of parents who smoke have an increased frequency of respiratory infections, increased respiratory symptoms,

and slightly smaller rates of increase of maturing lung function; (3) The simple separation of smokers and nonsmokers within the same air space may reduce, but does not eliminate, the exposure of nonsmokers to environmental tobacco smoke.

In 1984 alone, the economic burden to society from smoking was estimated at more than $53 billion.[45] The rate of absenteeism is approximately 50 percent higher for smokers. American businesses lose $26 billion in productivity annually because of smoking, and pay half of the $16 billion per year bill in smoking-related medical costs.

More than 37 million Americans are now former smokers. (See Figure 10.3.) Although the absolute number of smokers has remained almost constant from 1965 to 1985, the proportion of adult male smokers has declined from 52 percent in 1965 to 33 percent in 1985— and that for female smokers, from 34 percent to 28 percent.[45]

If present trends continue, in the year 2000, 22 percent, or 40 million of the adult population (20 percent men, 23 percent women) will be smokers.[46] (See Figure 10.4.) The smoking rates for adult males have consistently exceeded those for adult females. However, the percentage of smokers among high school

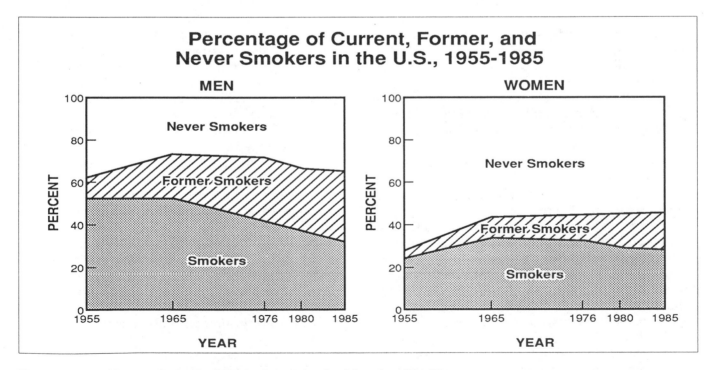

Figure 10.3 Smokers are increasingly becoming a minority. More than 37 million Americans are former smokers. *Source:* Office on Smoking and Health, U.S. Public Health Service, 1985.

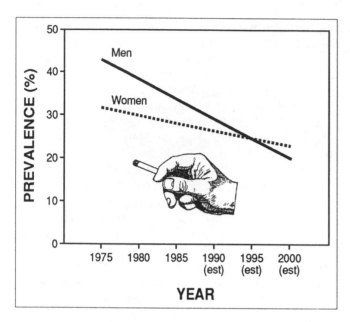

Figure 10.4 If present trends continue, a greater percentage of women than men will be smoking in the year 2000. *Source:* see reference 46.

senior girls is now greater than the percentage of boy smokers (20.5 percent vs. 16 percent). The proportion of black smokers tends to be higher than that of whites or Hispanics (37 percent vs. 32 percent vs. 26 percent, respectively). Annual per-capita consumption of cigarettes for adults increased steadily from 3597 in 1955 to a peak of 4345 in 1963, and then decreased to 3411 by 1984, the lowest since 1944.

The proportion of heavy smokers is of concern. Although aggregate per capita consumption of cigarettes has declined, among smokers, both male and female, a greater percentage of those who smoke are heavy smokers.[45] In 1965, 24 percent of male smokers consumed 25 or more cigarettes per day, compared with 31 percent in 1985; for females, the figures went from 13 percent to 23 percent.

Beyond high school, evidence suggests that the higher the level of education, the lower the likelihood of smoking. In general, smoking is inversely correlated to income level, with a substantially greater percentage of blue collar smokers than white collar smokers.[45] Data indicate that the younger the age of initiation, the greater the likelihood of smoking heavily later in life.

Two types of *smokeless tobacco*—snuff and chewing tobacco—are in current use.[61, 62] Snuff is a cured, finely ground tobacco that either can be taken nasally or, more commonly today, placed in small quantities between cheek and gum. Chewing tobacco comes in several forms, including loose-leaf, plug, and twist, all of which can be chewed directly and then spit out.

Surveys indicate that smokeless tobacco production has increased recently. A recent National Institutes of Health Consensus Conference on the health implications of smokeless tobacco use estimated that at least 12 million people over the age of 12 years in the U.S. used smokeless tobacco in 1985.[45]

The resurgence in popularity of smokeless tobacco can be linked to advertising campaigns by tobacco companies to promote users as "macho." Snuff and chewing tobacco are associated with a variety of serious adverse effects, especially oral cancer.[62] Smokeless tobacco may also affect reproduction, longevity, the cardiovascular system, and oral health (producing bad breath, abrasion of teeth, gum recession, periodontal bone loss, and tooth loss).

The declines in smoking since 1964 are beginning to be reflected in lower mortality rates for the leading smoking-related killers. Approximately one-fourth of the amazing decline in coronary heart disease mortality can be attributed to the reduction in cigarette smoking. Although the total number of lung cancer deaths in the United States increased from 18,313 in 1950 to an estimated 130,000 in 1986, recent statistics show a 4 percent drop from 1982 to 1983 in lung cancer incidence among white men (though this decreased incidence is not yet fully reflected in the death rate). In contrast, the death rate for lung cancer among women rose dramatically between 1960 and 1983, with a 6.2 percent average annual increase, and it now tops breast cancer as the leading cancer killer among women.[45]

Efforts to reduce tobacco consumption in the United States include public information/legislation (Public Law 89–92 for warning labels), community-based, worksite-based, physician, and school-based interventions, and taxation.[45, 63–65] A 1985 survey indicated that 92 percent of Americans understood that smoking increases the risk of emphysema, and 95 percent understood this about lung cancer, 80 percent about low birth weight, and 80 percent about cancer of the esophagus. In a recent national survey of worksite-based health promotion activities, roughly 27 percent of employers reported they had a smoking policy. A 1985 survey of major insurance providers found that 63 percent offered nonsmoking premium discounts on individual life insurance, and 25 percent provided nonsmoking premium discounts on both individual life and individual health insurance.[45]

The most significant trend in smoking cessation is an increasingly negative attitude toward cigarette smoking, as exemplified by the numerous ordinances and regulations that separate smokers and nonsmokers in restaurants, airplanes, schools, worksites, and other public places.[63] By 1985, sixteen states had legislation restricting smoking in government controlled offices, and at least ten states had laws requiring that companies with 50 or more employees establish policies about smoking in the workplace.[45] More than 35 states have passed some type of legislation to safeguard the rights of nonsmokers.

There is a shift in emphasis away from "smoking except where prohibited," to "no smoking except where allowed." Eighteen states now require elementary and secondary schools to include instruction on the dangers of tobacco use. The use of peer counselors in schools has proven effective in discouraging students from smoking.

Over 70 percent of patients, according to one Gallup poll, reported they would quit smoking cigarettes if their physician urged them to do so.[45] Yet only 25–30 percent of current smokers report receiving physician advice to quit. One analysis suggests that a third of a million Americans would quit smoking if the Federal excise tax were doubled.

Self-help in quitting smoking with no professional supervision shows a respectable 18 percent quit rate after one year.[63] When physicians provide more than advice or counseling to patients, one year quit rates rise from 6 percent to 22.5 percent. Physician intervention with cardiac patients results in one year quit rates of 43 percent. Using nicotine chewing gum to quit smoking produces a one-year quit rate of 11 percent, but this increases to 29 percent when using nicotine gum is combined with other treatments.

Nicotine is a powerfully addictive drug, six to eight times more addictive than alcohol.[66, 67] The 1988 Surgeon General's Report on the health consequences of smoking emphasized the addiction factor.[66] The three primary criteria for *drug dependence* are: highly controlled or compulsive use, psychoactive effects, and drug-reinforced behavior. The nicotine in cigarettes and other forms of tobacco meets these criteria.

The pharmacologic and behavioral processes that reinforce tobacco addiction are similar to those that reinforce addiction to drugs like heroin and cocaine. In one study of 1,000 people seeking treatment for alcohol or drug dependence, 57 percent said that cigarettes would be harder to quit using than their problem substance.[67] Cigarettes, however, were generally rated as less pleasurable than alcohol or drugs.

In spite of the progress to date, more than 50 million Americans still smoke. More effective incentives for quitting are needed.

Relationship to Exercise

The relationship between exercise and smoking is a complex one.[68–77] Many studies have shown that smoking before exercise decreases performance.[68, 69] In one study of eight adults who were smokers, smoking just two filter cigarettes led to elevated heart rates, and a decrease in $\dot{V}O_{2max}$ and breathing efficiency during graded exercise testing.[68]

Very few active people smoke. In the author's study of 2,300 Los Angeles marathon runners, only three percent were smokers. Dr. Koplan from the Centers for Disease Control reported that 81 percent of men and 75 percent of women runners who had smoked cigarettes had stopped smoking after beginning regular recreational running.[71] Framingham study data associated increased physical activity with fewer cigarettes smoked per day.[77] Some evidence suggests that craving for cigarettes is reduced during physical activity.[70]

However, other research data have not shown that people voluntarily increasing their physical fitness level are more likely than nonexercisers to reduce smoking.[73] More study is needed to determine the role of physical activity in reducing the desire to smoke cigarettes.[72]

Weight gain is a likely outcome of smoking cessation, and is often reported as a strong disincentive. Several epidemiological studies indicate that smokers weigh less than nonsmokers but eat more.[74–76] Figure 10.5 shows the results of a study of 13 sedentary female smokers.[74] They gained 2.2 kilograms of body weight (nearly five pounds) after 48 days of smoking cessation. Caloric intake increased by an average of 227 Calories a day. Of the three able to stop smoking for 413 days, weight gain averaged 8.2 kilograms (18 pounds). The ten returning to smoking returned to their starting weight.

One study of males has suggested that on the average a man who gives up smoking can expect to gain 2.3 kg, or to lose one kilogram after starting smoking.[76]

Research has shown that smoking 24 cigarettes a day increases 24-hour energy expenditure by 215 Calories or nearly 10 percent.[75] People who quit smoking should plan on both a reduction in caloric intake and an increase in physical activity.[76]

Hypertension

In most Western societies, average blood pressure increases with age. Figure 10.6 shows that in the United States, hypertension is twice as prevalent among the elderly as it is among the 35–44 age group.[13, 78] In a few societies (primitive tribal communities) there is little rise in blood pressure with age.[79, 80]

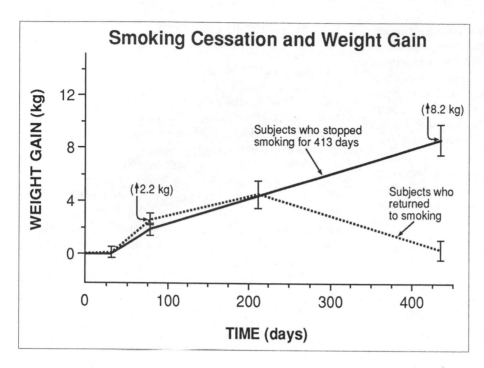

Figure 10.5 Mean weight gain for those who successfully quit smoking for 413 days and for those who returned to smoking. *Source:* see reference 74.

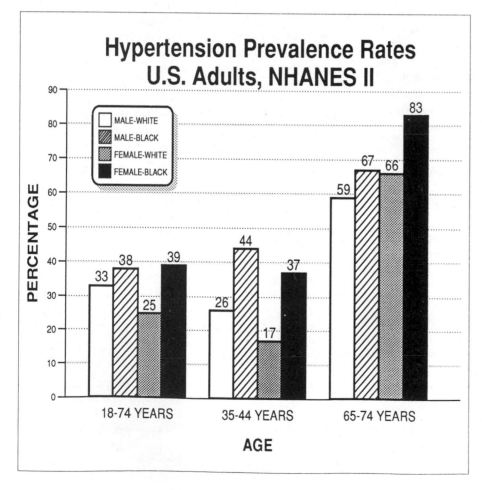

Figure 10.6 Hypertension is prevalent in 64 percent of the elderly (76 percent of blacks, 63 percent of whites). *Source:* National Health and Nutrition Examination II (1976–1980). See reference 13.

There is growing awareness by the American public of the importance of keeping blood pressure under control. The 1985 National Health Interview Survey showed that 92 percent of the public thought that high blood pressure was related to coronary heart disease, and 78 percent related high blood pressure to stroke. In addition, 73 percent of the population had had their blood pressure taken by a physician within the past year.[13]

Most hypertension experts now recommend that lifestyle measures (in particular, weight reduction and sodium and alcohol restriction) should be used both to prevent and to treat high blood pressure.[78, 81–90] If lifestyle measures fail to reduce blood pressure significantly, then drug therapy can be tried (if medically advisable).

There are several reasons for reserving drug therapy as a measure of last resort.[78, 81, 82, 89] There are potential from side effects of drugs, as well as possible unforeseen long-term adverse effects. For instance, there has been much speculation that the potentially adverse effects of diuretics in inducing low blood potassium and magnesium levels, cardiac arrhythmias, high LDL-C levels, or impaired glucose tolerance may actually offset their beneficial lowering of blood-pressure.

The problem of patient compliance, and the expense of therapy and its medical supervision are additional considerations.[82] More than 10 million hypertensive patients are currently receiving antihypertensive medications, at an estimated cost of approximately $2.5 billion, figures that exceed those for any other single disease.[83]

The 1988 Joint National Committee on Detection, Evaluation and Treatment of High Blood Pressure advocates a treatment strategy utilizing non-drug approaches as a first line of defense, backed up by a *step-care therapy* approach utilizing various drugs.[85] (See Figure 10.7.) [However, it is generally agreed that markedly elevated initial blood pressure readings (diastolic blood pressure 115 mm Hg or greater) may require immediate drug therapy.]

Nonpharmacologic Treatment Measures

Recent evidence suggests that various lifestyle-change measures, particularly weight reduction, salt restriction, and moderation of alcohol consumption, may lower elevated pressure and improve the efficacy of pharmacologic agents, if needed.[85] Such nonpharmacologic approaches are urged for both the prevention and treatment of high blood pressure; even when drugs are appropriate, lifestyle measures should continue.

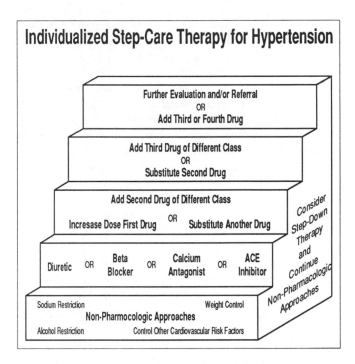

Figure 10.7 Non-pharmacologic approaches are recommended in the first instance for most hypertensives, with a step-care drug therapy approach for those who do not respond appropriately. *Source:* 1988 Report of the Joint National Committee on Detection, Evaluation, and Treatment of High Blood Pressure. See reference 85.

Based on currently available evidence, a practical lifestyle prescription for the reduction of high blood pressure includes the following:[85, 91]

- For the overweight, weight reduction should be the primary goal. Physical activity and Calorie restriction are both helpful. Physical activity has a moderate independent effect.

- For all hypertensives, dietary sodium should be restricted to a 2,000 mg level. All Americans are urged to consume no more than 3,300 mg a day.

- Alcohol intake should be less than two ounces per day. One standard alcoholic drink has 0.5 ounces of alcohol.

- Supplemental magnesium and calcium should only be given to those who are deficient.

- More fiber and less saturated fat may help lower blood pressure and are beneficial for lowering overall cardiovascular disease risk.

Weight Reduction

Weight reduction for hypertensives who are over their ideal weight can be a powerful means of reducing blood pressure.[11, 85, 90–96] Obesity is the environmental factor most often identified as contributing to hypertension.[96–99] There is a strong correlation between body weight and blood pressure and between increases in body weight and increases in blood pressure, particularly among children and young to middle-aged adults. Weight reduction by caloric restriction often results in a substantial decrease in blood pressure, even if ideal body weight is not achieved. (See Chapter 11 for a review of the association between obesity and cardiovascular disease).

One study showed that the majority of mildly overweight hypertensives who lost moderate amounts of body weight could control their blood pressure without medication.[98] Hypertensives who had been on blood pressure medication for five years (subjects of the Hypertension Detection and Follow-up Program) were taken off their drugs, and then randomly assigned to either a weight-loss group, sodium-restriction group, or control group. After 56 weeks, the weight-loss group (with an average weight loss of 10 pounds) was 3.43 times as successful in staying normotensive as the control group was. Most successful were the overweight, mild hypertensives who reduced their weight and the nonoverweight, mild hypertensives who restricted their sodium to 2.3 g of salt per day. (See Figure 10.8.)

Dietary Measures

Sodium is essential for a wide variety of functions in the body. Although needs vary from person to person, a minimum of 200 mg sodium per day is considered necessary for adults to maintain physiological balance.[39] (One teaspoon of salt = 2,000 mg sodium = 5 g salt (NaCl) = 85.5 mmol sodium). The Food and Nutrition Board, National Academy of Sciences, National Research Council considers 1100 to 3300 mg sodium (2.8–8.4 g salt) as a "safe and adequate" daily dietary intake for healthy adults. The average American ingests 4,000–6,000 mg sodium a day.[11]

In recent years, the American public has been encouraged to reduce sodium intake to help prevent hypertension.[11] Although this recommendation is considered controversial, most studies support the concept that high sodium intakes are associated with increased risk of high blood pressure.[11, 85, 90, 91, 100, 101] Hypertensives or those at risk for hypertension (which includes blacks, the elderly, and those with a family history of hypertension) are especially urged to limit sodium intake to 2,000 mg per day.[85, 90]

Potassium appears to help reduce blood pressure by increasing the amount of sodium excreted in the urine.[102] The *sodium to potassium ratio* (Na:K) has been explored as a potentially useful indicator of hypertension risk.[102, 103] The average Na:K ratio in the United States is 1.2–1.4, but 0.60 is recommended. To achieve such a ratio, the diet should contain more potassium and less sodium. Table 10.5 contrasts the sodium and potassium levels for various food groups.

There have been many studies looking at the relationship of *calcium* to blood pressure.[104–109] During the 1970s, some researchers found that the risk of heart disease was lower in areas with "hard" water (usually high in calcium).[109] Some researchers thought that perhaps the calcium in the hard water was lowering the blood pressure of people who drank it, reducing the risk of heart disease.

During the 1980s, some studies found that calcium was associated with lower blood pressure, but some did not.[104–108] Much more research is needed to settle this issue. For now, consuming at least the recommended dietary allowance (RDA) for calcium (800 mg), mainly through low-fat dairy products, seeds and nuts, leafy green vegetables, and dried fruit, is a good idea.

Alcohol

Epidemiologic studies have shown that people who regularly consume large amounts of alcohol (three or more drinks a day) have higher blood pressure than people who abstain or who drink only moderate amounts.[11, 110–115] Among heavy drinkers, the prevalence of high blood pressure is four times greater than for those who abstain.

In 1985 an estimated 10.6 million Americans were *alcohol dependent,* and 7.3 million more experienced some negative consequence of alcohol abuse such as arrest, accident, or impairment of health or job performance.[111, 116, 117] Alcohol-related problems include symptoms of alcohol dependence such as memory loss, inability to stop drinking until intoxicated, inability to cut down on drinking, binge drinking, and withdrawal symptoms.

The estimated per capita consumption of alcohol in the United States was 2.65 gallons in 1984. (See Figure 10.9.) Two-thirds of the adult U.S. population drink; however, the 10 percent of these who drink most heavily drink half of the total amount. In 1985, nearly five percent of high school seniors drank every day, down from seven percent in 1979.[111]

Heavy drinking has been consistently associated with increased risk of death from heart disease.[19, 111, 118] Ultrastructural changes in the heart tissue occur with chronic exposure to ethanol, with an associated increase in sudden death from abnormal heart arrhythmias.

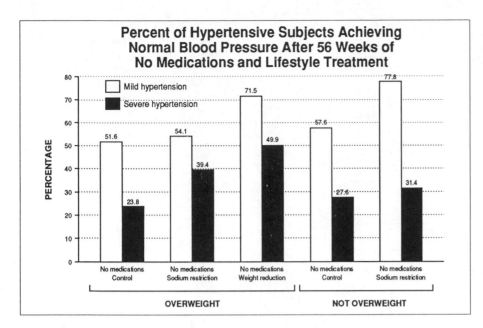

Percent of Hypertensive Subjects Achieving Normal Blood Pressure After 56 Weeks of No Medications and Lifestyle Treatment

Figure 10.8 Nearly three-fourths of overweight mild hypertensives and half of severe hypertensives who lost weight during a 56-week study were able to achieve normal blood pressure levels without medication. *Source:* see reference 98.

Ethanol use alters lipoprotein metabolism and blood lipid profiles, increasing high density lipoprotein cholesterol (HDL-C) and very low density lipoprotein (VLDL-C).[19, 119–122] HDL-C is inversely related to coronary heart disease, and some researchers feel that alcohol may reduce heart disease risk through its effects on HDL-C.[11]

The effect of alcohol on HDL-C depends on the amount consumed. Moderate daily consumption of ethanol has been found to increase HDL$_2$-C (the more protective HDL subfraction), whereas heavy alcohol consumption increases HDL$_3$-C (considered nonprotective against heart disease).[121] Alcohol consumption, however, is not as effective as aerobic exercise in elevating HDL-C.[122]

Evidence that moderate drinking has a protective effect against coronary heart disease is controversial.[111] Several studies have suggested that moderate alcohol

Table 10.5   Sodium and Potassium Levels for Various Food Groups

Low Sodium, High Potassium Foods

Fruits and Fruit Juices	Pineapple, grapefruit, pears, strawberries, watermelon, raisins, bananas, apricots, oranges, etc.
Low Sodium Cereals	Oatmeal (unsalted), Roman meal hot cereal, Shredded Wheat, etc
Nuts (Unsalted)	Hazel nuts, Macadamia, almonds, peanuts, cashews, coconut, etc.
Vegetables	Summer squash, zucchini, eggplant, cucumber, onions, lettuce, green beans, broccoli, etc.
Beans (Dry, Cooked)	Great North, lentils, lima beans, red kidney beans, etc.

High Sodium, Low Potassium Foods

Fats	Butter, margarine, salad dressings.
Soups	Onion soup, mushroom soup, chicken noodle soup, tomato soup, split pea soup, etc.
Breakfast Cereals	Corn flakes, Product 19, Wheaties, Total, Nutri-Grain, etc.
Breads	All varieties except for low sodium brands.
Processed Meats	Bacon, canned meats, sausages, etc.
Cheeses	Nearly all varieties except when specifically labeled as low sodium.

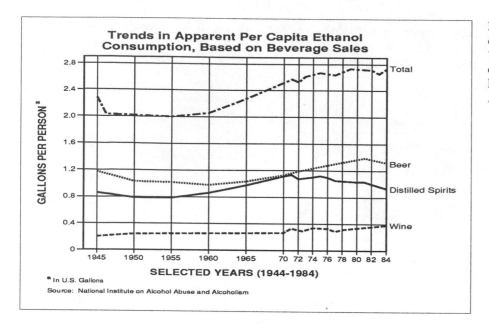

Figure 10.9 Per capita alcohol consumption rose strongly during the 1960s and 1970s, finally plateauing during the 1980s. *Source:* National Institute on Alcohol Abuse and Alcoholism. See reference 111.

consumption is associated with low death rates from cardiovascular disease,[11, 111, 123–126] but others do not support this contention.[127–130]

Even if moderate drinking were shown conclusively to reduce the risk of heart disease, recommendations to increase alcohol consumption would be ill-advised because of overriding considerations regarding other health concerns.[11, 111, 131–136] Nonsmokers who consume between one and three drinks each day have a 60 percent higher risk of oral cancer than nondrinkers. Among those who smoke between 20–39 cigarettes each day, those who consume between one and three drinks each day have triple the risk of oral cancer of nondrinkers who smoke the same amount.

Drinking less than one drink each day doubles the risk for hemorrhagic stroke, compared with not drinking at all.[130] One to three drinks per week increases the risk of breast cancer for women.[133–136] Excessive alcohol drinking is associated with increased risk of colorectal cancer.[132]

There are too many problems associated with drinking in our society to even think of recommending this approach for heart disease reduction. The cure would be far worse than the disease.

Role of Exercise

When a person walks briskly, cycles, jogs, or swims, it is generally agreed that systolic blood pressure and heart rate will increase, while diastolic blood pressure changes little. Following exercise, the blood pressure of hypertensive men will fall below pre-exercise values.[139, 140] One study showed that after a single, 10-minute bout of treadmill exercise, blood pressures of hypertensives fell below pre-exercise values (normotensives tend to be more resistant to postexercise hypotension). After five such 10-minute bouts (with 3 minutes between bouts for measurements), blood pressures were depressed for over 90 minutes.[139]

Two major epidemiological studies have now been conducted, researching the effects of fitness and habitual activity on the development of hypertension.[141, 142] Dr. Ralph Paffenbarger of Stanford University followed 15,000 Harvard male alumni for six to ten years (from the time they entered Harvard).[141] During the study period, 681 of the men developed severe hypertension (160/95 mm Hg). Alumni who did not engage in vigorous sports or other activity were at a 35-percent greater risk of hypertension than those who did.

The physical fitness status of 4,820 men and 1,219 women aged 20–65 years was assessed by maximal treadmill testing.[142] Participants had normal blood pressures at the start of the study, and were followed for an average of four years. After adjustment for important factors, the participants with low levels of physical fitness had a 52-percent greater risk of developing hypertension than the highly fit participants did.

Elevated blood pressures during graded exercise testing of people with normal blood pressures at rest have been found to be predictive of future problems with resting hypertension.[143, 144] (See Figure 10.10.) In one study, follow-up found a prevalence of hypertension among normotensive subjects with a hypertensive response to exercise testing 2.1 to 3.4 times higher than among those with a normotensive response.[143]

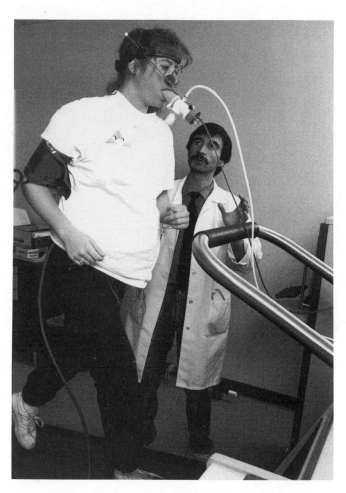

Figure 10.10 People with normal resting blood pressures who experience elevated blood pressure responses during graded exercise testing are at increased risk of developing future resting hypertension.

Several recent reviews have summarized the studies of effects of aerobic exercise training on the blood pressures of hypertensive people.[145–148] The vast majority of the studies indicate that exercise training is associated with lower diastolic pressures (ranging from 3–15 mm Hg) and lower systolic pressures (ranging from 5–25 mm Hg). Many of the studies reviewed, however, had poor designs, and more research is needed with control of various confounding factors.

In one study with an excellent design, 16 weeks of aerobic exercise by 44 hypertensives led to a mean reduction in diastolic blood pressure of 7.1 mm Hg.[149] The researchers concluded that the beneficial effect was in part mediated by an exercise-induced decrease in norepinephrine.

Exercise may decrease blood pressure through its effects on plasma catecholamines, suppressing the sympathetic nervous system. Exercise may also normalize kidney function, decrease insulin secretion (insulin tends to cause the kidney to retain sodium), and alter the sensitivity of blood vessel receptors.[147, 150–154] More study is needed to establish the mechanism behind this.

In summary, studies suggest that habitual activity and physical fitness may reduce the risk of developing hypertension (see Figure 10.11), and improve the control of high blood pressure among hypertensive people.[155]

Hypercholesterolemia

The body naturally synthesizes *cholesterol*, which is essential in the formation of bile acids (used in fat digestion). It is also an essential component of cell membranes, and is found in large amounts in the brain and nerve tissue. Cholesterol is found in all animal foods, but not in plant foods.[11] Egg yolks and organ meats such as liver and kidney are particularly rich in cholesterol.

Cholesterol and other fats such as *triglycerides* are insoluble in water (they tend to float). Cholesterol is found in every cell of the body, and has very important physiological functions. Cholesterol and other fats are transported between various tissues through the blood by particles called *lipoproteins*.

Figure 10.12 depicts average cholesterol levels for six age groups in the United States.[13] The average American male and female have serum cholesterol levels of 211 and 215 mg/dl respectively, a slight decrease from the levels of the 1960s.[156] (See Appendix B, Tables 60–62, for a complete table of serum cholesterol levels of Americans). (All Americans are urged to reduce their serum cholesterol levels to less than 200 mg/dl.)[157, 158]

Mean cholesterol levels rise with an increase in age, especially among American women. This age-related increase in serum cholesterol levels does not occur in all populations of the world. The Tarahumara Indians of Northern Mexico, for example, renown for their extraordinary physical fitness and endurance as long-distance runners, have body fat percentages 35 to 50 percent lower than those of American males, and serum cholesterol levels averaging only 136 mg/dl.[159] Hypertension, obesity, and the usual age-related rise in serum cholesterol are virtually absent among the Tarahumaras.[159]

Table 10.6 shows that approximately one-fourth of Americans have blood cholesterol levels above 240 mg/dl.[156] Based on MRFIT data, about 80 percent of middle-aged American men have cholesterol levels

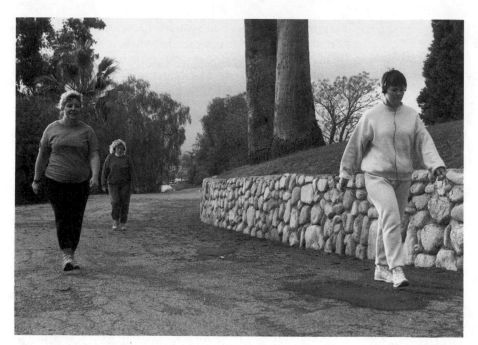

Figure 10.11 Regular exercise is associated with a lower risk of developing high blood pressure.

above 180 mg/dl, which is considered a more optimal serum cholesterol level.[23, 160]

The American public is becoming more knowledgeable about the importance of serum cholesterol levels to health. Between 1983 and 1986, the percentage of adults who believed that reducing high blood choles-

terol levels would have a substantial effect on heart disease increased from 64 to 72 percent.[161] In 1983, 35 percent of adults reported that they had had their cholesterol level checked versus 46 percent in 1986. By 1986, 23 percent of adults reported that they had made dietary changes specifically to lower their blood choles-

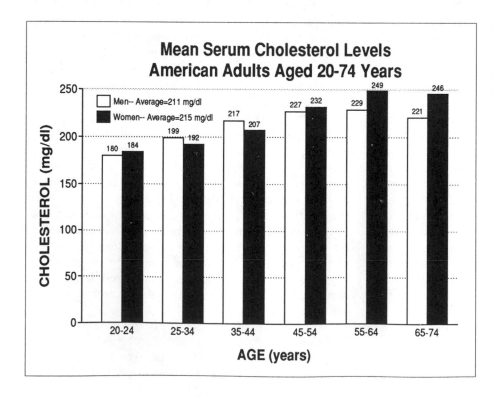

Figure 10.12 Serum cholesterol levels rise with increase in age. *Source:* National Health and Nutrition Examination Survey II (1976–1980). See reference 13.

Table 10.6   U.S. Prevalence of High Serum Cholesterol (≥240 mg/dl) by Age, Race, and Gender (Percent of each population)

Age	White Men	Black Men	White Women	Black Women
20-74	25.0	23.9	29.2	23.7
20-24	6.1	2.9	6.5	7.0
25-34	15.0	19.3	12.4	8.7
35-44	27.9	24.5	21.1	16.9
45-54	36.5	40.3	40.6	40.7
55-64	37.3	35.3	53.7	46.5
65-74	32.4	27.2	52.1	48.4

Source: National Center for Health Statistics; Fulwood R, Kalsbeck W, Rifkind B, Russell-Briefel R, Muesing R, LaRose J, Lippel K. Total Serum Cholesterol Levels of Adults 20-74 Years of Age: United States, 1976-80. Vital and Health Statistics, Ser. II, No. 236. DHHS Pub. No. (PHS) 86-1686. Public Health Service. Washington, DC; US Government Printing Office, May 1986.

terol level, up from 14 percent in 1983. In 1986, 64 percent of physicians surveyed thought that reducing high blood cholesterol levels would have a substantial effect on heart disease, up considerably from 39 percent in 1983.[162] The median range of blood cholesterol at which physicians counseled diet therapy was 240–259 mg/dl in 1986, down from 260–279 mg/dl in 1983.

Description of Lipoproteins

To transport the cholesterol and triglycerides, the body utilizes different protein packets called lipoproteins. There are three major lipoproteins in the fasting blood—*high density lipoprotein* (HDL), *low density lipoprotein* (LDL), and *very low density lipoprotein* (VLDL). Figure 10.13 outlines the protein and lipid composition of each lipoprotein.[163] HDL is the smallest and most dense lipoprotein, being nearly half protein. LDL carries the most cholesterol. VLDL is mostly triglyceride.

The protein part of the lipoprotein, which carries the lipids in the blood, is called *apoprotein*. Apoproteins are also very important in activating or inhibiting certain enzymes involved in the metabolism of fats. (They are identified by letters—HDL, for example, has several different apoproteins, the important ones being Apo A-1 and Apo A-II. LDL is high in Apo B.[163–171]

The HDL particle appears to act as a type of shuttle as it takes up cholesterol from the blood and body cells and transfers it to the liver, where it is used to form bile

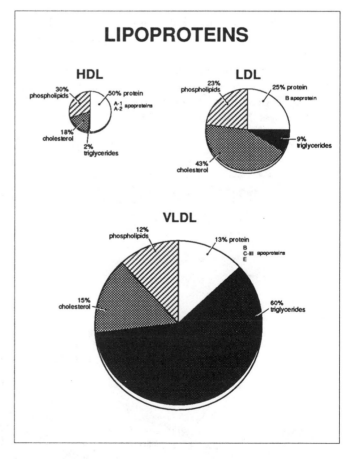

Figure 10.13   There are three different lipoproteins in fasting blood. *Source:* see reference 163.

acids.[172-174] The bile acids are involved in the digestion process, with some of them passing out with the stool, thus providing the body with a major route for excretion of cholesterol. HDLs have for this reason been called the "garbage trucks" of the blood system, collecting cholesterol and dumping it into the liver.

LDL, on the other hand, is formed after VLDL gives up its triglycerides to body cells. LDLs are very high in cholesterol, and take their cholesterol to various body cells, where it is deposited for cell functions. When excessively high, the cholesterol in the LDL contributes to the build up of atherosclerosis.[167-171] (See Figure 10.14.)

HDL cholesterol (HDL-C) concentration is thus emerging as an important measure of heart disease risk. In Framingham, Massachusetts, nearly 2,500 men and women, 49–82 years old, were observed for four years. High amounts of HDL-C were found to be associated with low heart disease risk.[172]

Table 10.7 summarizes the HDL-C levels of American adults.[174] Mean HDL-C levels are higher among women than men (8.9 mg/dl higher for whites, 4.4 mg/dl for blacks), and higher among blacks than whites. Age has little effect on HDL-C.[175-177] The National Cholesterol Education Program regards HDL-C levels below 35 mg/dl as an important risk factor. (See Box 10.2).

Because of the importance of HDL-C, the ratio of HDL-C to total cholesterol (*HDL-C/TC*) has been found to be highly predictive of heart disease.[173] CHD risk is 50 percent lower for those with HDL-C/TC ratios above

Table 10.7 HDL-Cholesterol (mg/dl) for Adults Age 20–74 Years by Gender and Race

	Mean	25th%	50th%	75th%
White Men	44.5	36.0	43.0	50.1
Black Men	51.9	40.1	49.0	59.0
White Women	53.4	44.0	51.1	61.1
Black Women	56.3	45.0	53.1	65.0

Source: The Second National Health and Nutrition Examination Survey. See reference 174.

0.30. To figure the HDL-C/TC, divide the HDL-C values by the TC value. For example, if your HDL-C is 55 mg/dl, and your TC is 180 mg/dl, then the HDL-C/TC is 55/180 or 0.31 (a good ratio). Table 10.8 summarizes the HDL-C/TC ratios of Americans.[173] Notice that females for all age groups have higher HDL-C/TC ratios, indicating lower risk of CHD. The HDL-C/TC ratio tends to decrease with age, primarily from the age-related increase in total cholesterol.

Most medical laboratories do not measure the LDL-C, but rather calculate it based on measurements of total cholesterol, HDL-C, and triglycerides. As shown in Figure 10.13, all three lipoproteins carry cholesterol. Thus the total cholesterol equals the cholesterol in the

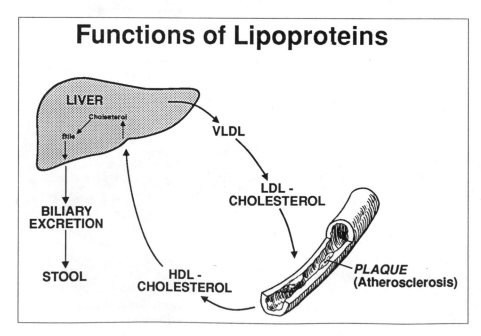

Figure 10.14 LDL and HDL have opposing functions. HDL takes cholesterol to the liver, where it is changed to bile and eventually excreted in the stool. This is the body's major method of reducing its cholesterol stores.

Table 10.8 High Density Lipoprotein Cholesterol (HDL-C) / Total Cholesterol (TC) Ratios (HDL-C/TC) of American Males and Females by Age Groups

Age		Percentile		
		10th (Poor)	50th (Average)	90th (Good)
5-19	Males	0.214–0.265	0.295–0.359	0.407–0.443
	Females	0.239–0.252	0.323–0.332	0.425–0.442
20-39	Males	0.144–0.189	0.213–0.282	0.300–0.393
	Females	0.188–0.224	0.296–0.329	0.419–0.428
40-59	Males	0.144–0.150	0.206–0.215	0.283–0.311
	Females	0.150–0.194	0.260–0.284	0.353–0.414
>60	Males	0.148–0.163	0.228–0.235	0.330–0.344
	Females	0.135–0.171	0.248–0.261	0.360–0.383

Source: Adapted from reference 173. Data from the Lipid Research Clinics Program.

LDL, HDL, and VLDL. In the indirect procedure, an estimate of the VLDL-C is made by multiplying triglycerides by 16 percent. The equation is as follows:[178]

LDL-C = {Total Cholesterol –

[HDL-C + (0.16 × Triglycerides)]}

For example, if the total cholesterol is 200 mg/dl, HDL-C is 50 mg/dl, and triglycerides are 100 mg/dl:

LDL-C = {200 – [50 + (0.16 × 100)]} = 134 mg/dl

Treatment of Hypercholesterolemia

Many studies have shown that when serum cholesterol levels are lowered, the incidence and death from CHD decreases.[19, 160, 179–183] The results of the Lipid Research Clinics Coronary Primary Prevention Trial (LRC-CPPT), organized by the National Heart, Lung, and Blood Institute, showed that a 50-percent reduction in CHD incidence can be predicted for those who reduce their plasma cholesterol levels 25 percent (a 2-percent drop in CHD for every 1-percent drop in serum cholesterol).[182] Using 30-year follow-up data from the Framingham study, death from heart disease increased nine percent for each 10 mg/dl increase in serum cholesterol for people under age 50.[179]

Data from 361,662 men age 35–57 in the Multiple Risk Factor Intervention Trial (MRFIT) clearly demon-strate that the relationship between serum cholesterol and risk of CHD death is continuous, graded, and strong over the entire range of the cholesterol distribution.[160] Figure 10.15 summarizes the results, showing that death rates for CHD climb steadily when serum cholesterol levels rise above 180 mg/dl. Thus the great majority of adults in the United States are at risk for CHD because their serum cholesterol levels are above 180 mg/dL.

These studies demonstrate that treatment of high blood cholesterol levels is important for reducing the risk of CHD. The National Cholesterol Education Program (NCEP) of the National Heart, Lung, and Blood Institute, National Institutes of Health, offers practical detection and treatment recommendations for health professionals,[156, 157] and is composed of a group of national experts in blood cholesterol control. Table 10.9 summarizes the major guidelines. (See Box 10.2 for a listing of the CHD risk factors.)

The next section of this Chapter outlines the pertinent dietary and lifestyle factors useful in conjunction with Table 10.9.

Diet and Other Lifestyle Measures

Several major organizations have recently published dietary recommendation consensus reports for both the prevention and treatment of hypercholesterol-

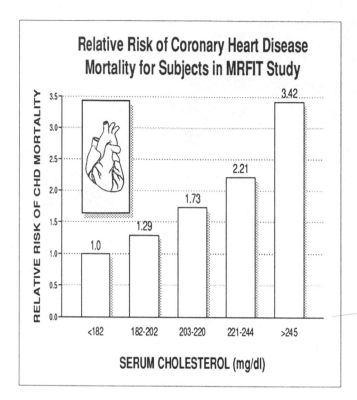

Figure 10.15 The risk of coronary heart disease begins at serum cholesterol levels above 180 mg/dl. *Source:* Data from the Multiple Risk Factor Intervention Trial (MRFIT). See reference 160.

Box 10.3   National Cholesterol Education Program/American Heart Association Guidelines for Dietary Prevention and Treatment of High Serum Cholesterol Levels and Coronary Heart Disease

- Total fat intake should be less than 30 percent of calories.
- Saturated fat intake should be less than 10 percent of calories.
- Polyunsaturated fat intake should not exceed 10 percent of calories.
- Cholesterol intake should not exceed 300 mg/day.
- Carbohydrate intake should constitute 50 percent or more of calories, with emphasis on complex carbohydrates.
- Protein intake should provide the remainder of the calories.
- Sodium intake should not exceed 3 g/day.
- Alcoholic consumption should not exceed 1–2 oz of ethanol per day. Two ounces of 100 proof whisky, 8 oz of wine, or 24 oz of beer each contain 1 oz of ethanol.
- Total calories should be sufficient to maintain the individual's recommended body weight.
- A wide variety of foods should be consumed.

Source; National Cholesterol Education Program (187) and the American Heart Association (188).

emia. These include the American Medical Association's Council on Scientific Affairs,[184] the American Heart Association (AHA),[185, 186] the National Cholesterol Education Program (NCEP),[157,158,187] the National Heart, Lung, and Blood Institute,[188] the Inter-Society Commission for Heart Disease Resources,[19] and the World Health Organization.[181]

The NCEP and AHA guidelines are the most recent, and are generally regarded as the present-day standard.[186,187] These are outlined in Box 10.3. In general, the guidelines urge Americans to consume less animal saturated fat and cholesterol and include more carbohydrates and fiber while moderating sodium, total caloric, and alcohol intake.

The effect of reducing dietary saturated fat and cholesterol on serum cholesterol can be estimated using the revised *Hegsted formula.* Through the 1950s and 1960s, Drs. Keys, Anderson, Grande, and Hegsted conducted scores of feeding experiments, which have produced high-quality information on the effects of dietary *saturated fats, polyunsaturated fatty acids* (PUFA), and cholesterol on serum cholesterol.[23,189–191] These studies are summarized in the famous "Hegsted Equation,"

which has been revised recently.[191] The revised Hegsted formula is outlined in Table 10.10, with an example for practical usage.

This equation is for the average person. People have been found to respond differently.[192–194] Overall, PUFA depress serum cholesterol levels, while dietary saturated fats and cholesterol increase serum cholesterol.

Table 10.11 summarizes the recent literature on the effects of diet on lipids and lipoproteins.[194–204] Not all saturated fats act alike; the medium-chain saturated fats have little effect on serum lipids.[204] The long-chain saturated fats, in general, tend to raise serum cholesterol and LDL-C levels.[196] *Monounsaturated fatty acids* (MUFA) were once thought to have little effect on serum cholesterol and lipoprotein levels. However,

Table 10.9 NCEP Guidelines

Initial Classification and Recommended Follow-Up Based on Total Cholesterol

Classification

<200 mg/dl	Desirable blood cholesterol
200-239 mg/dl	Borderline-high blood cholesterol
≥240 mg/dl	High blood cholesterol

Recommended Follow-Up

<200 mg/dl	Repeat within 5 years. Give diet and risk factor information.
200-239 mg/dl	A) *Without* definite CHD or 2 other CHD risk factors.* Give dietary information and recheck annually.
	B) *With* definite CHD or 2 other CHD risk factors. Lipoprotein analysis with further action based on LDL-C level.
≥240 mg/dl	Lipoprotein analysis with further action based on LDL-C level.

Classification and Treatment Decisions Based on LDL-Cholesterol

Classification

<130 mg/dl	Desirable LDL-C
130-159 mg/dl	Borderline-High-Risk LDL-C
≥160 mg/dl	High-Risk LDL-C

Recommended Treatment Decisions

<130 mg/dl	Repeat within 5 years. Give diet and risk factor information.
130-159 mg/dl	A) *Without* definite CHD or 2 other CHD risk factors. Give dietary information and recheck annually.
	B) *With* definite CHD or 2 other CHD risk factors. Extensive clinical and physical exams to determine possible causes. Initiate vigorous dietary and lifestyle therapy.
≥160 mg/dl	Drug therapy may need to be initiated, but only after vigorous dietary and lifestyle therapy has failed.

*See Box 10.2 for a listing of the risk factors used by NCEP. *Source:* National Cholesterol Education Program (NCEP). Report of the Expert Panel on Detection, Evaluation, and Treatment of High Blood Cholesterol in Adults. National Heart, Lung, and Blood Institute, U.S. Department of Health and Human Services, Public Health Service, National Institutes of Health. NIH Publication No. 88-2925, 1988.

several recent studies suggest that MUFA has the equivalent effect of PUFA in lowering LDL-C, with the added advantage of not causing a decrease in HDL-C like PUFA does.[197-199] The dominant effect of *fish oils* is to decrease triglycerides, having little effect on LDL-C or total cholesterol.[200-203]

To have a favorable HDL-C/TC ratio, the total cholesterol and LDL-C must be lowered and the HDL-C elevated through an application of both dietary and lifestyle factors. A summary of the important factors for elevating HDL-C is given in Box 10.4, and one for lowering LDL-C and total cholesterol, in Box 10.5. These factors are listed in order of approximate importance as summarized from the literature.[19, 172, 174-177, 180, 186, 187, 194, 205-219]

Serum triglycerides are also associated with heart disease risk, but not independently of LDL and HDL.[19, 220-223] The majority of long-term studies have shown no independent usefulness of triglyceride as a predictor of cardiovascular disease, after the effects of cholesterol and other heart disease risk factors have been accounted for statistically. In one 12-year follow-up study of 1,589 healthy men without known cardiovascular disease or hypercholesterolemia, no significant association was found between *hypertriglyceridemia* (values of 250–499 mg/dl) and cardiovascular death.[220]

Table 10.10 The Revised Hegsted Formula for Estimating Serum Cholesterol from Dietary Changes in Cholesterol and Fats

Estimated Decreases in Serum Cholesterol of Equal Calorie Reductions by Two-Thirds of Dietary Saturated Fat and Dietary Cholesterol

Change in Dietary Lipid	Estimated Decrease in Serum Cholesterol
Saturated fat reduced from 17% to 6% of Calories	24
Cholesterol reduced from 240 to 80 mg/1000 kcal	16

Note: Change in serum cholesterol = (2.16 × change in S) − (1.65 × change in P) + (0.097 × change in dietary cholesterol). S and P represent the percentages of total calories obtained from saturated and polyunsaturated fats, respectively, and C represents the intake of dietary cholesterol in milligrams per 1000 kcal. *Source:* see reference 191.

Box 10.4 Lifestyle Factors* that Increase High Density Lipoprotein Cholesterol (HDL-C). In order of approximate importance. Supporting references given in parentheses.

1. Weight reduction and leanness (172–177,218)

2. Aerobic exercise, at least 10 miles per week (174,177,205,215)

3. Smoking cessation (174,177,216)

4. Moderate alcohol consumption** (172–177)

*Other non-lifestyle factors that are important are being female and black. Age has little effect on HDL-C.
**This lifestyle factor, however, cannot be advised because of relationship to other more serious health problems.

Table 10.11 Lipid Classification

Saturated Fats		Monounsaturated Fats	Polyunsaturated Fats	
Medium Chain	Long Chain	High Oleic-w-9	High Linoleic-w-6	High Linolenic-w-3
C6-C12	C14-24*	Olive	Corn oil	Linseed
Kernel oils	Cocoa butter	Canola	Soy	Fish oils
Coconut	Dairy fats		Safflower	Salmon
Palm kernel	Lard		Sunflower	Maackerel
	Tallow			Tuna
	Palm oil			Anchovy
	Hydrogenated margarine, oil			
Little effect on lipids	Raise LDL-C, and TC	Decrease TC, LDL-C; No effect HDL-C	Decrease TC, LDL-C, and HDL-C	Decrease triglycerides; little effect on TC or LDL-C

Note: An exception is C18 (stearic acid) which does not raise serum cholesterol levels. *Source:* Adapted from: Babayan VK. Am J Clin Nutr 48:1520, 1988.

TC = total cholesterol. LDL-C = low density lipoprotein cholesterol. HDL-C = high density lipoprotein cholesterol.

> **Box 10.5   Lifestyle Factors* that Decrease Low Density Lipoprotein Cholesterol (LDL-C) and Total Cholesterol. In order of approximate importance. Supporting references given in parentheses.**
>
> 1. Decrease in dietary saturated fat intake (160, 186, 187, 188, 191, 196)
>
> 2. Decrease in body weight (180, 186, 187, 209)
>
> 3. Decrease in dietary cholesterol intake (157–160, 186, 191)
>
> 4. Increase in dietary polyunsaturated fatty acids (185–190)
>
> 5. Increase in carbohydrate and dietary water soluble fibers (especially fruits and vegetables) (194, 211, 219)
>
> 6. Increase in monounsaturated fatty acids (197–199)
>
> 7. Control of stress (213–215, 217)
>
> 8. Decrease in dietary caffeine, coffee consumption (206–208, 210, 211)
>
> ---
>
> *In Western countries, LDL-C and total cholesterol rise with age, but this is not considered to be an inevitable consequence of aging.

In other words, hypertriglyceridemia is a poor marker for cardiovascular risk. Optimal triglyceride values are less than 110 mg/dl. Endurance athletes often have values below 80 mg/dl.[205] Triglycerides can be lowered by losing weight, increasing aerobic exercise, and reducing alcohol intake.

Use of Drugs

The NCEP has urged the use of drugs when dietary and lifestyle changes have proved inadequate in lowering high serum total cholesterol or LDL-C levels. Table 10.12 outlines the expected results from use of several major cholesterol lowering medications.

Role of Exercise

Several reviews have summarized the effects of exercise on blood lipids and lipoproteins.[205, 224–229] Despite initial confusion due to poorly controlled studies, there is now a growing consensus. In general, men and women who participate in vigorous endurance-type exercise have plasma lipid and lipoprotein profiles consistent with lower risk for CHD.[228] See Figure 10.16.

The major differences between active people and matched physically inactive controls appear to be a lower plasma triglyceride concentration, and greater high-density lipoprotein mass.[230–244] Total cholesterol and LDL-C may be lower for some active people, but leanness and dietary quality appear to be much more important factors than physical activity. (See Figure 10.17.)

Exercise training studies suggest that 1,000 kcal/week of endurance type exercise (e.g., 10 miles of brisk walking and/or jogging) at moderate intensity is required to produce plasma lipid or lipoprotein changes. Above 1,000 kcal/week, a dose-response relationship exists, with greater changes occurring up to an expenditure of 4,500 kcal/week.[243]

The change in body weight that often occurs during exercise training is a possible confounder when the effects of exercise on blood lipids and lipoproteins are evaluated. As will be reviewed in Chapter 11, weight loss is associated with a dramatic improvement in the blood lipid profile—with weight loss, total cholesterol, LDL-C, and triglycerides decrease, while HDL-C increases.[245]

The independent effect of aerobic exercise during weight loss, however, is limited to improving the magnitude of change in the triglycerides and HDL-C, but not total cholesterol and LDL-C.[236, 240, 241, 246, 247] In a study by the author, total cholesterol and LDL-C fell 13 percent for both sedentary controls and exercising obese women after five weeks of a 1268-Calorie diet.[244] Exercise was found to have an independent effect only on triglycerides and HDL-C.

Although the association between regular endurance exercise and increased HDL-C and decreased triglycerides is now well established, the exact mechanism explaining these changes remains unsolved.[205] However, growing evidence points towards the interplay of three important enzymes: *lipoprotein lipase* (LPL), *hepatic lipase* (HL), and *lecithin: cholesterol acyltransferase* (LCAT).

HDL is not secreted by any of the body organs as a totally complete particle. Instead, it is assembled in the plasma from precursors from the small intestine and

Table 10.12   Cholesterol Lowering Medications

	Effects on Lipid/Lipoprotein Levels			Long-Term Reduction in	
	LDL-C	HDL-C	Triglyceride	CHD Risk	Safety
Nicotinic Acid (niacin)	15–30% dec	10–20% inc	15–40% dec	Yes	Yes
Cholestyramine (Questran)	15–30% dec	NC/inc	NC/inc	Yes	Yes
Gemfibrozil (Lopid)	0–15% dec	10–15% inc	15–40% dec	Yes	Yes
Lovastatin (Mevacor)	25–40% dec	10–15% inc	15–20% dec	NP	NP
Probucol (Lorelco)	10–15% dec	20–25% dec	NC	NP	NP

Note: dec = decrease; inc = increase; NC = no change; NP = not proven.   *Source:* Southern California Kaiser Permanente

liver, and from other circulating lipoproteins, especially the chylomicrons and VLDL. Lipoprotein lipase, an enzyme in the capillary walls of both muscle and fat tissue, breaks down the triglycerides in the passing lipoproteins, allowing body cells to take in fatty acids.[164–166,248,249] The chylomicrons and VLDL shrink, and give up various proteins, cholesterol, and phospholipids to incomplete HDL that have been formed from the liver and small intestine.

An enzyme from the liver, LCAT, "matures" the incomplete HDL by connecting fatty acids to the free cholesterol in the HDL particle. The incomplete HDL swells into a mature sphere (HDL$_3$). The LCAT enzyme then grabs more cholesterol from the tissues and other circulating lipoproteins to form even bigger HDL particles (HDL$_2$). Hepatic lipase, an enzyme localized in the cells surrounding liver sinusoid capillaries, irreversibly removes HDL$_2$ particles from the blood.[250] See Figure 10.18 for a summary of the actions of these three enzymes.

Those who are trained by regular aerobic exercise can have up to double the normal lipoprotein lipase activity in muscle and adipose tissue. This allows working muscles to use more fatty acids for fuel. Several researchers have reported that endurance athletes have nearly double the capacity for triglyceride clearance from the blood following meals than inactive people do, which is associated with increased HDL production.[251,252]

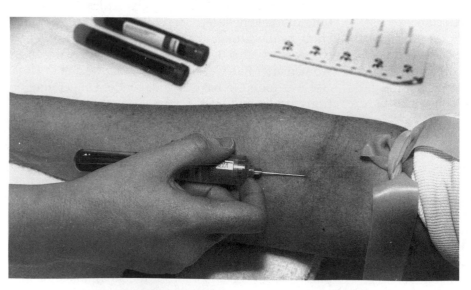

Figure 10.16 The blood lipid and lipoprotein profiles of active people are similar to those of people with lower risk for coronary heart disease.

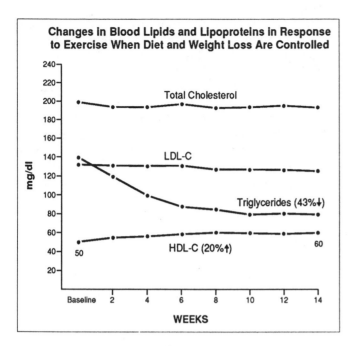

Figure 10.17 When potential changes in diet composition and body weight are controlled, aerobic exercise has little effect on total cholesterol and LDL-C, but major effects on triglycerides and HDL-C. *Source:* Data represent estimated changes based on review of literature.[230-247]

The activity of the LCAT enzyme is also increased in active people do. In one study, LCAT activity was reported to be 2 to 7 times higher among elite athletes than among sedentary controls.[253] Hepatic lipase activity decreases with regular training, allowing the HDL to stay in circulation longer.[254] Overall, the HDL-C concentration increases because of greater production (LPL and LCAT) and decreased removal (HL).[255]

Women, who have higher HDL-C levels than men, might realize this benefit through the effects of endogenous estrogen.[256] Estrogen appears to decrease the activity of hepatic lipase. As reviewed in Chapter 9, recent studies have shown that steroid use dramatically decreases HDL-C while increasing LDL-C.[257-259] Athletes who use steroids to build muscle tissue are thus placing themselves at higher risk of heart disease.

Several studies have shown that single bouts of exercise of moderate or greater duration result in immediate and significant elevations of plasma HDL-C among both men and women.[260-270] This is probably due to the LPL exercise-induced degradation of triglycerides.[266] Results from 9–12 km treadmill running tests show that HDL-C rises both during and immediately after the bout, with the increases greater (25 percent vs. 14 percent) with higher intensity running (90 percent vs. 60 percent $\dot{V}O_{2max}$).[269] In another study of 12 female marathon runners, HDL-C increased 23 percent immediately following their marathon run.[264]

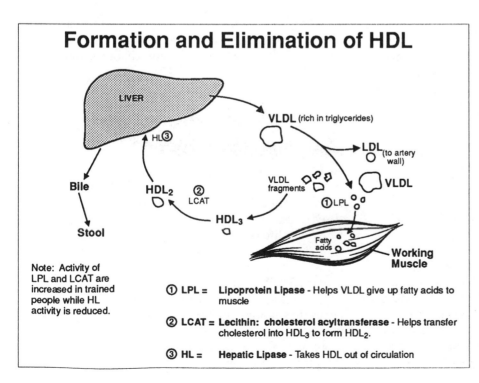

Figure 10.18 HDL is formed within the blood by the action of two key enzymes (lipoprotein lipase and lecithin: cholesterol acyltransferase) and then taken out of circulation by hepatic lipase. Active people tend to have higher LPL and LCAT and lower HL enzyme activity levels. See text for wide variety of references used for these figures.

These changes are transient, however, and return to baseline levels within several hours of the exercise bout.[270] It is likely that the chronically elevated HDL-C levels found in habitual exercisers are the cumulative result of regular acute stimulation.

Several published reports have suggested that weight training is associated with favorable changes in blood lipid and lipoprotein profiles.[271-273] However, the effects appear to be much smaller than those of aerobic exercise.[272, 274-275]

Exercise in the Prevention of Heart Disease

Epidemiological studies have left no doubt as to the existence of a strong inverse relationship between physical exercise and coronary heart disease risk. This is supported by several recent reviews.[1, 276-282]

Review of Major Studies

Forty-three studies of North American and European working-age men were recently reviewed by the Centers for Disease Control.[281] Not one of the studies reported a significantly greater risk of CHD for the more active participants. Sixty-eight percent of the studies reported a statistically significant association or graded response supporting the hypothesis that physical activity reduces risk of CHD. Methodologically superior studies were more likely to report an inverse association.

The relative risk of CHD associated with inactivity generally ranged from 1.5 to 2.4, similar to the relative risks of the better accepted risk factors such as hypertension (>150 mm Hg vs. ≤120 mm Hg = RR 2.1), hypercholesterolemia (>268 mg/dl vs. ≤218 mg/dl = RR 2.4), and cigarette smoking (≥ 1 pack / day vs. no smoking = RR 2.5).

The confounding factors of age, sex, blood pressure, smoking status, and total serum cholesterol were considered by many of the studies. Adjustments indicate that physical activity exerts an effect on CHD independent of these other risk factors. Table 10.13 summarizes some of the major studies reviewed in the Centers for Disease Control review[281] and other studies that have been published since this review.[283-290]

In general, these studies show that both physical fitness and physical activity (whether on the job or during leisure) are associated with decreased risk of CHD, and that regular physical activity should be promoted in CHD prevention as vigorously as blood pressure control, dietary modification to lower serum cholesterol, and smoking cessation.[281] Given the large proportion of sedentary people in the United States, the incidence of CHD attributable to insufficient physical activity is likely to be surprisingly large. Table 10.14 compares the relative prevalence of the major risk factors of CHD.[281]

Important details remain unclear.[281, 291-295] More information is needed on women and elderly men. Do people with other CHD risk factors benefit more from the physical activity? What biochemical or metabolic mechanisms mediate the effect? How rapidly do the benefits accrue (or diminish)? How important is the intensity of the physical activity?

Figure 10.19 shows that VO_{2max} may not be all important in reducing the risk of CHD. Active workers who burn many Calories throughout their work day have relatively low VO_{2max} values, compared with athletes, yet most studies show that they have a comparable risk of CHD.

Inverse Association with Risk Factors

The positive effect of physical activity on CHD risk is probably due to several factors.[296-313] Of particular interest is the evidence that regular physical activity is inversely associated with the primary risk factors of heart disease (and some of the secondary factors as well).[277, 278, 296-302] For whatever reasons, regular aerobic activity has been associated with decreased cigarette smoking, lower prevalence of high blood pressure, and a more favorable blood lipoprotein profile. In addition, exercise helps to control obesity, diabetes, and stress. (See Figure 10.20.)

Sports Medicine Insight
Cardiac Rehabilitation

In 1986, 284,000 coronary bypass surgeries were conducted in the United States.[2] *Cardiac rehabilitation* has been organized to help restore these and other heart disease patients to the most productive, active, and satisfying life possible.

The emphasis in cardiac rehabilitation is usually on lifestyle changes, as well as optimization of drug therapy.[314, 315] Exercise is considered the cornerstone of cardiac rehabilitation, but weight control, cessation of cigarette smoking, group therapy and family counseling, vocational counseling, a low-Calorie, low-fat diet, systematic follow-up examinations, and careful drug therapy are also important.[316]

Table 10.13 Relationship Between Physical Activity, Physical Fitness, and Coronary Heart Disease

Study Location	Subject Groups Compared	Relative Risk*
London postal, civil servants	Active postmen vs. sedentary	2.0
London transport busmen	Active conductors vs. drivers	2.3
US railroad workers	Active section men vs. clerks	2.0
North Dakota farmers	Active farmers vs. nonfarmers	1.8
Washington D.C. postal workers	Active carriers vs. clerks	2.8
Italy residents	Heavy workers vs. sedentary	3.1
Greek islands residents	Heavy workers vs. sedentary	2.0
San Francisco longshoremen	Heavy workers vs. light tasks	1.6
Harvard alumni	Heavy leisure exercise vs. light	1.6
Framingham, MA male residents	High vs. low amounts of exercise	1.9
Los Angeles firemen/policemen	Good vs. low physical fitness	2.4
Gothenberg, Sweden residents	Good vs. low physical fitness	2.3
North Karelia male residents	Heavy workers vs. light	1.6
Seattle residents	High intensity leisure vs. none	2.5
MRFIT study subjects (286)	Moderate exercise vs. little	1.4
Eastern Finland (287)	Active vs. sedentary	1.3
US railroad workers (288)	Good vs. low physical fitness	1.4
Honolulu heart study (289)	Active vs. inactive elderly	1.5
Lipid Research Clinic (290)	Good vs. poor physical fitness	3.0

Source: Adapted from Centers for Disease Control review article (281) plus references as noted.

Relative risk is the increase in coronary heart disease risk that inactive/low fitness subjects have relative to active/high fitness subjects. A relative risk of 1.4 means that inactive/low fitness subjects have a 40 percent increased risk of CHD as compared with active/high fitness subjects.

Table 10.14 A Comparison of the Prevalence of Several Major Risk Factors for Coronary Heart Disease

Risk Factor	Percent of U.S. Population
Cigarette Smoking	30%
Hypercholesterolemia (≥240 mg/dl)	25%
Hypertension (+140/90 mm Hg)	30%
Obesity (BMI≥27.2)	25%
Inactivity	60%
Irregular activity	33%
Completely sedentary	27%

Source: Adapted from reference 281.

Although as late as 1966 it was common practice to have the patient with acute myocardial infarction stay in bed a minimum of two to three weeks, today there is a careful three-to-four-phase program of exercise that begins with low-level ambulation within the first 24–48 hours after the heart attack, and then progressively increased physical activity to a level that is maintained for life.[317] Such programs are under the care of cardiologists and Exercise Specialists certified by the American College of Sports Medicine. (See Figure 10.21.)

While cardiac rehabilitation programs do help patients improve their functional aerobic capacity, studies have failed to establish that participants live longer or have fewer subsequent heart attacks.[318-321] However, when exercise is combined with proper diet and nonsmoking, there may be a reduction in mortality rates.[322]

Although cardiac rehabilitation has become increasingly popular, only 15 percent of eligible

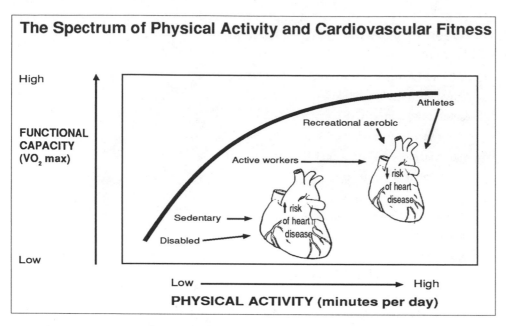

The Spectrum of Physical Activity and Cardiovascular Fitness

Figure 10.19 Very high $\dot{V}O_{2max}$ values are not necessary to reduce risk of CHD. However, at least moderate physical activity is important, and is usually associated with higher than average $\dot{V}O_{2max}$ values.

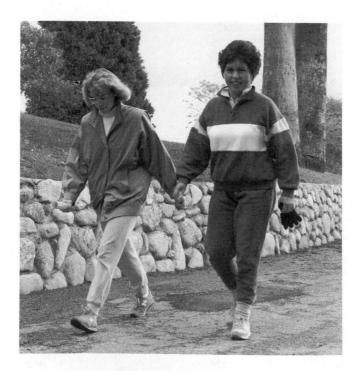

Figure 10.20 Regular physical activity is associated with a lower prevalence for most of the major risk factors of coronary heart disease.

candidates participate in supervised and monitored programs.[323] For a variety of reasons, these programs are not feasible for the vast majority of patients. Consequently, alternative approaches, including home-based programs, are being explored. Home-based programs can provide an opportunity for primary prevention for other family members and are usually more convenient.

Cardiac rehabilitation programs are safe. To determine the incidence of major cardiovascular complications in outpatient cardiac rehabilitation programs, data from 167 randomly selected cardiac rehabilitation programs were reviewed.[324] The programs reported that 51,303 patients exercised 2,351,916 hours during a four-year period. Twenty-one cardiac arrests (18 in which the patient was successfully resuscitated and three fatal) and 8 nonfatal myocardial infarctions were reported (8.9/1,000,000 patient hours of exercise for cardiac arrests, 1.3/1,000,000 for fatalities). The data indicate that cardiac rehabilitation programs have a low risk of major cardiovascular complications.

Summary

1. Death from heart disease (also called cardiovascular disease, CVD) is the leading killer among people in developed countries worldwide.

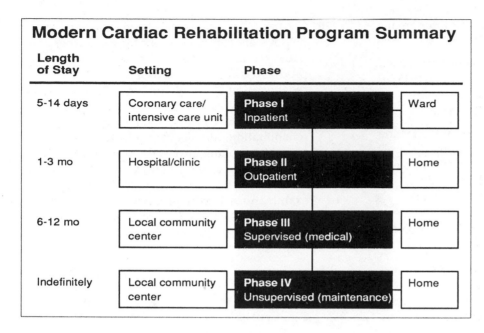

Modern Cardiac Rehabilitation Program Summary

Length of Stay	Setting	Phase	
5-14 days	Coronary care/ intensive care unit	**Phase I** Inpatient	Ward
1-3 mo	Hospital/clinic	**Phase II** Outpatient	Home
6-12 mo	Local community center	**Phase III** Supervised (medical)	Home
Indefinitely	Local community center	**Phase IV** Unsupervised (maintenance)	Home

Figure 10.21 There are four phases to the modern cardiac rehabilitation program. Participants include people who have CHD, people who have had a myocardial infarction (MI), those with coronary artery disease who have not had an MI, and surgery patients. Patients with no complications are expected to progress from phase I through phase III within one year after an acute cardiac event. Phase IV is designed for lifelong participation. Cardiac rehabilitation programs are found at many different sites, including hospitals, YMCAs, universities, community centers, and medical clinics. *Source:* Adapted from Wilson PK. Cardiac Rehabilitation: Then and Now. Physician Sportsmed 16(9):75–84, 1988.

2. Atherosclerosis is the underlying factor in 85 percent of CVD deaths. Coronary heart disease (CHD) is the major form of heart disease, and is caused by atherosclerosis and clotting in the coronary arteries.

3. An estimated 60 million Americans have hypertension (systolic BP $\geq$140 mm Hg and/or diastolic BP $\geq$90 mm Hg), making it the most prevalent form of CVD.

4. Nearly one million Americans die each year from CVD, representing 47 percent of all deaths. More than one half million die from heart attacks each year.

5. Since the mid-1960s, CHD deaths have dropped by more than 42 percent, and stroke deaths by more than 50 percent. More than 60 percent of the decline in CHD is related to changes in lifestyle.

6. Risk factors for heart disease include male sex, family history, cigarette smoking, hypertension, high serum cholesterol, low HDL-C, history of stroke or peripheral vascular disease, and severe obesity. The danger of heart attack increases with the number of risk factors.

7. Cigarette smoking is the most important of the known modifiable risk factors for CHD.

8. The relationship between exercise and smoking is complex. Many studies have shown that smoking before exercise adversely affects performance. Very few active people smoke. More study needs to be done to determine the role of physical activity in reducing the desire for cigarette smoking. Weight gain is a likely outcome of smoking cessation, and is related to the effect of smoking on 24-hour energy expenditure.

9. The 1988 Joint National Committee on Detection, Evaluation, and Treatment of High Blood Pressure has organized a treatment scheme emphasizing non-drug approaches (especially weight reduction, salt restriction, and moderation of alcohol consumption) as a first line of defense, and then a step-care therapy approach with various drugs to treat hypertension.

10. Heavy drinking has been consistently associated with increased risk of death from heart disease. Ethanol use alters lipoprotein metabolism and blood lipid profiles, increasing HDL-C and VLDL-C. Evidence that moderate drinking has a protective effect against coronary heart disease is controversial. Even if moderate drinking were shown conclusively to reduce the risk of heart disease, recommendations to increase alcohol consumption would be ill-advised because of other overriding health concerns.

11. Following a bout of aerobic exercise, blood pressures fall for at least 90 minutes. Studies have shown that both physical fitness and habitual aerobic activity are associated with a decreased risk of hypertension. Exercise training

is associated with lower blood pressures among hypertensive people.

12. Approximately one-fourth of Americans have blood cholesterol levels above 240 mg/dl. Death rates for CHD climb steadily when serum cholesterol levels rise above 180 mg/dl.

13. There are three major lipoproteins in the fasting blood: HDL, LDL, and VLDL. LDL and HDL have opposing functions. HDL takes cholesterol to the liver where it is changed to bile and eventually excreted in the stool. LDL takes cholesterol to the artery wall. HDL-C and the ratio of HDL-C to total cholesterol are important measures of heart disease risk.

14. The National Cholesterol Education Program (NCEP) guidelines for classification and treatment of hypercholesterolemia were reviewed. The NCEP dietary recommendations are based on reduction of dietary saturated fat and cholesterol, with increased intake of complex carbohydrate foods.

15. Box 10.4 summarizes the lifestyle factors that increase HDL-C; Box 10.5 summarizes the lifestyle factors that decrease LDL-C.

16. A consistent finding is that with weight loss, total cholesterol, LDL-C, and triglycerides decrease, while HDL-C increases. The independent effect of aerobic exercise during weight loss, however, is limited to improving the magnitude of change in the triglycerides and HDL-C, but not total cholesterol and LDL-C.

17. HDL is formed within the blood by the action of two key enzymes, LPL and LCAT, and then taken out of circulation by hepatic lipase. Active people tend to have higher LPL and LCAT and lower HL enzyme activity levels.

18. Epidemiological studies have left no doubt as to the existence of a strong inverse relationship between physical exercise and coronary heart disease risk. These observations suggest that in CHD prevention programs, regular physical activity should be promoted as vigorously as blood pressure control, dietary modification to lower serum cholesterol, and smoking cessation.

19. The favorable effect of physical activity in decreasing CVD is probably due to several factors. One of the major factors is that regular physical activity is associated with a reduction of the major risk factors of heart disease.

20. Cardiac rehabilitation has been organized to help restore coronary artery bypass surgery patients and other heart disease patients to productive life. The emphasis in cardiac rehabilitation is usually on lifestyle changes, as well as optimization of drug therapy. Exercise is considered the cornerstone of cardiac rehabilitation, but weight control, cessation of cigarette smoking, group therapy and family counseling, vocational counseling, a low-Calorie, low-fat diet, systematic follow-up examinations, and careful drug therapy are also important. There are four phases to the modern cardiac rehabilitation program.

References

1. Paffenbarger RA, Hyde RT. Exercise In the Prevention of Coronary Heart Disease. Prev Med 13:3–22, 1984.

2. American Heart Association. 1989 Heart Facts. Dallas: 7320 Greenville Avenue, Texas 75231.

3. Anderson WAD, Scotti TM. Synopsis of Pathology. St. Louis: C.V. Mosby Co., 1980.

4. Steinberg D, Parthasarathy S, Caren TE, Witztum JL. Beyond Cholesterol. N Eng J Med 320:915–924, 1989.

5. Ross R. The Pathogenesis of Atherosclerosis—An Update. N Eng J Med 314:488–500, 1986.

6. Welin L, Sv rdsudd K, Wilhelmsen L, et al. Analysis of Risk Factors for Stroke in a Cohort of Men Born in 1913. N Engl J Med 317:521–526, 1987.

7. American Heart Association. High Blood Pressure Fact Sheet. National Center, 7320 Greenville Ave., Dallas, TX 75231. 1986.

8. Anonymous. Years of Life Lost From Cardiovascular Disease. JAMA 256:2794, 1986.

9. Eichner ER. Exercise and Heart Disease: Epidemiology of the "Exercise Hypothesis." Amer J Med 75:1008–1023, 1986.

10. Enos WF, Holmes RH, Beyer J. Coronary Disease Among United States Soldiers Killed in Action in Korea. JAMA 152:1090–1093, 1953.

11. U.S. Department of Health and Human Services. The Surgeon General's Report on Nutrition and Health. DHHS (PHS) Publication No. 88–50211. U.S. Government Printing Office: Washington, DC, 1988.

12. Kuller LH, Perper JA, Dai WS, Rutan G, Traven N. Sudden Death and the Decline in Coronary Heart Disease Mortality. J Chron Dis 39:1001–1019, 1986.

13. National Center for Health Statistics: Health, United States, 1988. DHHS Pub. No. (PHS) 89–1232. Public Health Service. Washington. U.S. Government Printing Office, March, 1989.

14. U.S. Department of Health and Human Services. Public Health Service. Office of Disease Prevention and Health Promotion. Prevention '86/'87: Federal Programs and Progress. U.S. Government Printing Office: Washington, DC, 1987.

15. Ragland KE, Selvin S, Merrill DW. The Onset of Decline in Ischemic Heart Disease Mortality in the United States. Am J Epidemiol 127:516–531, 1988.

16. Sempos C, Cooper R, Kovar MG, McMillen M. Divergence of the Recent Trends in Coronary Mortality for the Four Major Race–Sex Groups in the United States. Am J Public Health 78:1422–1427, 1988.

17. Garraway WM, Whisnant JP. The Changing Pattern of Hypertension and the Declining Incidence of Stroke. JAMA 258:214–217, 1987.

18. Moser M, Rafter J, Gajewski J. Insurance Premium Reductions. JAMA 251:756–757, 1984.

19. Reports of Inter-Society Commission for Heart Disease Resources. Circulation 70:155A–205A, 1984.

20. Kottke TE, Puska P, et al. Projected Effects of High-Risk Versus Populations-Based Prevention Strategies in Coronary Heart Disease. Am J Epidemiol 121:697–704, 1985.

21. Goldman L, Cook EF. The Decline In Ischemic Heart Disease Mortality Rates. Ann Intern Med 101:825–836, 1984.

22. Goldberg RJ, Gore JM, Alpert JS, Dalen JE. Recent Changes in Attack and Survival Rates of Acute Myocardial Infarction (1975 through 1981). JAMA 255:2774–2779, 1986.

23. Stamler J, Shekelle R. Dietary Cholesterol and Human Coronary Heart Disease. Arch Pathol Lab Med 112:1032–1040, 1988.

24. Slattery ML, Randall DE. Trends in Coronary Heart Disease Mortality and Food Consumption in the United States Between 1909 and 1980. Am J Clin Nutr 47:1060–1067, 1988.

25. U.S. Department of Agriculture, Human Nutrition Information Service. 1985. Nationwide Food Consumption Survey, Continuing Survey of Food Intakes by Individuals: Women 19–50 Years and Their Children 1–5 Years, 1 Day, 1985. U.S. Dept. of Agric., Rpt. No 85–1. Men 19–50 Years, 1 Day, 1985. U.S. Dept. of Agric., Rpt. No 85–3.

26. National Cholesterol Education Program. Report of the Expert Panel on Detection, Evaluation, and Treatment of High Blood Cholesterol in Adults. National Heart, Lung, and Blood Institute, U.S. Department of Health and Human Services, Public Health Service, National Institutes of Health. NIH Publication No. 88–2925, 1988.

27. Buring JE, Evans DA, Fiore M, et al. Occupation and Risk of Death From Coronary Heart Disease. JAMA 258:791–792, 1987.

28. Jacobsen BK, Thelle DS. Risk Factors for Coronary Heart Disease and Level of Education. Am J Epidemiol 127:923–932, 1988.

29. Kaplan GA, Salonen JT, Cohen RD, et al. Social Connections and Mortality From All Causes and From Cardiovascular Disease: Prospective Evidence From Eastern Finland. Am J Epidemiol 128:370–380, 1988.

30. Nunes EV, Frank KA, Kornfeld DS. Psychologic Treatment for the Type A Behavior Pattern and for Coronary Heart Disease: A Meta-Analysis of the Literature. Psychosomatic Medicine 48:159, 1987.

31. Siegel JM. Type A Behavior: Epidemiologic Foundations and Public Health Implications. Annu Rev Public Health 5:343–367, 1984.

32. Shoham-Yakubovich I, Ragland DR, Brand RJ, Syme SL. Type A Behavior Pattern and Health Status After 22 Years of Follow-up in the Western Collaborative Group Study. Am J Epidemiol 128:579–588, 1988.

33. Appels A, Mulder P, van 'T Hof M, et al. A Prospective Study of the Jenkins Activity Survey as a Risk Indicator for Coronary Heart Disease in the Netherlands. J Chron Dis 40:959–965, 1987.

34. Karasek RA, Theorell T, Schwartz JE, et al. Job Characteristics in Relation to the Prevalence of Myocardial Infarction in the US Health Examination Survey (HES) and the Health and Nutrition Examination Survey (HANES). Am J Public Health 78:910–918, 1988.

35. Pieper C, LaCroix AZ, Karasek RA. The Relation of Psychosocial Dimensions of Work with Coronary Heart Disease Risk Factors: A Meta-Analysis of Five United States Data Bases. Am J Epidemiol 129:483–494, 1989.

36. Hager T. High-Risk "Heart" Families: A Genealogical Look. JAMA 250:1663–1664, 1983.

37. Perkins KA. Family History of Coronary Heart Disease: Is It An Independent Risk Factor? Am J Epidemiol 124:182–194, 1986.

38. Hunt SC, Blickenstaff K, Hopkins PN, et al. Coronary Disease and Risk Factors in Close Relatives of Utah Women With Early Coronary Death. West J Med 145:329–334, 1986.

39. Sorensen TIA, Nielsen GG, Andersen PK, Teasdale TW. Genetic and Environmental Influences on Premature Death in Adult Adoptees. N Engl J Med 318:727–732, 1988.

40. Tofler GH, Brezinski D, Schafer AI, et al. Concurrent Morning Increase in Platelet Aggregability and the Risk of Myocardial Infarction and Sudden Cardiac Death. N Engl J Med 316:1514–1518, 1987.

41. Muller JE, Ludmer PL, Willich SN, et al. Circadian Variation in the Frequency of Sudden Cardiac Death. Circulation 75:131–138, 1987.

42. Kannel WB, Wolf PA, Castelli WP, D'Agostino RB. Fibrinogen and Risk of Cardiovascular Disease. JAMA 258:1183–1186, 1987.

43. Leon AS. Age and Other Predictors of Coronary Heart Disease. Med Sci Sports Exerc 19:159–167, 1987.

44. U.S. Department of Health and Human Services, Public Health Service, Office On Smoking and Health. The Health Consequences of Smoking: Cardiovascular Disease, a Report of the Surgeon General. U.S. Government Printing Office, Washington, D.C., 1983.

45. McGinnis, JM. Tobacco and Health: Trends in Smoking and Smokeless Tobacco Consumption in the United States. Annu Rev Public Health 8:441–467, 1987.

46. Pierce JP, Fiore MC, Novotny TE, et al. Trends in Cigarette Smoking in the United States. JAMA 261:61–65, 1989.

47. Pierce JP, Fiore MC, Novotny TE, et al. Trends in Cigarette Smoking in the United States. JAMA 261:56–60, 1989.

48. Pierce JP, Fiore MC, Novotny TE, et al. Trends in Cigarette Smoking in the United States. JAMA 261:49–55, 1989.

49. Fielding JE. Banning Worksite Smoking. Am J Public health 76:957–959, 1986.

50. Department of Health and Human Services. Smoking and Health: A National Status Report. HHD/PHS/CDC-87–8396, 1986.

51. Office of Disease Prevention and Health Promotion and Office on Smoking and health, Public Health Service, U.S. Dept of Health and Human Services, 1985. A Decision Maker's Guide to Reducing Smoking at the Worksite. Office of Disease Prevention and Health Promotion, 2132 Switzer Building, 330 C Street, S.W., Washington, D.C., 20201.

52. Mattson ME, Pollack ES, Cullen JW. What Are the Odds that Smoking Will Kill You? Am J Public Health 77:425–431, 1987.

53. Warner KE. Health and Economic Implications of a Tobacco-Free Society. JAMA 258:2080–2086, 1987.

54. Wolf PA, D'Agostino RB, Kannel WB, et al. Cigarette Smoking As A Risk Factor for Stroke. JAMA 259:1025–1029, 1988.

55. Walker WJ, Brin BN. U.S. Lung Cancer Mortality and Declining Cigarette Tobacco Consumption. J Clin Epidemiol 41:179–185, 1988.

56. Humble CG, Samet JM, Pathak DR. Marriage to a Smoker and Lung Cancer Risk. Am J Public Health 77:598–602, 1987.

57. U.S. Department of Health and Human Services, Office on Smoking and Health. The Health Consequences of Involuntary Smoking: A Report of the Surgeon General. U.S. Government Printing Office, Washington, D.C., 1986.

58. Helsing KJ, Sandler DP, Comstock GW, Chee E. Heart Disease Mortality in Nonsmokers Living With Smokers. Am J Epidemiol 127:915–922, 1988.

59. Svendsen KH, Kuller LH, Martin MJ, Ockene JK. Effects of Passive Smoking in the Multiple Risk Factor Intervention Trial. Am J Epidemiol 126:783–795, 1987.

60. Eriksen MP, LeMaistre CA, Newell GR. Health Hazards of Passive Smoking. Annu Rev Public Health 9:47–70, 1988.

61. Council on Scientific Affairs. Health Effects of Smokeless Tobacco. JAMA 255:1038–1044, 1986.

62. Glover ED, Edmundson EW, Edwards SW, Schroeder KL. Implications of Smokeless Tobacco Use Among Athletes. Physician Sportsmed 14(12):95–105, 1986.

63. Schwartz JL. Review and Evaluation of Smoking Cessation Methods: The United States and Canada, 1978–1985. National Cancer Institute, U.S. Department of Health and Human Services, Public Health Service, National Institutes of Health. NIH Publication No. 87–2940, 1987.

64. Janz NK, Becker MH, Kirscht JP, et al. Evaluation of a Minimial-Contact Smoking Cessation Intervention in an Outpatient Setting. Am J Public Health 77:805–809, 1987.

65. Anda RF, Remington PL, Sienko DG, Davis RM. Are Physicians Advising Smokers to Quit? JAMA 257:1916–1919, 1987.

66. U.S. Department of Health and Human Services. The Health Consequences of Smoking: Nicotine Addiction. A Report of the Surgeon General, 1988. U.S. Department of Health and Human Services, Public Health Service, Office on Smoking and Health. DHHS Publication No. (PHS). Stock Number 017–001–00468–5.

67. Kozlowski LT, Wilkinson DA, Skinner W, et al. Comparing Tobacco Cigarette Dependence With Other Drug Dependencies. JAMA 261:898–901, 1989.

68. Rotstein A, Sagiv M. Acute Effect of Cigarette Smoking on Physiologic Response to Graded Exercise. Int J Sports Med 7:322–324, 1986.

69. Marti B, Abelin T, Minder CE, Vader JP. Smoking, Alcohol Consumption, and Endurance Capacity: An Analysis of 6,500 19-Year-Old Conscripts and 4,100 Joggers. Prev Med 17:79–92, 1988.

70. West R. Schneider N. Craving for Cigarettes. British J Addiction 82(4):407–415, 1987.

71. Koplan JP, Powell KE, et al. An Epidemiologic Study of the Benefits and Risks of Running. JAMA 248:3118–3121, 1982.

72. Blair SN, Jacobs DR, Powell. Relationships Between Exercise or Physical Activity and Other Health Behaviors. Public Health Rep 100:172–180, 1985.

73. Blair SN, Goodyear NN, Wynne KL, Saunders RP. Comparison of Dietary and Smoking Habit Changes In Physical Fitness Improvers and Nonimprovers. *Prev Med* 13:411–420, 1984.

74. Stamford BA, Matter S, Fell RD, et al. Effects of Smoking Cessation On Weight Gain, Metabolic Rate, Calorie Consumption, and Blood Lipids. Am J Clin Nutr 43:486–494, 1986.

75. Hofstetter A, Schutz Y, Jequier E, Wahren J. Increased 24-Hour Energy Expenditure in Cigarette Smokers. N Eng J Med 314:79–82, 1986.

76. Perkins KA, Eptstein LH, Marks BL, et al. The Effect of Nicotine on Energy Expenditure During Light Physical Activity. N Eng J Med 320:898–903, 1989.

77. Dannenberg AL, Keller JB, Wilson WF, Castelli WP. Leisure Time Physical Activity in the Framingham Offspring Study. Am J Epidemiol 129:76–88, 1989.

78. The Working Group on Hypertension in the Elderly. Statement on Hypertension in the Elderly. JAMA 256:70–74, 1986.

79. WHO Scientific Group. Primary Prevention of Essential Hypertension. Geneva: World Health Organization, 1983.

80. Salmond CE, Joseph JG, Prior IAM, et al. Longitudinal Analysis of the Relationship Between Blood Pressure and Migration. The Tokelau Island Migrant Study. Am J Epidemiol 122:291–301, 1985.

81. Abernethy JD. The Need to Treat Mild Hypertension: Misinterpretation of Results From the Australian Trial. JAMA 256:3134–3137, 1986.

82. Jacob RG, Shapiro AP, Reeves RA, et al. Relaxation Therapy for Hypertension: Comparison of Effects With Concomitant Placebo, Diuretic, and Beta-Blocker. Arch Intern Med 146:2335–2340, 1986.

83. Chobanian AV. Antihypertensive Therapy in Evolution. N Engl J Med 314:1701–1702, 1986.

84. Nonpharmacological Approaches to the Control of High Blood Pressure. Final Report of the Subcommittee on Nonpharmacological Therapy of the 1984 Joint National Committee on Detection, Evaluation, and Treatment of High Blood Pressure. Hypertension 8:444–467, 1986.

85. 1988 Joint National Committee. The 1988 Report of the Joint National Committee on Detection, Evaluation, and Treatment of High Blood Pressure. Arch Intern Med 148:1023–1038, 1988.

86. Labarthe DR. Mild Hypertension: The Question of Treatment. Annu Rev Public Health 7:193–215, 1986.

87. Caldwell JE. Diuretic Therapy and Exercise Performance. Sports Med 4:290–304, 1987.

88. Hypertension Detection and Follow-up Program Cooperative Group. Persistence of Reduction in Blood Pressure and Mortality of Participants in the Hypertension Detection and Follow-up Program. JAMA 259:2113–2122, 1988.

89. Aagaard GN. Hypertension: Indications, Goals, and Potential Risks of Drug Therapy. West J Med 141:476–480, 1984.

90. Houston MC. Sodium and Hypertension. Arch Intern Med 146:179–185, 1986.

91. Kaplan NM. Dietary Aspects of the Treatment of Hypertension. Annu Rev Public Health 7:503–519, 1986.

92. Kaplan NM. Non-Drug Treatment of Hypertension. Ann InternMed 102:359–373, 1985.

93. Dustan HP. Obesity and Hypertension. Ann Intern Med 103:1047–1049, 1985.

94. Pan WH, Nanas S, Dyer A, et al. The Role of Weight in the Positive Association Between Age and Blood Pressure. Am J Epidemiol 24:612–623, 1986.

95. Stamler R, Stamler J, Grimm R, et al. Nutritional Therapy for High Blood Pressure: Final Report of a Four-Year Randomized Controlled Trial—The Hypertension Control Program. JAMA 257:1484–1491, 1987.

96. Tuomilehto J, Pietinen P, Salonen JT, et al. Nutrition Related Determinants of Blood Pressure. Prev Med 14:413–427, 1985.

97. Wilber JA. The Role of Diet In the Treatment of High Blood Pressure. J Am Diet Assoc 80:25–29, 1982.

98. Langford HG, Blaufox MD, et al. Dietary Therapy Slows the Return of Hypertension After Stopping Prolonged Medication. JAMA 253:657, 1985.

99. Berchtold P, Sims EAH. Obesity and Hypertension: Conclusions and Recommendations. Int J Obes 5:183, 1981.

100. Weinberger MH, Cohen SJ, Miller JZ, et al. Dietary Sodium Restriction as Adjunctive Treatment of Hypertension. JAMA 259:2561–2567, 1988.

101. Miller JZ, Weinberger MH, Daugherty SA, et al. Heterogeneity of Blood Pressure Response to Dietary Sodium Restriction in Normotensive Adults. J Chron Dis 40:245–250, 1987.

102. Holbrook JT, et al. Sodium and Potassium Intake and Balance In Adults Consuming Self-Selected Diets. Am J Clin Nutr 40:786, 1984.

103. Khaw KT, Barrett-Connor E. Dietary Potassium and Stroke-Associated Mortality. N Engl J Med 316:235–240, 1987.

104. Schramm MM, Cauley JA, Sandler RB, Slemenda CW. Lack of an Association Between Calcium Intake and Blood Pressure in Postmenopausal Women. Am J Clin Nutr 44:505–511, 1986.

105. Karanja N, McCarron DA. Calcium and Hypertension. Annu Rev Nutr 6:475–494, 1986.

106. van Beresteyn ECH, Schaafsma G, de Waard H. Oral Calcium and Blood Pressure: A Controlled Intervention Trial. Am J Clin Nutr 44:883–888, 1986.

107. Lyle RM, Melby CL, Hyner GC, et al. Blood Pressure and Metabolic Effects of Calcium Supplementation in Normotensive White and Black Men. JAMA 257:1772–1776, 1987.

108. Lyle RM, Melby CL, Hyner GC. Metabolic Differences Between Subjects Whose Blood Pressure Did or Did Not Respond to Oral Calcium Supplementation. Am J Clin Nutr 47:1030–1035, 1988.

109. Council for Agricultural Science and Technology. Diet and Health, Report No. 111. 137 Lynn Ave, Ames, Iowa 50010–7120. 1987.

110. MacMahon SW. Alcohol Consumption and Hypertension. Hypertension 9:111–121, 1987.

111. Sixth Special Report to the U.S. Congress on Alcohol and Health. Alcohol, Drug Abuse, and Mental Health Association. National Institute on Alcohol Abuse and Alcoholism. DHHS (PHS) Publication No. (ADM) 87–1519. 1987.

112. Lang T, Degoulet P, Aime F, et al. Relationship Between Alcohol Consumption and Hypertension Prevalence and Control in a French Population. J Chron Dis 40:713–720, 1987.

113. Arkwright PD, et al. The Pressor Effect of Moderate Alcohol Consumption in Man: A Search for Mechanisms. Circulation 66:515–519, 1982.

114. Cooke KM, et al. Alcohol Consumption and Blood Pressure. Med J Australia 1:65–69, 1982.

115. Jackson R, Stewart A, Beaglehole R, Scragg R. Alcohol Consumption and Blood Pressure. Am J Epidemiol 122:1037–1044, 1985.

116. MacGregor RR. Alcohol and Immune Defense. JAMA 256:1474–1478, 1986.

117. AMA Council on Scientific Affairs. Alcohol and the Driver. JAMA 255:522–527, 1986.

118. Camacho TC, Kaplan GA, Cohen RD. Alcohol Consumption and Mortality in Alameda County. J Chron Dis 40:229–236, 1987.

119. Haskell WL, Camargo C, Williams PT, Vranizan KM. The Effect of Cessation and Resumption of Moderate Alcohol Intake on Serum High-Density-Lipoprotein Subfractions. A Controlled Study. N Eng J Med 310:805–810, 1984.

120. Camargo CA, et al. The Effect of Moderate Alcohol Intake On Serum Apolipoproteins A-I and A-II. JAMA 253:2854–2857, 1985.

121. Contaldo F, D'Arrigo E, Carandente V, et al. Short-term Effects of Moderate Alcohol Consumption on Lipid Metabolism and Energy Balance in Normal Men. Metabolism 38:166–171, 1989.

122. Hartung GH, Reeves RS, Foreyt JP, et al. Effect of Alcohol Intake and Exercise On Plasma High-Density Lipoprotein Cholesterol Subfractions and Apolipoprotein A-I In Women. Am J Cardiol 58:148–151, 1986.

123. Salonen JT, Puska P, Nissinen. Intake of Spirits and Beer and Risk of Myocardial Infarction and Death—A Longitudinal Study in Eastern Finland. J Chron Dis 36:533–543, 1983.

124. Heiss G, Johnson NH, et al. The Epidemiology of Plasma High Density Lipoprotein Cholesterol Levels—The Lipid Research Clinics Program Prevalence Study. Circulation 62:IV–116, 1980.

125. Stampfer MJ, Colditz GA, Willett WC, Speizer FE, Hennekens CH. A Prospective Study of Moderate Alcohol Consumption and the Risk of Coronary Disease and Stroke in Women. N Engl J Med 319:267–273, 1988.

126. Camargo CA, et al. The Effect of Moderate Alcohol Intake On Serum Apolipoproteins A-I and A-II. JAMA 253:2854–2857, 1985.

127. Kaufman DW, et al. Alcoholic Beverages and Myocardial Infarction In Young Men. Am J Epidemiol 121:548–554, 1985.

128. Poikolainen K, Simpura. One-Year Drinking History and Mortality. Prev Med 12:709–714, 1983.

129. Hamburg DA. Health and Behavior. Washington D.C.: National Academy Press, 1982.

130. Donahue RP, Abbott RD, Reed DM, Yano K. Alcohol and Hemorrhagic Stroke. JAMA 255:2311–2314, 1986.

131. Blume S, Levy RI, Kannel WB, Takamine J. The Risks of Moderate Drinking. JAMA 256:3213–3214, 1986.

132. Klatsky AL, Armstrong MA, Friedman GD, Hiatt RA. The Relations of Alcoholic Beverage Use to Colon and Rectal Cancer. Am J Epidemiol 128:1007–1015, 1988.

133. Hiatt RA, Klatsky A, Armstrong MA. Alcohol and Breast Cancer. Prev Med 17:683–685, 1988.

134. Longnecker MP, Berlin JA, Orza MJ, Chalmers TC. A Meta-Analysis of Alcohol Consumption in Relation to Risk of Breast Cancer. JAMA 260:652–656, 1988.

135. Graham S. Alcohol and Breast Cancer. N Engl J Med 316:1211–1212, 1987.

136. Schatzkin A, Jones DY, Hoover RN, et al. Alcohol Consumption and Breast Cancer in the Epidemiologic Follow-up Study of the First National Health and Nutrition Examination Survey. N Engl J Med 316:1169–1173, 1987.

137. Jacob RG, Shapiro AP, Reeves RA, et al. Relaxation Therapy for Hypertension: Comparison of Effects With Concomitant Placebo, Diuretic, and Beta-Blocker. Arch Intern Med 146:2335–2340, 1986.

138. Benson H. Systemic Hypertension and The Relaxation Response. N Engl J Med 296:1152–1156, 1977.

139. Bennett T, Wilcox RG, MacDonald. Post-Exercise Reduction of Blood Pressure in Hypertensive Men is Not Due to Acute Impairment of Baroflex Function. Clinical Sci 67:97, 1984.

140. Hagberg JM, Montain SJ, Martin WH. Blood Pressure and Hemodynamic Responses After Exercise in Older Hypertensives. J Appl Physiol 63:270–276, 1987.

141. Paffenbarger RS, Wing AL, Hyde RT, Jung DL. Physical Activity and Incidence of Hypertension in College Alumni. Am J Epidemiol 117:245–256, 1983.

142. Blair SN, Goodyear NN, Gibbons LW, et al. Physical Fitness and Incidence of Hypertension in Healthy Normotensive Men and Women. JAMA 252:487–490, 1984.

143. Benbassat J, Froom P. Blood Pressure Response to Exercise As a Predictor of Hypertension. Arch Intern Med 146:2053–2055, 1986.

144. Jette M, Landry F, Sidney K, Blumchen G. Exaggerated Blood Pressure Response to Exercise in the Detection of Hypertension. J Cardiopulmonary Rehabil 8:171–177, 1988.

145. Seals DR, Hagberg JM. The Effect of Exercise Training On Human Hypertension: A Review. Med Sci Sports Exerc 16:207, 1984.

146. Tipton CM. Exercise, Training, and Hypertension. IN: Terjung RL (ed). Exerc Sports Sci Rev 12:245–306, 1984.

147. Kenney WL, Zambraski EJ. Physical Activity in Human Hypertension. Sports Med 1:459, 1984.

148. McMahon M, Palmer RM. Exercise and Hypertension. Med Clin North Am 69:57–69, 1985.

149. Duncan JJ, Farr JE, Upton J, et al. The Effects of Aerobic Exercise on Plasma Catecholamines and Blood Pressure in Patients with Mild Essential Hypertension. JAMA 254:2609–2613, 1985.

150. Jennings G, Nelson L, Nestel P, et al. The Effects of Changes in Physical Activity On Major Cardiovascular Risk Factors, Hemodynamics, Sympathetic Function, and Glucose Utilization In Man: A Controlled Study of Four Levels of Activity. Circulation 73:30–40, 1986.

151. Report of the Second Task Force on Blood Pressure Control in Children—1987. Pediatrics 79:1–25, 1987.

152. Panico S, Celentano E, Krogh V, et al. Physical Activity and its Relationship to Blood Pressure in School Children. J Chron Dis 40:925–930, 1987.

153. Raglin JS, Morgan WP. Influence of Exercise and Quiet Rest on State of Anxiety and Blood Pressure. Med Sci Sports Exerc 19:456–463, 1987.

154. Strazzullo P, Cappuccio FP, Trevisan M, et al. Leisure Time Physical Activity and Blood Pressure in School-children. Am J Epidemiol 127:726–733, 1988.

155. Siscovick DS, Laporte RE, Newman JM. The Disease-Specific Benefits and Risks of Physical Activity and Exercise. Public Health Rep 100:180–188, 1985.

156. National Center for Health Statistics—National Heart, Lung, and Blood Institute Collaborative Lipid Group. Trends in Serum Cholesterol Levels Among U.S. Adults Aged 20 to 74 Years. JAMA 257:937–942, 1987.

157. National Cholesterol Education Program. Report of the Expert Panel on Detection, Evaluation, and Treatment of High Blood Cholesterol in Adults. National Heart, Lung, and Blood Institute, U.S. Department of Health and Human Services, Public Health Service, National Institutes of Health. NIH Publication No. 88–2925, 1988.

158. Ernst ND, Cleeman J, Mullis R, et al. The National Cholesterol Education Program: Implications for Dietetic Practitioners from the Adult Treatment Panel Recommendations. J Am Diet Assoc 88:1401–1411, 1988.

159. Connor WE, Cerqueira MT, Connor RW, Wallace RB, Malinow MR, Casdorph HR. The plasma lipids, lipoproteins, and diet of the Tarahumara Indians of Mexico. Am J Clin Nutr 31:1131–1142, 1978.

160. Stamler J, Wentworth D, Neaton JD. Is Relationship Between Serum Cholesterol and Risk of Premature Death From Coronary Heart Disease Continuous and Graded? Findings in 356,222 Primary Screenees of the Multiple Risk Factor Intervention Trial (MRFIT). JAMA 256:2823–2828, 1986.

161. Schucker B, Bailey K, Heimbach JT, et al. Change in Public Perspective On Cholesterol and Heart Disease: Results From Two National Surveys. JAMA 258:3527–3531, 1987.

162. Schucker B, Wittes JT, Cutler JA, et al. Changes in Physician Perspective on Cholesterol and Heart Disease. JAMA 258:3521–3526, 1987.

163. Haskell WL. The Influence of Exercise On the Concentrations of Triglyceride and Cholesterol in Human Plasma. Exerc Sports Sci Rev 12:205–244, 1984.

164. Tall AR, Small DM. Plasma High-Density Lipoproteins. N Eng J Med 299:1232–1236, 1978.

165. Krauss RM. Regulation of High Density Lipoprotein Levels. Med Clin North Am 66:403–430, 1982.

166. Eckel RH. Lipoprotein Lipose. N Engl J Med 320:1060–1068, 1989.

167. Simons LA, Gibson JC. Plasma Lipids and Lipoproteins. IN: Lipids: A Clinicians' Guide. Baltimore: University Park Press, 1980.

168. Patsch JR. Metabolic Aspects of Subfractions of Serum Lipoproteins. IN: Metabolic Risk Factors In Ischemic Cardiovascular Disease (Carlson LA, Pernow B: Eds). New York: Raven Press, 1982.

169. Kottle BA, Zinsmeister AR, Holmes DR, et al. Apoproteins and Coronary Artery Disease. Mayo Clin Proc 61:313–320, 1986.

170. Freedman DS, Srinivasan SR, Shear CL, et al. The Relation of Apolipoproteins A-1 and B in Children to Parental Myocardial Infarction. N Engl J Med 315:721–726, 1986.

171. Manninen V, Elo MO, Frick MH, et al. Lipid Alterations and Decline in the Incidence of Coronary Heart Disease in the Helsinki Heart Study. JAMA 260:641–651, 1988.

172. Castelli WP, Garrison RJ, Wilson PWF, et al. Incidence of Coronary Heart Disease and Lipoprotein Cholesterol Levels: The Framingham Study. JAMA 256:2835–2838, 1986.

173. Green MS, Heiss G, Rifkind BM, et al. The Ratio of Plasma High-Density Lipoprotein Cholesterol to Total and Low-Density Lipoprotein Cholesterol: Age-Related Changes and Race and Sex Differences in Selected North American Populations: The Lipid Research Clinics Programs Prevalence Study. Circulation 72:93–104, 1985.

174. Linn S, Fulwood R, Rifkind B, et al. High Density Lipoprotein Cholesterol Levels Among U.S. Adults by Selected Demographic and Socioeconomic Variables. Am J Epidemiol 129:281–294, 1989.

175. Diehl AK, Fuller JH, Mattock MB, et al. The Relationship of High Density Lipoprotein Subfractions to Alcohol Consumption, Other Lifestyle Factors, and Coronary Heart Disease. Atherosclerosis 69:145–153, 1988.

176. Meilahn EN, Kuller LH, Stein EA, et al. Characteristics Associated with Apoprotein and Lipoprotein Lipid Levels in Middle-Aged Women. Arteriosclerosis 8:515–520, 1988.

177. Patterson CC, McCrum E, McMaster D, et al. Factors Influencing Total Cholesterol and High-Density Lipoprotein Cholesterol Concentrations in a Population at High Coronary Risk. Acta Med Scand Suppl 728:150–158, 1988.

178. DeLong DM, Delong ER, Wood PD, et al. A Comparison of Methods for the 178. Estimation of Plasma Low- and Very Low-Density Lipoprotein Cholesterol. JAMA 256:2372–2377, 1986.

179. Anderson KM, Castelli WP, Levy D. Cholesterol and Mortality: 30 Years of Follow-up From the Framingham Study. JAMA 257:2176–2180, 1987.

180. Levy RI. Cholesterol and Cardiovascular Disease: No Longer Whether, But Rather When, In Whom, and How? Circulation 72:686–691, 1985.

181. World Health Organization. Prevention of Coronary Heart Disease. Geneva: World Health Organization, 1982.

182. Lipid Research Clinics Program: The Lipid Research Clinics Coronary Primary Prevention Trial Results, I and II: JAMA 251:351–374, 1984.

183. Borhani NO. Prevention of Coronary Heart Disease in Practice: Implications of the Results of Recent Clinical Trials. JAMA 254:257–262, 1985.

184. AMA Council on Scientific Affairs. JAMA 250:1873, 1983.

185. American Heart Association Special Report. Recommendations for Treatment of Hyperlipidemias in Adults. Circulation 69:1065A, 1984.

186. American Heart Association. Position Statement: Dietary Guidelines for Healthy American Adults: A Statement for Physicians and Health Professionals by the Nutrition Committee. Circulation 77:721A–724A, 1988.

187. Adult Treatment Panel, National Cholesterol Education Program (National Cholesterol Education Program Expert Panel, National Heart, Lung, and Blood Institute: Report of the National Cholesterol Education Program Expert Panel on Detection, Evaluation, and Treatment of High Blood Cholesterol in Adults. Arch Intern Med 148:36–69, 1988.

188. Consensus Conference. Lowering Blood Cholesterol to Prevent Heart Disease. JAMA 253:2080–2086, 1985.

189. Keys A, Anderson JT, Grand F. Serum Cholesterol Response to Changes in the Diet. The Effect of Cholesterol in the Diet. Metabolism 14:759–765, 1965.

190. Keys A, et al. Serum Cholesterol Response to Changes in the Diet. IV. Particular Saturated Fatty Acids in the Diet. Metabolism 14:776–787, 1965.

191. Hegsted DM. Serum-Cholesterol Response to Dietary Cholesterol: A Re-evaluation. Am J Clin Nutr 44:299–305, 1986.

192. Vorster HH, Silvis N, Venter CS, et al. Serum Cholesterol, Lipoproteins, and Plasma Coagulation Factors in South African Blacks on a High-Egg but Low-Fat Intake. Am J Clin Nutr 46:52–57, 1987.

193. Grundy SM, Vega GL. Plasma Cholesterol Responsiveness to Saturated Fatty Acids. Am J Clin Nutr 47:822–824, 1988.

194. Kris-Etherton PM, Krummel D, Russell ME, et al. The Effect of Diet on Plasma Lipids, Lipoproteins, and Coronary Heart Disease. J Am Diet Assoc 88:1373–1400, 1988.

195. Bonanome A, Grundy SM. Effect of Dietary Stearic Acid on Plasma Cholesterol and Lipoprotein Levels. N Engl J Med 318:1244–1248, 1988.

196. Glueck CJ, Gordon DJ, Nelson JJ, et al. Dietary and Other Correlates of Changes in Total and Low Density Lipoprotein Cholesterol in Hypercholesterolemic Men: the Lipid Research Clinics Coronary Primary Prevention Trial. Am J Clin Nutr 44:489–500, 1986.

197. Baggio G, Pagnan A, Muraca M, et al. Olive-Oil-Enriched Diet: Effect on Serum Lipoprotein Levels and Biliary Cholesterol Saturation. Am J Clin Nutr 47:960–964, 1988.

198. Grundy SM, Florentin L, Nix D, Whelan MF. Comparison of Monounsaturated Fatty Acids and Carbohydrates for Reducing Raised Levels of Plasma Cholesterol in Man. Am J Clin Nutr 47:965–969, 1988.

199. Mattson FH. A Changing Role for Dietary Monounsaturated Fatty Acids. J Am Diet Assoc 89:387–391, 1989.

200. Failor RA, Childs MT, Bierman EL. The Effects of w3 and w6 Fatty Acid-Enriched Diets on Plasma Lipoproteins and Apoproteins in Familial Combined Hyperlipidemia. Metabolism 37:1021–1028, 1988.

201. Harris WS, Dujovne CA, Zucker M, Johnson B. Effects of a Low Saturated Fat, Low Cholesterol Fish Oil Supplement in Hypertriglyceridemic Patients. Ann Int Med 109:465–470, 1988.

202. Schectman G, Kaul S, Cherayil GD, et al. Can the Hypotriglyceridemic Effect of Fish Oil Concentrate Be Sustained? Ann Int Med 110:346–352, 1989.

203. Yetiv JZ. Clinical Applications of Fish Oils. JAMA 260:665–670, 1988.

204. Babayan VK. Am J Clin Nutr 48:1520, 1988.

205. Haskell WL. The Influence of Exercise On the Concentrations of Triglyceride and Cholesterol in Human Plasma. Exerc Sports Sci Rev 12:205–244, 1984.

206. LaCroix AZ, Mead LA, Liang KY, et al. Coffee Consumption and the Incidence of Coronary Heart Disease. N Engl J Med 315:977–982, 1986.

207. LeGrady D, Dyer AR, Shekelle RB, et al. Coffee Consumption and Mortality in the Chicago Western Electric Company Study. Am J Epidemiol 126:803–812, 1987.

208. Rosenberg L, Palmer JR, Kelly JP, Kaufman DW, Shapiro S. Coffee Drinking and Nonfatal Myocardial Infarction in Men Under 55 Years of Age. Am J Epidemiol 128:570–578, 1988.

209. Kromhout D. Body Weight, Diet, and Serum Cholesterol in 871 Middle-Aged Men During 10 Years of Follow-Up (the Zutphen Study). Am J Clin Nutr 38:591–598, 1983.

210. Kark JD, Friedlander Y, Kaufman NA, Stein Y. Coffee, Tea, and Plasma Cholesterol: The Jerusalem Lipid Research Clinic Prevalence Study. Br Med J 291:699, 1985.

211. Aro A, Tuomilehto J, Kostiainen E, Uusitalo U, Pietinen P. Boiled Coffee Increases Serum Low Density Lipoprotein Concentration. Metabolism 36:1027–1030, 1987.

212. Fisher M, Levine PH, Weiner B, et al. The Effect of Vegetarian Diets on Plasma Lipid and Platelet Levels. Arch Intern Med 146:1193–1197, 1986.

213. Freedman DS, Srinivasan SR, Shear CL, et al. The Relation of Apolipoproteins A-1 and B in Children to Parental Myocardial Infarction. N Engl J Med 315:721–726, 1986.

214. Pieper C, LaCroix AZ, Karasek RA. The Relation of Psychosocial Dimensions of Work with Coronary Heart Disease Risk Factors: A Meta-Analysis of Five United States Data Bases. Am J Epidemiol 129:483–494, 1989.

215. Cooper KH. Controlling Cholesterol. New York: Bantam Books, 1988.

216. de Parscau L, Fielding CJ. Abnormal Plasma Cholesterol Metabolism in Cigarette Smokers. Metabolism 35:1070–1073, 1986.

217. Weidner G, Sexton G, McLellarn R, et al. The Role of Type A Behavior and Hostility in an Elevation of Plasma Lipids in Adult Women and Men. Psychosom Med 49:136, 1987.

218. Wood PD, Stefanick ML, Dreon DM, et al. Changes in Plasma Lipids and Lipoproteins in Overweight Men During Weight Loss Through Dieting As Compared With Exercise. N Engl J Med 319:1173–1179, 1988.

219. ADA Reports. Position of The American Dietetic Association: Health Implications of Dietary Fiber. J Am Diet Assoc 88:216–221, 1988.

220. Barrett-Connor E, Khaw KT. Borderline Fasting Hypertriglyceridemia: Absence of Excess Risk of All-Cause and Cardiovascular Disease Mortality in Healthy Men without Hypercholesterolemia. Prev Med 16:1–8, 1987.

221. Austin MA. Plasma Triglyceride as a Risk Factor for Coronary Heart Disease. Am J Epidemiol 129:249–259, 1989.

222. Cambien F, Acqueson A, Richard JL, et al. Is the Level of Serum Triglyceride a Significant Predictor of Coronary Death in "Normocholesterolemia" Subjects? Am J Epidemiol 124:624–632, 1986.

223. Schaefer EJ, Rees DG, Siquel EN. Nutrition, Lipoproteins, and Atherosclerosis. Clin Nutr 5:99–111, 1986.

224. Haskell WL. Exercise-Induced Changes in Plasma Lipids and Lipoproteins. Prev Med 13:23–26, 1984.

225. Tran VZ, Weltman A, Glass GV, Mood DP. The Effects of Exercise On Blood Lipids and Lipoproteins: A Meta-Analysis of Studies. Med Sci Sports Exerc 15:393–402, 1983.

226. Hartung GH. Diet and Exercise in the Regulation of Plasma Lipids and Lipoproteins in Patients At Risk of Coronary Disease. Sports Med 1:413–418, 1984.

227. Wood PD, Terry RB, Haskell WL. Metabolism of Substrates: Diet, Lipoproteins Metabolism, and Exercise. Fed Proc 44:358–363, 1985.

228. Williams PT, Krauss RM, Wood PD, et al. Lipoprotein Subfractions of Runners and Sedentary Men. Metabolism 35:45–52, 1986.

229. Goldberg L, Elliot DL. The Effect of Physical Activity on Lipid and Lipoprotein Levels. Med Clin N Amer 69:41–55, 1985.

230. Baker TT, Allen D, Lei KY, Willcox KK. Alterations in Lipid and Protein Profiles of Plasma Lipoproteins in Middle-Aged Men Consequent to an Aerobic Exercise Program. Metabolism 35:1037–1043, 1986.

231. Cook TC, Laporte RE, Washburn RA, et al. Chronic Low Level Physical Activity as a Determinant of High Density Lipoprotein Cholesterol and Subfractions. Med Sci Sports Exerc 18:653–657, 1986.

232. Schwartz RS. The Independent Effects of Dietary Weight Loss and Aerobic Training on High Density Lipoproteins and Apolipoprotein A-1 Concentrations in Obese Men. Metabolism 36:165–171, 1987.

233. Gordon DJ, Leon AS, Ekelund LG, et al. Smoking, Physical Activity, and Other Predictors of Endurance and Heart Rate Response to Exercise in Asymptomatic Hypercholesterolemic Men. Am J Epidemiol 125:587–600, 1987.

234. Hespel P, Lignen P, Fagard R, et al. Changes in Plasma Lipids and Apoproteins Associated with Physical Training in Middle-Aged Sedentary Men. Am Heart J 115:786–792, 1988.

235. Hanefeld M, Fischer S, Julius U, et al. More Exercise for the Hyperlipidemic Patients? Ann Clin Res 20:77–83, 1988.

236. Schwartz RS. The Independent Effects of Dietary Weight Loss and Aerobic Training on High Density Lipoproteins and Apolipoprotein A-I Concentrations in Obese Men. Metabolism 36:165–171, 1987.

237. Durstine JL, Pate RR, Sparling PB, et al. Lipid, Lipoprotein, and Iron Status of Elite Women Distance Runners. Int J Sports Med 8 (suppl):119–123, 1987.

238. Cauley JA, La Porte RE, Sandler RB, Orchard TJ, Slemenda CW, Petrinin AM. The Relationship of Physical Activity to High Density Lipoprotein Cholesterol in Postmenopausal Women. J Chron Dis 39:687–697, 1986.

239. Jobin J, Lupien PJ, Moorjani S, et al. Association of High Density Lipoprotein Fractions with Leisure-Time Physical Activity in Middle-Aged Men. IN: Dotson CO, Humphrey JH (eds). Exercise Physiology: Current Selected Research. New York: AMS Press, Inc., 1988.

240. Tran ZV, Weltman A. Differential Effects of Exercise On Serum Lipid and Lipoprotein Levels Seen With Changes In Body Weight. JAMA 254:919–924, 1985.

241. Sopko G, Leon AS, et al. The Effects of Exercise and Weight Loss on Plasma Lipids in Young Obese Men. Metabolism 34:227–235, 1985.

242. Lampman RM, Santinga JT, et al. Effect of Exercise Training on Glucose Tolerance, In Vivo Insulin Sensitivity, Lipid and Liproprotein Concentrations in Middle-Aged Men With Mild Hypertriglyceridema. Metabolism 34:205, 1985.

243. Glatter TR. Hyperlipidemia. Postgrad Med 76:49–59, 1984.

244. Nieman DC, Register UD, Lindsted K, Dizon G, De Guia E, Haig J. Effect of Exercise on Serum Lipid and Lipoprotein Levels Seen with Changes in Body Weight. Fed Proc 45:704, 1986 (abstract). Am J Clin Nutr (in press).

245. Stevenson DW, Darga LL, Spafford TR, et al. Variable Effects of Weight Loss on Serum Lipids and Lipoproteins in Obese Patients. Int J Obes 12:495–502, 1987.

246. Schwartz RS. The Independent Effects of Dietary Weight Loss and Aerobic Training on High Density Lipoproteins and Apolipoprotein A-I Concentrations in Obese Men. Metabolism 36:165–171, 1987.

247. Tran ZV, Weltman A. Differential Effects of Exercise on Serum Lipid and Lipoprotein Levels Seen With Changes in Body Weight. JAMA 254:919–924, 1985.

248. Nikkila EA, Kuusi T, Taskinen MR. Role of Lipoprotein Lipase and Hepatic Endothelial Lipase in the Metabolism of High Density Lipoproteins: A Novel Concept on Cholesterol Transport in HDL Cycle. IN: Metabolic Risk Factors In Ischemic Cardiovascular Disease (Carlson LA, Pernow B: Eds). New York: Raven Press, 1982.

249. Kuusi T, et al. Plasma High Density Lipoproteins HDL2, HDL3, and Postheparin Plasma Lipases in Relation to Parameters of Physical Fitness. Atherosclerosis 41:209–219, 1982.

250. Nicoll A, Miller NE, Lewis B. High-Density Lipoprotein Metabolism. Adv Lipid Res 17:53–96, 1980.

251. Sady SP, Cullinane EM, Saritelli A, et al. Elevated High-Density Lipoprotein Cholesterol in Endurance Athletes is Related to Enhanced Plasma Triglyceride Clearance. Metabolism 37:568–572, 1988.

252. Cohen JC, Noakes TD, Benade AJS. Postprandial Lipemia and Chylomicron Clearance in Athletes and in Sedentary Men. Am J Clin Nutr 49:443–447, 1989.

253. Tsopanakis C, Kotsarellis D, Tsopanakis A. Plasma Lecithin: Cholesterol Acyltransferase Activity in Elite Athletes From Selected Sports. Eur J Appl Physiol 58:262–265, 1988.

254. Herbert PN, Bernier DN, et al. High-Density Lipoprotein Metabolism in Runners and Sedentary Men. JAMA 252:1034–1037, 1984.

255. Peltonen P, et al. Changes in Serum Lipids, Lipoproteins, and Heparin Releasable Lipolytic Enzymes During Moderate Physical Training in Man: A Longitudinal Study. Metabolism 30:518–525, 1981.

256. Hazzard WR, Haffner SM, et al. Preliminary Report: Kinetic Studies on the Modulation of High-Density Lipoproteins, Apolipoprotein, and Subfraction Metabolism by Sex Steroids in a Postmenopausal Woman. Metabolism 33:779, 1984.

257. Webb OL, Laskarzewski PM, Glueck CJ. Severe Depression of High-Density Lipoprotein Cholesterol Levels in Weight Lifters and Body Builders by Self-Administered Exogenous Testosterone and Anabolic-Androgenic Steroids. Metabolism 33:971, 1984.

258. Hurley BF, Seals DR, et al. High-Density-Lipoprotein Cholesterol in Bodybuilders v Powerlifters. JAMA 507–513, 1984.

259. Cohen JC, Faber WM, Benada AJS, Noakes TD. Altered Serum Lipoprotein Profiles in Male and Female Power Lifters Ingesting Anabolic Steroids. Physician Sportsmed 14(6):131–136, 1986.

260. Hartung GH. Diet and Exercise in the Regulation of Plasma Lipids and Lipoproteins in Patients At Risk of Coronary Disease. Sports Med 1:413–418, 1984.

261. Kuusi T, Kostiaimen E, Vartiainen E, et al. Acute Effects of Marathon Running on Levels of Serum Lipoproteins and Androgenic Hormones in Healthy Males. Metabolism 33:527–531, 1984.

262. Dufaux B, Order U, Muller R, Hollmann W. Delayed Effects of Prolonged Exercise on Serum Lipoproteins. Metabolism 35:105–109, 1986.

263. Zuliani U, Bonetti A, Cerioli G, Catopano A, Zeppilli P. Plasma Lipids, Lipoproteins and Apoproteins B and A-1 Before and After A 24-Hour Endurance Race In Cross Country Skiers. J Sports Med 26:8–10, 1986.

264. Skinner ER, Black D, Maughan RJ. Variability in the Response of Different Male Subjects to the Effect of Marathon Running on the Increase in Plasma High Density Lipoprotein. Eur J Appl Physiol 54:488–493, 1985.

265. Kantor MA, Cullinane EM, Sady SP, Herbert PN, Thompson PD. Exercise Acutely Increases High Density

Lipoprotein-Cholesterol and Lipoprotein Lipase Activity in Trained and Untrained Men. Metabolism 36:188–192, 1987.

266. Schlierf G, Dinsenbacher A, Kather H, et al. Mitigation of Alimentary Lipemia by Postprandial Exercise—Phenomena and Mechanism. Metabolism 36:726–730, 1987.

267. Skinner ER, Watt C, Maughan RJ. The Acute Effect of Marathon Running on Plasma Lipoproteins in Female Subjects. Eur J Appl Physiol 56:451–456, 1987.

268. Haskell WL. Exercise-Induced Changes in Plasma Lipids and Lipoproteins. Prev Med 13:23–26, 1984.

269. Hicks AL, MacDougall JD, Muckle TJ. Acute Changes in High-Density Lipoprotein Cholesterol With Exercise of Different Intensities. J Appl Physiol 63:1956–1960, 1987.

270. Berger GMB, Griffiths MP. Acute Effects of Moderate Exercise on Plasma Lipoprotein Parameters. Int J Sports Med 8:336–341, 1987.

271. Clarkson PM, Hintermister R, Fillyaw M, et al. High Density Lipoprotein Cholesterol in Young Adult Weight Lifters, Runners, and Untrained Subjects. Hum Biol 53:251–257, 1981.

272. Tsopanakis C, Kotsarellis D, Tsopanakis AD. Lipoprotein and Lipid Profiles of Elite Athletes in Olympic Sports. Int J Sports Med 7:316–321, 1986.

273. Hurley BF, Hagberg JM Goldberg AP, et al. Resistive Training Can Reduce Coronary Risk Factors Without Altering VO2 max or Percent Body Fat. Med Sci Sports Exerc 20:150–154, 1988.

274. Fang CL, Sherman WM, Crouse SF, Tolson H. Exercise Modality and Selected Coronary Risk Factors: A Multivariate Approach. Med Sci Sports Exerc 20:455–462, 1988.

275. Kokkinos PF, Hurley BF, Vaccaro P, et al. Effects of Low- and High-Repetition Resistive Training on Lipoprotein-Lipid Profiles. Med Sci Sports Exerc 20:50–54, 1988.

276. Siscovick DS, Laporte RE, Newman JM. The Disease-Specific Benefits and Risks of Physical Activity and Exercise. Public Health Rep 100:180–188, 1985.

277. Laporte RE, Adams LL, et al. The Spectrum of Physical Activity, Cardiovascular Disease and Health: An Epidemiologic Perspective. Am J Epidemiol 120:507–517, 1984.

278. Poole GW. Exercise, Coronary Heart Disease and Risk Factors: A Brief Report. Sports Med 1:341–349, 1984.

279. Paffenbarger RS, et al. Physical Activity As An Index of Heart Attack Risk in College Alumni. Am J Epidemiol 108:161–174, 1978.

280. Leon AS. Physical Activity Levels and Coronary Heart Disease. Med Clin North Am 69:3–19, 1985.

281. Powell KE, Thompson PD, Caspersen CJ, Kendrick JS. Physical Activity and the Incidence of Coronary Heart Disease. Annu Rev Public Health 8:253–287, 1987.

282. Eichner ER. Exercise and Heart Disease: Epidemiology of the "Exercise Hypothesis." Amer J Med 75:1008–1023.

283. Sobolski J, Kornitzer M, Backer GD, et al. Protection Against Ischemic Heart Disease in the Belgian Physical Fitness Study: Physical Fitness Rather Than Physical Activity? Am J Epidemiol 125:601–610, 1987.

284. Mundal R, Erikssen J, Rodahl K. Assessment of Physical Activity by Questionnaire and Personal Interview With Particular Reference to Fitness and Coronary Mortality. Eur J Appl Physiol 56:245–252, 1987.

285. Scragg R, Stewart A, Jackson R, Beaglehole R. Alcohol and Exercise in Myocardial Infarction and Sudden Coronary Death in Men and Women. Am J Epidemiol 126:77–85, 1987.

286. Leon AS, Connett J, Jacobs DR, Rauramaa R. Leisure-Time Physical Activity Levels and Risk of Coronary Heart Disease and Death: The Multiple Risk Factor Intervention Trial. JAMA 258:2388–2395, 1987.

287. Salonen JT, Slater JS, Tuomilehto J, Rauramaa R. Leisure Time and Occupational Physical Activity: Risk of Death from Ischemic Heart Disease. Am J Epidemiol 127:87–94, 1988.

288. Slattery ML, Jacobs DR. Physical Fitness and Cardiovascular Disease Mortality: The US Railroad Study. Am J Epidemiol 127:571–580, 1988.

289. Donahue RP, Abbott RD, Reed DM, Yano K. Physical Activity and Coronary Heart Disease in Middle-Aged and Elderly Men: The Honolulu Heart Program. Am J Public Health 78:683–685, 1988.

290. Ekelund LG, Haskell WL, Johnson JL, et al. Physical Fitness As A Predictor of Cardiovascular Mortality in Asymptomatic North American Men: The Lipid Research Clinics Mortality Follow-Up Study. N Engl J Med 319:1379–1384, 1988.

291. Morris JN, et al. Vigorous Exercise In Leisure-Time: Protection Against Coronary Heart Disease. Lancet 2:1207, 1980.

292. Paffenbarger RS. Physical Activity and Fatal Heart Attack: Protection or Selection. IN: Exercise in Cardiovascular Health and Disease (Amsterdam EA, Wilmore JH, DeMaria AN: Eds). New York: Yorke Medical Books, 1977.

293. Paffenbarger RS, Hyde RT, Wing AL, Steinmetz CH. A Natural History of Athleticism and Cardiovascular Health. JAMA 252:491–495, 1984.

294. Siscovick DS, Weiss NS, et al. The Incidence of Primary Cardiac Arrest During Vigorous Exercise. N Eng J Med 311:874–877, 1984.

295. Siscovick DS, Weiss NS, et al. Habitual Vigorous Exercie and Primary Cardiac Arrest: Effect of Other Risk Factors on the Relationship. J Chron Dis 37:625–631, 1984.

296. Siscovick DS, Laporte RE, Newman JM. The Disease-Specific Benefits and Risks of Physical Activity and Exercise. Public Health Rep 100:180–188, 1985.

297. Folsom AR, Caspersen CJ, et al. Leisure Time Physical Activity and Its Relationship to Coronary Risk Factors In A Population-Based Sample. Am J Epidemiol 121:570–579, 1985.

298. Blair SN. Physical Activity Leads to Fitness and Pays Off. Physician Sportsmed 13:153–157, 1985.

299. Patton JF, Vogel JA, Bedynek JL, Alexander D, Albright R. Aerobic Capacity and Coronary Risk Factors in a Middle-Aged Army Population. J Cardiopulmonary Rehabil 6:491–498, 1986.

300. Sallis JF, Patterson TL, Buono MJ, Nader PR. Relation of Cardiovascular Fitness and Physical Activity to Cardiovascular Disease Risk Factors in Children and Adults. Am J Epidemiol 127:933–941, 1988.

301. Tell GS, Vellar OD. Physical Fitness, Physical Activity, and Cardiovascular Disease Risk Factors in Adolescents: The Oslo Youth Study. Prev Med 17:12–24, 1988.

302. Gibbons LW, Blairs SN, Cooper KH, Smith MS. Association Between Coronary Heart Disease Risk Factors and Physical Fitness in Healthy Adult Women. Circulation 67:977–983, 1983.

303. Scheuer J. Effects of Physical Training on Myocardial Vascularity and Perfusion. Circulation 66:491–495, 1982.

304. Pearl PM. The Effects of Exercise on the Development and Function of the Coronary Collateral Circulation. Sports Med 4:86–94, 1987.

305. Kavanagh T. Does Exercise Improve Coronary Collaterization? A New Look at an Old Belief. Physician Sportsmed 17(11):96–114, 1989.

306. Dix CJ, Hassall DG, Bruckdorfer R. The Increased Sensitivity of Platelets to Prostacyclin In Marathon Runners. Thromb Haemostas (Stuttgart) 51:385–387, 1984.

307. Eichner ER. Coagulability and Rheology: Hematologic Benefits From Exercise, Fish, and Aspirin. Implications for Athletes and Nonathletes. Physician Sportsmed 14(10):102–110, 1986.

308. Ferguson EW, Bernier LL, Batna GR, et al. Effects of Exercise and Conditioning On Clotting and Fibrinolytic Activity in Men. J Appl Physiol 62:1416–1421, 1987.

309. Kramsch DM, et al. Reduction of Coronary Atherosclerosis By Moderate Conditioning Exercise in Monkeys On An Atherogenic Diet. N Eng J Med 305:1483–1488, 1981.

310. Hubbard JD, Inkeles S, Barnard RJ. Nathan Pritikin's Heart. N Eng J Med 313:52, 1985.

311. Kramsch DM, et al. Reduction of Coronary Atherosclerosis By Moderate Conditioning Exercise in Monkeys On An Atherogenic Diet. N Eng J Med 305:1483–1488, 1981.

312. Arntzenius AC, et al. Diet, Lipoproteins, and the Progression of Coronary Atherosclerosis. N Eng J Med 312:805–811, 1985.

313. Superko HR. The Role of Diet, Exercise, and Medication in Blood Lipid Management of Cardiac Patients. Physician Sportsmed 16(11):65–82, 1988.

314. Pollock ML, Wilmore JH, Fox SM. Exercise In Health and Disease. Philadelphia: W. B. Saunders Co., 1984.

315. Wilson PK. Cardiac Rehabilitation: Then and Now. Physician Sportsmed 16(9):75–84, 1988.

316. Ben-Ari E, Kellermann JJ, Fisman EZ, Pines A, Peled B, Drory Y. Benefits of Long-Term Physical Training in Patients After Coronary Artery Bypass Grafting—A 58-Month Follow-up and Comparison With a Nontrained Group. J Cardiopulmonary Rehabil 6:165–170, 1986.

317. Wilson PK, Fardy PS, Froelicher VF. Cardiac Rehabilitation, Adult Fitness, and Exercise Testing. Philadelphia: Lea and Febiger, 1981.

318. Wilhelmsen L, Sanne H, Elmfeldt D, et al. A Controlled Trial of Physical Training After Myocardial Infarction. Effects On Risk Factors, Non-fatal Reinfarction and Death. Prev Med 4:491–508, 1975.

319. Rechnitzer PA, et al. Relation of Exercise to the Recurrence Rate of Myocardial Infarction in Men. Am J Cardiol 51:65–69, 1983.

320. Hagberg JM, Ehsani AA, Holloszy JO. Effect of 12 Months of Intense Exercise Training on Stroke Volume in Patients With Coronary Artery Disease. Circulation 67:1194–1199, 1983.

321. Shephard RJ. Does Cardiac Rehabilitation After Myocardial Infarction Favorably Affect Prognosis? Physician Sportsmed 16(6):116–127, 1988.

322. Kallio V, et al. Reduction In Sudden Death by a Multifactorial Intervention Programs After Acute Myocardial Infarction. Lancet 11:1091–1094, 1979.

323. Fardy PS. Home-Based Cardiac Rehabilitation. Physician Sportsmed 15(12):89–94, 1987.

324. Van Camp SP, Peterson RA. Cardiovascular Complications of Outpatient Cardiac Rehabilitation Programs. JAMA 256:1160–1163, 1986.

Physical Fitness Activity 10.1— Heart Chec Plus

For this physical fitness activity, you will be determining your overall coronary heart disease risk by answering the questions in the Heart Chec Plus questionnaire (Figure 10.22) and taking several tests, including resting blood pressure, height and weight, frame size, and blood lipid profile. The blood lipid tests (total cholesterol, HDL-C, triglycerides, and glucose) can be taken from a local medical clinic. After filling in the questionnaire data, a computer software program called Heart Check Plus from Wellsource Inc., should be used to calculate your final risk profile score. This is an excellent computer software program, and can be ordered from the following address:

Wellsource
15431 Southeast 82nd Drive, Suite D
P.O. Box 569
Clackamas, OR 97015

HEART CHEC PLUS
QUESTIONNAIRE

INSTRUCTION

Heart Chec is a coronary risk screening and education program for the prevention of heart disease. Several health tests will be made including: blood test for total cholesterol, HDL cholesterol, blood fats (triglycerides) and blood sugar levels, a blood pressure check, and height and weight analysis. A health and lifestyle history is also taken to identify other risk factors. All information is kept confidential and is used only for developing the coronary risk profile.

The test data is then entered into a computer that develops a personal coronary risk profile, calculates your probability of developing coronary heart disease in the next eight years, and makes recommendations on how you may reduce your risk of heart disease. A group evaluation will be presented to explain your test results and answer any questions you may have.

INFORMED CONSENT AND RELEASE

I understand the purpose of this coronary risk evaluation program and do willingly consent to have my blood drawn and other tests performed for the purpose of developing a coronary risk profile with recommendations. I release the sponsoring organization(s) and personnel involved from any responsibility or liability for any injury or health consequence that may occur from my participation in this program. I further assume all responsibility for obtaining medical or other professional help for any health problem(s) identified in this program.

Participant _____

Witness _____

Date _____

BIOGRAPHICAL DATA

Name (print) _____

Address _____

City _____

State _____ Zip _____

_____-_____-_____ Phone

_____-_____-____ Date

2 1 M 1 F Sex

3 _____ Age

4 1 Yes 1 No Have you had any food or drink (other than water) in the last 14 hours? Describe

_____

5 How long has it been since you had a thorough physical exam?
1 Less than one year
1 One to two years
1 Three to five years
1 Six to ten years
1 Ten to twenty years
1 More than twenty years

DISEASES

Check those diseases that apply to you or your family history.

Family History	Personal History	
6 1	22 1	Asthma
7 1	23 1	Emphysema
8 1	24 1	Cirrhosis
9 1	25 1	Diabetes
10 1	26 1	Gout
11 1	27 1	Heart Disease
12 1	28 1	Heart Attack
13 1	29 1	High blood pressure
14 1	30 1	Kidney disease
15 1	31 1	Lung disease
16 1	32 1	Nervous breakdown
17 1	33 1	Overweight
18 1	34 1	Peptic ulcer
19 1	35 1	Stroke
20 1	36 1	Thyroid, low
21 1	37 1	Thyroid, high

* If you do have a family history of heart disease, how many blood relatives died before the age of 60? _____

SYMPTOMS

Do you encounter pain or discomfort in the chest after:
38 1 Yes 1 No Exercise
39 1 Yes 1 No Exposure to cold
40 1 Yes 1 No Eating
41 1 Yes 1 No When nervous or tense

Are you bothered by:
42 1 Yes 1 No Shortness of breath after climbing a flight of stairs
43 1 Yes 1 No Dizziness
44 1 Yes 1 No Chronic cough
45 1 Yes 1 No Pain in legs when walking or climbing stairs
46 1 Yes 1 No Excessive thirst and urination

Figure 10.22 Heart Chec Plus Questionnaire

MEDICATIONS

Check those medications you <u>currently</u> are taking.

47 1 Birth control pills
48 1 Hormones
49 1 Thyroid
50 1 Blood pressure medicine
51 1 Heart medicine
52 1 Other

EXERCISE STATUS

53 1 Yes 1 No Does your employment require vigorous, sustained physical activity?

54 How often do you engage (for 20 minutes or more) in vigorous, aerobic exercise such as walking, jogging, cycling, swimming, active sports, etc.?
1 Don't exercise regularly
1 1 time a week
1 2 times a week
1 3 times a week
1 4 times a week
1 5 times a week
1 6+ times a week

STRESS/RELAXATION STATUS

55 1 Yes 1 No Do you frequently experience severe nervous tension?
56 1 Yes 1 No Do you often experience excessive stress and pressures?
57 1 Yes 1 No Are you generally considered highly competitive and hard driving?
58 1 Yes 1 No Do you take time to relax regularly and do things you enjoy?
59 1 Yes 1 No Do you take regular vacations?
60 1 Yes 1 No Do you get 7-8 hours sleep per night?

SMOKING STATUS

61 How much do you smoke?
1 Never smoked
1 Stopped smoking more than 10 years ago
1 Stopped smoking less than 10 years ago
1 Smoke 1 pack a day
1 Smoke 2 packs a day
1 Smoke 3 or more packs a day

DRINKING STATUS

62 How often do you drink alcoholic beverages?
1 Don't drink
1 Have 1-2 drinks a session
1 Have 3-4 drinks a session
1 Have 5-6 drinks a session
1 Have 7 or more drinks a session

63 How often do you drink coffee, cola, and other caffeinated beverages?
1 Don't drink these
1 Drink 1-2 cups a day
1 Drink 3-4 cups a day
1 Drink 5-6 cups a day
1 Drink 7 or more cups a day

EATING HABITS

64 1 Yes 1 No I usually eat a good breakfast.
65 1 Yes 1 No I often snack between meals.
66 1 Yes 1 No I often eat my main meal after 7 p.m.
67 1 Yes 1 No I eat a vegetarian diet (no meat, fish, or fowl).
68 1 Yes 1 No I use shortening as the primary fat in cooking.
69 1 Yes 1 No Primarily, I use butter for a spread.
70 1 Yes 1 No Primarily, I use whole milk.
71 1 Yes 1 No Primarily, I use whole wheat bread and cereal products.
72 1 Yes 1 No I salt food freely.

NUTRITION DATA

Enter the **number** of servings eaten.

73 ____ Usual # of desserts a week (cookies, candy, pop, cake, pie, ice cream, etc.)
74 ____ Usual # of servings of meat a week
75 ____ Usual # of servings of fish or fowl a week
76 ____ Usual # of servings of organ meat or shellfish a week
77 ____ Usual # of servings of cream, toppings, or cheese a week
78 ____ Usual # of eggs eaten a week (including those used in cooking and in prepared foods)
79 ____ Usual # of servings of deep fried food a week (French fries, doughnuts, potato chips)

HEALTH SCREENING DATA

To be filled in by test personnel only.

80 ____ Height in inches (No shoes; 5' = 60")
81 ____ Weight in pounds (Light clothing)
82 ____ Frame size (S = small, M = medium, L = large)
83 ____ Resting heart rate per minute
84 ____ Systolic blood pressure (sitting)
85 ____ Diastolic blood pressure
86 ____ Total cholesterol mg/dl
87 ____ HDL mg/dl (high density lipoproteins)
88 ____ Triglycerides mg/dl
89 ____ Glucose mg/dl
90 ____ ECG results
1 = Normal
2 = Borderline
3 = Abnormal (LVH, ST segment depression, significant Q waves)
4 = Not done
Comments:

Chapter 11

Physical Activity and Obesity

"The success of a weight loss program should be measured by the type of weight which is lost and the overall health status of the individual rather than the total weight loss."[1]

Obesity in America

Thin is in, yet as we shall see in this section, Americans are among the fattest people in the world. Despite our thin standards of beauty, society at the same time promotes "fat" ways of living and a sedentary lifestyle.

As defined in Chapter 5, obesity is a condition of excess body fat. (See Figure 11.1.) National studies of Americans during the last 30 years show that many are overweight and obese. Obesity affects about 34 million adults ages 20 to 74, with the highest rates among the poor and minority groups.[2] For adult men and women, 24.4 and 26.7 percent, respectively, are considered obese (defined in most national studies as a body mass index greater than approximately 27 kg/m^2, or 20 percent overweight).[2-7] The Government's year 2000 goal is to reduce the prevalence of obesity in the U.S. adult population to no more than 20 percent.

Figure 11.2 shows that the prevalence of obesity is very high for black females—nearly 50 percent. There was little change in the incidence of obesity between 1960 and 1980.[2,4-6]

Although approximately one in four Americans is considered obese, a majority of American adults weigh more than they should. Among those over 40, 80 percent of men and 70 percent of women are more than 10 percent overweight.[8] The average U.S. female is now 64 inches tall, weighing 142 pounds. This is 16 pounds more than is recommended. The average U.S. male is 69.5 inches tall, and weighs in at 173 pounds, 12 pounds more than is recommended.

Some people insist that America no longer be called "the land of the free" but instead "the land of the fat." Apparently the United States has a greater percentage of overweight people than either Canada or Britain.[9] (See Figure 11.3.)

National surveys also reveal that a large number of our children and teenagers are obese.[10, 11] Among American children and youth 6 to 17 years of age, 28.9 percent of the boys and 25.2 percent of the girls are considered obese. When comparing current figures with those from 1965, the percentage of obese children 6 to 11 years in the 1980s is approximately 54 percent higher, and among youth 12 to 17 years of age, 39 percent higher. (See Figure 11.4.)

Figure 11.5 shows that both males and females differ in their degree of fatness during various stages of the life-cycle.[12, 13] Males experience a decrease in fatness at puberty, while females experience an increase. Peak fatness for both sexes occurs at age 50, followed by a decrease.

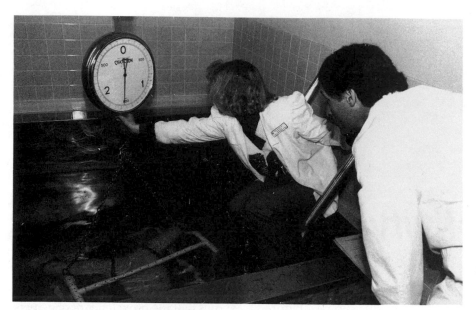

Figure 11.1 Obesity is defined as a condition of excess body fat. This is best measured using underwater weighing techniques as described in Chapter 5.

The 1985 National Health Interview Survey revealed that obesity is more prevalent among married than unmarried, Black than White, lower than higher income, and lower than the higher educated.[14] In other words, obesity is more prevalent among the lower socio-economic status groups in the United States.

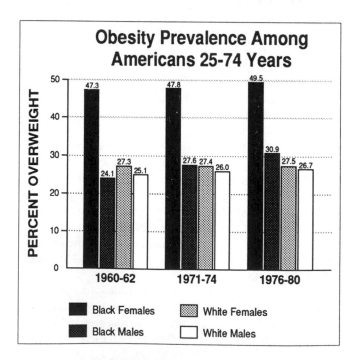

Figure 11.2 Close to one out of four American adults is considered obese—but the prevalence of obesity is much higher among black females. *Source:* see reference 2.

Disadvantages of Obesity

Researchers have estimated that altogether, adult Americans carry an excess of 2.3 billion pounds of fat.[15] These Calories represent the energy potential of 1–3 billion gallons of gasoline. This American tendency to store excess energy as fat is associated with many health problems[15–37]—in fact, it constitutes one of the more important medical and public health problems of our time.[16] Hippocrates said it long ago: "When more food than is proper has been taken, it occasions disease."

The National Institutes of Health has summarized the large number of health problems associated with obesity.[7] There are at least seven major health problems.[15–37]

- **A Psychological Burden:** As noted earlier, in setting standards of beauty, Americans think thin—but they live fat. Some have called our era the "age of Caloric anxiety." Because of the strong pressures from society to be thin, obese people often suffer feelings of guilt, depression, anxiety, and low self-esteem. In terms of suffering, this may be the greatest burden of obesity, especially among adolescents.[34]

- **Increased High Blood Pressure:** High blood pressure is three times as common among the obese as it is among normal-weight people.[23, 27, 28, 33] Recent studies are showing that even among schoolchildren, increases in obesity are associated with corresponding increases in blood pressure.[24, 27]

- **Increased Levels of Cholesterol and Other Lipids in the Blood:** the obese, including children, are

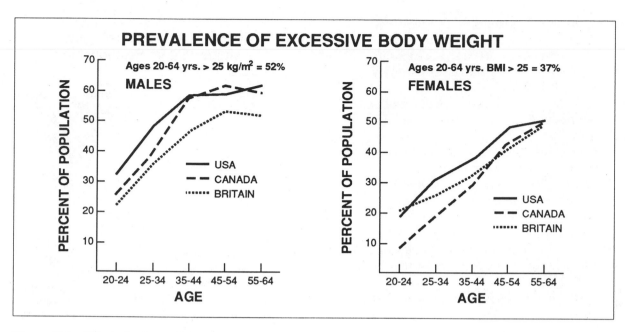

Figure 11.3 When obesity is defined as a body mass index greater than 25 kg/m², a greater percentage of American adults are obese than those of either Canada or Britain. *Source:* see reference 9.

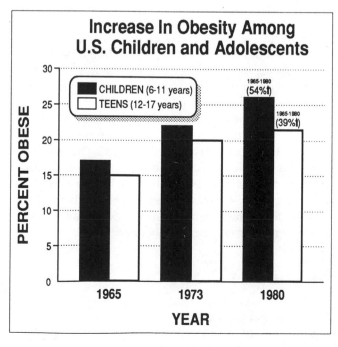

Figure 11.4 Prevalence of obesity among U.S. children and adolescents rose strongly between 1965 and 1980. *Source:* see reference 10.

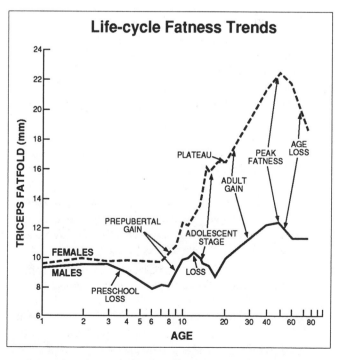

Figure 11.5 Males and females experience different trends in fatness with an increase in age. *Source:* see reference 13.

more likely to have higher blood cholesterol, triglyceride, and LDL-C levels, and lower HDL-C levels.[27–31,33] The prevention of obesity in early life may be important in reducing the risk of coronary heart disease in later life.

■ **Increased Diabetes:** The prevalence of diabetes is nearly three times as high among the obese.[7,23,33] Weight loss by *Type II diabetics* often results in dramatic improvements in their blood glucose and insulin levels. (See Chapter 14.)

■ **Increased Cancer:** The American Cancer Society study involving one million men and women showed that obese males had a higher mortality rate from cancer of the colon, rectum, and prostate. Obese females had a higher mortality rate from cancer of the gallbladder, bile ducts, breast, uterus, and ovaries.[7,17,26,33]

■ **Increased Early Death:** Hippocrates, the ancient Greek physician, once noted that "sudden death is more common in those who are naturally fat than in the lean." Several modern studies have confirmed the wisdom of Hippocrates. Various studies in the United States and elsewhere have confirmed the association between obesity and mortality rates.[7,15,25,26,30,35–37] (See Figure 11.6.) The overall relationship is represented by a J-shaped curve, with the lowest mortality for both men and women occurring among people somewhat below the average body mass index.

Mortality from lung cancer and digestive diseases increases with decreasing fatness, while mortality from heart disease, cancer, and diabetes increases with increasing fatness.[15] Minimum mortality is associated with a body weight at least 10 percent below the average for Americans, after adjustment for cigarette smoking.[25,32] If the American population lost its excess body mass, it would reduce mortality by 15 percent, corresponding to three years of added life expectancy.[15]

The American Cancer Society followed 750,000 men and women for 12 years and found that those at least 40 percent over average weight had death rates from all causes nearly twice those of average-weight people.[25] (See Table 11.1.)

■ **Increased Heart Disease:** Obese people have more of the typical risk factors for *heart disease* (high blood pressure and serum cholesterol levels), and they die from it at a higher rate.[7,26,30,33,37] It has been estimated that if everyone were at optimal weight there would be 25 percent less *coronary heart disease* and 35 percent less *congestive heart failure* and *stroke*.[15]

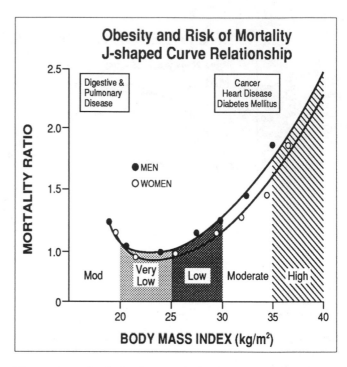

Figure 11.6   As the body mass index increases, mortality from heart disease, cancer, and diabetes also increases. Individuals with digestive diseases and pulmonary diseases (most due to cigarette smoking) that lead to loss of body weight tend to die early. *Source:* see reference 15.

Recent information is showing that it makes a difference where the excess fat is deposited, with respect to medical complications.[33,38–48] The obese people most vulnerable to heart disease, high blood pressure and cholesterol, diabetes, and early death tend to have more of their fat deposited in abdominal areas rather than the hip and thigh areas.

In other words, health risks are greater for those who have most of their body fat in the upper body, especially the trunk and abdominal areas. This is called *android obesity* in comparison to *gynoid obesity* (characterized by deposition of body fat in the hips and thighs). (See Figure 11.7.) This can be measured by looking at the ratio of waist-to-hip circumferences. (See Chapter 5.) A high ratio predicts more complications from obesity.

Theories of Obesity

Explaining why so many Americans weigh more than they should has been a source of confusion to researchers and the public alike. Currently, most theories of obesity fall into three categories: genetic and parental influences, high energy intake, and low energy expenditure.[49–52] (See Figure 11.8.)

Table 11.1 Mortality Rates for Obese Versus Normal-Weight Men and Women*

	Women		Men	
	120–129%	140%+	120–129%	140%+
All causes of death	1.29	1.89	1.27	1.87

Source: See reference 25.

*Mortality rate of 1.0 equals death rate for normal-weight people.

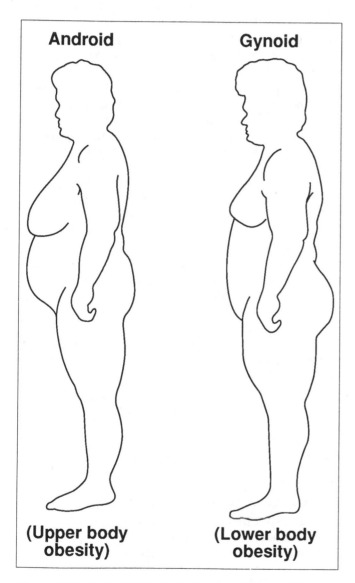

Figure 11.7 Android obesity is characterized by high amounts of body fat in the trunk and abdominal areas, and is associated with increased medical complications. Gynoid obesity is characterized by high amounts of body fat in the hip and thigh areas.

The development of obesity involves a prolonged period in which energy intake exceeds energy expenditure. Beyond that, however, the relative importance of persistent overeating, abnormally low energy expenditure, or both, and the influence of heredity remains controversial.

Genetic and Parental Influences

Several studies have suggested that genetic and parental factors are important in explaining why some find it difficult to avoid obesity.[53–56] A recent study comparing adult fraternal and identical twins found that the body weights of the identical twins were much closer together than the body weights of the fraternal twins were.[54]

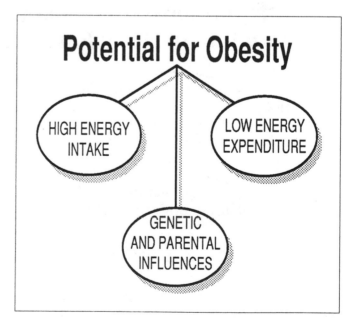

Figure 11.8 The theories of obesity fall into three categories.

A study of adults who had been adopted before the age of one revealed that despite being brought up by their adoptive parents, their body weights were still very similar to those of their real parents.[55]

In perhaps the best study yet on the role genetics play in obesity, 1698 members of 409 families were studied, including spouses, foster parents-adopted children, siblings by adoption, first-degree cousins, uncles/aunts-nephews/nieces, parents-natural children, full siblings, dizygotic twins, and monozygotic twins.[56] Biological inheritance was found to account for only 25 percent of the variance in fat mass. (See Figure 11.9.) Thus nongenetic influences such as lifestyle and environmental and cultural factors were shown to be more important.

These studies do demonstrate, however, that some people are more prone to obesity than others because of genetic factors. Such people have to be unusually careful with their dietary and exercise habits to counteract these inherited tendencies.

Another apparently genetic factor relates to the number of fat cells in the body. Fat cell number can increase two to three-fold as a result of overeating, and once formed, the extra fat cells cannot be removed by the body.[49, 57] This is called *hyperplasia obesity*. This can happen anytime during the life-span, but infants seem to be particularly susceptible, when their fat cells are still dividing. (Figure 11.10)

Infants who form extra fat cells when overnourished tend to remain overfat as children.[58-60] And obese children and teenagers can remain obese as adults. In one study, 36 percent of obese adults had been overly heavy as infants, with twice as many of the obese women reporting they had been obese as children.[58]

High Energy Intake

There is some evidence that obese people tend to consume more Calories than normal-weight people, choosing larger portions of rich foods that are high in fats and sugars.[15,61-63] Some researchers, however, have reported the opposite—that obese people do not eat more.[64,65] But obese people may underreport the actual amount of food they eat, especially any food eaten during binge eating.[66-68] In one study, nearly half of obese women were found to have a serious problem with *binge eating*, compared to only 10 to 15 percent of normal weight women.[69]

There is good reason to believe that the abundant availability of tasty, calorically rich foods, especially those high in fat, is the primary reason why so many Americans are overweight.[15, 57, 70-78] The average American consumes nearly 40 percent of Calories as fat, much higher than the 25 to 30 percent recommended. In the laboratory much evidence has accumulated from studies with rats and other animals that this amount of dietary fat can itself be a cause of obesity.[57]

The most commonly used dietary means of inducing obesity in rats is to feed them a high-fat diet.[49, 57] When the fat content of the rat diet (which in standard chows is 2–6 percent) is increased to 30–60 percent, rats typically become obese. The rats appear to enjoy the extra dietary fat so much that they consume more Calories than normal.

Rats also become very obese on "supermarket diets"—such foods as chocolate chip cookies, salami, cheese, marshmallows, milk chocolate, peanut butter, and sweetened whole milk.[49]

Most studies have shown that naturally lean people have a very difficult time gaining weight on low-fat regimens, but gain easily when the diet is high in fat.[70-79]

In one study, 24 women consumed a progression of three 2-week diets that derived 15–20 percent, 30–35 percent, and 45–50 percent, respectively, of Calories from fat.[72] The diets were similar in appearance and taste, but differed in the amount of high-fat ingredients used. The mean daily intakes on the low-, medium-, and high-fat diets, respectively, were 2,087, 2,352, and 2,714

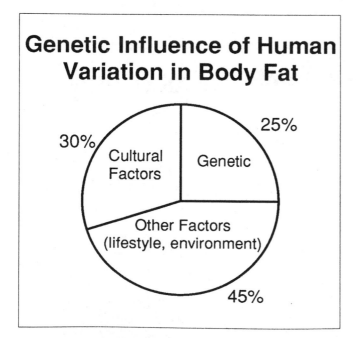

Genetic Influence of Human Variation in Body Fat

25% Genetic
30% Cultural Factors
Other Factors (lifestyle, environment)
45%

Figure 11.9 Genetic influences on obesity are considered less important than nongenetic influences such as cultural, environmental, and lifestyle factors. *Source:* see reference 56.

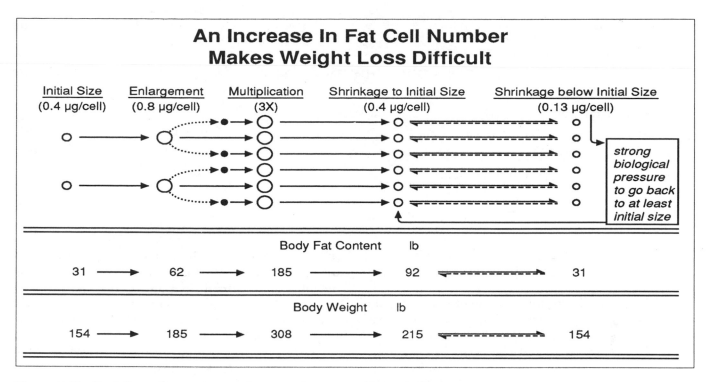

Figure 11.10 Fat cell number can increase because of overnourishment during any time of life, and this increase is irreversible. In the sample case outlined in this figure, once cell number increases, it is nearly impossible to reduce body weight back to normal because of strong biological pressures to keep fat cells at near normal size. *Source:* see reference 49.

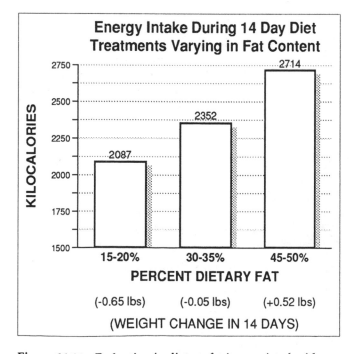

Figure 11.11 Reduction in dietary fat is associated with a lower caloric intake and weight loss. *Source:* see reference 72.

Calories. (See Figure 11.11.) The women spontaneously consumed 27 percent fewer Calories on the low-fat diet compared to the high-fat diet, resulting in significant changes in body weight.

Thus the habitual consumption of low-fat diets may be an effective approach to weight control. It has promise not offered by traditional restrictive diets because there are no strict limitations on the quantity of food consumed.

The importance of a low-fat, high-carbohydrate, high-fiber diet for both prevention and treatment of obesity cannot be emphasized enough.[75-79] In another study, obese and non-obese people were allowed to eat until satisfied under two different conditions.[77] In Phase 1 of the study, only low-Calorie, high-carbohydrate, high-fiber foods were offered. In Phase 2, only high-Calorie, high-fat, low-fiber foods were allowed. Researchers found that both the obese and the non-obese groups prolonged their eating time by 33 percent and felt satisfied after only consuming 1,570 Calories per day in Phase 1 of the diet (whole grains, vegetables, salads, fruits, low-fat dairy products). During Phase 2, however, they felt satisfied only after consuming 3,000

Table 11.2 The Effects of a Low Versus High Energy Diet on Energy Intake

	Low Energy Diet	High Energy Diet
Fiber	7 grams/1,000 kcal	1 gram/1,000 kcal
Energy Intake (kcal/day)	1,570	3,000
Satiety Score*	5.1	5.5
Total Eating Time (min/day)	69	52

*Scale of 0 (extremely hungry) to 10 (full to nausea)

Source: see reference 77.

Calories per day. It appears that the human body can avoid obesity if the fat content of the diet is low. (See Table 11.2.)

Why does dietary fat promote obesity so easily among both rats and humans? One explanation is that the body uses less Calories to process dietary fat than to process dietary carbohydrate. Figure 11.12 shows that if a person consumes 100 extra Calories from dietary fat (for example, one tablespoon of butter), only three Calories are used by the body to transform the butter into body fat. However, 100 extra Calories of carbohydrate require 23 Calories to make the transformation. In other words, a given caloric quantity of excess dietary fat is more fattening than a calorically comparable quantity of excess carbohydrate.[71]

Another study has shown that when obese women are given 2,000 Calories of carbohydrate all at once (one huge meal), only 20 Calories are actually stored as fat.[70] The body has a difficult time turning the carbohydrate into fat, and when it does, the majority of the fat is used for metabolism.[73] This is vitally important information. The message is this—pasta, potatoes, and bread do not make people nearly as fat as the high fat sauce, sour cream, and margarine used with them!

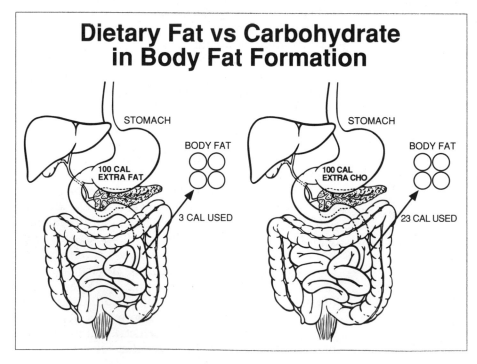

Figure 11.12 The body converts dietary fat into body fat more efficiently than it converts dietary carbohydrate into body fat. *Source:* see reference 71.

Low Energy Expenditure

All humans expend energy in three ways—through the *resting metabolic rate*, physical activity, and digesting and metabolizing food *(thermic effect of food)*.[71, 76] (See Figure 11.13.)

Resting Metabolic Rate

The largest number of Calories expended by most people (except for athletes who train several hours a day) is from the *resting metabolic rate* (RMR). This represents the energy expended by the body to maintain life and normal body functions, such as respiration and circulation. The resting metabolic rate of the average 154-pound male amounts to approximately 1,600 Calories per day, or 60 to 75 percent of total daily energy expenditure. This is a considerable amount of energy, equivalent to jogging 16 miles!

The RMR is best measured by collecting and analyzing expired air *(indirect calorimetry)* several hours after eating. RMR can also be estimated through the use of equations. Table 11.3 summarizes some of the more commonly used equations.[80-82]

Amazingly enough, an obese person actually has a higher RMR than a normal weight person.[71,76,83-87] This is because the RMR is closely tied to the amount of lean body weight (nonfat tissue such as muscle and bone). Obese people, because of the extra weight they must carry, have more lean body weight—resulting in a higher RMR.

Obese people have daily RMRs approximately 500 Calories higher than those of non-obese people.[88, 89] However, when obese people lose their excess weight, RMR tends in drop and with some (especially those who have been severely obese), RMR may be 15–20 percent below that of normal weight people of similar heights and weights.[33, 90, 91] The factors behind the lower than normal RMR in the post-obese are unknown.

The excess weight of mildly and moderately obese people is approximately 25 percent lean body tissue and 75 percent fat.[33] With each kilogram of body weight loss, the RMR drops approximately 20 Calories per day. A loss of 20 kilograms will reduce RMR by approximately 400 Calories per day.

Physical Activity

All *physical activity*, all muscular movement, expends Calories. The average sedentary person usually expends only 300–800 Calories a day in physical activity, most of this from informal, unplanned types of movement. On the other hand, top athletes usually match their RMR energy expenditure through hard, intense exercise. For optimal health, most physical fitness experts recommend burning at least 200 to 400 Calories per day through planned exercise. (See Chapter 8.)

Table 11.4 outlines the average energy expenditure of a moderately active person. Most Americans fall far short of this level. Physical Fitness Activity 11.1 will help you determine how many Calories you expend each day.

Do the obese exercise more or less than normal-weight people? Although measurement of physical activity is extremely difficult, most studies show that both obese children and adults are less active than normal weight people.[15, 16, 49, 52, 88, 93–100] Overweight girls have been found to be less active than lean ones while playing sports.[96] For example, obese adolescent girls when swimming spend less time actually moving their arms and legs and more time standing and floating than normal-weight girls. While playing tennis, obese girls have been found to be inactive 77 percent of the time

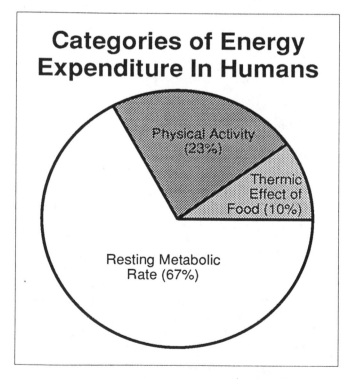

Figure 11.13 Approximately 67 percent of human energy expenditure is from the resting metabolic rate. Sedentary people expend about 23 percent of their energy in miscellaneous physical activity, and another 10 percent metabolizing and digesting food. *Source:* see references 71 and 76.

Table 11.3 Equations for Estimating Resting Metabolic Rate

1. *Equations by Owens* (80)

Males

Resting Metabolic Rate (kcal/day) = 879 + 10.2 (kg) (SD = 215)

Females

Resting Metabolic Rate (kcal/day) = 795 + 7.18 (kg)

kg (body weight in kilograms)

2. *Revised Harris-Benedict Equations* (81)

Males

Resting Metabolic Rate (kcal/day) = 88.362 + (4.799 × ht) + (13.397 × kg) - (5.677 × age)

Females

Resting Metabolic Rate (kcal/day) = 447.593 + (3.098 × ht) + 9.247 × kg) - 4.330 × age)

ht (height in centimeters); kg (weight in kilograms)

3. *World Health Organization Equations* (82)

Age range (years)	Equation for kcal/day Resting Metabolic Rate	Standard deviation (actual vs predicted)
Males		
18-30	15.3 (kg) + 679	151
30-60	11.6 (kg) + 879	164
> 60	13.5 (kg) + 487	148
Females		
18-30	14.7 (kg) + 496	121
30-60	8.7 (kg) + 829	108
> 60	10.5 (kg) + 596	108
kg (body weight in kilograms)		

compared with 56 percent of the time for normal-weight girls.

Obese men informally walk an average of 3.7 miles per day compared to 6 miles per day for those of normal weight; obese women walk 2 miles per day compared to 4.9 miles per day for normal-weight women.[97] The obese have been found to stay in bed longer, and spend 17 percent less time on their feet than normal weight people.[98] When given a choice of an escalator or stairs, the obese are more likely than the lean to take the escalator.[15]

The amount of time spent watching television has been associated with an increased prevalence of obesity for both children and adults.[94,95,99] In one national study, twice as many teens who watched more than 5 hours of television per day were obese compared to teens who watched less than one hour per day.[99] (See Figure 11.14.)

The researchers suggested that TV watching decreased the opportunity for exercise, and also prompted more snacking because of all the food advertisements.

Children 4 to 8 years of age have been found to have increased body fat levels if daytime activity is less than normal.[100] Even with infants, a low level of physical activity is an important factor in predicting rapid weight gain during the first year of life.[52]

Thus there appears to be a tendency for obese people to be less physically active than normal-weight people. However, because they weigh more, the obese expend more Calories when they do engage in physical activity. In other words, even though obese people tend to engage in less physical activity than lean people, they expend more energy in the course of that activity. The end result is that daily energy expenditure from physical activity is little different between the obese and the

Table 11.4 Examples of Daily Energy Expenditures of Moderately Active Adults

Activity Category	Time (hours)	Man (155 lbs) Rate (kcal/min)	Man (155 lbs) Total (kcal)	Woman (115 lbs) Rate (kcal/min)	Woman (115 lbs) Total (kcal)
Sleeping, reading	8	1.0–1.2	540	0.9–1.1	440
Very light activity (seated and standing activities)	12	1.3–2.5	1300	1.2–2.0	900
Light activity (walking 2.5-3 mph)	3	2.5–4.9	600	2.0–3.9	450
Moderate activity (walking 3.5-4.0 mph)	1	5.0–7.4	300	4.0–5.9	240
Heavy activity	0	7.5–12.0		6.0–10.0	
Totals	**24**		**2740**		**2030**

Note: The average American male and female are not this active. Dietary intake studies show a caloric intake of 2,560 and 1,588 for males and females (ages 19–50) respectively.

Source: National Research Council, National Academy of Sciences, 1980.

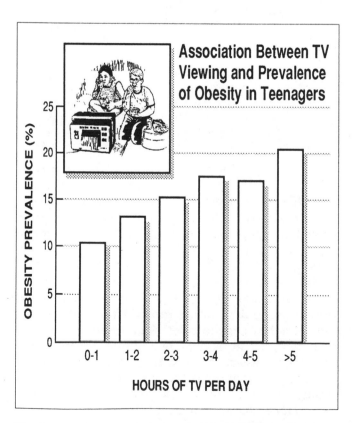

Figure 11.14 The prevalence of obesity among teenagers who watch television more than five hours per day is double that of teenagers viewing less than one hour a day. *Source:* see reference 99.

non-obese.[86, 88] For this reason, most experts feel that overeating is a more important factor than inactivity in accounting for the large number of obese people in developed countries.[15] Nonetheless, most experts agree that increased physical activity is necessary for the overall success of a weight control program.

Thermic Effect of Food

The *thermic effect of food* (TEF) is the increase in energy expenditure above the RMR that can be measured for several hours after a meal. (See Figure 11.15.) In other words, as your body digests, absorbs, transports, metabolizes, and stores the food you eat, energy is required.[71, 76] The TEF is higher after carbohydrate and protein meals than it is after fat meals.[87, 101–103] The average person's TEF is about 7 to 10 percent of total ingested Calories, or about 120 to 170 Calories per day for women, and about 180 to 260 Calories per day for men.[86] For example, if you eat a meal containing 800 Calories, your body uses 56 to 80 Calories just to process the meal.

The TEF has been found to be higher with larger meals.[104] For normal people, the TEF raises the energy expenditure of the body 43 percent over the RMR one hour after a 1,500 kcal meal; after a 1000 kcal meal, there is a 25 percent increase over the RMR.[37] As you can see from Figure 11.15, the TEF peaks about 60–90 minutes following a meal and lasts up to 4–6 hours.[49]

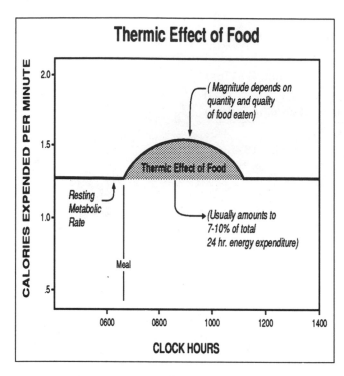

Figure 11.15 The thermic effect of food (TEF) is the energy expended for the digestion, absorption, transport, metabolism, and storage of food. *Source:* see reference 102.

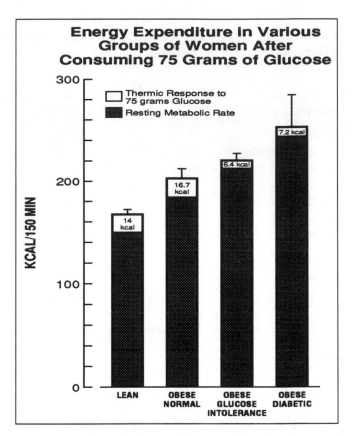

Figure 11.16 Although the thermic effect of food was reduced slightly for obese subjects with diabetic tendencies, the total energy expended during the 150 minutes following ingestion of 200 Calories of glucose was much higher for the obese than the lean due to their higher resting metabolic rates (larger lean body masses). *Source:* see reference 107.

Do the obese expend fewer Calories in digesting and metabolizing their food than normal-weight people? Most researchers have concluded that obese people have a slightly lower TEF, especially if they are diabetic.[83, 105–109] However, the difference is too small in terms of actual Calories to be important. In addition, most obese people have higher RMR, due to their increased muscle mass, more than making up for the small decrease in TEF.[107] (See Figure 11.16.)

Table 11.5 summarizes the information of this section on energy expenditure, comparing obese and non-obese people. The 177 people in this study varied widely in weight and degree of obesity. In general, obese people were found to expend more energy each day than non-obese people, despite lower levels of physical activity. This was due primarily to higher RMR.[86]

Treatment of Obesity

Three aspects of obesity combine to make it a compelling public health problem: its association with increased chronic disease, widespread prevalence, and resistance to change.

Weight management, however, has proven very difficult for most obese people. Most studies show that the majority of people entering weight management programs return to their starting weight within two years.[110]

It's been said that obesity is harder to treat than alcoholism. Many alcoholics can learn to live entirely without alcohol, but you can't abstain from eating—the obese face the more difficult task of continuing to consume food, but in moderation. Human nature being what it is, it is easier "not to at all," than to "a little bit."

Table 11.6 outlines the three classifications of obesity, and the basic type of treatment now recommended for each. Notice that the large majority of obese people are "mildly obese," and most of the ensuing discussion will deal with this classification. Treatment schemes for "severe" and "moderate" obesity will be reviewed first.

Table 11.5 Energy Expenditure in 177 Humans (Obese and Nonobese) Studied in a Respiratory Chamber (Average Weight = 97 kg; range = 41-178 kg)

Variable	Average (kcal/day)	Range (kcal/day)	Obese vs Lean
24 hour energy expenditure	2,292	1,371–3,615	Increased
All types of physical activity	348	138–685	Decreased
Resting metabolic rate	1,813	1,102–2,935	Increased
Thermic Effect of Food	165	–258–476	Little difference

Source: see reference 86.

*Increased means increased in an obese person in comparison to a lean person.

Severe Obesity

As noted in Table 11.6, *severe obesity* is defined as weighing more than double the ideal weight. Severe obesity is associated with serious medical complications.

Until recently, severely obese people were rarely able to lose weight and keep it off. The advent of surgical treatments for obesity in the past 30 years has dramatically changed this picture. Large amounts of weight (up to 200 lb) can now be lost and the loss maintained by severely obese patients. The surgery involves radically reducing the volume of the stomach to less than 50 ml. Some surgeons call this *gastric stapling,* others, "gastric reduction procedures."[111-114] (See Figure 11.17.)

Only certain people are allowed to undertake this type of surgery.[114] To be cleared for surgery, the patient must show a history of repeated failures to lose weight by acceptable nonsurgical methods, be severely obese (more than 100 percent overweight for at least three years), and be experiencing some medical complica-tions from the obesity. There must be a commitment by the patient, surgeon, and hospital to comprehensive, lifelong follow-up.[115]

Weight reduction is dramatic and long-term, with an expected weight loss of close to half the excess weight.[114-118] Patients go through drastic forced changes in eating habits. The reduced 50-ml stomach requires them to eat less during each meal, more often, and without any liquids at meal time.

For most, the loss in weight and improvement in eating habits leads to an improvement in blood lipids, glucose, and overall health.[114-116, 119] However, a sub-group of patients respond poorly to the surgery, in terms of failure to lose substantial weight, moderate to life-threatening medical complications, and emotional trauma.[120-121] Complications occur in 5–10 percent of cases, with mortality running at 0–3 percent.

Although severely obese subjects tend to lose more weight with gastric reduction surgery than with the very-low-Calorie diet (VLCD), there are fewer

Table 11.6 Treatment for Obesity

| Type | Classification of Obesity | | |
	Mild	Moderate	Severe
% Overweight	20–40%	41–100%	>100%
Sample Weights for 140 lb Ideal	168–196 lb	197–280 lb	>280 lb
Body Mass Index	25–30 kg/m^2	30–35 kg/m^2	>35 kg/m^2
Prevalence	90.5%	9.0%	0.5%
Treatment	Behavior Therapy (Diet, Exercise, Behavior Therapy)	VLCD and Behavior Therapy*	Gastric Surgery

* = Very-low-Calorie diet under medical supervision only.

Sources: adapted from reference 33, 49.

Gastric Reduction Surgery

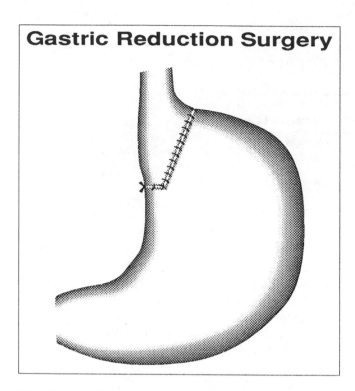

Figure 11.17 Gastric reduction surgery reduces the volume of the stomach, resulting in dramatic changes in eating habits. *Source:* see references 111–114.

complications with the latter.[121] Gastric reduction surgery should only be resorted to after nonsurgical techniques have failed.

Moderate Obesity

Moderate obesity, defined as being 41–100 percent overweight, characterizes about 9 percent of the obese population.[49] The extent of body fat excess warrants special measures under medical supervision. Treatment for moderate obesity should include special dietary counseling, with behavior modification, in medical clinics.

Moderately obese people have at least 50 pounds of excess fat tissue—enough to call for the maximum rate of weight reduction consistent with safety and reasonable comfort. Fasting is attractive to some patients, but this method raises problems of safety, comfort, and effectiveness.[50] With fasting, 40 to 50 percent of the weight loss comes from the lean body weight, compromising health and personal appearance. On the other hand, conventional reducing diets of 1,200–1,500 Calories produce too slow a weight loss to be practical. A compromise between the two, the very-low-Calorie diet, has recently proven very effective (for weight loss) and safe.[50, 122–137]

Also called the protein-sparing modified fast, the *very-low-Calorie diet* (VLCD) provides 400–700 Calories per day. Special supplements provide ample protein to help avoid loss of muscle tissue. Patients can use either a regimen of 100% special formula beverages, or a combination of natural foods such as fish, fowl, or lean meat, along with mineral and vitamin supplements. All patients should receive 1.5 L water and appropriate mineral and vitamin supplementation to insure RDA standards are met.[132] A small amount of carbohydrates can be added to diminish ketosis.

During rapid weight loss, sudden death from various complications can occur.[128, 133] For this reason, very-low-Calorie diets should only be used by moderately obese people under the supervision of a physician, hospital, or clinic actively engaged in the study and use of such diets. Most manufacturers of other types of VLCD have been reluctant to furnish them directly to the public, and limit distribution to physicians, hospitals, and clinics to ensure proper supervision. A careful clinical and biological checkup, and ongoing monitoring are necessary to insure against kidney dysfunction, infection, and other problems.[132] When VLCD are administered this way, they are generally safe.[49, 127]

Patients tend to lose 3 to 5 pounds a week on the VLCD, and reflect marked improvements in their blood lipid profiles.[131, 135] Unfortunately, however, losses usually are poorly maintained.

In one study of 400 patients, half of the patients who started the VLCD program did not complete treatment.[136] Patients who completed treatment lost a mean of 84 percent of their excess weight, but regained an average of 59 percent to 82 percent by the 30-month follow-up.

In another study of 4,026 obese patients in the Optifast (420 Calories protein supplement) treatment program, 25 percent of patients dropped out within the first 3 weeks.[135] Of the patients remaining in the program, 68 percent lost weight, but did not reach their goal. Of this group, recidivism was extremely high, with only 5–10 percent maintaining weight loss after 18 months. Thirty-two percent of the patients successfully attained the goal weight. Of this group, 30 percent of women and 58 percent of men maintained weight loss to within 10 pounds of posttreatment weight for at least 18 months.

Mild Obesity

Mild obesity, defined as being 20–40 percent overweight, is by far the most common form, characterizing 90.5 percent of the obese.[49] Since the ultimate goal of a weight-reduction program is to lose weight and maintain the loss, a nutritionally balanced, low-energy diet that is applicable to the patient's lifestyle is most appropriate. A comprehensive weight-reduction program that incorporates diet, exercise, and behavior modification is more likely to lead to long-term weight control.[138]

For most mildly obese people, a weight loss of about one percent of total body weight per week is optimal.[33] For example, if a person weighs 150 pounds, the goal should be to lose no more than 1.5 pounds each week. Another goal is to lose primarily fat tissue, while protecting the lean body weight.

As will be summarized later, one pound of body fat is equal to approximately 3,500 Calories. To lose 1.5 pounds of body fat, 5,250 Calories must be lost—750 Calories a day for a week. A combination of diet and exercise is generally most effective, as well as best for general health.

Conservative treatment for mild obesity involves three elements:[138–141]

1. Diet
   The caloric intake should be reduced, preferably by reducing the fat content of the diet, while increasing the complex carbohydrates.

2. Exercise
   Energy expenditure should be increased 200 to 400 Calories per day by increasing all forms of physical activity.

3. Behavior modification
   Several techniques have proved effective, including:

   a. Self-monitoring: Diet diaries are kept, recording food amounts consumed and the circumstances surrounding the eating.

   b. Control of the events that precede eating: Identification of the circumstances that elicit eating and overeating.

   c. Development of techniques to control the act of eating: Typical behavior modification techniques are used. (See section near end of chapter.)

   d. Reinforcement through use of rewards: A system of formal rewards facilitates progress.

   e. Cognitive restructuring: learning to counter negative thoughts, and to use thinking processes as a tool.

Diet

Very-low-Calorie diets are not recommended for the mildly obese, because the crux of long-term weight control is behavior change, and that is difficult to accomplish when one is on a highly specialized dietary regimen. When the daily caloric intake falls below 1,200, unless specialized supplements are used, the diet usually contains insufficient amounts of the various vitamins and minerals,[1,49,50,138,139] and the overall nutritional status of the individual can be easily compromised. In addition, unless there is special supplementation and close medical supervision, diets containing less than 1,200 Calories per day result in high amounts of muscle tissue loss, and can cause life-threatening complications.

At any given time, 2.5 million Americans are estimated to be dieting to lose weight.[142] The 1985 National Health Interview Survey estimated that 27 percent of males and 46 percent of females were trying to lose weight.[2] Only 27 and 21 percent of adult women and men, respectively, who were overweight were both dieting and exercising to lose weight (the 1990 goal is 50 percent).

In response to the American preoccupation with weight loss, a multi-billion dollar industry dedicated to selling "quick and easy" weight loss has sprung up. A proliferation of diet books and products utilizing false and misleading concepts are now available. Box 11.1 outlines several criteria that the National Council Against Health Fraud recommends to evaluate the validity and effectiveness of weight loss programs.[143]

Health fraud can be defined as the promotion, for financial gain, of fraudulent or unproven devices, treatments, services, plans, or products (including, but not limited to, diets and nutritional supplements) that alter or claim to alter the human condition.[144] Those who promote medical remedies that do not work or have not been proven to work are called "quacks." The cost of quackery and fraud escalated from a yearly estimate of $1–$2 billion 25 years ago to $10–$25 billion by 1984. The following techniques characterize quacks and their claims:

- The claims sound too good to be true—but they are what people want to be told.

- Quacks may belittle the regular food supply, established medicine, and scientifically based nutrition and regulation by the government under the guise that people should have "freedom of choice."

- Quacks may use case histories, testimonials, and subjective evidence in an attempt to justify their claims.

Box 11.1   Guidelines for Evaluating Commercial Weight-Loss Promotions.

Commercial weight-loss or control programs that do the following should be disparaged:

1. Promise or imply dramatic, rapid weight-loss (i.e., substantially more than one-percent of total body weight per week).

2. Promote diets that are extremely low in Calories (i.e., below 800 Calories per day; 1200-Calorie-per-day diets are preferred) unless under the supervision of competent medical experts.

3. Attempt to make clients dependent upon special products rather than teaching them how to make good choices from the conventional food supply (this does not condemn the marketing of low-calorie convenience foods, which may be chosen by consumers).

4. Do not encourage permanent, realistic lifestyle changes including regular exercise and the behavioral aspects of eating wherein food may be used as a coping device (i.e., programs should focus upon changing the *causes* of overweight rather than simply the *effect,* which is the overweight itself).

5. Misrepresent salespeople as "counselors" supposedly qualified to give guidance in nutrition and/or general health. Even if adequately trained, such "counselors" would still be objectionable because of the obvious conflict-of-interest that exists when providers profit directly from the products they recommend and sell.

6. Require large sums of money at the start or require that clients sign contracts for expensive, long-term programs. Such practices too often have been abused as salespeople focus attention upon signing up new people rather than delivering continuing, satisfactory service to consumers. Programs should be on a pay-as-you-go basis.

7. Fail to inform clients about the risks associated with weight-loss in general, or the specific program being promoted.

8. Promote unproven or spurious weight-loss aids such as human chorionic gonadotrophin hormone, starch blockers, diuretics, sauna belts, body wraps, passive exercise, ear stapling, acupuncture, Electric Muscle Stimulating devices, spirulina, amino acid supplements (e.g., arginine, ornithine), glucomannan, and so forth.

9. Claim that "cellulite" exists in the body.

10. Claim that the use of an appetite suppressant or methylcellulose (a "bulking agent") enables a person to lose body fat without restricting the customary Caloric intake.

11. Claim that a weight-control product contains a unique ingredient or component.

Source: see reference 143.

To judge the reliability of books and articles, ask these questions:

- What are the author's qualifications?
- What evidence does the author supply for any claims that are made?
- Why was it published? Is the author or company trying to sell you something?
- How is the information reviewed in newsletters by knowledgeable professionals?

Based on reviews of some of the most common published diets, the author has established a system of ratings.[50, 145-148] (See Figure 11.18.) Of the diets, those with an excellent rating conform to the U.S. Dietary Goals and Recommended Dietary Allowances. These diets are recommended because they follow principles advocated for a healthy lifestyle.

Diets with a poor rating tend to either be too high in fat and cholesterol or deficient in several important minerals and vitamins. Some of the poor diets are also based on unproven and misleading information. These "novelty" diets promote certain nutrients, foods, or combinations of foods as having unique, magical, or previously undiscovered fat-loss qualities.

Weight reduction is considered a therapeutic success if weight loss is maintained with no expense to overall health. The criteria used to achieve this goal require that the weight-reduction diet should: (1) satisfy all nutrient needs except energy, (2) conform to

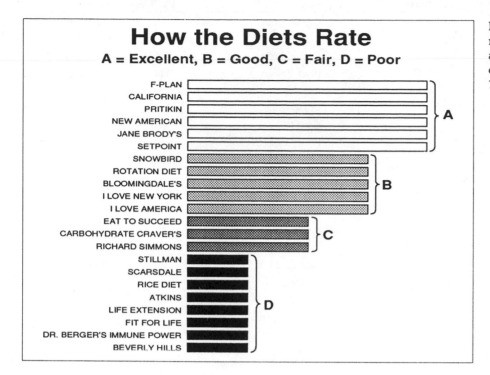

Figure 11.18 Diets with an excellent rating tend to follow principles advocated for a healthy and balanced diet. *Source:* see references 50, 145–148).

individual tastes and habits, (3) minimize hunger and fatigue, (4) be readily obtainable and socially acceptable, (5) favor the establishment of a changed eating pattern, and (6) be conducive to the improvement of overall health.[145]

The whole concept of dieting can be criticized on psychological grounds, for going on a diet implies going off it, and the resumption of old eating habits.[49] For this reason, one can argue that the most effective diet is not a diet at all, but rather, a gradual change in eating patterns and a shift to foods that the person can continue to eat indefinitely. This means increasing the intake of complex carbohydrates, particularly fruits, vegetables, legumes, and cereals, and decreasing the intake of fats and refined sugars. This course of action probably gives the best chance of maintaining the lowered weight, and it is an eminently safe one. One should never lose weight by any method that cannot be included permanently in a healthy lifestyle.

In other words, the same diet that is being recommended for the treatment and prevention of cardiovascular disease and diabetes should be used in preventing and treating obesity. This diet is high in carbohydrate, but low in fat. Whole grains, vegetables, and fruits are emphasized, and low-fat meats and dairy products are recommended.

Thus, in light of current evidence, the most important dietary habit for both preventing and treating obesity is a strong emphasis on low-caloric density foods high in complex carbohydrates and dietary fiber and low in fat. Table 11.7 compares the caloric content of common foods and shows that vegetables and fruits have the lowest number of Calories, while high-fat and sugar, low-fiber foods contain the most.

As stated previously, obese people tend to take in less Calories when consuming high-fiber, high-carbohydrate foods, and still tend to feel satisfied. The dietary fiber and water in the fruits and vegetables take up room in the stomach, apparently helping to reduce the hunger drive more quickly as the stomach fills with food.[149]

The Wrong Way to Lose Weight with Diet

Various potions have been advocated for weight reduction. As you read the following list, and compare it with Box 11.1, you should understand why most experts classify the advocacy of these items as weight control quackery.[150]

1. **Starch blockers:** This enzyme inhibitor is supposed to block the digestion and absorption of ingested carbohydrate. Several studies have now shown these to be not only ineffective, but also possibly risky. In addition, they have been declared illegal as unapproved drugs. Starch blockers tie into that common American myth that carbohydrates are responsible for obesity.

Table 11.7 Calories Found in One Cup Portions of Food

Food	Calories Per Cup	Ranking	Food	Calories Per Cup	Ranking
Vegetable Oils	1927		Grape Juice	155	
Shortening	1812		Whole Milk	150	
Margarine	1616		Oatmeal (Cooked)	145	**Moderately Low**
Butter	1600	**Very High in**	Plain Yogurt	144	**(Juices, Soups,**
Mayonnaise	1582	**Calories**	Pineapple Juice	139	**Cereals, Milk)**
Peanut Butter	1520	**(Fats)**	Crabmeat	135	
Salad Dressing, Blue Cheese	1234		Corn (Cooked)	134	
Honey	1040		Peas (Cooked)	126	
Cake Icing	1035		Low-Fat Milk	121	
Nuts, Macadamia	940		White Bread	120	
Jams/Preserves	880		Apple Juice	116	
Chocolate Candy	860		Orange Juice	112	
Peanuts, Oil Roasted	840	**High**	Rice Krispies	112	
Sunflower Seeds	821	**(Nuts, Seeds**	Corn Chex	111	
Cashews	787	**and Sugar)**	Non-Fat Milk	86	
Almonds	766		Oranges	85	
White Sugar	720		Pumpkin	83	
Granola	595		Winter Squash	79	
Sour Cream	493		Pineapple	77	
Dates	489		Blackberries	74	**Low**
Walnuts	486		Apples	64	**(Non-Fat Milk,**
Dried Pears	472	**Moderately**	Grapes	58	**Fruits)**
Coconut	466	**High**	Onions	58	
Cheddar Cheese	455	**(Dried Fruit,**	Cantaloupe	57	
Raisins	434	**Cheese, Flour)**	Beets (Cooked)	52	
Flour (Wheat, Enriched)	420		V-8 Juice	51	
Grape Nuts	407		Watermelon	50	
CornedBeef Hash	400		Carrots	48	
Prunes	385		Broccoli (Cooked)	46	
Ice Cream (16% Fat)	349		Strawberries	45	
Sweet Potato	344		Green Beans	44	
Pork (Lean, Roasted)	341		Kale (Cooked)	41	
Ricotta Cheese (Skim Milk)	340		Kohlrabi (Raw)	38	
Ice Cream (10% Fat)	269		Summer Squash (Cooked)	36	
Turkey	262		Sprouted Mung Beans	32	**Very Low**
Ham (Roasted)	249	**Moderate**	Zucchine (Cooked)	28	**(Vegetables)**
Soybeans (Cooked)	234	**(Legumes, Some**	Collards (Cooked)	27	
Brown Rice (Cooked)	232	**Dairy Products,**	Cauliflower (Raw)	24	
Cottage Cheese (4%, Large Curd)	232	**Rice)**	Cabbage (Raw)	22	
Yogurt (Fruit Flavored)	231		Celery	18	
Red Kidney Beans (Cooked)	230		Mushrooms (Raw)	18	
Spanish Rice	213		Cucumber	14	
Lentils (Cooked)	210		Spinach (Raw)	12	
Macaroni (Cooked)	190		Romaine Lettuce	8	
Whole Wheat Cereal (Cooked)	180	**Moderately**	Iceberg Lettuce	7	
Wheat Chex	169	**Low (Juices,**	Swiss Chard (Raw)	6	
Tomato Soup (With Milk)	160	**Soups, Cereals, Milk)**			

Source: USDA Food Composition Tables (Handbook No. 8 series).

As discussed already, fat is the prime culprit, not carbohydrates.

2. **Bulk producers:** Examples are methycellulose (found in Metamucil) and glucomannan, which absorb liquid in the stomach, creating a feeling of fullness. Glucomannan is chemically extracted from konjac tubers (underground vegetables from Japan), and is supposed to absorb liquid, forming a high-fiber gel that produces a feeling of fullness to help switch off the hunger drive. There is no scientific evidence that such bulk-producing products effectively cause weight loss or do anything other than create the feeling of fullness of ordinary bulky foods such as whole grains, apples, carrots, and other fruits and vegetables. They can cause problems such as esophageal obstruction, caused by swelling of the tablets during ingestion.[151]

3. **Spirulina:** This is a dark green powder or pill derived from algae. Claims have been made that phenylalanine, an amino acid found in spirulina (and in most other protein sources) "acts on the brain's appetite center to switch off your hunger pangs . . . " The Food and Drug Administration (FDA) is not aware of any evidence that phenylalanine is safe and effective as an appetite suppressant.

4. **Benzocaine:** This is the active ingredient in AYDS candy and dietetic lozenges and gum. Benzocaine is a topical anesthetic said to work by "numbing" the tongue, reducing the ability to taste foods. According to the AMA Drug Evaluations, "there are no conclusive data to support benzocaine's effectiveness as an anorexiant."

5. **Phenylpropanolamine (PPA):** This is the active ingredient in most nonprescription weight-control products, such as Dexatrim, Appedrine, Control, Dietac, Prolamine, and Adrinex. PPA is related to amphetamines and has similar side effects, including nervousness, insomnia, headaches, nausea, tinnitus (ringing in the ears), and elevated blood pressure. Although PPA may be somewhat effective for short-term weight loss, PPA and comparable appetite suppressants have not proved effective for long-term weight control, and there has been evidence of harmful side-effects.

6. **Growth hormone releasers:** Various products such as Lipogene-GH, Nite Diet, Dream Away, Nite Time Diet, and HGH-3X are sold with the claim that if they are taken before retiring, weight loss will occur overnight because of the increased release of growth hormone from the amino acids arginine and ornithine contained in the products. In other words, these amino acids stimulate human growth hormone, causing you to "burn fat while you sleep." Unfortunately, research has not supported this attractive theory (submitted by Pearson and Shaw in their book, *Life Extension*).

7. **Cholecystokinin (CCK):** CCK is a hormone involved in digestion (especially of fat). Producers of CCK claim that it will reduce hunger and cause sudden and dramatic weight loss. No CCK product has been approved by the FDA for public sale for any purpose.

8. **DHEA:** This unapproved drug is derived from human urine and other sources. Manufacturers tout DHEA as a "natural" weight-loss product. DHEA is known chemically as dehydroepiandrosterone or dehydroandrosterone. The FDA has not received any data to substantiate the claims for DHEA, and has written the manufacturers telling them to stop selling it.

9. **Grapefruit pills:** For decades grapefruit has been promoted as having special fat burning properties. Grapefruit pills contain grapefruit extract, diuretics, and bulk-forming agents; some contain phenylpropanolamine (PPA) along with herbs or other ingredients. The FDA has not approved the sale of these products, and is unaware of any valid medical evidence that they are safe or effective. The U.S. Postal Service has taken action to bar use of the mails by one grapefruit pill supplier, Citrus Industries, marketer of the Grapefruit Super Pill.

Exercise

As we shall see in this section, in the "battle of the bulge" two weapons are needed—both diet and exercise. However, research is pointing towards control of caloric intake as the more powerful of the two.[33]

Current Issues Regarding Exercise and Weight Loss

There are several issues regarding the role of aerobic exercise in weight loss. These are summarized in Box 11.2. Each of these will be explained in turn, with the benefits reviewed later in this chapter.

Box 11.2 Current Issues Regarding the Role of Exercise in Weight Loss

Does an aerobic exercise program—

1. accelerate weight loss significantly when combined with a reducing diet?
2. cause the resting metabolic rate to stay elevated for a long time after the bout, burning many extra calories?
3. counter the diet-induced decrease in resting metabolic rate?
4. counter the diet-induced decrease in fat-free mass?
5. lead to a chronic decrease in appetite?
6. augment the thermic effect of food?

Current Issue #1: Does aerobic exercise accelerate weight loss significantly when combined with a reducing diet?

Table 11.8 summarizes the results of ten well-designed studies that measured the effects of aerobic exercise on body composition changes during reducing diets.[152-161]

In general, moderate amounts of aerobic exercise (2–7 hours per week) when combined with a reducing diet add little to the diet-induced weight loss.[152-169] In order for aerobic exercise to have a major effect on reduction of body weight, daily exercise sessions need to be long in duration and high in intensity.[170] Many reviewers have concluded that moderate amounts of aerobic exercise alone (without dietary intervention) are largely ineffective in promoting weight loss.[16, 153, 154, 163, 170-172]

Figure 11.19 summarizes the findings of a five-week study by the author.[152] Participants were fed 1,268 Calories a day in a research kitchen and randomly assigned to either an exercise group (five 45-minute brisk walking sessions per week) or a non-exercise group. Both groups averaged 5.5 kilograms (12 pounds) of weight loss after five weeks. Figure 11.20 summarizes a 12-week study in which exercise participants walked/jogged 30 minutes five times a week.[153] Exercise alone had no effect on weight loss, and contributed little to the weight loss effect of the reducing diet (1,200 Calories a day).

Why does aerobic exercise have so little effect in accelerating weight loss during a reducing diet? There are several reasons:

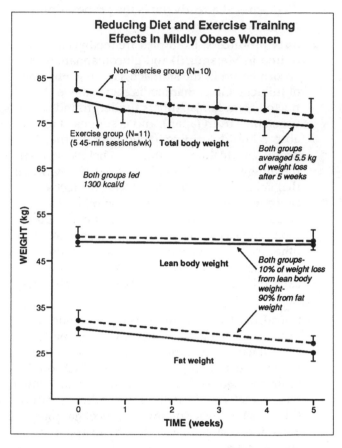

Figure 11.19 Aerobic exercise did not accelerate weight loss in this group of mildly obese women on a 1,268-Calorie diet. *Source:* see reference 152.

- The *net energy expenditure* of moderate aerobic exercise sessions is small. The net energy cost of exercise equals the Calories expended during the exercise session in excess of the Calories expended by the person's resting metabolism and other activities he might have engaged in had he not been formally exercising.[152, 173] This is outlined in Table 11.9.

- Some exercisers tend to reward themselves by resting more after the session is over for the rest of the day. Thus the total 24-hour energy expenditure on exercise days may be little different than that on non-exercise days.[152]

- Many obese people cannot engage in large amounts of exercise without injury. Large amounts of exercise are needed to have a significant impact on weight loss, but the risk of musculoskeletal injury limits the amount of exercise that can be engaged in.[50]

Table 11.8   Review of Studies Where Subjects on Reducing Diets Were Randomly Assigned to Aerobic Exercise and Nonexercise Groups

			Changes in Weight, Exercise vs. Dieting Sedentary Group			
Reference	Diet (calories/ day)	Exercise (hrs/wk)	Length of Study (wks)	Body Wt (lbs)	Fat Wt (lbs)	Lean Wt (lbs)
Nieman (152)	1268	3.8	5	NS	NS	NS
Hagan (153)	1200	2.5	12	–5.5	–3.3	–2.2
Van Dale (154)	767	2.7	12	NS	NS	NS
Hill (155)	800	5.0	5	NS	–3.7	+2.9
Phinney (156)	720	7.0	4	NS	NA	NA
Katch (157)	1200	2.5	20	NS	NS	NS
Van Dale (158)	800	4.0	14	8.6	7.5	NS
Hammer (159)	800/1450	3.8	16	NS	NS	NS
Warwick (160)	800	14.0	3.5	NS	NA	NA
Lennon (161)	1500	3.0	12	NS	NS	NS

NS = not significant

NA = information not available

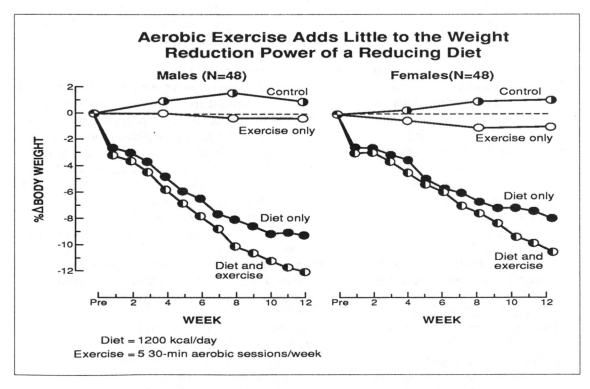

Figure 11.20   Exercise alone had no effect on weight loss, and contributed little to the weight loss effect of the reducing diet (1,200 Calories a day) on this group of 48 males and 48 females. *Source:* see reference 153.

Table 11.9   The Net Energy Cost of a 3-Mile Walk in 45 Minutes by a 70-Kilogram Man

Factor	Calories Expended
Gross Energy Expenditure of 3-Mile Walk	215 Calories
Resting Metabolic Rate for 45 Minutes	–50 Calories
Energy Expenditure for Mild Physical Activity the Person Might Have Engaged in Had He Not Been Formally Walking	–50 Calories
Net Energy Expenditure for 3-Mile Walk	115 Calories

Current Issue #2: Does aerobic exercise cause the resting metabolic rate to stay elevated for a long time after the bout, burning many extra Calories?

In general, most researchers have found that the amount energy expended after aerobic exercise is small unless there has been exercise of unusual duration and intensity.[174–181] For example, cycling 80 minutes at 70 percent $\dot{V}O_{2max}$ expended 125 extra Calories during 12 hours of recovery. Few obese people would be capable of exercising at these intense levels.

Moderate amounts of exercise result in very small post-exercise energy expenditures. Jogging two miles at 12 minutes per mile raises RMR for only 31 minutes, with about 10 extra Calories expended.[176] When the pace is increased to 8.5 minutes per mile, RMR is increased for 48 minutes, with 15 extra Calories expended.

Figure 11.21 shows the results of one study in which participants cycled at 70 percent $\dot{V}O_{2max}$ for varying durations of time.[177] Researchers concluded that in general, 15 extra Calories are burned during recovery for every 100 Calories expended during exercise.

Current Issue #3: Does aerobic exercise counter the diet-induced decrease in resting metabolic rate?

Most studies do not support the concept that aerobic training counters the usual 10–20 percent diet-induced reduction in resting metabolic rate.[1, 152, 154–158, 171, 182–184] For example, in one study, 12 mildly obese women were put on 530-Calorie diets for 28 days, and an exercise program (3 sessions/week, 30–45 minutes at 60 percent $\dot{V}O_{2max}$). RMR dropped 16 percent despite the exercise program.[182]

In another study, half of 13 mildly obese participants in a four-week VLCD (720 Calories/day) regimen exercised a total of 27 hours at 50 percent $\dot{V}O_{2max}$.[156] RMR actually dropped more in the exercise group than in the sedentary group (10 percent for both groups in the first week, but then a further 17 percent in the exercise group). Apparently the exercise session prompted energy conservation, decreasing the RMR.

Current Issue #4: Does aerobic exercise counter the diet-induced decrease in fat-free mass?

Analysis of Table 11.8 shows that in general, the combination of a moderate aerobic exercise program with a reducing diet does little to protect lean body mass during weight reduction.[152–155, 157–159, 161] As explained earlier, the excess weight of the obese is about 75 percent fat and 25 percent fat free mass.[33] Thus during weight reduction, some loss of lean body mass is expected and probably desirable.

During weight loss, the percentage lost as lean body mass increases in proportion to the severity of the caloric deficit. During total fasting, the body weight that is lost is close to 50 percent fat and 50 percent lean body mass.[185] During a VLCD (with appropriate protein intake), the proportions improve to 75 percent fat and 25 percent fat free mass.[186] During a 1,200–1,500-Calorie diet, the proportions improve even more to 90 percent fat and 10 percent fat free mass.[152] Moderate aerobic exercise has little effect on these proportions.

Weight training during weight loss, however, does provide sufficient stimulus to the fat free mass to afford protection.[187, 188] In one eight-week study of 40 obese women, adding weight training exercise to a 1,200–1,500-Calorie diet (three sets, 10 repetitions of eight different exercises, three sessions per week) did improve maintenance of lean body weight relative to that of those who dieted without such exercise.[188] (See Figure 11.22.) Adding weight training to the diet program did not increase the rate of weight loss, however. Weight training sessions resulted in a net energy expenditure of only 139 Calories/session.

Current Issue #5: Does aerobic exercise lead to a chronic reduction in appetite?

Although it is true that intense aerobic exercise reduces the desire to eat over the short-term,[189] the majority of studies show that caloric intake is usually increased or unchanged in response to long-term exercise training programs.[163, 190, 191] When energy intake is

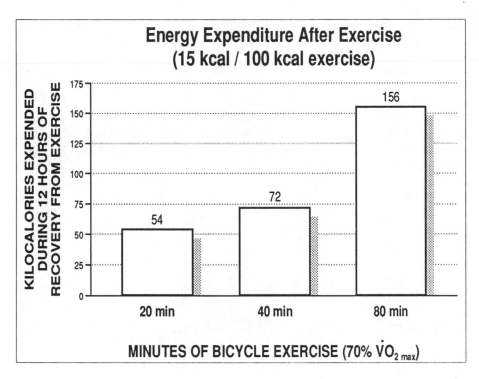

Figure 11.21 Energy expenditure after heavy bicycle exercise (70 percent $\dot{V}O_{2max}$) results in approximately 15 extra Calories expended during recovery for every 100 Calories expended during the exercise. *Source:* see reference 177.

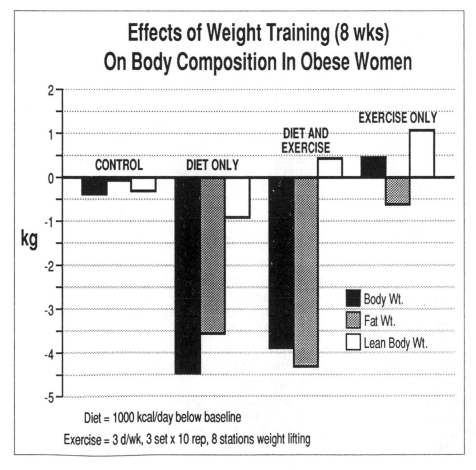

Figure 11.22 Weight training during a 1,200–1,500 Calorie diet can counter the usual diet-induced loss of lean body mass. *Source:* see reference 188.

increased, it is usually below the increased expenditure, however, with a negative energy balance and loss of body fat.[191] In other words, there does appear to be an acute exercise response of reduced food intake: in the long term active people eat more yet stay leaner than sedentary controls. It is possible that a certain level of physical activity is necessary before the body can precisely control food intake to match energy expenditure.

However, the obese may respond differently to exercise than normal-weight people.[192, 193] While highly trained athletes and lean people usually increase energy intake in response to increased physical activity, untrained obese people commonly do not change energy intake when they become involved in exercise training. For the obese, food-related cues seem more important than exercise-generated signals.

Few studies have investigated the effects of exercise on changes in food selection, and the results have been inconsistent.[191] (See Chapter 9.)

Current Issue #6: Does aerobic exercise augment the thermic effect of food?

As described earlier, RMR is elevated for several hours after a meal because of the thermic effect of food (TEF). Some researchers have suggested that aerobic exercise, either before[194] or after[195–197] eating, may augment the TEF.

However, the best designed studies have failed to support this proposition.[198–200] In one of the best studies (of obese women), the thermogenic response to a 700–1,000 Calorie meal was not affected by moderate exercise (24 minutes, averaging 300 kgm/min on a bicycle) following the meal.[198] Even in studies in which an effect has been found, the increase in TEF has represented less than 15 extra Calories, hardly enough to have a meaningful impact on obesity.[194]

Studies are mixed on the effects of physical fitness on TEF. While one study has shown that TEF is lower for people with high $\dot{V}O_{2max}$ levels,[201] two others have shown the opposite.[202, 203] More research is needed in this area.

Benefits of Exercise for Weight Loss

Despite the questions raised by these issues, however, moderate aerobic exercise contributes several benefits for weight loss. (See Figure 11.23.) Box 11.3 summarizes five benefits of aerobic exercise.[1, 16, 33, 49, 50, 138, 152, 154, 170]

The improvement in $\dot{V}O_{2max}$ following moderate aerobic exercise has been found to vary from 10–25 percent of baseline levels after 5–15 weeks of exercise.[152–154, 158–162, 169, 183] In a study of mildly obese women by the author, $\dot{V}O_{2max}$ improved 21 percent after just five weeks of brisk walking.[152] (See Figure 11.24.)

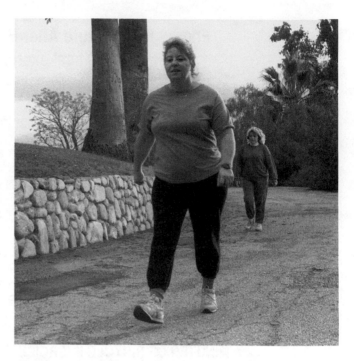

Figure 11.23 Moderate aerobic exercise such as brisk walking is associated with several important benefits for the obese.

Box 11.3 Benefits of Moderate Aerobic Exercise for the Obese

Moderate aerobic exercise by the obese is associated with:

1. Improved cardiorespiratory endurance ($\dot{V}O_{2max}$).1[52–154, 158–162, 169, 183] (See Chapter 7.)

2. Improved blood lipid profile, in particular decreased triglycerides and increased HDL-C, with weight loss more responsible for decreases in total cholesterol and LDL-C.[163, 174, 208–213] (See Chapter 10.)

3. Improved psychological state, especially increased general well-being and vigor and decreased anxiety and depression.[49, 50, 174, 204, 212, 215–218] (See Chapter 13.)

4. Enhanced group social support, which may improve chances of long-term maintenance of weight loss.[49, 50, 204, 219]

5. Decreased risk of obesity-related diseases (e.g., diabetes, heart disease, hypertension.[49, 50, 174, 204–207] (See Chapters 10 and 14.)

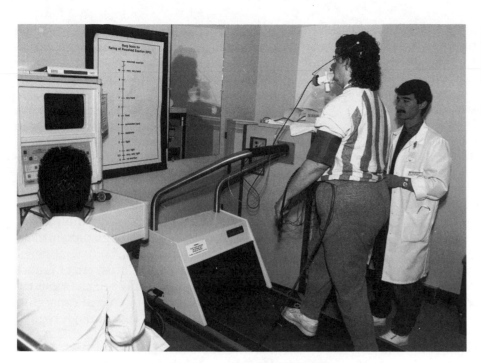

Figure 11.24 After just five weeks of brisk walking, the $\dot{V}O_{2max}$ of a group of mildly obese women improved 21 percent. *Source:* see reference 152.

Weight loss usually is associated with an improvement in blood lipid profile. (See Chapter 10.) Researchers consistently find that with weight loss, total cholesterol, LDL-C, and triglyceride levels decrease, while HDL-C levels increase.[208] The independent effect of aerobic exercise, however, is limited to improving the magnitude of change in the triglycerides and HDL-C, but not total cholesterol and LDL-C.[209-211] In a study by the author, total cholesterol and LDL-C fell 13 percent for both sedentary controls and exercising obese women after five weeks of a 1,268-Calorie diet.[152, 209] Exercise was found to have an independent effect only on triglycerides and HDL-C.

In addition to the physiological benefits, there is strong, mounting evidence associating exercise with feelings of well-being, reduced anxiety and depression, an increase in self-esteem, and elevated mood.[215-217] This supports the practice of including exercise with weight loss programs, particularly to counter the feelings of depression and irritability common during weight loss.

In most obesity studies, participants exercise together. Preliminary results suggest that the social interaction during the weeks of exercising may enhance long-term maintenance of weight loss. In one recent study, researchers examined the effect of exercise in a VLCD program in combination with behavioral techniques, nutrition education, and group therapy.[207]

After four months of treatment with the VLCD, the addition of an exercise component did not signifi-cantly increase weight loss (17.5 kg for nonexercisers, 21.8 for exercisers). At the two year follow-up, however, nonexercisers had regained 95.8 percent of the four-month weight loss, exercisers 58.2 percent. Thus, structured exercise may provide ancillary benefits such as increased group cohesiveness, communication, and opportunities for information-sharing that persist for months after the program is over.

As discussed at the beginning of this chapter, obesity is associated with many complications, such as heart disease, diabetes, high blood pressure, and high blood cholesterol levels. There is now strong evidence that exercise can help to counter each of these. (See Chapters 10 and 14.)

So in summary, moderate aerobic exercise during weight reduction helps to improve one's general health status, but the real power behind weight loss comes from a reduction of Calories (in particular, dietary fat). The success of a weight loss program should be measured not only by the total amount of weight lost, but also the quality of the weight loss and final health status.[1] A moderate reduction in Calories promotes loss of fat weight while sparing the lean body weight; aerobic exercise improves fitness and general health status.

Exercise Precautions for the Obese

There are several exercise precautions for the obese, and their importance increases with the increasing degree of obesity.[220] These include providing for heat intolerance, difficulty in breathing, movement restriction, musculoskeletal pain and injury, local muscular weakness, and balance-anxiety.

In addition, the obese are at higher risk for cardiovascular disease, diabetes, and hypertension. However, if the exercise leader is careful to follow appropriate American College of Sports Medicine screening procedures (Chapter 3), has adequately prepared for emergencies, and emphasizes low-to-moderate intensity *non-weight-bearing activities* (such as bicycling, swimming, water exercises, and brisk walking), exercise programs for the severely obese can be conducted safely.

Enhancing Opportunities for Exercise

Social reinforcement, and compliance are enhanced through group participation in activities which are recreational, fun, varied, and which offer the participant a feeling of personal success.[221] Regimented calisthenics are not generally advisable. On the other hand, music, games, and social interaction will improve compliance.

Another key principle is that exercise need not be formal to be beneficial. It can take place at different times of the day, as a part of regular daily activities (like climbing stairs or walking to a neighbor's house), and as such is often more attractive to the obese, who want to avoid being noticed during exercise.

Methods that Don't Work

The obese person is particularly vulnerable to the countless fraudulent exercise devices and techniques that are constantly promoted,[221] including:

Mechanical Vibration and Fat Loss: Passive exercise devices include roller machines, oscillating tables, passive motion tables, and massagers that do all the work while shaking, rolling, and moving body parts. Such gadgets have been hailed as effortless exercise devices that take off or redistribute fat. However, mechanically vibrating body fat is the same as shaking beef fat in a bag—the fat is still all there after the shaking stops.

Continuous Passive Motion (CPM) tables are motorized machines that continuously move isolated muscle groups through their range of motion without requiring any effort by the user. Originally developed as therapeutic tools for polio victims, CPM tables are now appearing in health salons across the United States and promoted for losing inches and gaining fitness without sweating or lifting a finger.[222] CPM machines can be helpful for therapy and rehabilitation, but not for losing body fat or improving cardiorespiratory fitness.

Weight-Reducing Clothing: Special weight-reducing clothing, including heated belts, rubberized suits, and oilskins, primarily cause dehydration. Although circumference measures or scale weight may temporarily decrease, body fat does not. Rubberized suits are potentially dangerous because they block body heat loss and sweat evaporation.

Cellulite Cures: Cellulite is the term used to describe unsightly fat tissue that causes the overlying skin to appear dimpled like an orange peel.[223] Supposedly, 80 percent of all women and 10 percent of all men have cellulite deposits located primarily in the thigh, buttocks, and knee areas. Proponents claim that cellulite is fat trapped in abnormal and chronically inflamed connective tissue, with impeded blood and lymph access. Exorbitant fees are often charged for high protein diets, massage, sauna, special skin creams, body wrappings, or pseudoelectric devices used to "break up or reduce cellulite deposits." Cellulite is simply subcutaneous fat, packaged somewhat differently in normal connective tissue. The only real cure is fat loss through regular aerobic exercise and improved diet.

Electrical Muscle Stimulators (EMS)—EMS devices are claimed to provide "all the figure-toning of 3,000 sit-ups without moving an inch." Other claimed benefits include face lifts without surgery, slimming and trimming, weight loss, bust development, spot reducing, and removal of cellulite. The Food and Drug Administration considers such claims for EMS devices to be fraudulent.

Spot Reducing—The concept of spot reduction is based on the widely held belief that it is possible to selectively "burn off" fat from specific areas of the body by exercising nearby muscles. For example, some people believe that doing sit-ups burns abdominal fat. Research, however, has shown that the concept of spot reduction is false. In one study, participants performed a total of 5,000 sit-ups over a 27-day period. Fat tissue biopsies revealed that sit-ups did not selectively reduce fat cell size in the abdominal area.[224]

Specific calisthenics may help tone the muscles in a certain area, but they do not help melt away the fat.[225] If spot reducing really worked, then fat people who chewed gum would have thin faces! Interestingly, aerobic exercise appears to selectively burn more fat from abdominal areas than other body areas.[226] Obviously, the best way to decrease abdominal fat is to consume less Calories than are expended.

Behavior Modification

Behavior modification is one of the most widely used treatments for obesity.[49] Well over 100 studies have been published testing the effectiveness of behavior modifi-

Table 11.10 Behavioral Principles of Weight Control

Stimulus Control

Shopping	Shop for food after eating
	Shop from a list
	Avoid ready-to-eat foods
	Don't carry more cash than is needed for list
Plans	Plan ahead to limit food intake
	Substitute exercise for snacking
	Eat meals at scheduled times
	Don't accept food offered by others
Activities	Store food out of sight
	Eat all food in the same place
	Remove food from inappropriate home storage areas
	Keep serving dishes off the table
	Use smaller dishes and utensils
	Avoid being the food server
	Leave the table immediately after eating
Holidays, Parties	Plan eating habits before parties
	Eat a low-calorie snack before parties
	Practice polite ways to decline food
Eating Behavior	Put fork down between mouthfuls
	Chew thoroughly before swallowing
	Pause in the middle of the meal
	Do nothing else while eating (e.g., reading, TV)
Reward	Solicit help from family and friends (praise)
	Use self-monitoring records as the basis for rewards
	Plan specific rewards for specific behaviors
Self-Monitoring	Keep diet diary that includes time and place of eating, type and amount of food, who is present, and how you feel
Nutrition Education	Use diet diary to identify problem areas
	Make small changes that you can maintain
	Learn nutritional values of foods
	Decrease fat and increase complex carbohydrate intake
Physical Activity	Increase routine, informal activity (e.g., increase use of stairs)
Informal Activity	Keep a record of distance walked/day
	Begin a moderate exercise program
Formal Exercise	Keep a formal record
	Increase the exercise gradually
Cognitive Restructuring	Avoid setting unreasonable goals
	Think about progress, not shortcomings
	Avoid imperatives like "always' and "never"
	Counter negative thoughts with reasoned ones
	Set weight goals that are reasonable
	Realize that when any event takes place, the mind has the power to decide what reaction should take place (negative reactions can be controlled

Source: Adapted from reference 227.

cation. It has proven to be more effective than any other studied treatment.

Behavior modification considers in great detail the eating behavior to be changed, events which trigger the eating, and its consequences (e.g., feelings, rewards).[227]

Behavior modification goes beyond merely educating the obese about diet and exercise—knowledge alone is usually insufficient to help the majority of people improve their behavior.[228-230] One study found that obese and overweight people knew more than normal-weight people about nutrition, health care, and exercise.[228] In other words, nutrition and fitness knowledge is not necessarily related to good weight control.

The primary behavior to be changed is eating, and a number of techniques are typically employed to slow the rate of eating and allow body signals to indicate satisfaction. Focus is placed on events that trigger eating, such as shopping for food, or keeping high-fat foods in the house. Patients are taught to remove various stimuli that prompt eating from their environment, with rewards for learning the proper behaviors. Table 11.10 outlines some of the more common techniques.

A Practical Summary

Let's suppose that a friend of yours should weigh 120 pounds but weighs 144 pounds instead. The 24 extra pounds of weight classifies your friend as mildly obese. Of these 24 pounds, 75 percent (or 18 pounds) is probably excess body fat, 25 percent extra lean body weight. As you remember, obese people tend to have higher lean body weights because of the extra muscle built up to carry around the excess weight.

Before counseling your friend to make various lifestyle changes, you would do well to first have her keep a diet diary. By identifying the circumstances surrounding her eating, and her associated feelings, she can decide how to control some of these circumstances. In addition, a reward system can be set up.

For example, if you find that your friend's primary problem is eating snacks high in fats (potato chips or salted nuts) while studying or doing homework assignments, perhaps low-Calorie snacks like fresh fruit or veggies could be substituted. If the snacking stems from anxiety over school work, a 10-minute brisk walk before each study session might help reduce this anxiety. If your friend manages to make two behavioral change (low-Calorie snacks and brisk walking), there might be a pre-arranged reward, such as a new music tape or a special outfit.

The over-all goal must be permanent exercise and dietary lifestyle changes.[231] Any long-term program must start with a plan, including a time frame for reaching goals like achieving ideal weight. Because your friend has 18 pounds of excess fat, a 63,000-Calorie deficit will be needed (18 pounds × 3,500 Calories/pound).

It is important to remember that the mildly obese should not lose more than one percent of their body weight per week. Weight losses greater than one percent of body weight are poorly maintained, and may cause mental depression and decreased motivation.

One percent of your friend's weight would mean no more than 1 to 1-1/2 pounds per week. One pound of body fat loss per week means a daily deficit of 500 Calories (500 × 7 = 3500). If your friend starts walking three miles every day, this would represent close to 115 additional Calories. On the eating side, a good focus is to reduce fat—for both caloric reduction and general health. The equivalent of four tablespoons of fat each day would represent 400 Calories (one tablespoon of fat has 100 Calories).

In practice, this could be achieved in the usual case by using low-fat or nonfat dairy products, only lean cuts of meat, reducing use of visible fats (margarines, salad dressing, mayonnaise, oil, sour cream, etc.), and substituting low-Calorie spreads (e.g., low-fat yogurts, low-Calorie fruit jams, low-fat cheese spreads, etc). There should also be a switch to more fruits, salads, steamed vegetables, and whole grain products.

The net 500-Calorie deficit would mean that in one week close to one pound of fat would be lost. By 18 weeks, if the exercise and low-fat diet is continued, the excess body fat (18 pounds) and lean body weight (6 pounds) should be gone—permanently—if the new exercise and eating behaviors are permanent.

The primary weapons in this battle of the bulge—daily exercise and a low-fat diet—will also help you to feel better, improve your health status, and help prevent other health problems.

Sports Medicine Insight
Eating Disorders: Bulimia and Anorexia Nervosa

Our unresolved paradox is that our food-laden, sedentary society holds in high esteem the thin and beautiful. On the one hand our magazine covers, movie stars, and athletic heroes advance the concept that thin is in. But on the other hand we are led (often through advertising) to believe that technological labor-saving devices and sumptuous foods rich in fats and sugars are desirable benefits of upper-class living.

Out of this quandary has emerged a sector of our population that are extremely disordered in their eating habits—the bulimics and the anorexics. *Bulimia* and *anorexia nervosa* have several characteristics that have been summarized by the American Psychiatric Association. (See Box 11.4.)

Among college students nationwide, 1–2 percent of women and 0.1–0.2 percent of men are classified as bulimic (using the DSM IIIR diagnostic criteria).[232–235] However, symptoms of bulimia and anorexia, such as binge eating, induced vomiting, and an extreme fear of gaining weight are present in alarming numbers of college students. For example, in one study, 23 percent of college women and 14 percent of college men reported episodes of binge eating at least once a week. In addition, 28 percent of the women and 7 percent of the men stated that they were "often" to "always" terrified of gaining weight.[232]

A startling number of adolescents are practicing unhealthful behaviors to regulate body weight.[236, 237] In one study of tenth-grade students, 13 percent reported the use of vomiting, laxatives, or diuretics to control their weight.[237] These students expressed an abnormal concern with their weight, frequently dieted, and experienced guilt following periods of excessive eating.

There are many published reports of the abnormal weight-control behaviors of athletes, especially ballet dancers, gymnasts, runners, and swimmers.[238, 239] At one competitive swimming camp, researchers found that of the 900 swimmers ages 9 to 18, 15.4 percent of the girls and 3.6 percent of the boys used a variety of abnormal weight-loss techniques to meet the demands of their sport.[238] Girls in particular were likely to misperceive themselves as overweight.

Weight patterns of athletes can be grouped into three categories.[239] There are sports such as baseball where maintenance of low weight is not important. The second category involves sports with specific weight divisions such as wrestling or boxing. Weight fluctuations can be rapid, frequent (15 times per season), and large (one survey found that the weight of 41 percent fluctuated 5.0 to 9.1 kg every week of the season, with an average end-of-season weight gain of from 2 to 20.5 kg). The third category involves sports in which low weights

---

Box 11.4   Defining Bulimia and Anorexia Nervosa

Bulimia:

1. There are recurrent episodes of binge-eating (rapid consumption of a large amount of food in a short period of time, often less than two hours).

2. During the eating binges there is a feeling of lack of control over the eating behavior.

3. The individual regularly engages in either self-induced vomiting, use of laxatives, or rigorous dieting or fasting in order to counteract the effects of the binge-eating.

4. There are a minimum average of two binge-eating episodes per week for at least three months.

Anorexia nervosa:

1. There is an intense fear of becoming obese, even when underweight.

2. There is a disturbance in the way in which one's body weight, size or shape is perceived. For example, one claims to "feel fat" even when extremely thin, or believes that one area of the body is "too fat" even when obviously underweight.

3. There is a refusal to maintain body weight over a minimal normal weight for age and height. For example, weight loss is so severe that weight is more than 25 percent below normal. In a growing child, there is a failure to make expected weight gains, leading to body weights 15 percent below expected.

4. With females, there is an absence of at least three consecutive menstrual cycles ("amenorrhea").

are the norm, such as distance running, gymnastics, figure skating, and ballet. Low weights in this category are necessary for optimal performance and appearance, and participants are often willing to utilize abnormal weight-control behaviors to attain the necessary weight for competition.

Binge eating and the various forms of purging (vomiting, laxative and diuretic use) can cause serious medical problems,[237,240] including stomach dilation and rupture, infection of the lung from vomitus, low body levels of chloride and potassium ions, infection and rupture of the esophagus, enlargement of the salivary glands, and tooth erosion and loss. Death is frighteningly common among anorexics—who can literally starve themselves to death. Karen Carpenter, a famous pop singer of the 1970s, died from complications related to her battles with anorexia.

Bulimic symptoms are more common among those with a history of weight problems. In addition, 30 to 50 percent of anorexics develop bulimia.[241] One of the main features of anorexia nervosa, the morbid fear of becoming fat, is also central to bulimia.

What can be done to help the anorexic or bulimic? Most experts feel they need specialized professional help—generally in eating disorder clinics. These clinics usually have a staff of professionals, including physicians, psychologists, dietitians, and nurses to meet the varied needs of people with eating disorders.[242] Often bulimics and anorexics have very deep seated emotional problems at the foundation of their eating problems. Long-term professional care is necessary.

Summary

1. In this chapter, emphasis was placed on describing the various theories of obesity, and how this major health problem can be treated.

2. The majority of American adults weight more than they should, and approximately one-fourth of all children, youth, and adults are obese.

3. There are many disadvantages associated with obesity, including several diseases such as cancer, diabetes, and heart disease. Obesity is associated with early death.

4. Three major theories of obesity were discussed, with emphasis placed on the importance of genetic and parental influences, dietary factors (especially excess dietary fat), and insufficient energy expenditure.

5. Some people are more prone to obesity than others, and need to be unusually careful in their dietary and exercise habits.

6. When humans eat diets high in fat, excess body fat is formed more easily than it is with a high-carbohydrate, high-fiber diet. Including more fruits, vegetables, legumes, and whole grains in the diet while moderating high-fat, low-fiber foods such as oils, margarine, butter, cheese, and fatty meats is probably the most important measure for controlling obesity.

7. Although obese people have higher resting metabolic rates than normal-weight people because of their extra lean body weight, they tend to exercise less than lean people. However, most studies have found that overeating is more prominent than underexercising in explaining obesity.

8. Following a meal, energy is expended by the body to process the food. This is called the thermic effect of food. Some obese people may have a slightly lower than average thermic effect of food, but this does not appear to be a major factor explaining why people gain excess weight.

9. Obesity is very difficult to treat. There are three classifications of obesity, and each requires different approaches.

10. Severe obesity is defined as weighing more than double the ideal weight. In certain cases, gastric reduction surgery is recommended.

11. Moderate obesity is defined as being 41–100 percent overweight. Because of the high amounts of excess body fat, the very-low-Calorie diet can be effective, but should only be administered under medical supervision.

12. The majority of obese people are mildly obese (20–40 percent overweight). For them, a weight loss of about one percent total body weight per week is optimal—utilizing a combination of improved diet, increased exercise, and appropriate behavioral modification.

13. To lose one pound of fat, an excess of 3,500 Calories must be expended.

14. The caloric intake should be reduced, generally best done by reducing the fat content of the diet and increasing the complex carbohydrate content. Weight watchers must beware of the many "quick and easy" weight loss methods.

15. Six issues regarding the role of physical activity in weight reduction were reviewed, including the theories that aerobic exercise: accelerates weight loss significantly when combined

with a reducing diet; causes the resting metabolic rate to stay elevated for a long time after the exercise bout, burning extra Calories; counters the diet-induced decrease in resting metabolic rate; counters the diet-induced decrease in fat-free mass; leads to a chronic decrease in appetite; augments the thermic effect of food.

16. The are several important benefits of exercise for the obese, including these effects of moderate aerobic activity: improved cardiorespiratory endurance; improved blood lipid profile; improved psychological state; group social support which may enhance long-term maintenance of weight loss; and decreased risk of obesity-related diseases.

17. Moderate aerobic exercise during weight reduction helps to improve one's general health status, but the real power behind weight loss comes from a reduction in dietary Calories. The success of a weight loss program should be measured not only by the total amount of weight lost, but also by the quality of the weight loss, and final health status.

18. Behavior modification consists of various procedures to help change eating behavior, events which trigger eating, and the consequences.

19. Bulimia and anorexia nervosa are two unhealthy and sometimes life-threatening eating disorders. Bulimics consume large amounts of food within short periods of time, and then engage in various purging techniques. People with anorexia nervosa have disturbed perceptions of their body images, which tend to prompt excessive weight loss. Long-term professional care is necessary.

References

1. Belko AZ, Van Loan M, Barbieri TF, Mayclin P. Diet, Exercise, Weight Loss, and Energy Expenditure in Moderately Overweight Women. Int J Obes 11:93–104, 1987.

2. National Center for Health Statistics: Health, United States, 1987. DHHS Pub. No. (PHS) 88–1232. Public Health Service. Washington. U.S. Government Printing Office, Mar. 1988.

3. Forman MR, Trowbridge FL, Gentry EM, et al. Overweight Adults in the United States: The Behavioral Risk Factor Surveys. Am J Clin Nutr 44:410–416, 1986.

4. Harlan WR, Landis JR, Flegal KM, Davis CS, Miller ME. Secular Trends in Body Mass in the United States, 1960–1980. Am J Epidemiol 128:1065–1074, 1988.

5. Flegal KM, Harlan WR, Landis JR. Secular Trends in Body Mass Index and Skinfold Thickness With Socioeconomic Factors in Young Adult Men. Am J Clin Nutr 48:544–551, 1988.

6. Flegal KM, Harlan WR, Landis JR. Secular Trends in Body Mass Index and Skinfold Thickness With Socioeconomic Factors in Young Adult Women. Am J Clin Nutr 48:535–543, 1988.

7. National Institutes of Health. Consensus Development Conference Statement. Health Implications of Obesity. February 11–13, 1985. Ann Intern Med 103:981–1077, 1985.

8. Simopoulos AP. Obesity and Body Weight Standards. Annu Rev Public Health 7:481–492, 1986.

9. Millar WJ, Stephens T. The Prevalence of Overweight and Obesity in Britain, Canada. and United States. Am J Public Health 77:38–41, 1987.

10. Gortmaker SL, Dietz WH, Sobol AM, Wehler CA. Increasing Pediatric Obesity in the United States. Am J Dis Child 141:535–540, 1987.

11. Ross JG, Pate RR, Lohman TG, Christenson GM. Changes in the Body Composition of Children. JOPERD November/December, 1987. pp. 74–77.

12. Lohman TG. The Use of Skinfold to Estimate Body Fatness On Children and Youth. JOPERD November/December, 1987, pp. 98–102.

13. Garn SM, Clark DC. Trends in Fatness and the Origins of Obesity. Pediatrics 57:443–456, 1976.

14. National Center for Health Statistics, C. A. Schoenborn. 1988. Health Promotion and Disease Prevention: United States, 1985. Vital and Health Statistics. Series 10, No. 163. DHHS Pub. No. (PHS) 88–1591. Public Health Service. Washington: U.S. Government Printing Office.

15. Bray GA, Gray DS. Obesity. Part I—Pathogenesis. West J Med 149:429–441, 1988.

16. Pacy PJ, Webster J, Garrow JS. Exercise and Obesity. Sports Med 3:89–113, 1986.

17. Lew EA, Garfinkel L. Variations in Mortality by Weight Among 750,000 Men and Women. J Chronic Dis 32:563–576, 1979.

18. Burton BT, Foster WR. Health Implications of Obesity: An NIH Consensus Development Conference. J Am Diet Assoc 85:1117–1121, 1985.

19. Garfinkel L. Overweight and Cancer. Ann Int Med 103:1034–1036, 1985.

20. Garrison RJ, Castelli WP. Weight and Thirty-Year Mortality of Men in the Framingham Study. Ann Int Med 103:1006–1009, 1985.

21. Lew EA. Mortality and Weight: Insured Lives and the American Cancer Society Studies. Ann Int Med 103:1024–1029, 1985.

22. Hubert HB, et al. Obesity As An Independent Risk Factor for Cardiovascular Disease: A 26-year Follow-up of Participants in the Framingham Heart Study. Circulation 67:968–977, 1983.

23. Seidell JC, de Groot LCPGM, van Sonsbeek JLA, et al. Associations of Moderate and Severe Overweight With Self-Reported Illness and Medical Care in Dutch Adults. Am J Public Health 76:264, 1986.

24. Clarke WR, Woolson RF, Lauer RM. Changes In Ponderosity and Blood Pressure In Childhood: The Muscatine Study. Am J Epidemiol 124:195–206, 1986.

25. Manson JE, Stampfer MJ, Hennekens CH, Willett WC. Body Weight and Longevity: A Reassessment. JAMA 257:353–358, 1987.

26. Simopoulos AP. Obesity and Carcinogenesis: Historical Perspective. Am J Clin Nutr 45:271–276, 1987.

27. Smoak CGG, Burke GL, Webber LS, et al. Relation of Obesity to Clustering of Cardiovascular Disease Risk Factors in Children and Young Adults. Am J Epidemiol 125:364–372, 1987.

28. Hubert HB, Eaker ED, Garrison RJ, Castelli WP. Life-Style Correlates of Risk Factor Change in Young Adults: An Eight-Year Study of Coronary Heart Disease Risk Factors in the Framingham Offspring. Am J Epidemiol 125:812–831, 1987.

29. Jacobsen BK, Thelle DS. The Tromso Heart Study: Food Habits, Serum Total Cholesterol, HDL Cholesterol, and Triglycerides. Am J Epidemiol 125:622–630, 1987.

30. Hubert HB. The Importance of Obesity In the Development of Coronary Risk Factors and Disease: The Epidemiologic Evidence. Annu Rev Public Health 7:493–502, 1986.

31. Nanas S, Pan WH, Stamler J, et al. The Role of Relative Weight in the Positive Association Between Age and Serum Cholesterol in Men and Women. J Chron Dis 40:887–892, 1987.

32. Albanes D, Jones Y, Micozzi MS, Mattson ME. Associations Between Smoking and Body Weight in the U.S. Population: Analysis of NHANES II. Am J Public Health 77:439–444, 1987.

33. Jéquier E. Energy, Obesity, and Body Weight Standards. Am J Clin Nutr 45:1035–1047, 1987.

34. Stallings VA, Archibald EH, Pencharz PB, et al. One-year follow-up of weight, total body potassium, and total body nitrogen in obese adolescents treated with the protein-sparing modified fast. Am J Clin Nutr 48:91–94, 1988.

35. Harris T, Cook EF, Garrison R, et al. Body Mass Index and Mortality Among Nonsmoking Older Persons: The Framingham Heart Study. JAMA 259:1520–1524, 1988.

36. Hoffmans MDAF, Kromhout D, De Lezenne Coulander C. The Impact of Body Mass Index of 78,612 18-Year Old Dutch Men on 32-Year Mortality From All Causes. J Clin Epidemiol 41:749–756, 1988.

37. Hamm P, Shekelle RB, Stamler J. Large Fluctuations in Body Weight During Young Adulthood and Twenty-Five-Year Risk of Coronary Death in Men. Am J Epidemiol 129:312–318, 1989.

38. Haffner SM, Stern MP, Hazuda HP, Pugh J, Patterson JK. Do Upper-Body and Centralized Adiposity Measure Different Aspects of Regional Body-Fat Distribution?: Relationship to Non-Insulin-Dependent Diabetes Mellitus, Lipids, and Lipoproteins. Diabetes 36:43–51, 1987.

39. Fujioka S, Matsuzawa Y, Tokunaga K, Tarui S. Contribution of Intra-Abdominal Fat Accumulation to the Impairment of Glucose and Lipid Metabolism in Human Obesity. Metabolism 36:54–59, 1987.

40. Reichley KB, Mueller WH, Hanis CL, et al. Centralized Obesity and Cardiovascular Disease Risk in Mexican Americans. Am J Epidemiol 125:373–386, 1987.

41. Gillum RF. The Association of Body Fat Distribution With Hypertension, Hypertensive Heart Disease, Coronary Heart Disease, Diabetes and Cardiovascular Risk Factors in Men and Women Aged 18–79 Years. J Chron Dis 40:421–428, 1987.

42. Rimm AA, Hartz AJ, Fischer ME. A Weight Shape Index for Assessing Risk of Disease in 44,820 Women. J Clin Epidemiol 41:459–465, 1988.

43. Barakat HA, Burton DS, Carpenter JW, Holbert D, Israel RG. Body Fat Distribution, Plasma Lipoproteins and the Risk of Coronary Heart Disease of Male Subjects. Int J Obes 12:473–480, 1988.

44. Soler JT, Folsom AR, Kushi LH, et al. Association of Body Fat Distribution with Plasma Lipids, Lipoproteins, Apolipoproteins A1 and B in Postmenopausal Women. J Clin Epidemiol 41:1075–1081, 1988.

45. Krotkiewski M, Bjorntorp P, Sjostrom L, Smith U. Impact of Obesity on Metabolism in Men and Women. J Clin Invest 72:1150–1162, 1983.

46. Lapidus L, et al. Distribution of Adipose Tissue and Risk of Cardiovascular Disease and Death: A 12-Year Follow Up Of Participants In the Population of Women in Gothenburg, Sweden. BMJ 289:1257–1261, 1984.

47. Bjorntorp P. Regional Patterns of Fat Distribution. Ann Int Med 103:994–995, 1985.

48. Ohlson LD, Larsson B, Svardsudd L, et al. The Influence of Body Fat Distribution on the Incidence of Diabetes Mellitus. Diabetes 34:1055–1058, 1985.

49. Stunkard AJ. Eating and Its Disorders. New York: Raven Press, 1984.

50. Frankle RT, Yang MU. Obesity and Weight Control: The Health Professional's Guide to Understanding and Treatment. Rockville, Maryland: Aspen Publishers, Inc., 1988.

51. Nash JD. Eating Behavior and Body Weight: Physiological Influences. Am J Health Promotion 1:5–15, 1987.

52. Roberts SB, Savage J, Coward WA, et al. Energy Expenditure and Intake of Infants Born to Lean and Overweight Mothers. N Engl J Med 318:461–466, 1988.

53. Mayer J. Genetic Factors in Human Obesity. Ann NY Acad Sci 131:412 421, 1965.

54. Stunkard AJ, Foch TT, Hrubec Z. A Twin Study of Human Obesity. JAMA 256:51–54, 1986.

55. Stunkard AJ, Sorensen TIA, Hanis C, et al. An Adoption Study of Human Obesity. N Engl J Med 314:193–198, 1986.

56. Bouchard C, Pérusse L, Leblanc C, et al. Inheritance of the Amount and Distribution of Human Body Fat. Int J Obes 12:205–215, 1988.

57. Corbett SW, Stern JS, Keesey RE. Energy Expenditure in Rats With Diet-Induced Obesity. Am J Clin Nutr 44:173–180, 1986.

58. Freedman DS, Shear CL, Burke GL, et al. Persistence of Juvenile-Onset Obesity over Eight Years: The Bogalusa Heart Study. Am J Public Health 77:588–592, 1987.

59. Patterson RE, Typpo JT, Typpo MH, Krause GF. Factors Related to Obesity in Preschool Children. J Am Diet Assoc 86:1376–1381, 1986.

60. Sorensen TIA, Sonne-Holm S. Risk in Childhood of Development of Severe Adult Obesity: Retrospective, Population-Based Case-Cohort Study. Am J Epidemiol 127:104–113, 1988.

61. de Boer JO, van Es AJH, van Raaij MA, Hautvast JGAJ. Energy Requirments and Energy Expenditure of Lean and Overweight Women, Measured by Indirect Calorimetry. Am J Clin Nutr 46:13–21, 1987.

62. Romieu I, Willett WC, Stampfer MJ, et al. Energy Intake and Other Determinants of Relative Weight. Am J Clin Nutr 47:406–412, 1988.

63. Bray GA. The Energetics of Obesity. Med Sci Sports Exerc 15:32–40, 1983.

64. Braitman LE, Adlin EV, Stanton JL. Obesity and Caloric Intake: The National Health and Nutrition Examination Survey of 1971–1975 (HANES I). J Chron Dis 38:727–739, 1985.

65. Baecke JAH, Stavern WAV, Burema J. Food Consumption, Habitual Physical Activity, and Body Fatness In Young Dutch Adults. Am J Clin Nutr 37:287–294, 1983.

66. Willett W, Stampfer MJ. Total Energy Intake: Implications for Epidemiologic Analyses. Am J Epidemiol 124:17–27, 1986.

67. Kromhout D, Saris WHM, Horst CH. Energy Intake, Energy Expenditure, and Smoking in Relation to Body Fatness: the Zutphen Study. Am J Clin Nutr 47:668–674, 1988.

68. Lissner L, Habicht JP, Strupp BJ, et al. Body Composition and Energy Intake: Do Overweight Women Overeat and Underreport? Am J Clin Nutr 49:320–325, 1989.

69. Marcus MD, Wing RR, Lamparski DM. Binge Eating and Dietary Restraint in Obese Patients. Addictive Behaviors 10:163–168, 1985.

70. Acheson KJ, Schutz Y, Bessard T, Flatt JP, Jequier E. Carbohydrate Metabolism and De Novo Lipogenesis in Human Obesity. Am J Clin Nutr 45:78–85, 1987.

71. Sims EAH, Danforth E. Expenditure and Storage of Energy in Man. J Clin Invest 79:1019–1025, 1987.

72. Lissner L, Levitsky DA, Strupp BJ, et al. Dietary Fat and the Regulation of Energy Intake in Human Subjects. Am J Clin Nutr 46:886–892, 1987.

73. Tremblay A, Plourde G, Despres JP, Bouchard C. Impact of Dietary Fat Content and Fat Oxidation on Energy Intake in Humans. Am J Clin Nutr 49:799–805, 1989.

74. Dreon DM, Frey-Hewitt B, Ellsworth N, Williams PT, Terry RB, Wood PD. Dietary Fat:Carbohydrate Ratio and Obesity in Middle-Aged Men. Am J Clin Nutr 47:995–1000, 1988.

75. Flatt JP, Ravussin E, Acheson KJ, Jequier E. Effects of Dietary Fat on Postprandial Substrate Oxidation and on Carbohydrate and Fat Balance. J Clin Invest 76:1019–1024, 1985.

76. Danforth E. Diet and Obesity. Am J Clin Nutr 41:1132–1145, 1985.

77. Duncan KH, Bacon JA, Weinsier RL. The Effects of High and Low Energy Density Diets On Satiety, Energy Intake, and Eating Time of Obese and Nonobese Subjects. Am J Clin Nutr 37:763–767, 1983.

78. Schneeman BO. Effects of Nutrients and Nonnutrients on Food Intake. Am J Clin Nutr 42:966–972, 1985.

79. Stevens dJ, Levitsky DA, VanSoest PJ, et al. Effect of Psyllium Gum and Wheat Bran on Spontaneous Energy Intake. Am J Clin Nutr 46:812–817, 1987.

80. Owen OE, Holup ML, D'Alessio DA, et al. A Reappraisal of the Caloric Requirements of Men. Am J Clin Nutr 46:875–885, 1987.

81. The Harris Benedict Equation Reevaluated: Resting Energy Requirements and the Body Cell Mass. Am J Clin Nutr 40:168–182, 1984.

82. Report of a Joint FAO/WHO/UNU Expert Consultation. Energy and Protein Requirements. World Health Organization, 1985.

83. Jequier E, Schutz Y. Long-term Measurements of Energy Expenditure In Humans Using A Respiration Chamber. Am J Clin Nutr 38:989–998, 1983.

84. Ravussin E, Burnand B, Schutz Y, Jequier E. Twenty-four-hour Energy Expenditure and Resting Metabolic Rate In Obese, Moderately Obese, and Control Subjects. Am J Clin Nutr 35:566–573, 1982.

85. Epstein LH, Wing RR, Cluss P, et al. Resting Metabolic Rate in Lean and Obese Children: Relationship to Child and Parent Weight and Percent Overweight Change. Am J Clin Nutr 49:331–336, 1989.

86. Ravussin E, Lillioja S, Anderson TE, Christin L, Bogardus C. Determinants of 24-hour Energy Expenditure in Man. J Clin Invest 78:1568–1578, 1986.

87. Lean MEJ, James WPT. Metabolic Effects of Isoenergetic Nutrient Exchange Over 24 Hours in Relation to Obesity in Women. Int J Obesity 12:15–27, 1988.

88. Blair DB, Buskirk ER. Habitual Daily Energy Expenditure and Activity Levels of Lean and Adult-Onset and Child-Onset Obese Women. Am J Clin Nutr 45:540–550, 1987.

89. de Boer JO, van Es AJH, van Raaij MA, Hautvast JGAJ. Energy Requirments and Energy Expenditure of Lean and Overweight Women, Measured by Indirect Calorimetry. Am J Clin Nutr 46:13–21, 1987.

90. Geissler CA, Miller DS, Shah M. The Daily Metabolic Rate of the Post-Obese and the Lean. Am J Clin Nutr 45:914–920, 1987.

91. Weigle DS, Sande KJ, Iverius PH, Monsen ER, Brunzell JD. Weight Loss Leads to a Marked Decrease in Nonresting Energy Expenditure in Ambulatory Human Subjects. Metabolism 37:930–936, 1988.

92. Ravussin E, Lillioja S, Knowler WC, et al. Reduced Rate of Energy Expenditure As a Risk Factor for Body-Weight Gain. N Engl J Med 318:467–472, 1988.

93. Tryon WW. Activity as a Function of Body Weight. Am J Clin Nutr 46:451–455, 1987.

94. Tucker LA. The Relationship of Television Viewing to Physical Fitness and Obesity. Adolescence 21:797–806, 1986.

95. Tucker LA, Freidman GM. Television Viewing and Obesity in Adult Males. Am J Public Health 79:516–518, 1989.

96. Bullen BA, Reed RB, Mayer J. Physical Activity of Obese and Nonobese Adolescent Girls Appraised by Motion Picture Sampling. Am J Clin Nutr 14:211–223, 1964.

97. Chirico AM, Stunkard AJ. Physical Activity and Human Obesity. N Eng J Med 263:935–940, 1960.

98. Bloom WL, Eidex MF. Inactivity as a Major Factor in Adult Obesity. Metabolism 16:679–684, 1967.

99. Dietz WH, Gortmaker SL. Do We Fatten Our Children at the Television Set? Obesity and Television Viewing in Children and Adolescents. Pediatrics 75:807–812, 1985.

100. Berkowitz RI, et al. Physical Activity and Adiposity: A Longitudinal Study From Birth to Childhood. J Pediatr 106:734–737, 1985.

101. Nair KS, Halliday D, Garrow JS. Thermic Response to Isoenergetic Protein, Carbohydrate, or Fat Meals in Lean and Obese Subjects. Clin Sci 65:307–312, 1983.

102. Horton ES. Introduction: An Overview of the Assessment and Regulation of Energy Balance In Humans. Am J Clin Nutr 38:972–977, 1983.

103. Schwartz RS, Ravussin E, et al. The Thermic Effect of Carbohydrate Versus Fat Feeding In Man. Metabolism 34:285–293, 1985.

104. Hill JO, et al. Meal Size and Thermic Response to Food in Male Subjects as a Function of Maximum Aerobic Capacity. Metabolism 33:743–749, 1984.

105. Segal KR, Gutin B, Nyman AM, Pi-Sunyer FX. Thermic Effect of Food at Rest, During Exercise, and After Exercise In Lean and Obese Men of Similar Body Weight. J Clin Invest 76:1107–1112, 1985.

106. Schutz Y, et al. Decreased Glucose-Induced Thermogenesis After Weight Loss In Obese Subjects: A Predisposing Factor for Relapse of Obesity. Am J Clin Nutr 39:380–387, 1984.

107. Nair KS, Webster J, Garrow JS. Effect of Impaired Glucose Tolerance and Type II Diabetes on Resting Metabolic Rate and Thermic Response to a Glucose Meal in Obese Women. Metabolism 35:640–644, 1986.

108. Zed C, James WPT. Dietary Thermogenesis in Obesity: Fat Feeding at Different Energy Intakes. Int J Obes 10:375–390, 1986.

109. Vernet O, Christin L, Schutz Y, Danforth E, Jequier F. Enteral Verus Parenteral Nutrition: Comparison of Energy Metabolism in Lean and Moderately Obese Women. Am J Clin Nutr 43:194–209, 1986.

110. Brownell KD. The Psychology and Physiology of Obesity: Implications for Screening and Treatment. J Am Diet Assoc 84:406–414, 1984.

111. Priddy MLB. Gastric Reduction Surgery: A Dietitian's Experience and Perspective. J Am Diet Assoc 85:455–458, 1985.

112. Olsson SA, Petersson BG, et al. Effects of Weight Reduction After Gastroplasty On Glucose and Lipid Metabolism. Am J Clin Nutr 40:1273–1280, 1985.

113. Kral JG. Morbid Obesity and Related Health Risks. Ann Int Med 103:1043–1047, 1985.

114. Van Itallie TB, Gray GA, Conner WE, et al. Guidelines for Morbid Obesity. Am J Clin Nutr 42:904–905, 1985.

115. Graney AS, Smith LB, Hammer KA. Gastric Partition ing for Morbid Obesity. J Am Diet Assoc 86:630–635, 1986.

116. Jimenez JG, Fong BS, Julien P, et al. Weight Loss in Massive Obesity: Reciprocal Changes in Plasma HDL Cholesterol and HDL Binding to Human Adipocyte Plasma Membranes. Metabolism 37:580–586, 1988.

117. Naslund I, Jarnmark I, Andersson H. Dietary Intake Before and After Gastric Bypass and Gastroplasty for Morbid Obesity in Women. Int J Obes 12:503–513, 1988.

118. McFarland RJ, Ang L, Parker W, et al. The Dynamics of Weight Loss After Gastric Partition for Gross Obesity. Int J Obes 13:81–88, 1989.

119. Hale PJ, Singh BM, Crase J, et al. Following Weight Loss in Massively Obese Patients Correction of the Insulin Resistance of Fat Metabolism is Delayed Relative to the Improvement in Carbohydrate Metabolism. Metabolism 37:411–417, 1988.

120. Lovig T, Haffner FW, Nygaard K, Stadaas JO. Gastric Banding for Morbid Obesity: Early Results. Int J Obes 11:377–384, 1987.

121. Andersen T, Stokholm KH, Backer OG, Quaade F. Long-Term (5-Year) Results After Either Horizontal Gastroplasty or Very-Low-Calorie Diet for Morbid Obesity. Int J Obes 12:277–284, 1988.

122. Lockwood DH, Amatruda JM. Very Low Calorie Diets In the Management of Obesity. Annu Rev Med 35:373–381, 1984.

123. Timmons KH, Slaten BL, Svacha AJ. Metabolic Effects of Liquid Protein. J Am Diet Assoc 82:53–57, 1983.

124. Roberts HJ. The Hazards of Very-Low-Calorie Dieting. Am J Clin Nutr 41:171–172, 1985.

125. Wadden TA, Stunkard AJ, Brownell KD, Day SC. A Comparison of Two Very-Low-Calorie Diets: Protein-Sparing-Modified Fast Versus Protein-Formula-Liquid Diet. Am J Clin Nutr 41:533–539, 1985.

126. Wadden TA et al. The Cambridge Diet: More Mayhem? JAMA 250:2833–2834, 1983.

127. Wadden TA, Stunkard AJ, Brownell KD. Very Low Calorie Diets: Their Efficacy, Safety, and Future. Ann Int Med 99:675–683, 1983.

128. Van Itallie TB, Yang MU. Cardiac Dysfunction In Obese Dieters: A Potentially Lethal Complication of Rapid, Massive Weight Loss. Am J Clin Nutr 39:695–702, 1984.

129. Hoffer LJ, Bistrian BR, et al. Metabolic Effects of Carbohydrate in Low-Calorie Diets. Metabolism 33:820–825, 1984.

130. Brown MR, Klish WJ, et al. A High Protein, Low Calorie Liquid Diet In the Treatment of Very Obese Adolescents: Long-Term Effect on Lean Body Mass. Am J Clin Nutr 38:20–31, 1983.

131. Henry RR, Wiest-Kent TA, Scheafter L, et al. Metabolic Consequences of Very-Low-Calorie Diet Therapy in Obese Non-Insulin-Dependent Diabetic and Nondiabetic Subjects. Diabetes 35:155–164, 1986.

132. Apfelbaum M, Fricker J, Igoin-Apfelbaum L. Low- and Very-Low-Calorie Diets. Am J Clin Nutr 45:1126–1134, 1987.

133. Young EA, Ramos R, Harris MM. Gastrointestinal and Cardiac Response to Low-Calorie Semistarvation Diets. Am J Clin Nutr 47:981–988, 1988.

134. Stallings VA, Archibald EH, Pencharz PB. Potassium, Magnesium, and Calcium Balance in Obese Adolescents on a Protein-Sparing Modified Fast. Am J Clin Nutr 47:220–224, 1988.

135. Kirschner MA, Schneider G, Ertel NH, Gorman J. An Eight-Year Experience With a Very-Low-Calorie Formula Diet for Control of Major Obesity. Int J Obes 12:69–80, 1988.

136. Hovell MF, Koch A, Hofstetter R, et al. Long-Term Weight Loss Maintenance: Assessment of a Behavioral and Supplemented Fasting Regimen. Am J Public Health 78:663–666, 1988.

137. Wadden TA, Stunkard AJ, Day SC, Gould RA, Rubin CJ. Int J Obes 11:239–249, 1987.

138. Council on Scientific Affairs. Treatment of Obesity in Adults. JAMA 260:2547–2551, 1988.

139. Stunkard AJ. Conservative Treatments for Obesity. Am J Clin Nutr 45:1142–1154, 1987.

140. Brownell KD, Steen SN. Modern Methods for Weight Control: The Physiology and Psychology of Dieting. Physician Sportsmed 15(12):122–137, 1987.

141. Brownell KD. Public Health Approaches to Obesity and Its Management. Annu Rev Public Health 7:521–533, 1986.

142. Arrington R, Bonner J, Stitt KR. Weight Reduction Methods of College Women. J Am Diet Assoc 85:483–484, 1985.

143. National Council Against Health Fraud. NCAHF Guidelines for Evaluating Commercial Weight-Loss Promotions. NCAHF Newsletter (March/April):1, 1987.

144. ADA Reports. Position of The American Dietetic Association: Identifying Food and Nutrition Misinformation. J Am Diet Assoc 88:1589–1591, 1988.

145. Rock CL, Coulston AM. Weight-Control Approaches: A Review by the California Dietetic Association. J Am Diet Assoc 88:44–48, 1988.

146. Trubo R. Fad Diets: Sorting Through the Misinformation. Medical World News, August 11, 1986, pp. 44–59.

147. Johnson J. Dieting by the Book. Vibrant Life, January/February 1987, 17–26.

148. Fisher MC, Lachance PA. Nutrition Evaluation of Published Weight-Reducing Diets. J Am Diet Assoc 85:450–454, 1985.

149. Geliebter A, Westreich S, Gage D. Gastric Distention by Balloon and Test-Meal Intake In Obese and Lean Subjects. Am J Clin Nutr 48:592–594, 1988.

150. Willis J. The Fad-Free Diet: How To Take Weight Off (And Keep It Off) Without Getting Ripped Off. FDA Consumer July/August 1985, pp. 26–29.

151. Henry DA. Glucomannan and Risk of Oesophageal Obstruction. Br Med J 292:591–592, 1986.

152. Nieman DC, Haig JL, De Guia ED, et al. Reducing Diet and Exercise Training Effects on Resting Metabolic Rates in Mildly Obese Women. J Sports Med 28:79–88, 1988.

153. Hagan RD, Upton SJ, Wong L, Whittam J. The Effects of Aerobic Conditioning and/or Caloric Restriction in Overweight Men and Women. Med Sci Sports Exerc 18:87–94, 1986.

154. Van Dale D, Saris WHM, Schoffelen PFM, Ten Hoor F. Does Exercise Give An Additional Effect in Weight Reduction Regimens? Int J Obes 11:367–375, 1987.

155. Hill JO, Sparling PB, Shields TW, Heller PA. Effects of Exercise and Food Restriction on Body Composition and Metabolic Rate in Obese Women. Am J Clin Nutr 46:622–630, 1987.

156. Phinney SD, LaGrange BM, O'Connell M, Danforth E. Effects of Aerobic Exercise on Energy Expenditure and Nitrogen Balance During Very Low Calorie Dieting. Metabolism 37:758–765, 1988.

157. Katch V, Becque MD, Marks C, Moorehead C, Rocchini A. Basal Metabolism of Obese Adolescents: Inconsistent Diet and Exercise Effects. Am J Clin Nutr 48:565–569, 1988.

158. van Dale D, Saris WHM. Repetitive Weight Loss and Weight Regain: Effects on Weight Reduction, Resting Metabolic Rate, and Lipolytic Activity Before and After Exercise and/or Diet Treatment. Am J Clin Nutr 49:409–416, 1989.

159. Hammer RL, Barrier CA, Roundy ES, Bradford JM, Fisher AG. Calorie- Restricted Low-Fat Diet and Exercise in Obese Women. Am J Clin Nutr 49:77–85, 1989.

160. Warwick PM, Garrow JS. The Effect of Addition of Exercise to a Regime of Dietary Restriction on Weight Loss, Nitrogen Balance, Resting Metabolic Rate and Spontaneous Physical Activity in Three Obese Women in a Metabolic Ward. Int J Obes 5:25–32, 1981.

161. Lennon D, Nagle F, Stratman F, et al. Diet and Exercise Training Effects on Resting Metabolic Rate. Int J Obes 9:39–47, 1985.

162. Pavlou KN, Steffee WP, Lerman RH, Burrows BA. Effects of Dieting and Exercise on Lean Body Mass, Oxygen Uptake, and Strength. Med Sci Sports Exerc 17:466–471, 1985.

163. Wood PD, Stefanick ML, Dreon DM, et al. Changes in Plasma Lipids and Lipoproteins in Overweight Men During Weight Loss Through Dieting As Compared With Exercise. N Engl J Med 319:1173–1179, 1988.

164. Atomi Y, Miyashita M. Influences of Weight Reduction on Aerobic Power and Body Composition of Middle-Aged Women. J Sports Med 27:501–509, 1987.

165. Zuti WB, Golding LA. Comparing Diet and Exercise As Weight Reduction Tools. Physician Sportsmed 4(1):49–53, 1976.

166. Dudleston AK, Bennion M. Effect of Diet and/or Exercise on Obese College Women. J Am Diet Assoc 56:126–129, 1970.

167. Johnson CC, Stone MH, Lopez-S, A, et al. Diet and Exercise in Middle-Aged Men. J Am Diet Assoc 81:695–701, 1982.

168. Gwinup G. Weight Loss Without Dietary Restriction: Efficacy of Different Forms of Aerobic Exercise. Am J Sports Med 15:275–279, 1987.

169. Belko AZ, Van Loan M, Barbieri TF, Mayclin P. Diet, Exercise, Weight Loss, and Energy Expenditure in Moderately Overweight Women. Int J Obes 11:93–104, 1987.

170. Hagan RD. Benefits of Aerobic Conditioning and Diet for Overweight Adults. Sports Med 5:144–155, 1988.

171. Heymsfield SB, Casper K, Hearn J, Guy D. Rate of Weight Loss During Underfeeding: Relation to Level of Physical Activity. Metabolism 38:215–223, 1989.

172. Hamborg B. Obesity and Physical Activity. Scand J Med (Suppl) 29:217–220, 1982.

173. Garrow JS. Thermogenesis and Obesity in Man. IN: Bjorntorp P, Cairella M, Howard AN (eds). Recent Advances in Obesity Research: III. Proceedings of the 3rd International Congress on Obesity, 8–11 October 1980. London: John Libbey and Co., LD., 208–213, 1981.

174. Brehm BA. Elevation of Metabolic Rate Following Exercise: Implications for Weight Loss. Sports Med 6:72–78, 1988.

175. Maehlum S, Grandmontagne M, Newsholme EA, Sejersted OM. Magnitude and Duration of Excess Postexercise Oxygen Consumption in Healthy Young Subjects. Metabolism 35:425–429, 1986.

176. Brehm BA, Gutin B. Recovery Energy Expenditure for Steady State Exercise in Runners and Nonexercisers. Med Sci Sports Exerc 18:205–210, 1986.

177. Bahr R, Ingnes I, Vaage O, et al. Effect of Duration of Exercise On Excess Postexercise O_2 Consumption. J Appl Physiol 62:485–490, 1987.

178. Akabas SF, Colt E, Pi-Sunyer FX. Lack of Sustained Increase in $\dot{V}O_2$ Following Exercise in Fit and Unfit Subjects. Am J Clin Nutr 41:545–549, 1985.

179. Poehlman ET, Melby CL, Badylak SF, Calles J. Aerobic Fitness and Resting Energy Expenditure in Young Adult Males. Metabolism 38:85–90, 1989.

180. Hermansen L, et al. Postexercise Elevation of Resting Oxygen Uptake: Possible Mechanisms and Physiological Significance. IN: Physiological Chemistry of Training and Detraining (Marconnet/Poortmans/Hermansen: eds). Basel: S. Karger, 1984.

181. Bielinski R, Schutz Y, Jequier E. Energy Metabolism During the Postexercise Recovery in Man. AJCN 42:69–82, 1985.

182. Mathieson RA, Walberg JL, Gwazdauskas FC, et al. The Effect of Varying Carbohydrate Content of a Very-Low-Caloric Diet on Resting Metabolic Rate and Thyroid Hormones. Metabolism 35:394–398, 1986.

183. Henson LC, Poole DC, Donahoe CP, Heber D. Effects of Exercise Training on Resting Energy Expenditure During Caloric Restriction. Am J Clin Nutr 46:893–899, 1987.

184. Geissler CA, Miller DS, Shah M. The Daily Metabolic Rate of the Post-Obese and the Lean. Am J Clin Nutr 45(5):914–20, 1987.

185. Garrow JS. Energy Balance In Man—An Overview. Am J Clin Nutr 45:1114–1119, 1987.

186. Brown MR, Klish WJ, et al. A High Protein, Low Calorie Liquid Diet in the Treatment of Very Obese Adolescents: Long-Term Effect on Lean Body Mass. Am J Clin Nutr 38:20–31, 1983.

187. Donnelly JE, Jacobsen DJ. Body Composition Changes With Very Low Calorie Diet and Exercise. Med Sci Sports Exerc 19:S69, 1987.

188. Ballor DL, Katch VL, Becque MD, Marks CR. Resistance Weight Training During Caloric Restriction Enhances Lean Body Weight Maintenance. Am J Clin Nutr 47:19–25, 1988.

189. Wilmore JH. Appetite and Body Composition Consequent to Physical Activity. Res Quart Exerc Sport 54:415–425, 1983.

190. Thompson DA, Wolfe LA, Eikelboom R. Acute Effects of Exercise Intensity on Appetite in Young Men. Med Sci Sports Exerc 20:222–227, 1988.

191. Titchenal CA. Exercise and Food Intake: What is the Relationship? Sports Med 6:135–145, 1988.

192. Pi-Sunyer FX, Woo R. Effect of Exercise On Food Intake In Human Subjects. Am J Clin Nutr 42:983–990, 1985.

193. Woo R, Pi-Sunyer FX. Effect of Increased Physical Activity on Voluntary Intake In Lean Women. Metabolism 34:836–840, 1985.

194. Young JC, Treadway JL, Balon TW, et al. Prior Exercise Potentiates the Thermic Effect of a Carbohydrate Load. Metabolism 35:1048–1053, 1986.

195. McDonald RB, Wickler S, Horwitz B, Stern JS. Meal-Induced Thermogenesis Following Exercise Training in the Rat. Med Sci Sports Exerc 20:44–49, 1988.

196. Segal KR, Gutin B. Thermic Effects of Food and Exercise In Lean and Obese Women. Metabolism 32:581–589, 1983.

197. Welle S. Metabolic Responses to a Meal During Rest and Low-Intensity Exercise. Am J Clin Nutr 40:990–994, 1984.

198. Schutz Y, Bessard T, Jéquier E. Exercise and Postprandial Thermogenesis in Obese Women Before and After Weight Loss. Am J Clin Nutr 45:1424–1432, 1987.

199. Belko AZ, Barbieri TF, Wong EC. Effect of Energy and Protein Intake and Exercise Intensity on the Thermic Effect of Food. Am J Clin Nutr 43:863–869, 1986.

200. Pacy PJ, Barton N, Webster JD, Garrow JS. The Energy Cost of Aerobic Exercise in Fed and Fasted Normal Subjects. Am J Clin Nutr 42:764–768, 1985.

201. Tremblay A, Despres JP, Bouchard C. The Effects of Exercise-Training on Energy Balance and Adipose Tissue Morphology and Metabolism. Sports Med 2:223–233, 1985.

202. Tremblay A, Cote J, LeBlanc J. Diminished Dietary Thermogenesis in Exercise-Trained Human Subjects. Eur J Appl Physiol 52:1–4, 1983.

203. Hill JO, et al. Meal Size and Thermic Response to Food in Male Subjects as a Function of Maximum Aerobic Capacity. Metabolism 33:743–749, 1984.

204. Thompson JK, Blanton P. Energy Conservation and Exercise Dependence: A Sympathetic Arousal Hypothesis. Med Sci Sports Exerc 19:91–99, 1987.

205. Neufeld ND, Ezrin C, Corbo L, Long D, Bush MA. Effects of caloric Restriction and Exercise on Insulin Receptors in Obesity: Association With Changes in Membrane Lipids. Metabolism 35:580–587, 1986.

206. Schneider SH, Khachadurian AK, Amorosa LF, et al. Abnormal Glucoregulation During Exercise in Type II (Non-Insulin-Dependent) Diabetes. Metabolism 36:1161–1166, 1987.

207. Sikand G, Kondo A, Foreyt JP, et al. Two-Year Follow-up of Patients Treated With a Very-Low-Calorie Diet and Exercise Training. J Am Diet Assoc 88:487–488, 1988.

208. Stevenson DW, Darga LL, Spafford TR, et al. Variable Effects of Weight Loss on Serum Lipids and Lipoproteins in Obese Patients. Int J Obes 12:495–502, 1987.

209. Nieman DC, Register UD, Lindsted K, Dizon G, De Guia E, Haig J. Effect of Exercise on Serum Lipid and Lipoprotein Levels Seen with Changes in Body Weight. Fed Proc 45:704, 1986 (abstract). Am J Clin Nutr (in press).

210. Schwartz RS. The Independent Effects of Dietary Weight Loss and Aerobic Training on High Density Lipoproteins and Apolipoprotein A-I Concentrations in Obese Men. Metabolism 36:165–171, 1987.

211. Tran ZV, Weltman A. Differential Effects of Exercise on Serum Lipid and Lipoprotein Levels Seen With Changes in Body Weight. JAMA 254:919–924, 1985.

212. Lampman RM, Schteingart DE, Foss ML. Exercise as a Partial Therapy for the Extremely Obese. Med Sci Sports Exerc 18:19–24, 1985.

213. Kromhout D. Body Weight, Diet, and Serum Cholesterol in 871 Middle-Aged Men During 10 Years of Follow-Up (the Zutphen Study). Am J Clin Nutr 38:591–598, 1983.

214. Cramer SR, Nieman DC, Lee JW. The Effects of Moderate Exercise Training on Psychological Well-Being and Mood State in Women. (Manuscript under review.)

215. Stephens T. Physical Activity and Mental Health in the United States and Canada: Evidence from Four Population Surveys. Prev Med 17:35–47, 1988.

216. Hughes JR. Psychological Effects of Habitual Aerobic Exercise: A Critical Review. Prev Med 13:66–78, 1984.

217. Ross CE, Hayes D. Exercise and Psychologic Well-Being in the Community. Am J Epidemiol 127:762–771, 1988.

218. Mellin LM, Slinkard LA, Irwin CE. Adolescent Obesity Intervention: Validation of the SHAPEDOWN Program. J Am Diet Assoc 87:333–338, 1987.

219. Sikand G, Kondo A, Foreyt JP, et al. Two-Year Follow-up of Patients Treated With a Very-Low-Calorie Diet and Exercise Training. J Am Diet Assoc 88:487–488, 1988.

220. Foss ML. Exercise Concerns and Precautions for the Obese. IN: Nutrition and Exercise In Obesity Management (Storlie J, Jordan HA: Eds). New York: Spectrum Publications, 1984.

221. Franklin BA. Myths and Misconceptions in Exercise for Weight Control. IN: Nutrition and Exercise in Obesity Management (Storlie J, Jordan HA: Eds). New York: Spectrum Publications, 1984.

222. Gauthier MM. Continuous Passive Motion: The No-Exercise Exercise. Physician Sportsmed 15(8):142–148, 1987.

223. Fenner L. Cellulite: Hard to Budge Pudge. FDA Consumer, May 1980.

224. Katch FI, Clarkson PM, et al. Effects of Sit Up Exercise Training On Adipose Cell Size and Adiposity. Res Quart Exerc Sports 55:242–247, 1984.

225. Frankle RT, Yang MU. Obesity and Weight Control: The Health Professional's Guide to Understanding and Treatment. Rockville, Maryland: Aspen Publishers, Inc., 1988.

226. Despres JP, Bouchard C, et al. Effects of Aerobic Training On Fat Distribution In Male Subjects. Med Sci Sports Exerc 17:113–118, 1985.

227. Stunkard AJ, et al. What Is Behavior Therapy? A Very Short Description of Behavioral Weight Control. Am J Clin Nutr 41:821–823, 1985.

228. Burns CM, Richman R, Caterson ID. Nutrition Knowledge in the Obese and Overweight. Int J Obes 11:485–492, 1987.

229. Green LW. Modifying and Developing Health Behavior. Annu Rev Public Health 5:215–236, 1984.

230. Holli BB. Using Behavior Modification in Nutrition Counseling. J Am Diet Assoc 88:1530–1536, 1988.

231. American College of Sports Medicine. Position Statement On Proper and Improper Weight Loss Programs. Med Sci Sports Exerc 17:1984.

232. Zuckerman DM, Colby A, Ware NC, Lazerson JS. The Prevalence of Bulimia Among College Students. Am J Public Health 76:1135–1137, 1986.

233. Schotte DE, Stunkard AJ. Bulimia vs Bulimic Behaviors on a College Campus. JAMA 258:1213–1215, 1987.

234. Drewnowski A, Hopkins SA, Kessler RC. The Prevalence of Bulimia Nervosa in the U.S. College Student Population. Am J Public Health 78:1322–1325, 1988.

235. Kurtzman FD, Yager J, Landsverk J, Wiesmeier E, Bodurka DC. Eating Disorders Among Selected Female Student Populations at UCLA. J Am Diet Assoc 89:45–53, 1989.

236. Killen JD, Taylor CB, Telch MJ, et al. Depressive Symptoms and Substance Use Among Adolescent Binge Eaters and Purgers: A Defined Population Study. Am J Public Health 77:1539–1541, 1987.

237. Killen JD, Taylor CB, Telch MJ, et al. Self-Induced Vomiting and Laxative and Diuretic Use Among Teenagers. JAMA 255:1447–1449, 1986.

238. Dummer GM, Rosen LW, Heusner WW, et al. Pathogenic Weight-Control Behaviors of Young Competitive Swimmers. Physician Sportsmed 15(5):75–86, 1987.

239. Brownell KD, Steen SN, Wilmore JH. Weight Regulation Practices in Athletes: Analysis of Metabolic and Health Effects. Med Sci Sports Exerc 19:546–556, 1987.

240. Casper RC. The Pathophysiology of Anorexia Nervosa and Bulimia Nervosa. Annu Rev Nutr 6:299–316, 1986.

241. Swift WJ, Ritzholz M, Kalin NH, Kaslow N. A Follow-up Study of Thirty Hospitalized Bulimics. Psychosom Med 49:45, 1987.

242. Position of The American Dietetic Association: Nutrition Intervention in the Treatment of Anorexia Nervosa and Bulimia Nervosa. J Am Diet Assoc 88:68–71, 1988.

Physical Fitness Activity 11.1: Calculating Your Energy Expenditure

In this physical fitness activity, you will be calculating your average daily Calorie expenditure. As you may remember from your study of this chapter, during any given 24-hour period, the majority of your energy expenditure (if you are no more than moderately active) comes from your resting metabolic rate, with smaller amounts from physical activity and the energy used in digesting and metabolizing your food.

Table 11.11 outlines a method for determining the number of Calories burned each day, combining RMR and physical activity. Notice that Category 1 represents the energy you expend during sleeping or resting in bed, or in other words, your resting metabolic rate. Categories 2 through 9 represent different forms of physical activity, with Category 9 being the most intense.

The average female in the United States burns only 1,500 to 2,000 total Calories per day, and the average male, 2,300 to 3,000 Calories per day. Those spending more time in Categories 6 through 9 will burn more than these amounts.

Estimate the number of Calories you burn in a given day by averaging the number of hours you spend in each activity category. Make sure that your hour total equals 24! Review Table 11.4 to help you estimate the number of hours you might spend in each category.

Multiply the number of hours by the Calorie/kg factor and then your weight (in kilograms). The final step is to total the Calories you have estimated in the final column. Your final result should be close to the estimated amount of Calories you consume each day.

Table 11.11 Calculating Energy Expenditure

Directions: Estimate the average number of hours you spend in each category. Multiply the calorie/kg factor times the hours/day and then by your body weight. Put the total number of calories calculated for each category in the calorie/category blank.

Category	Average Hours/Day		Calorie/Kg Per Hour		Body Wt (kg)		Calorie/ Category
1	_____	×	1.04	×	_____	=	_____
2	_____	×	1.52	×	_____	=	_____
3	_____	×	2.28	×	_____	=	_____
4	_____	×	2.76	×	_____	=	_____
5	_____	×	3.36	×	_____	=	_____
6	_____	×	4.80	×	_____	=	_____
7	_____	×	5.60	×	_____	=	_____
8	_____	×	6.00	×	_____	=	_____
9	_____	×	8.00	×	_____	=	_____
Totals	24					=	Total (24 hour energy expenditure)

Category 1   Sleeping; resting in bed.

Category 2   Sitting; eating; listening; writing; etc.

Category 3   Light activity while standing; washing, shaving, combing hair, cooking.

Category 4   Slow walking; driving; dressing; showering.

Category 5   Light manual work (floor sweeping, window washing, driving a truck, painting, waiting on tables, nursing chores, house chores, electrical work, walking at moderate pace).

Category 6   Leisure activities and sports in a recreational environment (baseball, golf, volleyball, canoeing or rowing, archery, bowling, slow cycling, table tennis, etc.).

Category 7   Manual work at moderate pace (mining, carpentry, house building, snow shoveling, loading and unloading goods).

Category 8   Leisure and sport activities of higher intensity, but not competitive (canoeing, bicycling at less than 10 mph, dancing, skiing, badminton, gymnastics, moderate paced swimming, tennis, brisk walking, etc.).

Category 9   Intense manual work, high intensity sport activities or sport competition (tree cutting, carrying heavy loads, jogging and running (faster than 12 minutes a mile), racquetball, swimming, cross country skiing, mountain biking, etc.).

Source: Adapted from: Bouchard C, et al. A Method to Assess Energy Expenditure In Children and Adults. Am J Clin Nutr 37:461–467, 1983.

Physical Fitness Activity 11.2:
Weight Management Counseling

In this physical fitness activity, we will review your ability to determine appropriate weight loss goals for people who are mildly obese. Before answering the questions below, you should review the Practical Summary (page 344) one more time.

Our hypothetical person weighs 224 pounds; his ideal weight is 166 pounds. He needs to lose 58 pounds, which means that he is 35 percent overweight (which puts him into the mildly obese classification). Of these 58 pounds, 75 percent is excess body fat (43.5 pounds). The other 25 percent (14.5 pounds) is excess lean body weight, mainly muscle from carrying around his 224 pounds.

Question #1

If he has 43.5 extra pounds of body fat, how many excess Calories does he have stored in his fat tissues?

_____ Calories

Question #2

What is the maximum amount of weight he should lose per week?

_____ pounds per week.

This represents how many Calories of exercise and/or less food per week?

_____ Calories per week

Question #3

Based on the practical summary at the end of this chapter, outline below your dietary and exercise recommendations.

Exercise: How many miles of walking per day? (Use ACSM walking equation, and then subtract RMR and caloric expenditure for mild activity.)

_____ miles of walking per day

Diet: How many Calories less dietary fat per day?

_____ Calories of fat per day less

Other Recommendations?

_____

_____

_____

_____

_____

Chapter 12

Physical Activity and Aging

"All parts of the body which have a function, if used in moderation and exercised in labors in which each is accustomed, become thereby healthy, well-developed and age more slowly, but if unused and left idle they become liable to disease, defective in growth, and age quickly."—Hippocrates

Statistics and Trends

The fastest growing minority in the United States today is the *elderly*—those who reach or pass the age of 65.[1] Figure 12.1 shows that there are now nearly 30 million elderly people in the United States, a figure which will climb to 64.6 million, or 21 percent of the population, by the year 2030. The 65 and over group is growing twice as fast as the rest of the population.[2-8] The baby boom is being replaced by the senior citizen explosion.

Consider these statistics:[1-8]

- It is difficult to comprehend that in 1900, only 25 percent of American individuals lived beyond age 65, while in 1985, approximately 70 percent survived age 65, and 30 percent lived to be 80 or more. If present trends continue, within the next 10 or 20 years almost half of deaths will occur after age 80.[1] In the past five years, intense interest has been focused on the 85-and-older population (termed the "very old").[5] This is projected to be the fastest growing population segment over the next 25 years, expected to increase from 2.7 million in 1985 to approximately 7 million by the year 2015.

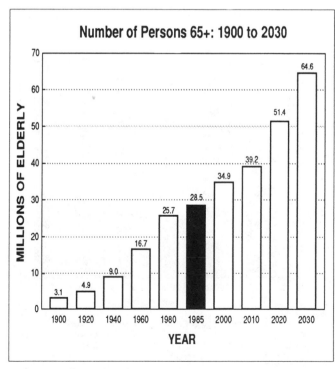

Figure 12.1 About 12 percent, or one in eight Americans are now 65 years of age or older. By the year 2030, one in five Americans will be elderly. *Source:* see reference 1.

359

▪ Length of life has increased remarkably during the 20th century. (See Figure 12.2.) *Life expectancy* at birth (the number of years a newborn baby can expect to live) reached a new high of 74.8 years in 1986.[4,8] Increases in life expectancy at birth during the first half of this century occurred mainly because of reductions in infant and childhood mortality. These reductions meant that more Americans survived to middle age. By contrast, increases in longevity in recent years have largely resulted from decreasing mortality from chronic diseases (primarily heart disease and stroke) among the middle-aged (45–64) and elderly populations (65–84).[4]

▪ Life expectancy at age 65 has increased dramatically within the last 25 years. From 1900 to 1960, life expectancy at age 65 improved only 2.4 years as compared with 2.4 years from 1960 to 1985.[3] People who are 65 years of age can now expect to live 16.7 more years, to the ripe old age of nearly 82, higher than ever before. (See Figure 12.2.)

Although these trends are generally welcome, concern has been expressed by some leaders about several issues.

▪ The central issue raised by increasing longevity is that of net gain in active functional years versus total years of disability and dysfunction. Present data are weak, but suggest that for each good, active, functional year gained, we add about 3.5 compromised years.[1] Whereas approximately two-thirds of the elderly perceive their health as "good" or "excellent," 50 percent have arthritis, 39 percent are hypertensive, 30 percent have a hearing impairment, 26 percent have heart disease, 17 percent have a deformity or orthopedic impairment, 15 percent have chronic problems with their sinuses, 10 percent have vision problems, and 9 percent have diabetes.[3] (See Figure 12.3.)

▪ Cardiovascular diseases (diseases of the heart and stroke combined) and cancers account for 72 percent of all deaths among the elderly. The number one cause of death is heart disease, accounting for 42.5 percent, with cancer second at 20 percent. Cancer deaths are increasing in this group at a rate of nearly 1 percent per year.

▪ *Osteoporosis*, defined as decrease in bone density, is widespread among the elderly. One third of women over 65 develop fractures of their spinal

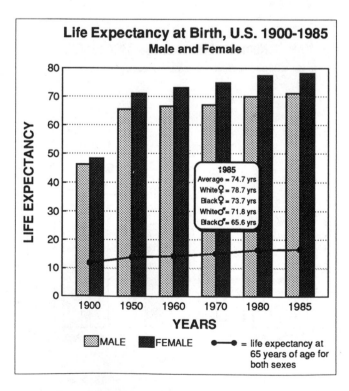

Figure 12.2 Life expectancy at birth has increased nearly 60 percent, whereas life expectancy at age 65 has increased 40 percent since the year 1900. *Source:* see reference 4.

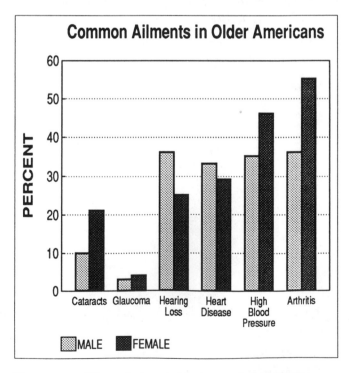

Figure 12.3 The majority of elderly people have at least one chronic disease and many have multiple problems. *Source:* National Institutes on Aging. FDA Consumer / October, 1988. (See also reference 3.)

bones, and by extreme old age, one of every three women and one of every six men will have had a hip fracture. (This will be discussed in more detail later in this chapter.) The projected number of hip fractures per year in the U.S. is projected to rise threefold between 1980 and 2040.[1] (See Figure 12.4.)

- In 1980 the number of cases of *senile dementia* was estimated at 2 million, with a mean age of 80. Projections for the year 2000 estimate the number will rise to 3.8 million, and by 2050, to 8.5 million. Senile dementia of the Alzheimer's type is now considered to be the most common acquired progressive brain syndrome.[9] Four percent of the American population is affected by the age of 65, and 20 percent of people 80 years and older develop *Alzheimer's disease.* The disease progresses from short-term memory loss to a final stage requiring total care.

- The forecasted increase in people 85 years of age and older may lead to a large increase in use of nursing homes in the future. One study showed that by the year 2012, state Medicaid nursing home payments will increase 280 percent to $6.3

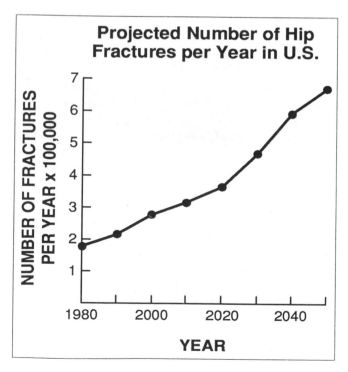

Projected Number of Hip Fractures per Year in U.S.

Figure 12.4 The number of hip fractures is projected to rise dramatically as the U.S. population ages. *Source:* National Center for Health Statistics and U.S. Bureau of the Census projections. See reference 1.

billion annually.[5,6] Financing the health care of the elderly in the future is a serious concern.

Despite the dramatic increase in the life expectancy of Americans, the United States still ranks behind 11 other nations in male life expectancy at birth.[4] The average life expectancy at birth is about 72 years in the developed countries, but only 55 years in the developing countries, largely because of their high infant mortality rates.[7]

The Aging Process

Aging refers to the normal yet irreversible biological changes that occur throughout a person's lifetime.[10] The aging process takes place at all ages, but for those over 65, it often becomes more manifest, with significant changes in quality of life. (See Box 12.1.)

BOX 12.1 The Aging Process

"You'll know you're old when everything hurts and what doesn't hurt doesn't work; when you get winded playing chess; when you stoop to tie your shoelaces and ask yourself, 'What else can I do while I'm down here?'; when everybody goes to your birthday party and stands around the cake just to get warm."—George Burns

---

In December 1987, Anna Williams died in a nursing home in Wales. At age 114, she was believed to be the oldest human on earth. Scientists think that 115–120 years is probably the upper limit of human longevity.[11] What factors are responsible for the aging process? There are two major theories of aging.[11-13]

"Error" theories speculate that with advancing age, we become less able to repair damage caused by internal malfunctions or external assault to the body. Various biochemical and hormone changes with aging may finally lead to death. The immune system is less effective in the elderly. The body may be less able to combat infection or destroy abnormal body cells.

"Program" theories of aging suggest that an internal clock starts ticking at conception and is programmed to run just so long. Some researchers feel that human cells can only divide a certain number of times and then stop, leading to death.

As a person ages, many changes take place in the body:[14-19]

- **Loss of taste and smell:** The elderly often complain of a decreased ability to taste and enjoy food. Taste buds decrease in number and size, affecting sweet and salty tastes in particular. About 40 percent of people 80 years or older appear to have difficulty identifying common substances by smell.

- **Periodontal (bone area around the teeth) bone loss:** The majority of the elderly suffer bone loss and disease in the tissues around the teeth as they grow older. As a result, 50 percent of the population over 60 have lost all of their teeth and about 65 percent have lost all teeth in at least one arch. The end result of this is obvious—older people tend to choose foods that are easy to chew, leading to a reduced consumption of fresh fruit and vegetables high in dietary fiber.

- **Decrease in gastrointestinal function:** With an increase in age, the stomach cells are less able to secrete digestive juices, interfering with the digestion of protein and vitamin B-12. The small intestine becomes less capable of absorbing some nutrients, and there may also be a reduced ability of the intestine to move its contents through the digestive tract, resulting in constipation.

- **Loss in visual and auditory function:** Visual function starts to decline around the age of 45, and worsens gradually thereafter. After age 80, less than 15 percent of the population has 20/20 vision. Gradual hearing loss generally begins at about age 20, and has been estimated to affect as many as 66 percent of people reaching 80.

- **Decrease in lean body weight:** As a person ages, body fat increases, while muscle and bone (or lean body weight) decreases. This leads to a decrease in energy expended during rest, partially explaining why the elderly consume less Calories than younger people.

- **Loss of bone mineral mass:** As discussed previously, loss of bone (osteoporosis) is an almost universal phenomenon with increasing age. The resulting fractures often mend with difficulty, resulting in long periods of decreased physical activity and social interaction.

- **Mental impairment:** As stated above, senility, also called senile dementia or organic brain syndrome, affects about 60 percent of the elderly. Some of the problems associated with senile dementia include impairment of memory, judgment, feelings, personality, and ability to speak. Senile dementia of the Alzheimer's type accounts for at least half of all dementia in old age.

- **Decreased ability to metabolize drugs:** The elderly have a decreased ability to absorb, distribute, metabolize, and excrete both prescription and nonprescription drugs. The majority of the elderly are on more than one prescription drug, and these can interact with each other, affecting nutritional status.

- **High prevalence of chronic disease:** As discussed earlier, up to 85 percent of the elderly suffer from at least one chronic disease. A variety of diseases are more common among the elderly, including diabetes, cancer, heart disease, high blood pressure, stroke, and arthritis.

- **Neuromuscular changes:** Reaction time, ability to balance, and strength of muscles, tendons, and ligaments decrease with aging, limiting normal activity for many. Accidents increase, and the ability to shop for and prepare food may be hampered.

- **Urinary incontinence:** Up to 20 percent of the elderly living at home and 75 percent of those in long-term-care facilities cannot control the muscle that controls urination. This can lead to social isolation, embarrassment, and the decision to live in a nursing home environment.

- **Decrease in liver and kidney function:** The size and function of the liver and kidneys decrease steadily with age, making the removal of metabolic waste products more difficult.

- **Decrease in heart and lung fitness:** With aging, there is a decrease on the order of 8–10 percent per decade in the ability of the heart and lungs to supply oxygen to the muscles. Most of this is due to the decreasing physical activity of the elderly. This will be discussed in detail in the next section.

Exercise and Aging

Figure 12.5 summarizes the physiological changes that take place in the human body with aging. Interestingly, many of the changes that accompany aging are similar to those associated with inactivity and weightlessness.[19–22] In this section, we shall review evidence that much of the deterioration attributed to aging can be explained by the fact that people tend to exercise less as they age.

All living cells, tissues, and organs participate in an aging or "disuse syndrome" when their particular activity is impaired. As Figure 12.5 shows, the identifying characteristics of both aging and the disuse syn-

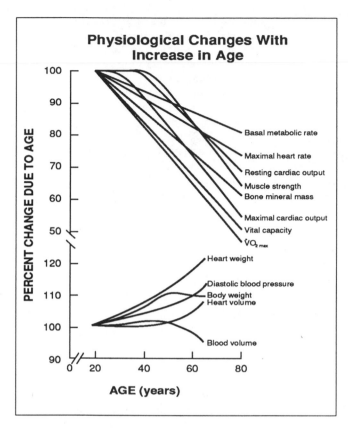

Figure 12.5 Aging is accompanied by a decrease in cardiorespiratory and musculoskeletal function. Many of these changes also occur during the transition from a trained to an untrained state. *Source:* adapted from 20–23.

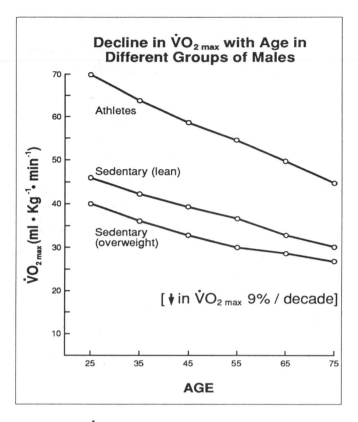

Figure 12.6 $\dot{V}O_{2max}$ decreases by about 9 percent per decade for males. *Source:* Adapted from reference 24.

drome are a decrease in cardiorespiratory function, obesity, musculoskeletal fragility, and premature aging.

$\dot{V}O_{2max}$ *and the Aging Process*

Most researchers that have evaluated the effects of aging on the cardiorespiratory system have focused on work capacity, or $\dot{V}O_{2max}$. The ability of the body to take in oxygen, transport it, and use it for oxidation of fuel is seen by many as the single best variable for defining the overall functional changes that occur with aging .[23]

$\dot{V}O_{2max}$ normally declines 8–10 percent per decade for both males and females after 25 years of age.[19–73] (See Figures 12.6 and 12.7.) From cross-sectional data, the rate of decline in $\dot{V}O_{2max}$ for sedentary men is 0.40–0.45 ml·kg⁻¹·min⁻¹ per year starting at age 25 (9 percent per decade). For sedentary women, the absolute rate of decline may be somewhat less, about 0.35–0.40 ml·kg⁻¹·min⁻¹ per year (which is still 9 percent per decade).[28]

Why does this decrease in $\dot{V}O_{2max}$ take place? Declining physical activity is probably responsible for at least half of it.[21, 22, 24, 64] As discussed in Chapter 1, results from the 1985 National Health Interview Survey show that the percent of U.S. elderly who exercise appropriately is half that of adults 18–29 years of age. Even if regular physical activity and body composition are kept constant, however, deterioration from the aging process itself still results in a decline in $\dot{V}O_{2max}$ of roughly 5 percent per decade.

Several researchers suggest that the age-related decline in maximal heart rate may be a major factor explaining this.[19, 24, 26, 27] In one study,[27] a lower maximal heart rate was solely responsible for differences in $\dot{V}O_{2max}$ between older and younger endurance athletes, because maximal stroke volume and maximal $\bar{a} - \bar{v}O_2$ differences were similar. (See Figure 12.8.)

Even intensive training during middle-age does not appear to prevent the maximal heart rate from decreasing.[62] Loss of muscle mass with aging may be another important factor explaining the decrease in $\dot{V}O_{2max}$.[19]

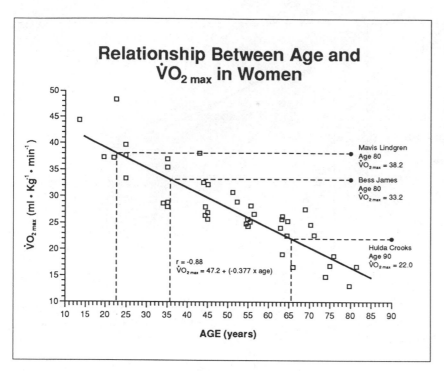

Figure 12.7 In this figure, the author[28] has plotted the $\dot{V}O_{2max}$ test results of 18 studies of a total of 1,159 women of widely varying ages.[33-49] $\dot{V}O_{2max}$ is negatively correlated with age for women (r = 0.88) ($\dot{V}O_{2max}$ = 47.20 + (−0.377 × age). Between the ages of 15 and 85, $\dot{V}O_{2max}$ appears to decrease 0.38 ml · kg⁻¹· min⁻¹ per year or 9.1 percent per decade for women. This decrease is similar to that reported for men.

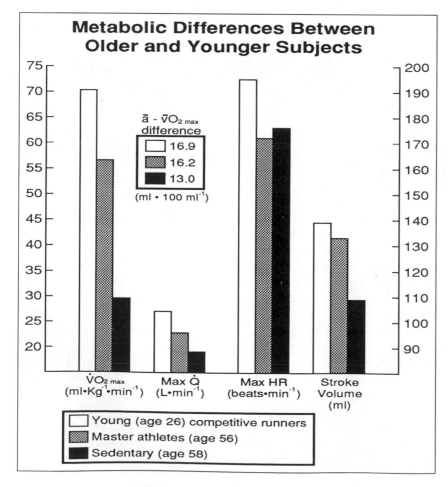

Figure 12.8 In this study of master athletes (average age 56 years), their lower maximal heart rates appeared to be the most important factor explaining why their $\dot{V}O_{2max}$ values were lower than those of younger athletes. Other cardiorespiratory parameters like stroke volume and $\bar{a} - \bar{v}O_2$ difference were not significantly different for older and younger athletes. *Source:* see reference 27.

Recapturing $\dot{V}O_{2max}$

Is it possible for elderly people to "recapture" lost $\dot{V}O_{2max}$ capacity? Despite the inevitable decrease in maximal heart rate and $\dot{V}O_{2max}$ with age, some men and women in their sixties and seventies are able, by means of exercise training, to increase their $\dot{V}O_{2max}$ above that of healthy untrained young people.[20, 24] Healthy men in their 50s who begin exercising vigorously have been reported to have $\dot{V}O_{2max}$ values 20–30 percent higher than that of young sedentary men. Middle-aged and old-master athletes who train for competition have $\dot{V}O_{2max}$ values 50 percent above that of ex-athletes of the same age who have stopped training.[25]

The author has been studying three elderly women, Hulda Crooks, Bess James, and Mavis Lindgren, for several years. (See Figures 12.9, 12.10, 12.11.) The results of this research are summarized in Table 12.1 and Figure 12.7. All three of these women have similar stories.

In 1962, at age 66, encouraged by her friends, Hulda climbed Mt. Whitney (14,495') for the first time. Training year-round for her annual Mt. Whitney climb, Hulda by age 91 had conquered the mountain 23 times. (See Figure 12.9.) She has also hiked the entire 212 miles of the John Muir trail, and since the age of 81 has climbed 88 of the highest peaks in southern California, including Mt. San Gorgonio (11,500'). Hulda also became the oldest woman in history to climb Mt. Fuji in Japan at the age of 91.

Hulda walks about three miles a day, and in her 90th year walked 1,200 miles. During the months preceding her Mt. Whitney climb, she develops her legs and heart by vigorously climbing stairs. Hulda is also a vegetarian and completely avoids alcohol and tobacco.

Bess James didn't start regular exercise until after she retired. At age 67 she began a regular walking program, and slowly progressed to 5 miles a day. At age 69 she began jogging; it took six months before she could jog one mile nonstop, and one year before she could jog 6 miles nonstop. She found that running made her feel better and helped her avoid breathlessness when climbing stairs. At age 70, she ran her first marathon, and has run 15 marathons between the ages of 70 and 80. (See Figure 12.10.) Her best marathon time came in 1982 (5 hours even). Bess runs 30–40 miles a week, consumes a high-carbohydrate diet, and avoids all alcohol and tobacco products.

Called "Amazing Mavis" by *Sports Illustrated* and many of her admirers, Mavis Lindgren is the hardworking owner of many national and world age-group records for various running events from the 10K to the 26.2-mile marathon. Mavis is a true "late-bloomer," having endured and overcome an unhealthy past.

As a child in Canada, she suffered through whooping cough and pneumonia, and experienced annual bouts of severe bronchitis throughout her adulthood. It wasn't until her early 60s, that Mavis, 20 pounds overweight, decided to begin walking faithfully every day. Slowly she increased her walking distance, and after

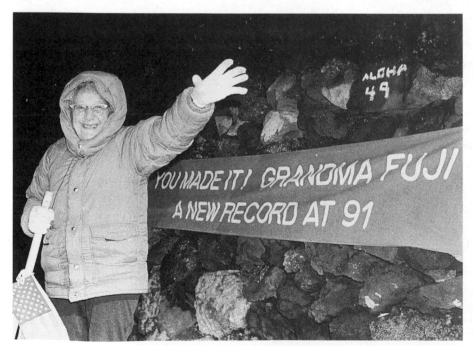

Figure 12.9 At age 91, Hulda Crooks conquered Mt. Whitney for the 23rd time since age 66, and became the oldest woman in history to climb Mt. Fuji.

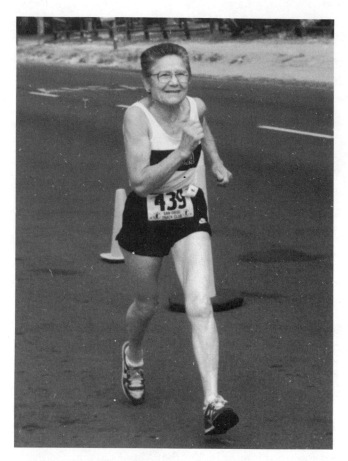

Figure 12.10 Bess James at age 79 ran the Los Angeles Marathon in 5 hours and 45 minutes.

several weeks began adding more and more jogging steps to her exercise routine.

As the months rolled by, Mavis experienced a rebirth of health, and as walking became easier, discovered that she also loved to run. After a long period of adaptation, she found herself running five miles, six days per week, and enjoying it. She maintained this regimen for several years. At the age of 70 in 1977, the running world discovered Mavis, thanks in great part to the persuasiveness of her son, a medical doctor who realized her unusual potential and urged her to double her training for marathon running.

Mavis found that she enjoyed the challenge of marathon running, and between 1977 and 1989 raced in 52 marathons, resetting her own age-group world record four different times (her age-group world record is 4 hours and 34 minutes). In the fall of 1984, Mavis also established a world best time for women over the age of 70 in the 10-kilometer (6.2-mile) event, racing to a 57-minute, 34-second finish. Mavis is also a vegetarian, avoids all alcohol and tobacco products, and runs 40–50 miles a week. (See Figure 12.11.)

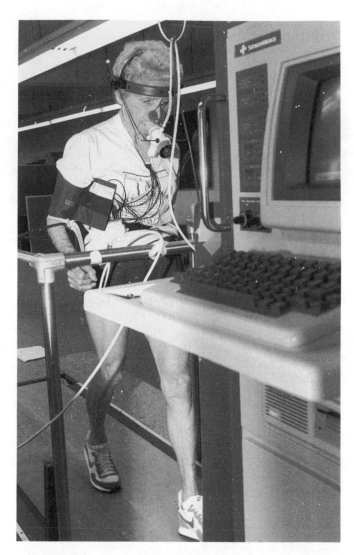

Figure 12.11 At the age of 80 years, Mavis Lindgren had the $\dot{V}O_{2max}$ capacity of a woman nearly 60 years younger than herself.

The results reflected in Table 12.1 and Figure 12.7 demonstrate that even when regular exercise is started late in life, many years worth of $\dot{V}O_{2max}$ can be recaptured. Mavis at age 80 had the $\dot{V}O_{2max}$ capacity of a woman nearly 60 years younger than herself. Bess at age 80 had the cardiorespiratory system of a woman nearly 45 years younger than herself, and Hulda at age 90 had one of a woman nearly 25 years younger than herself.

Can $\dot{V}O_{2max}$ be Maintained Despite Aging?

Can a regular program of exercise lessen the functional changes that normally occur as a person ages? In other

Table 12.1 Research Results on Three Elderly Women

Subject Characteristics

Subject	Age (yr)	Height (in)	Weight (lb)	Resting BP (mm Hg)	Miles/Wk Training
Hulda Crooks	90	61	120	115/60	15–20 (walking)
Bess James	80	60	108	100/60	30–40 (running)
Mavis Lindgren	80	62	103	110/70	40–50 (running)

Maximal Graded Exercise Test Results

Subject	$\dot{V}O_{2max}$ (ml/kg/min)	$\dot{V}_{Emax}$ (L/min)	$\dot{B}_{Rmax}$ (breaths/min)	R_{max}	$\dot{H}R_{max}$ (beats/min)
Hulda Crooks	22.6	53	40	1.3	130
Bess James	33.2	64	46	1.3	168
Mavis Lindgren	38.2	78	49	1.4	157

Skinfolds (mm) / Blood Lipid Profile (mg/dl)

Subject	Triceps	Suprailium	Thigh	Cholesterol	HDL-C	LDL-C	Triglyceride
Hulda Crooks	16	20	16	225	53	148	121
Bess James	18	4	15	231	66	139	131
Mavis Lindgren	13	3	9	225	66	142	87

Dietary Assessment Results

Subject	Kilocalories	%Pro	%Fat	%CHO	RDA met except for*
Hulda Crooks	1700	16	25	59	Zn
Bess James	1600	15	19	66	Zn, B-12
Mavis Lindgren	1700	12	34	54	Zn, B-12

*Two-thirds Recommended Dietary Allowance (RDA) met for major vitamins and minerals except those listed.

words, can regular exercise reverse or counter the aging process? The data suggest that the overall rate of loss is similar for active and inactive people, but that at any given age, the active conserve more function. (See Figure 12.6.) In other words, older athletes have higher $\dot{V}O_{2max}$ values than their sedentary counterparts, but they experience a steady decline in functional capacity at much the same rate.

Some researchers have suggested that even if physical activity and body composition are kept constant, deterioration caused by the aging process itself results in a decline in $\dot{V}O_{2max}$ of roughly 5 percent per decade.[24] However, other researchers have shown that intensive training can counter the drop in $\dot{V}O_{2max}$ for at least 10 years during middle age.[61, 62, 65–68] Researchers from San Diego followed a group of active men (ages 45 to 55) for 10 years, and found no loss in $\dot{V}O_{2max}$ as a result of exercising three hours per week at 86-percent capacity. It took this amount of activity, however, to counter the usual age related decrease in $\dot{V}O_{2max}$. However, after 20 years of follow-up with the same group of men, despite remaining active 3 to 4 days a week, $\dot{V}O_{2max}$ declined from 44.4 to 38.9 ml·kg⁻¹·min⁻¹ (12 percent or 0.27 ml·kg⁻¹·min⁻¹ per year).[73]

Data from another 10-year study of 24 master track athletes showed that athletes who maintained intensive training (35 miles/week) during the 10-year period were able to maintain a $\dot{V}O_{2max}$ of 54 ml·kg⁻¹·min⁻¹.[62] Athletes who remained active, but less intensively (24 miles/wk), experienced a 12.6-percent decrease in $\dot{V}O_{2max}$ (from 52.5 to 45.9 ml·kg⁻¹·min⁻¹). Maximal heart rate for all master athletes showed a consistent 7 beats/min drop over the 10-year follow-up period. The researchers concluded that physical training in itself does not maintain the maximal heart rate.

So in summary, although intensive exercise may forestall the drop in $\dot{V}O_{2max}$ during middle-age, eventually the aging process appears to dominate, and there will be a drop in $\dot{V}O_{2max}$. When the $\dot{V}O_{2max}$ is high early in life, as is the case with former endurance athletes, even intensive training will not sustain it at the same level in later years. (See Figure 12.6.) Within the age range of 60–65 years, data suggest that some reduction in $\dot{V}O_{2max}$ is inevitable even if very intensive training is maintained.[26, 62]

Figure 12.12 plots 46 of the 26.2-mile marathons Mavis Lindgren has run between the ages of 70 and 82 years. Despite maintaining a training regimen of 40–60 miles per week during this 12-year span, her marathon times have become progressively slower. Probably the most important factor affecting this decline is that although the quantity of training has remained the same, the intensity of her training sessions has probably diminished over time.

Physical Training by the Elderly

Cardiorespiratory Training

Whether older people respond to physical training to the same degree as their younger counterparts is not certain.[19] Several studies suggest that elderly people can respond to physical training over an 8–20 week period in a manner expected of younger subjects.[29,38,52–55,57–61,69] For the elderly, lower intensities of training can be effective in the early stages, probably because of the low initial level of fitness.[69]

In general, aerobic capacity can be improved at nearly all ages except perhaps after age 75.[19] Dr. Pollock of Florida State University has shown that men 49–65 years of age responded to an endurance training program (3 sessions per week, walk-jog, 30–45 minutes, for 20 weeks) with an increase of 19 percent in $\dot{V}O_{2max}$, the relative values being what would be expected of younger men, with the absolute values somewhat lower.[26] (See Figure 12.13.)

With extreme aging, however, the ability to engage in physical exercise declines.[30, 31, 49, 70] Training the cardiorespiratory system of the elderly is possible only when adequate intensity, frequency, and duration of effort is made.

The elderly are frequently divided into three approximate groupings: the *young old*, or those 65–74 years of age; *old old*, or 74–84 years of age; and *very old*, or greater than 84 years of age.[71] The question of whether regular cardiorespiratory exercise can improve aerobic

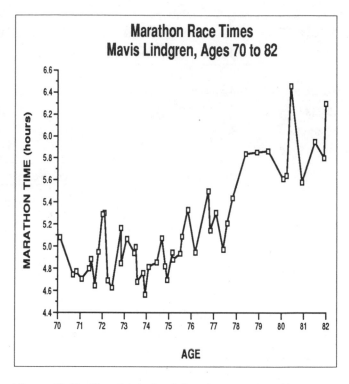

Figure 12.12 Despite maintaining the quantity of her training between the ages of 70 and 82 years, Mavis Lindgren has experienced a progressive increase in her marathon race times.

power for old old to very old people has received little attention. Several studies have shown that regular cardiorespiratory exercise by the old old to very old may have little effect on aerobic power or other metabolic parameters.[28, 56] At this extreme age, the aging process may dominate so powerfully that few improvements in cardiorespiratory fitness are possible. In addition, health problems and a lack of motivation often prevent many people over the age of 75 from engaging in appropriate amounts of exercise.

Musculoskeletal Training

Strength seems to peak in the third decade, followed by a plateau through approximately the age of 50, followed in turn by a 20-percent loss of strength by age 65, and progressing further as age increases.[19] Much of this is due to the loss of muscle mass. Resistance training can result in increased strength for both elderly men and women.[54, 72] However, hypertrophy is decreased, and (more importantly) ability to recruit motor units is increased.[19] Joint flexibility can also be improved when elderly people engage in appropriate range of motion exercise.[54, 74]

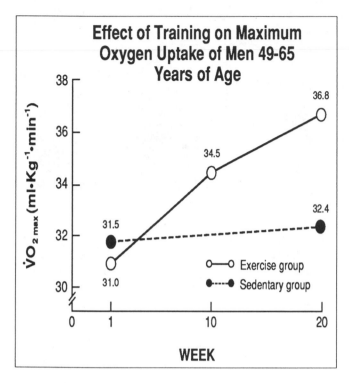

Figure 12.13 Middle-aged men respond to exercise training to an extent similar to that of younger men. *Source:* adapted from: Pollock ML. J Am Geriatr Soc 24:97–104, 1976.

Body Composition Changes

Aging brings the accumulation of fat and a substantial loss of muscle mass.[19] Loss of muscle mass can be as high as 10–12 percent, and can occur with no appreciable loss in overall body mass. Weight gain generally continues unchecked from age 25 to age 50. A gain in body fat of approximately 27 pounds is likely from age 20 to age 55, with a concomitant loss of 7 pounds of lean tissue. Men in their 80s can lose another 20 pounds of muscle mass, while gaining 7 pounds of body fat after age 55.

However, elderly people can have a level of body fatness similar to that of younger people if they remain consistently physically active and control food intake throughout life.[19, 28, 53] In one study of 13 male and 25 female elderly people, four one-hour exercise sessions per week led to significant reductions in body fat.[53]

Although short-term reductions in body fat are possible, however, regular exercise may not completely counter the usual age-related changes in body composition. In the study of master athletes discussed earlier in this chapter,[62] fat weight increased an average of about 2.5 pounds during a 10-year period, while fat-free weight dropped 3–6 pounds despite heavy training.[62]

Their aerobic training (about 30 miles per week of running) did not appear to protect fat-free weight. It many be necessary to add strength training to exercise regimens of adults as they age to maintain fat-free weight.

Exercise Prescription Guidelines for the Elderly

The American Medical Association, Council on Scientific Affairs, has developed recommendations for physicians when counseling the elderly to start exercise programs.[75]

- Stress the importance of exercise for elderly patients, explaining in detail its physiological and psychological benefits.

- Obtain a complete and reliable medical history and perform a physical examination, employing exercise testing for quantification of cardiovascular and physical fitness as appropriate, before the specific exercise prescription.

- Maintain an active interest in their exercise practices with appropriate follow-up.

- Encourage all patients to establish an exercise program as a lifetime commitment in preparation for their later years.

- Walking, with gradual progression, is a most convenient and adaptable form of exercise for the elderly. Other everyday activities such as climbing stairs and gardening are encouraged.

In general, the same basic principles used for younger adults can be applied, but with greater caution and slower progression. Older people can improve their fitness, but do need more time for adaptation, along with the realization that on the average, training for younger people produces higher absolute values.[26]

With an increasingly older population there is an urgent need for health practices that can prolong adult vigor and hopefully delay the onset and progression of chronic diseases.[76] In an aging society, prolonging active life expectancy, not just disabled existence, is an important goal. Medicated survival by the elderly is not the goal, and exercise is one factor, along with other lifestyle habits, that can improve the quality of life.

Physical Activity and Life Expectancy

Can regular exercise lengthen life expectancy? Dr. Ralph Paffenbarger of Stanford University showed that Harvard alumni whose weekly energy output in walking, stair climbing, and active sports totaled at least 2,000 Calories a week experienced a 28-percent reduction in all-cause death rates.[77] For those expending 3,500 Calories a week in exercise, death rates were an amazing 50 percent lower. Life expectancy was 2.15 years greater for those who expended more than 2,000 Calories a week compared with those who expended less than 500 Calories a week.

This has the same statistical impact (in epidemiological research terms) of removing cancer from the United States. In practical terms, because even sedentary people burn 1,000 Calories a week in physical activity, this improvement in longevity can be gained by walking or jogging 8–10 miles a week.[78]

A summary of the literature on the effects of exercise on longevity in animals showed an increase in life expectancy when exercise was initiated early in life.[79] However, when exercise has been started late in life, there has been little effect on the survival of old rats. Another study suggests that there has been an improvement in the longevity of rats who voluntarily ran one to four miles each day in activity wheels.[80] However, the active rats did not show the true increase in life-span experienced by the food-restricted sedentary rats.[80]

Perhaps the major benefit of exercise for the elderly is that it can help improve their motility and quality of life. Exercise can contribute to vigor and vitality, and can counteract the decrease in function and other troublesome symptoms of old age.

In the Sports Medicine Insight at the end of this chapter, the relationship of other health habits such as diet to life expectancy will be reviewed. In general, regular physical activity can have a beneficial impact on life expectancy by reducing the effects of chronic diseases such as heart disease, obesity, and diabetes.[78] However, there is little or no evidence to support the contention that physical activity can lengthen the *lifespan* (the maximal obtainable age of a particular member of the species).

Osteoporosis

Osteoporosis is an age-related disorder characterized by decreased bone mass and increased susceptibility to fractures.[81–87] (See Figure 12.14.) Osteoporosis is classified as either primary or secondary. There are two types of *primary osteoporosis:* Type I osteoporosis (postmenopausal), which is the accelerated decrease in bone mass that occurs when estrogen levels fall after menopause; and Type II osteoporosis (age-related), which is the inevitable loss of bone mass with age experienced by both men and women. *Secondary osteoporosis* may de-

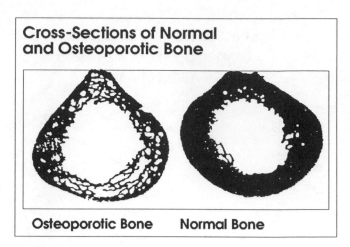

Figure 12.14 Osteoporosis is characterized by a decrease in the amount of bone, often so severe that it leads to fractures after even minimal trauma.

velop at any age as a consequence of hormonal, digestive, and metabolic disorders, as well as a loss of bone mineral mass from prolonged bedrest and weightlessness (space flight).[82]

Osteoporosis afflicts 15–20 million Americans over the age of 45, each year causing an estimated 1.3 million fractures.[81–83] Loss of bone mineral content (BMC) is an almost universal phenomenon with increasing age among white men and women in the United States. (See Figure 12.15.) Among those who live to be 90, 32 percent of women and 17 percent of men will have suffered hip fractures, leading to death in 12–20 percent of the cases and to long-term nursing home care for many of those who survive.[82] The cost of osteoporosis in the United States has been estimated at $7–10 annually.[83]

Risk Factors

Without effective preventive measures, the costs of osteoporosis are bound to increase along with the rapid increase in the number of older Americans.[83, 84] (See Figures 12.1, 12.4.) Prevention is important to counter both the financial burden and the limited effectiveness of treatment once fractures have occurred.

We don't really know why some people develop osteoporosis and others do not. Bone mineral content (BMC) varies considerably among women; the BMC of vertebrae can vary 40 percent among 25-year-olds and 70 percent among 80-year-olds.[87] Aging itself, the loss of sex hormones at menopause, and genetics all play a role.[83] Recent studies are also showing that BMC is lower among relatives of osteoporotic patients than among those with no family history of osteoporosis.[88, 89]

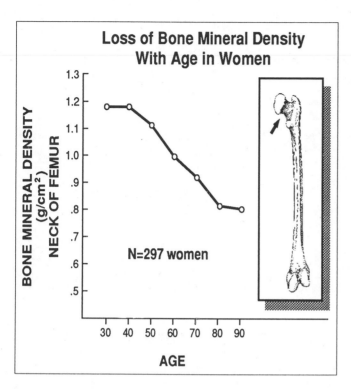

Figure 12.15 Age-related bone loss among U.S. women. *Source:* Data from: Melton LJ. J Clin Epidemiol 41:985–994, 1988.

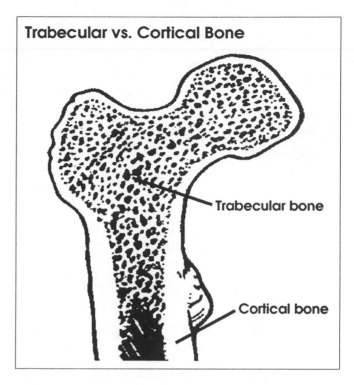

Figure 12.16 Cortical bone is the compact bone in the shaft. Trabecular bone is the spongy internal bone usually at the end.

Table 12.2 summarizes the scientific validity of the various risk factors for osteoporosis.[90]

Bone is a spongy protein matrix in which crystals of calcium and phosphorus salts are embedded.[83, 87] From birth until death, bone tissue is continually being formed, broken down, and reformed in a process called remodeling. The cells that break down bone are called *osteoclasts*, and those that build bone are called *osteoblasts*.

Peak bone mass is achieved at about age 35 for *cortical* bone (compact outer shaft bone), and earlier for *trabecular* bone (spongy, internal end bone). (See Figure 12.16.) Once peak bone mass is reached, osteoclast activity is greater than osteoblast activity, and adults begin to slowly lose bone mass.[87]

Bone mass is approximately 30 percent higher among men than women and approximately 10 percent higher among blacks than whites. Over their lifetimes, women lose about 35 percent of their cortical bone and 50 percent of their trabecular bone, whereas men lose about two-thirds of these amounts. Although bone mass is an important factor explaining why some develop osteoporosis and bone fractures and others do not,[91, 92] differences in bone architecture and structure also appear to be important.[83, 86]

At menopause, women normally have an accelerated loss of bone mineral mass (2.5–5 percent per year) for several years.[81] The result is that by age 65, 50 percent of all women have a bone mineral density below the normal fracture threshold of a 20-year-old woman.

Testing for osteoporosis is more widely available now, with costs ranging from $40–$300 depending on the method.

The role of dietary calcium in determining peak bone mass is uncertain.[83–85, 93–96] Some studies have suggested that when calcium intake has been appropriate, a greater bone mass is developed in early adulthood, decreasing the risk of age-related bone loss. When calcium intake is too low early in life (probably below 500 mg a day), peak bone mass may be lower than what is considered optimal.

For example, people with a lifelong low intake of dairy products because of *lactase deficiency* have an increased incidence of osteoporosis.[82] American women (ages 19–50 years) average 650 mg of dietary calcium a day, men, 920 mg.[97] These amounts are close to the 800 mg Recommended Dietary Allowance. In general, a lifetime of adequate calcium intake, coupled with adequate levels of serum estrogens appear to maximize bone density after menopause.[98]

Table 12.2   Scientific Validity of the Risk Factors of Osteoporosis

Well Established	Moderate Evidence	Inconclusive Evidence
Obesity (–)	Alcohol (+)	Moderate exercise
Black ethnicity (–)	Cigarette smoking (+)	Asian ethnicity
Age (+)	Heavy exercise (–)	Parity
Removal of ovaries (+)	Low dietary calcium (+)	Diabetes
(premenopausal)		Thiazide diuretic use
Use of steroids (+)		Progestin use
Estrogen use (–)		Using water fluoride
Bedrest (+)		Caffeine use

(+) = increased risk; (–) = decreased risk

Source: adapted from reference 90.

At present, studies of the effect of calcium supplementation on age-related bone loss are inconclusive.[83, 93–95] Some studies have shown that calcium supplementation can suppress bone loss, others have not. This relationship is complicated by the fact that age itself may influence both the intestinal absorption of calcium and the skeleton's ability to utilize the calcium. Decreases in the ability of the intestine to absorb calcium may begin as early as age 30 for some or as late as age 60 for others.

There is a potential risk of kidney stones with excessive calcium supplementation.[99] The rate of absorption of elderly osteoporotic women can be improved by giving vitamin D supplements.[100] In general, the postmenopausal women most likely to benefit from calcium supplementation are those who otherwise have low calcium intakes.[94]

It is recommended that women at high risk for osteoporosis increase their calcium intake by consuming calcium-rich foods—which include low-fat dairy products, leafy green vegetables, and nuts and seeds.[81] Other important lifestyle habits for decreasing the risk of osteoporosis include avoiding cigarette smoking, restricting alcohol, and engaging in regular physical activity.[83]

At present, estrogen replacement therapy is the best known safeguard against osteoporosis for postmenopausal women.[93, 96] Although this treatment has been associated with increased risk of developing endometrial and other cancers, many physicians believe the association is relatively weak, especially at lower doses, and prescribe estrogen in the belief that the risk of osteoporosis is much more significant.

Role of Physical Activity

Although there have been a growing number of research reports exploring the relationship between physical activity and BMC,[101–125] more rigorous studies are needed.[83, 112] The 1987 National Osteoporosis Foundation/National Institutes of Health conference[112] and the 1988 Surgeon General's Report[83] were both reserved in their support of exercise for preventing osteoporosis. There have been few well-designed studies confirming that exercise can have a significant and lasting effect on building and maintaining peak bone mass. One complicating factor is the extent to which exercise may reduce the incidence of fractures simply by reducing the likelihood of falls, and/or the severity of consequent injuries.[112]

There is good data to support the fact that humans lose bone mass rapidly when gravitational or muscular stress on the legs is reduced, as it is with weightlessness, bed rest, or spinal cord injury.[101, 114] A healthy person confined to bed rest for 4 to 36 weeks can lose an average of 1 percent of his bone mineral content per week. On the other hand, when gravity stress or muscle movement stress is applied to the bone, the pressure will produce an electric current (piezoelectric effect). This tends to build up the bone mineral mass.[101]

There is also substantial data showing that athletes have a greater bone density than sedentary people.[102, 115–119] The density appears to be related to the amount of stress exerted on the bones by the particular athletic activity. Walking, running, and racket sports maintain leg and spinal bone mass more effectively than such non-weight-bearing activities as bicycling and swimming. In descending order, the athletes with the greatest bone mineral mass are weight lifters, shot-putters and discus throwers, runners, soccer players, and finally, swimmers.[101]

For example, Figure 12.17 shows that spinal BMC is significantly higher for those participating in both aerobic (>40 miles/wk running or >6 hours/wk aerobic exercise classes) and weight-bearing regimens (>6 hours/wk rigorous weight lifting) than for sedentary people or people participating only in aerobic activity.[118]

Other studies have shown that competitive masters swimmers have significantly greater bone mineral content than non-athletes.[119] People with higher $\dot{V}O_{2max}$ values have greater bone mass in the femoral neck, lumbar spine, and forearm.[116] A significant relationship has been found between lifetime physical activity and bone area among postmenopausal women.[115] Significantly higher BMC has been measured among women who maintain an active lifestyle, particularly during their premenopausal years.[117]

Some researchers feel these differences may arise from factors of heredity and self-selection. In other words, people who tend to do well in sports competition tend to have strong, dense bones to begin with. Although this may be true to a certain extent, studies comparing the active and inactive arms of tennis players show differences in bones density.[101] For example, in one study comparing the bone density of ten professional tennis players with that of non-athletes, density was 15 percent higher in players' nondominant arm and 39 percent higher in their dominant arm.[121]

While it is well-known that gravity and muscle force exerted on the bone will increase bone size and density, and that inactivity caused by weightlessness and bed rest will lead to bone loss, there has been controversy over whether exercise can delay bone aging.[103] Recently, however, several excellent studies have provided preliminary evidence that exercise may help counter bone mineral mass loss among women.[105, 106, 108, 122, 123]

In one three-year study of 30 elderly women (mean age 81), half participated in a 40-minute program three times a week, and half engaged in no formal exercise. The sedentary control group had a bone mineral content loss of 3.28 percent during the 36 months, while the physical activity group had a 2.29 percent gain.[105]

In another study, of 3–4 years of regular exercise for 200 women ages 35–65,[106] two-thirds exercised for 135 minutes per week, whereas one-third remained sedentary. After 3 years, bone mineral mass decreased 7.2 percent among the sedentary group, but only 3.0 percent among the exercising women.

In another study, postmenopausal women who exercised at 70–90 percent $\dot{V}O_{2max}$ (jogging, stair climbing, walking) for 50–60 min, three times weekly for 17 months, increased their lumbar bone mineral content six percent, which then fell by five percent after 13 months of no exercise; this compared to a one percent loss for a matched sedentary group.[123] (See Figure 12.18.)

The Surgeon General has concluded that "until better information becomes available, 3 to 4 hours of weight-bearing exercise per week is potentially beneficial to the skeleton and could represent a safe, low-cost method for maintaining bone mass."[83]

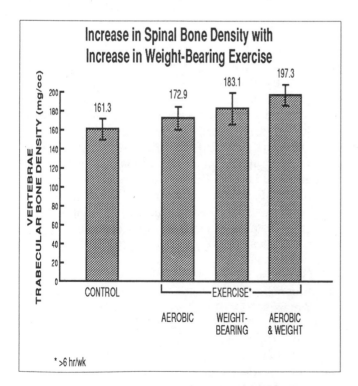

Figure 12.17 People who add weight training to their aerobic routines tend to have greater spinal bone mineral content than sedentary people or people who engage in aerobic activity alone. *Source:* see reference 118.

Sports Medicine Insight
Relationship Between Health Habits and Aging

The topic of "life extension," or "maximum life span" has been receiving a lot of attention recently. Several bestselling books have promoted various theories and

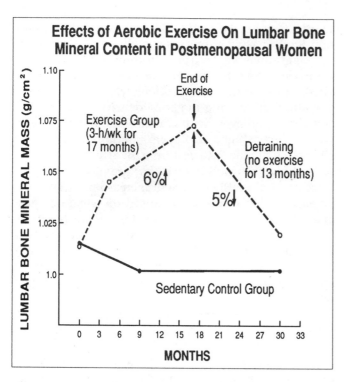

Figure 12.18 Three hours of aerobic exercise per week increased the lumbar BMC of postmenopausal women three percent within 4.5 months and six percent after 17 months. After 13 months of sedentary living, their BMC fell five percent. *Source:* see reference 123.

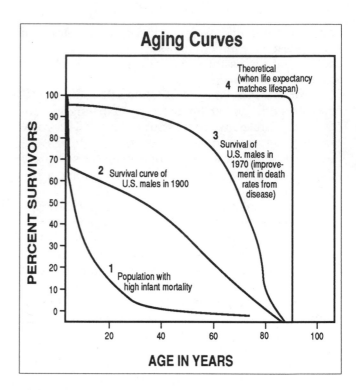

Figure 12.19 Four survival curves based on infant mortality and chronic disease death rates. *Source:* see reference 127.

ideas for enhancing longevity. Americans appear more eager than ever to seek out ways to ensure a longer life.[126]

As explained in this chapter, life expectancy is the average number of years of life expected for a population at a specific age, usually at birth. Life-span is the maximum age obtainable by a particular member of the species.[79]

Aging is a very complex phenomenon. It is a continuum that begins at birth and involves both psychological and physical factors, influenced by lifestyle, environment, and heredity. The emphasis of many researchers today is not so much on "life extension"—the addition of years to the life-span of the human species—as on a search for methods that will allow us to approach our true biogenetic potential for longevity. In other words (as discussed in this chapter), the central issue is that of net gain in active functional years, relative to years of disability and dysfunction.

Figure 12.19 demonstrates four "survival curves." For a population with high infant mortality, the percent of survivors by age 40 is very small. The second curve depicts U.S. males survivals in 1900. Life expectancy

was only about 47 years at birth, largely because infant mortality rates were still very high. The third curve shows that by 1970, the percentage of survivors at age 40 was much improved, largely because of much lower infant mortality rates and a decrease in death rates from chronic disease, primarily heart disease.

To reach theoretical curve number four, where life expectancy matches potential life-span, both infant mortality and chronic diseases will have to be totally controlled.[127] Our future challenge consists of practicing and discovering lifestyle techniques that will remove the obstacle of chronic disease (heart disease, cancer, diabetes, obesity, etc.), allowing us to live out our true life-span.

Health habits are clearly identified as strong factors influencing life expectancy and quality of life during old age.[126-136] Dr. Breslow of UCLA, for example, in his famous study of over 6,000 people in the San Francisco Bay area[128, 132] showed a dramatic difference in death rate between those who followed seven simple health habits (never smoked, moderate alcohol consumption, daily breakfast, no snacking, 7–8 hours of sleep per night, regular exercise, ideal weight) and those who did not. (See Figure 12.20.) Those who were active and never smoked had standardized mortality

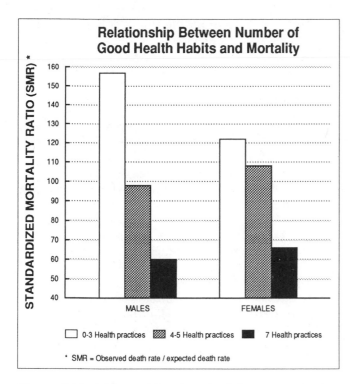

Relationship Between Number of Good Health Habits and Mortality

STANDARDIZED MORTALITY RATIO (SMR) *

☐ 0-3 Health practices   ▨ 4-5 Health practices   ■ 7 Health practices

* SMR = Observed death rate / expected death rate

Figure 12.20 Males and females who follow seven simple health practices have approximately half the mortality of people with 0–3 of these health habits. *Source:* see reference 128.

ratios (SMR—the rate of observed deaths/rate of expected deaths) 2.6 times lower than sedentary smokers (67 vs. 175). People following all seven health habits had standardized mortality ratios two times lower than people with no more than three habits (63 vs. 131 for the entire group, males and females combined).

Seventh-Day Adventists (SDA) are among the most researched populations in the world. Since the 1950s, researchers in Australia, Norway, Japan, Poland, New Zealand, the Caribbean Islands, the United States, and the Netherlands have published more than 140 scientific papers on tens of thousands of Seventh-Day Adventists.[133–136] Their unique lifestyle has been associated with dramatic increases in life expectancy resulting primarily from greatly reduced death rates from cardiovascular disease and cancer, the leading killers in Western countries.

SDA are a small, conservative, evangelical denomination with about 5 million members worldwide. Many follow a unique lifestyle. Church policy dictates that members abstain completely from smoking and the use of alcoholic beverages. Since the late 1800s, the church has highly recommended, but not required, that members follow other unique dietary practices, including a lacto-ovo-vegetarian diet, and the avoidance of coffee and tea, hot condiments and spices, and highly refined foods. A wide variety of fruits, vegetables, whole grains, nuts, and low-fat dairy products are advocated. Adventists also believe that a firm trust in God, use of pure water and air, moderate exposure to sunlight, participation in daily exercise such as brisk walking, and the development of mental abilities through formal education are important for health.

Depending on the country studied, SDA males have been found to live 4.2 to 9.5 years longer than their non-SDA male counterparts, and SDA females 1.9 to 4.6 years longer.[136] Dr. Hans Waaler, who studied SDA in Norway, explained that "in order for the population in general to achieve the same duration of life, one would have to, for instance, completely eliminate ischemic heart disease."[136]

Summary

1. The ranks of the aged are increasing rapidly, as heart disease and stroke continue to decrease. The fastest growing minority in the United States today is the elderly.

2. The average baby born today can expect to live to age 74.7. Increases in life expectancy at birth during the first half of this century occurred mainly because of reductions in infant mortality, and recently because of decreasing mortality from chronic diseases.

3. Prominent aging-related concerns include the quality of life in old age, the high prevalence of chronic diseases, osteoporosis, and senile dementia among the elderly, and the financial impact.

4. Aging refers to the normal yet irreversible biological changes that occur during the total years that a person lives. There are several theories of aging, including the "error" and "program" hypotheses. As a person ages, many changes take place in the body (summarized in the text).

5. There is great similarity between the physiological changes that accompany aging and those that accompany inactivity. The identifying characteristics of both aging and the disuse syndrome are a decrease in cardiorespiratory function, obesity, musculoskeletal fragility, and (among the inactive) premature aging.

6. Most researchers that have evaluated the effects of aging on the cardiorespiratory system have focused on work capacity, or $\dot{V}O_{2max}$. $\dot{V}O_{2max}$

normally declines 8–10 percent per decade for both males and females after 25 years of age.

7. Declining physical activity is probably responsible for at least half of the drop in $\dot{V}O_{2max}$ with age. The age-related decline in maximal heart rate may be a major factor. Even intensive training during middle-age does not appear to prevent the maximal heart rate from decreasing as one ages.

8. The elderly can recapture decades worth of $\dot{V}O_{2max}$ with appropriate (gradual) training.

9. The data suggest that the overall rate of loss of cardiorespiratory function is similar for active and inactive people, but that at any given age the active conserve more function.

10. Whether older people respond to physical training to the same degree as their younger counterparts is not certain. Several studies suggest the elderly can respond to physical training over an 8–20 week period in a manner expected of younger people.

11. In general, the same basic exercise prescription principles used for younger adults can be applied for the elderly, but with greater caution and slower progression.

12. Regular physical activity can have a beneficial impact on life expectancy by reducing the life-shortening effects of the various chronic diseases. However, there is little or no evidence to support the contention that physical activity can lengthen the potential life-span (the maximum age obtainable by a particular member of the species).

13. Osteoporosis is characterized by decreased bone mass and increased susceptibility to fractures. The mainstays of treatment include estrogen replacement, adequate lifelong calcium intake, and appropriate exercise.

14. Exercise helps build up bone mineral mass by inducing electric currents in the bone. Weightlessness and bed rest can cause a dramatic loss in bone mass. Cross-sectional studies show that athletes have denser bones than sedentary people. Preliminary studies show that postmenopausal women can retard bone mineral mass loss, or even increase bone density with appropriate exercise.

15. Health habits are clearly identified as a strong factor in life expectancy. However, there is no research support for the ability of lifestyle habits to lengthen the life-span.

References

1. Brody JA, Brock DB, Williams TF. Trends in the Health of the Elderly Population. Annu Rev Public Health 8:211–234, 1987.

2. U.S. Bureau of the Census, Current Population Reports, Series P-23, No. 128, America in Transition: An Aging Society, U.S. Government Printing Office, Washington, D.C., 1983.

3. Fowles DG. A Profile of Older Americans. Program Resources Department, American Association of Retired Persons. Administration on Aging, U.S. Department of Health and Human Services. 1985.

4. National Center for Health Statistics: Health, United States, 1988. DHHS Pub. No. (PHS) 89–1232. Public Health Service. Washington. U.S. Government Printing Office, March 1989.

5. Ray WA, Federspiel CF, Baugh DK, Dodds S. Impact of Growing Numbers of the Very Old on Medicaid Expenditures for Nursing Homes: A Multi-State, Population-Based Analysis. Am J Public Health 77:699–703, 1987.

6. Board of Trustees Report. A Proposal for Financing Health Care of the Elderly. JAMA 256:3379–3382, 1986.

7. Mahler H. Present Status of WHO's Initiative, "Health for All By the Year 2000." Annu Rev Public Health 9:71–97, 1988.

8. U.S. Department of Health and Human Services. Public Health Service. Office of Disease Prevention and Health Promotion. Prevention '86/'87: Federal Programs and Progress. U.S. Government Printing Office: Washington, D.C., 1987.

9. Claggett MS. Nutritional Factors Relevant to Alzheimer's Disease. J Am Diet Assoc 89:392–396, 1989.

10. American Dietetic Association Reports. Nutrition, Aging, and the Continuum of Health Care: Technical Support Paper. J Am Diet Assoc 87:345–347, 1987.

11. Flieger K. Why Do We Age? FDA Consumer, October 1988, pp. 20–25.

12. Taubman LB. Theories of Aging. Resident & Staff Physician April:31–37, 1986.

13. Saxon SV, Etten MH. Physical Change and Aging. New York: Tiresias Press, 1978.

14. Rowe JW. Health Care of the Elderly. N Engl J Med 312:827–835, 1985.

15. Shephard RJ. Nutrition and the Physiology of Aging, in: Young EA (ed). Nutrition, Aging, and Health. New York: Alan R. Liss, Inc., 1986.

16. Institute of Food Technologists' Expert Panel on Food Safety & Nutrition. Food Tech September:81–88, 1986.

17. Crapo PA. Nutrition in the Aged, In: Schrier RW (editor). Clinical Internal Medicine in the Aged. Philadelphia: W.B. Saunders Co., 1982.

18. Kelsey JL, Hochberg MC. Epidemiology of Chronic Musculoskeletal Disorders. Annu Rev Public Health 9:379–401, 1988.

19. Stamford BA. Exercise and the Elderly. Exerc Sport Sci Rev 16:341–379, 1988.

20. Bortz WM. Disuse and Aging. JAMA 248:1203–1208, 1982.

21. Smith EL, Gilligan C. Physical Activity Prescription for the Older Adult. Physician Sportsmed 11:91–101, 1983.

22. Bortz WM. The Disuse Syndrome. West J Med 141:691–694, 1984.

23. Bruce RA. Exercise, Functional Aerobic Capacity, and Aging—Another Viewpoint. Med Sci Sports Exerc 16:8–13, 1984.

24. Heath GW, Hagberg JM, Ehsani AA, Holloszy JO. A Physiological Comparison of Young and Older Endurance Athletes. J Appl Physiol 51:634–640, 1981.

25. Holloszy JO. Exercise, Health, and Aging: A Need For More Information. Med Sci Sports Exerc 15:1–5, 1983.

26. Rivera AM, Pels AE, Sady SP, et al. Physiological Factors Associated With the Lower Maximal Oxygen Consumption of Master Runners. J Appl Physiol 66:949–954, 1989.

27. Hagberg JM. A Hemodynamic Comparison of Young and Old Endurance Athletes During Exercise. J Appl Physiol 58:2041–2046, 1985.

28. Nieman DC, Pover NK, Segebartt KS, Arabatzis K, Johnson M, Dietrich SJ. Hematological, Anthropometric, and Metabolic Comparisons Between Active and Inactive Healthy Old Old to Very Old Women. (Manuscript under review.)

29. Adams G, de Vries H. Physiological Effects of an Exercise Training Regimen Upon Women Aged 52 to 79. J Gerontol 28:50–55, 1973.

30. Shephard R. Nutrition and the Physiology of Aging, in Young EA (ed): Nutrition, Aging, and Health. (Alan R. Liss Inc., New York, 1986), pp. 1–23.

31. Harris R, Harris S. Physical Activity, Aging and Sports. Center for the Study of Aging, Albany, New York, 1989.

32. Hodgson J, Buskirk E. Physical Fitness and Age, With Emphasis on Cardiovascular Function in the Elderly. J Am Geriatr Soc 25:385–392, 1977.

33. Plowman S, Drinkwater B, Horvath S. Age and Aerobic Power in Women: a Longitudinal Study. J Geront 34:512–520, 1979.

34. Asmussen E, Fruensgaard K, Norgaard S. A Follow-up Longitudinal Study of Selected Physiologic Functions in Former Physical Education Students—After Forty Years. J Amer Geriat Soc 23:442–450, 1975.

35. Astrand I. Aerobic Work Capacity in Men and Women With Special Reference to Age. Acta Physiol Scand (Suppl)49(169):1–92, 1960. See also: Astrand I. Reduction in Maximal Oxygen Uptake With Age. J Appl Physiol 35:649–654, 1973.

36. Atomi Y, Miyashita M. Maximal Aerobic Power of Japanese Active and Sedentary Adult Females of Different Ages, 20 to 62 years. Med Sci Sports Exerc 6:223–225, 1974.

37. Vogel J, Potton J, Mello R, Daniels W. An Analysis of Aerobic Capacity in a Large United States Population. J Appl Physiol 60:494–500, 1986.

38. Suominen H, Heikkinen E, Parkatti T. Effect of Eight Weeks' Physical Training on Muscle and Connective Tissue of the M. Vastus Lateralis in 69-year-old Men and Women. J Gerontol 32:33–37, 1977.

39. Barry A, Webster G, Daly J. Validity and Reliability of a Multistage Exercise Test for Older Men and Women. J Geront 24:284–291, 1969.

40. Smahel O, Tlusty L. Physical Fitness in Old Age. I. Aerobic Capacity and the Other Parameters of Physical Fitness Followed by Means of Graded Exercise in Ergometric Examination of Elderly Individuals. Respiration 26:161–181, 1969.

41. Benestad A, Halvorsrud J, Andersen K. The Physical Fitness of Old Norwegian Men and Women. Acta Med Scand 183:73–78, 1968.

42. Brown J, Shephard R. Some Measurements of Fitness in Older Female Employees of a Toronto Department Store. Canad Med Ass J 97:1208–1213, 1967.

43. Daly J, Barry A, Birhead N. The Physical Working Capacity of Older Individuals. J Gerontol 23:134–139, 1968.

44. Sidney K, Shephard R. Maximum and Submaximum Exercise Tests in Men and Women in the Seventh, Eighth, and Ninth Decades of Life. J Appl Physiol 43:280–287, 1977.

45. Drinkwater B, Horvath S, Wells C. Aerobic Power of Females, Ages 10 to 68. J Geront 30:385–394, 1975.

46. Foster V, Hume G, Dickinson A, Chatfield S, Byrnes W. The Reproducibility of $\dot{V}O_{2max}$, Ventilatory, and Lactate Thresholds in Elderly Women. Med Sci Sports Exerc 18:425–430, 1986.

47. Hossack K, Bruce R. Maximal Cardiac Function in Sedentary Normal Men and Women: Comparison of Age-Related Changes. J Appl Physiol 53:799–804, 1982.

48. Kilbom A. Physical Training With Submaximal Intensities in Women: Reaction to Exercise and Orthostasis. Scand J Clin Lab Invest 28:141–161, 1971.

49. Profant G, Early R, Nilson K, Kusumi F, Hofer V, Bruce R. Responses to Maximal Exercise in Healthy Middle-Aged Women. J Appl Physiol 33:595–599, 1972.

50. Posner J, Gorman K, Klein H, Woldow A. Exercise Capacity in the Elderly. Am J Cardiol 57:52C–58C, 1986.

51. Niinimaa V, Shephard R. Training and Oxygen Conductance in the Elderly. I. The Respiratory System. J Gerontol 33:354–361, 1978.

52. Seals D, Hurley B, Schultz J, Hagberg J. Endurance Training in Older Men and Women II. Blood Lactate Response to Submaximal Exercise. J Appl Physiol 57:1030–1033, 1984.

53. Sidney K, Shephard R, Harrison J. Endurance Training and Body Composition of the Elderly. Am J Clin Nutr 30:326–333, 1977.

54. Morey MC, Cowper PA, Feussner JR, et al. Evaluation of a Supervised Exercise Program in a Geriatric Population. J Am Geriatr Soc 37:348–354, 1989.

55. de Vries H. Physiological Effects of an Exercise Training Regimen Upon Men Aged 52 to 88. J Gerontol 25:325–336, 1970.

56. Benestad A. Trainability of Old Men. Acta Med Scand 178:321–327, 1965.

57. Stamford B. Physiological Effects of Training Upon Institutionalized Geriatric Men. J Gerontol 27:451–455, 1972.

58. Barry A, Daly J, Pruett E, Steinmetz J, Page H, Birkhead N, Rodahl K. The Effects of Physical Conditioning on Older Individuals. I. Work Capacity, Circulatory-Respiratory Function, and Work Electrocardiogram. J Gerontol 21:182–191, 1966.

59. Tzankoff S, Robinson S, Pyke F, Brawn C. Physiological Adjustments to Work in Older Men As Affected by Physical Training. J Appl Physiol 33:346–350, 1972.

60. Badenhop D, Cleary P, Schaal S, Fox E, Bartels R. Physiological Adjustments to Higher- or Lower-Intensity Exercise in Elders. Med Sci Sports Exerc 6:496–502, 1983.

61. Kasch FW, Wallace JP. Physiological Variables During 10 Years of Endurance Exercise. Med Sci Sports Exerc 8:5–8, 1976.

62. Pollock ML, Foster C, Knapp D, Rod JL, Schmidt DH. Effect of Age and Training on Aerobic Capacity and Body Composition of Master Athletes. J Appl Physiol 62:725–731, 1987.

63. Larson EB, Bruce RA. Health Benefits of Exercise in an Aging Society. Arch Intern Med 147:353–356, 1987.

64. Meredith CN, Zackin MJ, Frontera WR, Evans WJ. Body Composition and Aerobic Capacity in Young and Middle-Aged Endurance-Trained Men. Med Sci Sports Exerc 19:557–563, 1987.

65. Barnard RJ, Grimditch GK, Wilmore JH. Physiological Characteristics of Sprint and Endurance Masters Runners. Med Sci Sports Exerc 11:167–171, 1979.

66. Legwold G. Masters Competitors Age Little In Ten Years. Physician Sportsmed 10:27, 1982.

67. Pollock ML, Gushiken TT. Aerobic Capacity and the Aged Athlete. In: Butts NK, Gushiken TT, Zarins B (eds): The Elite Athlete. New York: Spectrum Publications, Inc., 1985.

68. Hagberg JM, Yerg JE, Seals DR. Pulmonary Function in Young and Older Athletes and Untrained Men. J Appl Physiol 65:101–105, 1988.

69. Gaesser GA, Belman MJ. Effects of Low- and High-Intensity Walking Training on Exercise Capacity of Elderly Subjects. Med Sci Sports Exerc 19:S46, 1987.

70. Himann JE, Cunningham DA, Rechnitzer PA, Paterson DH. Age-Related Changes in Speed of Walking. Med Sci Sports Exerc 20:161–166, 1988.

71. Zauber N, Zauber A. Hematologic Data of Healthy Very Old People. JAMA 257:2181–2184, 1987.

72. Frontera WR, Meredith CN, O'Reilly KP, et al. Strength Conditioning in Older Men: Skeletal Muscle Hypertrophy and Improved Function. J Appl Physiol 64:1038–1044, 1988.

73. Kasch FW, Wallace JP, Van Camp SP, Verity L. A Longitudinal Study of Cardiovascular Stability in Active Men Aged 45 to 65 Years. Physician Sportsmed 16(1):117–126, 1988.

74. Bassey EJ, Morgan K, Dallosso HM, Ebrahim SBJ. Flexibility of the Shoulder Joint Measured as Range of Abduction in a Large Representative Sample of Men and Women over 65 Years of Age. Eur J Appl Physiol 58:353–360, 1989.

75. Council and Scientific Affairs. Exercise Programs for the Elderly. JAMA 252:544–546, 1984.

76. Larson EB, Bruce RA. Health Benefits of Exercise in an Aging Society. Arch Intern Med 147:353–356, 1987.

77. Paffenbarger PS, Hyde RT, Wing AL, et al. Physical Activity, All-Cause Mortality, and Longevity of College Alumni. N Eng J Med 314:605–613, 1986.

78. Heyden S, Fodor GJ. Does Regular Exercise Prolong Life Expectancy? Sports Med 6:63–71, 1988.

79. Schneider EL, Reed JD. Life Extension. N Eng J Med 312:1159–1168, 1985.

80. Holloszy JO, Smith EK, Vining M, Adams S. Effect of Voluntary Exercise On Longevity of Rats. J Appl Physiol 59:826–831, 1985.

81. National Institutes of Health, Consensus Conference. Osteoporosis. JAMA 252:799–802, 1984.

82. Riggs BL, Melton LJ. Involutional Osteoporosis. N Engl J Med 314:1676–1685, 1986.

83. U.S. Department of Health and Human Services. The Surgeon General's Report on Nutrition and Health. DHHS (PHS) Publication No. 88–50211. U.S. Government Printing Office: Washington, D.C., 1988.

84. Resnick NM, Greenspan SL. "Senile" Osteoporosis Reconsidered. JAMA 261:1025–1029, 1989.

85. Rodysill KJ. Postmenopausal Osteoporosis—Intervention and Prophylaxis: A Review. J Chron Dis 40:743–760, 1987.

86. Johnston CC, Slemenda C. Osteoporosis: An Overview. Physician Sportsmed 15(11):65–68, 1987.

87. Wardlaw G. The Effects of Diet and Life-Style on Bone Mass in Women. J Am Diet Assoc 88:17–25, 1988.

88. Lutz J. Bone Mineral, Serum Calcium, and Dietary Intakes of Mother/Daughter Pairs. Am J Clin Nutr 1986;44:99–106.

89. Evans RA, Marel GM, Lancaster EK, et al. Bone Mass Is Low in Relatives of Osteoporotic Patients. Ann Int Med 109:870–873, 1988.

90. Peck WA, Riggs BL, Bell NH, et al. Research Directions in Osteoporosis. Am J Med 84:275–282, 1988.

91. Melton LJ, Kan SH, Frye MA, et al. Epidemiology of Vertebral Fractures in Women. Am J Epidemiol 129:1000–1011, 1989.

92. Melton LJ, Kan SH, Wahner HW, Riggs BL. Lifetime Fracture Risk: An Approach to Hip Fracture Risk Assessment Based on Bone Mineral Density and Age. J Clin Epidemiol 41:985–994, 1988.

93. Riis B, Thomsen K, Christiansen C. Does Calcium Supplementation Prevent Postmenopausal Bone Loss? N Engl J Med 316:173–7, 1987.

94. Dawnson-Hughes B, Jacques P, Shipp C. Dietary Calcium Intake and Bone Loss from the Spine in Health Postmenopausal Women. Am J Clin Nutr 46:685–687, 1987.

95. Spencer H, Kramer L. Osteoporosis, Calcium Requirement, and Factors Causing Calcium Loss. Clin Geriatr Med 3:389–402, 1987.

96. Kiel DP, Felson DT, Anderson JJ, et al. Hip Fracture and the Use of Estrogens in Postmenopausal Women: The Framingham Study. N Engl J Med 317:1169–1174, 1987.

97. U.S. Department of Agriculture, Human Nutrition Information Service. 1985. Nationwide Food Consumption Survey, Continuing Survey of Food Intakes by Individuals: Women 19–50 Years and Their Children 1–5 Years, 1 Day, 1985. U.S. Dept. of Agric., Rpt. No 85–1. Men 19–50 Years, 1 Day, 1985. U.S. Dept. of Agric., Rpt. No 85–3.

98. Cauley JA, Gutai JP, Kuller LH, et al. Endogeneous Estrogen Levels and Calcium Intakes in Postmenopausal Women: Relationships with Cortical Bone Measures. JAMA 260:3150–3155, 1988.

99. Walden O. The Relationship of Dietary and Supplemental Calcium Intake to Bone Loss and Osteoporosis. J Am Diet Assoc 89:397–400, 1989.

100. Francis RM, Peacock M. Local Action of Oral 1,25–Dihydroxycholecalciferol on Calcium Absorption in Osteoporosis. Am J Clin Nutr 46:315–318, 1987.

101. Smith EL. How Exercise Helps Prevent Osteoporosis. Contemporary OB/GYN: Active Woman, May, 1985.

102. Brewer V, Meyer BM, et al. Role of Exercise In Prevention of Involutional Bone Loss. Med Sci Sports Exerc 15:445–449, 1983.

103. Falch JA. The Effect of Physical Activity on the Skeleton. Scand J Soc Med [Suppl.] 29:55–58, 1982.

104. Aloia JF, Cohn SH, et al. Prevention of Involutional Bone Loss by Exercise. Ann Int Med 89:3, 1978.

105. Smith EL, Reddan W, Smith PE. Physical Activity and Calcium Modalities for Bone Mineral Increase in Aged Women. Med Sci Sports Exerc 13:60–64, 1981.

106. Smith EL, Smith PE, Ensign CJ, et al. Bone Involution Decrease in Exercising Middle-aged Women. Calcif Tissue Res 36:S129, 1984.

107. Lutter JM. Mixed Messages About Osteoporosis in Female Athletes. Physician Sportsmed 11:154–165, 1983.

108. Krolner B, Toft B, et al. Physical Exercise As Prophylaxis Against Involutional Vertebral Bone Loss: A Controlled Trial. Clin Sci 64:541, 1983.

109. Yeater RA, Martin RB. Senile Osteoporosis: The Effects of Exercise. Postgrad Med 75:147–163, 1984.

110. Drinkwater BL, Nilson K, Chesnut CH, et al. Bone Mineral Content of Amenorrheic and Eumenorrheic Athletes. N Eng J Med 311:277–281, 1984.

111. Marcus R, Cann C, et al. Menstrual Function and Bone Mass in Elite Women Distance Runners. Ann Int Med 102:158–163, 1985.

112. Block JE, Smith R, Black D, Genant HK. Does Exercise Prevent Osteoporosis? JAMA 257:3115–3117, 1987.

113. Montoye HJ. The 1987 C. H. McCloy Research Lecture: Better Bones and Biodynamics. Res Quart Exerc Sport 58:334–348, 1987.

114. Smith EL, Gilligan C. Effects of Inactivity and Exercise on Bone. Physician Sportsmed 15(11):91–104, 1987.

115. Kriska AM, Sandler RB, Cauley JA, et al. The Assessment of Historical Physical Activity and Its Relation to Adult Bone Parameters. Am J Epidemiol 127:1053–1063, 1988.

116. Pocock NA, Eisman JA, Yeates MG, et al. Physical Fitness Is a Major Determinant of Femoral Neck and Lumbar Spine Bone Mineral Density. J Clin Invest 78:618–621, 1986.

117. Stillman RJ, Lohman TG, Slaughter MH, Massey BH. Physical Activity and Bone Mineral Content in Women Aged 30 to 85 Years. Med Sci Sports Exerc 18:576–580, 1986.

118. Block JE, Genant HK, Black D. Greater Vertebral Bone Mineral Mass in Exercising Young Men. West J Med 145:39–42, 1986.

119. Orwoll BE, Ferar JL, Oviatt Sk, et al. The Effect of Swimming Exercise on Bone Mineral Content. Clin Res 35:194A, 1987.

120. Myburgh KH, Noakes TD, Roodt M, Hough FS. Effect of Exercise on the Development of Osteoporosis in Adult Rats. J Appl Physiol 66:14–19, 1989.

121. Pirnay F, Bodeux M, Crielaard JM, Franchimont P. Bone Mineral Content and Physical Activity. Int J Sports Med 8:331–335, 1987.

122. Snow-Harter C. Biochemical Changes in Postmenopausal Women Following A Muscle Fitness Program. Physician Sportsmed 15(8):90–96, 1987.

123. Dalsky GP, Stocke KS, Ehsani AA, et al. Weight-Bearing Exercise Training and Lumbar Bone Mineral Content in Postmenopausal Women. Ann Internal Med 108:824–828, 1988.

124. Lindberg JS, Powell MR, Hunt MM, et al. Increased Vertebral Bone Mineral in Response to Reduced Exercise in Amenorrheic Runners. West J Med 146:39–42, 1987.

125. Bilanin JE, Blanchard MS, Russek-Cohen E. Lower Vertebral Bone Density in Male Long Distance Runners. Med Sci Sports Exerc 21:66–70, 1989.

126. Rowe JW. Health Care of the Elderly. N Eng J Med 312:827–835, 1985.

127. Morrison SD. Nutrition and Longevity. Nutr Rev 41:133–142, 1983.

128. Enstrom JE, Kanim LE, Breslow L. The Relationship Between Vitamin C Intake, General Health Practices, and Mortality in Alameda County, California. Am J Public Health 76:1124–1130, 1986.

129. Paganini-Hill A, Ross RK, Henderson BE. Prevalence of Chronic Disease and Health Practices in a Retirement Community. J Chronic Dis 39(9):699–707, 1986.

130. Kaplan GA, Seeman TE, Cohen RD, Knudsen LP, Guralnik J. Mortality Among the Elderly in the Alameda County Study: Behavioral and Demographic Risk Factors [published erratum appears in Am J Public Health 77(7):818, 1987]. Am J Public Health 77(3):307–312, 1987.

131. Freis J. Aging, Natural Death, and the Compression of Morbidity. N Eng J Med 33:130–135, 1980.

132. Belloc NB, Breslow L. Relationship of Physical Health Status and Health Practices. Prev Med 1:409, 1972. (See also: Prev Med 9:469, 1980.)

133. Snowdon DA. Epidemiology of Aging: Seventh-day Adventists—A Bellwether for Future Progress. In: Intervention in the Aging Process, Part A: Quantification, Epidemiology, and Clinical Research. New York: Alan R. Liss Publishers, 1983.

134. Phillips RL, Kuzma JW, et al. Influence of Selection Versus Lifestyle on Risk of Fatal Cancer and Cardiovascular Disease Among Seventh-day Adventists. Am J Epidemiol 112:296–314, 1980.

135. Kahn HA, Phillips RL, Snowdon DA, Choi W. Association Between Reported Diet and All-Cause Mortality. Am J Epidemiol 119:775–787, 1984.

136. Nieman DC, Stanton HJ. The Adventist Lifestyle—A Better Way to Live. Vibrant Life, March/April, pp. 14–18, 1988.

Physical Fitness Activity 12.1— Calculating Your Health Age

In this physical fitness activity you will be answering questions from the health risk appraisal program "Healthier People" from The Carter Center Health Risk Appraisal Project. A computer software program to calculate your "risk age" from this questionnaire can be ordered from:

Edwin B. Hutchins, Ph.D., Program Director
Emory University
The Carter Center Health Risk Appraisal Project
1989 North Williamsburg Drive
Suite E
Decatur, GA 30033
(404) 321–4104

The printout from the computer software program will give your present "risk age" and a target "risk age." The Health Risk Appraisal will then list factors that you can change to lower your risk.

THE CARTER CENTER OF EMORY UNIVERSITY

Healthier People
Health Risk Appraisal

No. _____

Detach this coupon and put it in a safe place.
You will need it to claim your appraisal results.

✄ —

Healthier People
Health Risk Appraisal
The Carter Center of Emory University

No. _____

_____

Health Risk Appraisal is an educational tool. It shows you choices you can make to keep good health and avoid the most common causes of death for a person your age and sex. This Health Risk Appraisal is not a substitute for a check-up or physical exam that you get from a doctor or nurse. It only gives you some ideas for lowering your risk of getting sick or injured in the future. It is NOT designed for people who already have HEART DISEASE, CANCER, KIDNEY DISEASE, OR OTHER SERIOUS CONDITIONS. If you have any of these problems and you want a Health Risk Appraisal anyway, ask your doctor or nurse to read the report with you.

DIRECTIONS: To keep your answers confidential DO NOT write your name or any identification on this form. Please keep the coupon with your participant number on it. You will need it to claim your computer report. To get the most accurate results answer as many questions as you can and as best you can. If you do not know the answer leave it blank. Questions with a ★ (star symbol) are important to your health, but are not used by the computer to calculate your risks. However, your answers may be helpful in planning your health and fitness program.

Please put your answers in the empty boxes. (Examples: ☒ or ☐125)

1. SEX	1 ☐ Male 2 ☐ Female
2. AGE	☐ Years
3. HEIGHT (Without shoes) (No fractions)	☐ Feet ☐ Inches
4. WEIGHT (Without shoes) (No fractions)	☐ Pounds
5. Body frame size	1 ☐ Small 2 ☐ Medium 3 ☐ Large
6. Have you ever been told that you have diabetes (or sugar diabetes)?	1 ☐ Yes 2 ☐ No
7. Are you now taking medicine for high blood pressure?	1 ☐ Yes 2 ☐ No
8. What is your blood pressure now?	☐ / ☐ Systolic (High number) / Diastolic (Low number)
9. If you *do not* know the numbers, check the box that describes your blood pressure.	1 ☐ High 2 ☐ Normal or Low 3 ☐ Don't Know
10. What is your TOTAL cholesterol level (based on a blood test)?	☐ mg/dl
11. What is your HDL cholesterol (based on a blood test)?	☐ mg/dl
12. How many cigars do you usually smoke per day?	☐ cigars per day
13. How many pipes of tobacco do you usually smoke per day?	☐ pipes per day
14. How many times per day do you usually use smokeless tobacco? (Chewing tobacco, snuff, pouches, etc.)	☐ times per day

Health Risk Appraisal is an educational tool. It shows you choices you can make to keep good health and avoid the most common causes of death for a person your age and sex. This Health Risk Appraisal is not a substitute for a check-up or physical exam that you get from a doctor or nurse. It only gives you some ideas for lowering your risk of getting sick or injured in the future. It is NOT designed for people who already have HEART DISEASE, CANCER, KIDNEY DISEASE, OR OTHER SERIOUS CONDITIONS. If you have any of these problems and you want a Health Risk Appraisal anyway, ask your doctor or nurse to read the report with you.

Your report may be picked up at _____ on _____.

- -

15. CIGARETTE SMOKING
How would you describe your cigarette smoking habits?

1 ☐ Never smoked   ☛ Go to 18
2 ☐ Used to smoke   ☛ Go to 17
3 ☐ Still smoke   ☛ Go to 16

16. STILL SMOKE
How many cigarettes a day do you smoke?
☛ GO TO QUESTION 18

☐ cigarettes per day ☛ Go to 18

17. USED TO SMOKE
a. How many years has it been since you smoked cigarettes fairly regularly?

☐ years

b. What was the average number of cigarettes per day that you smoked in the 2 years before you quit?

☐ cigarettes per day

18. In the next 12 months how many thousands of miles will you probably travel by each of the following? (NOTE: U.S. average = 10,000 miles)
    a. Car, truck, or van:
    b. Motorcycle:

☐ ,000 miles
☐ ,000 miles

19. On a typical day how do you USUALLY travel?
    (Check one only)

1 ☐ Walk
2 ☐ Bicycle
3 ☐ Motorcycle
4 ☐ Sub-compact or compact car
5 ☐ Mid-size or full-size car
6 ☐ Truck or van
7 ☐ Bus, subway, or train
8 ☐ Mostly stay home

20. What percent of the time do you usually buckle your safety belt when driving or riding?

☐ %

21. On the average, how close to the speed limit do you usually drive?

1 ☐ Within 5 mph of limit
2 ☐ 6-10 mph over limit
3 ☐ 11-15 mph over limit
4 ☐ More than 15 mph over limit

22. How many times in the last month did you drive or ride when the driver had perhaps too much alcohol to drink?

☐ times last month

23. How many drinks of alcoholic beverages do you have in a typical week?

☛ (MEN GO TO QUESTION 33)

(Write the number of each type of drink)
☐ Bottles or cans of beer
☐ Glasses of wine
☐ Wine coolers
☐ Mixed drinks or shots of liquor

WOMEN
24. At what age did you have your first menstrual period?

☐ years old

25. How old were you when your first child was born?

☐ years old
(If no children write 0)

26. How long has it been since your last breast x-ray (mammogram)?

1 ☐ Less than 1 year ago
2 ☐ 1 year ago
3 ☐ 2 years ago
4 ☐ 3 or more years ago
5 ☐ Never

27. How many women in your natural family (mother and sisters only) have had breast cancer?

☐☐☐ women

28. Have you had a hysterectomy operation?

1 ☐ Yes
2 ☐ No
3 ☐ Not sure

29. How long has it been since you had a pap smear test?

1 ☐ Less than 1 year ago
2 ☐ 1 year ago
3 ☐ 2 years ago
4 ☐ 3 or more years ago
5 ☐ Never

★ 30. How often do you examine your breasts for lumps?

1 ☐ Monthly
2 ☐ Once every few months
3 ☐ Rarely or never

★ 31. About how long has it been since you had your breasts examined by a physician or nurse?

1 ☐ Less than 1 year ago
2 ☐ 1 year ago
3 ☐ 2 years ago
4 ☐ 3 or more years ago
5 ☐ Never

★ 32. About how long has it been since you had a rectal exam?

1 ☐ Less than 1 year ago
2 ☐ 1 year ago
3 ☐ 2 years ago
4 ☐ 3 or more years ago
5 ☐ Never

☞ *(WOMEN GO TO QUESTION 34)*

MEN
★ 33. About how long has it been since you had a rectal or prostate exam?

1 ☐ Less than 1 year ago
2 ☐ 1 year ago
3 ☐ 2 years ago
4 ☐ 3 or more years ago
5 ☐ Never

★ 34. How many times in the last year did you witness or become involved in a violent fight or attack where there was a good chance of a serious injury to someone?

1 ☐ 4 or more times
2 ☐ 2 or 3 times
3 ☐ 1 time or never
4 ☐ Not sure

★ 35. Considering your age, how would you describe your overall physical health?

1 ☐ Excellent
2 ☐ Good
3 ☐ Fair
4 ☐ Poor

★ 36. In an average week, how many times do you engage in physical activity (exercise or work which lasts at least 20 minutes without stopping and which is hard enough to make you breathe heavier and your heart beat faster)?

1 ☐ Less than 1 time per week
2 ☐ 1 or 2 times per week
3 ☐ At least 3 times per week

★ 37. If you ride a motorcycle or all-terrain vehicle (ATV) what percent of the time do you wear a helmet?

1 ☐ 75% to 100%
2 ☐ 25% to 74%
3 ☐ Less than 25%
4 ☐ Does not apply to me

★ 38. Do you eat some food every day that is high in fiber, such as whole grain bread, cereal, fresh fruits or vegetables?   1 ☐ Yes   2 ☐ No

★ 39. Do you eat foods every day that are high in cholesterol or fat, such as fatty meat, cheese, fried foods, or eggs?   1 ☐ Yes   2 ☐ No

★ 40. In general, how satisfied are you with your life?
1 ☐ Mostly satisfied
2 ☐ Partly satisfied
3 ☐ Not satisfied

★ 41. Have you suffered a personal loss or misfortune in the past year that had a serious impact on your life? (For example, a job loss, disability, separation, jail term, or the death of someone close to you.)
1 ☐ Yes, 1 serious loss or misfortune
2 ☐ Yes, 2 or more
3 ☐ No

★ 42a. Race
1 ☐ Aleutian, Alaska native, Eskimo or American Indian
2 ☐ Asian
3 ☐ Black
4 ☐ Pacific Islander
5 ☐ White
6 ☐ Other
7 ☐ Don't know

★ 42b. Are you of Hispanic origin such as Mexican-American, Puerto Rican, or Cuban?   1 ☐ Yes   2 ☐ No

★ 43. What is the highest grade you completed in school?
1 ☐ Grade school or less
2 ☐ Some high school
3 ☐ High school graduate
4 ☐ Some college
5 ☐ College graduate
6 ☐ Post graduate or professional degree

★ 44. What is your job or occupation?   (Check only one)
1 ☐ Health professional
2 ☐ Manager, educator, professional
3 ☐ Technical, sales or administrative support
4 ☐ Operator, fabricator, laborer
5 ☐ Student
6 ☐ Retired
7 ☐ Homemaker
8 ☐ Service
9 ☐ Skilled crafts
10 ☐ Unemployed
11 ☐ Other

★ 45. In what industry do you work (or did you last work)?   (Check only one)
1 ☐ Electric, gas, sanitation
2 ☐ Transportation, communication
3 ☐ Agriculture, forestry, fishing
4 ☐ Wholesale or retail trade
5 ☐ Financial and service industries
6 ☐ Mining
7 ☐ Government
8 ☐ Manufacturing
9 ☐ Construction
10 ☐ Other

Chapter 13

Physical Activity and Psychological Health

"My body must be set a-going if my mind is to work."—Jean Jacques Rousseau

Introduction: Fact or Fancy?

John came home feeling tense, anxious, and irritable. He was a manager for a large business firm and had spent all day, unsuccessfully, trying to mend sharp differences between two of his key department heads. After fighting traffic for 45 minutes on the way home, he felt he needed to clear his mind. Slipping on his well-worn jogging shoes, John went out for a 30-minute jog through the dirt trails behind his house. By the time he returned home, he felt completely different. His mind felt relaxed, his mood was elevated, and all his built-up tension was erased. After stretching and showering, John enjoyed the evening with his family.

Donna felt depressed. She had just received a low C grade on her first biochemistry test, and as a freshman medical student, she was extremely worried about her chances of staying in the program. Pulling on her jacket, she went out for a 40-minute brisk walk on the hilly roads near her school. By the time Donna returned to her dorm room, her spirits were lifted, her depression was gone, and she sat down at her desk with renewed determination to keep pressing on with her studies.

Is this fact or fancy? Is it really true that exercise can help alleviate mental anxiety, depression, and other problems? Does the motion of the body influence the mind?

Defining the Magnitude of the Problem

As discussed in Chapter 1, the promotion of physical activity is public policy in both the United States and Canada. While directed primarily at the reduction of cardiovascular diseases, obesity, and other chronic diseases, this policy could conceivably also have some beneficial effects on the population's mental health. Even a small effect could have a significant impact, because mental health problems and stress are so widespread in most Western countries.[1]

In the United States, for example, 19 percent of the population (nearly 30 million Americans) is affected by one or more mental disorders during any given six-month period, and 32 percent within a lifetime.[2, 3] The direct costs of mental health care in the United States are more than $22 billion per year. Anxiety disorders are the most prevalent of all mental illnesses, and affective disorders, including depression, are also highly prevalent. Numerous studies have shown that, at any one time, between 9 and 20 percent of the U.S. population have depressive symptoms.[2]

In 1985, the U.S. Public Health Service conducted the National Health Interview Survey, which included questions on the amount of stress experienced in the past 2 weeks and the effect of stress on health.[4] About one-half of U.S. adults reported experiencing at least a moderate amount of stress during the past two weeks. (See Figure 13.1.)

Despite this relatively high prevalence of stress, however, only 11 percent of adults had sought help in the past year for a personal or emotional problem.[4] Obviously a large percentage of the population could benefit by using various stress management techniques. (See Sports Medicine Insight, end of this chapter.)

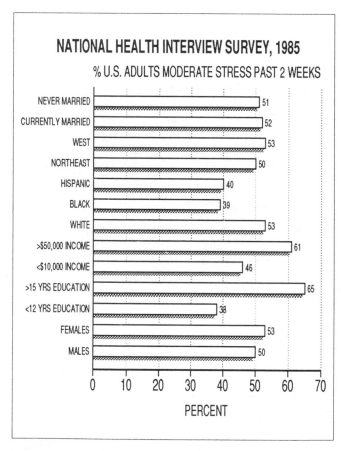

Figure 13.1 About one-half of U.S. adults reported experiencing at least a moderate amount of stress in the 2 weeks preceding the 1985 National Health Interview Survey. This prevalence varied according to race, income level, and education. *Source:* National Center for Health Statistics, C. A. Schoenborn. 1988. Health Promotion and Disease Prevention: United States, 1985. Vital and Health Statistics. Series 10, No. 163. DHHS Pub. No. (PHS) 88–1591. Public Health Service. Washington: U.S. Government Printing Office.

Relationship Between Psychological Health and Disease

For a long time researchers have known that psychological states can have a profound effect on one's physical health. Many studies have shown that being chronically anxious, depressed, or emotionally distressed is associated with deterioration of health.[5]

Repressed feelings of loss, denial, depression, inflexibility, conformity, lack of social ties, high levels of anxiety and dissatisfaction, and many life-changing events are associated with increased cancers, heart disease, and infection.[5] For example, a study that tracked middle-aged men in the Western Electric Company for 20 years found a positive association between increased incidence of psychological depression and mortality from cancer.

Data from national surveys suggest that marital happiness contributes far more to over-all happiness than any other variable, including satisfaction with work and friendships.[6,7,8] Divorced and separated people have poorer mental and physical health. Marital disruption is the single most powerful sociodemographic predictor of physical illness, with those who are separated having about 30 percent more acute illnesses and physician visits than those remaining married. Depression of immune function has also been associated with marital discord.[6,7]

A number of other studies have found bereavement and a lack of social and community ties to be associated with an overall increase in mortality.[9,10] In a study of 95,647 widowed individuals, mortality during the first week following widowhood was more than twice the norm, especially from cardiovascular disease, violent causes, and suicides.[11] Dr. Ruberman of New York has reported that heart disease patients classified as socially isolated (few contacts with friends, relatives, church or club groups) and having a high degree of life stress had more than four times the risk of dying from heart disease of men with low levels of isolation and stress.[12] This supports the statement made by William Harvey in 1628:

> "Every affection of the mind that is attended with either pain or pleasure, hope or fear, is the cause of an agitation whose influence extends to the heart."

Dr. George Vaillant of Harvard University studied the 40-year history of 204 men and found that poor mental health was associated with increased disease and death after allowing for the effects of drug abuse, obesity, or family history of long life.[13] Concluded Vaillant: "Good mental health facilitates our survival."

Since the 1950s, Friedman and Rosenman and their followers have argued energetically that people with the Type-A personality are at higher risk for coronary disease.[14] Type-A behavior is defined by a multitude of attributes, including hard-driving effort, striving for achievement, competitiveness, aggressiveness, haste, impatience, restlessness, alertness, and hurried motor movements.[15] Those classed as Type-A individuals find it difficult to relax, and are very time-conscious.

Many of the earlier studies supported the hypothesis that Type A individuals were more prone to cardiovascular disease.[14, 16, 17] However, a number of studies since the early 80s have not supported the hypothesis, including the Framingham Heart Study, the Honolulu Heart Study, the Multiple Risk Factor Intervention Trials, the Rotterdam Coronary Heart Disease Study, the Aspirin Myocardial Infarction Study, and the Beta-Blocker Heart Attack Trial.[14–20]

The hostility component of Type-A behavior may be most predictive of cardiovascular disease.[21, 22] It appears that cultural, social, and psychological factors may also be important.[18] Some researchers have reported that, paradoxically, many people derive more good than harm from Type-A behavior patterns. This is because Type-A behavior is associated with success, productivity, and a sense of satisfaction in life.

Relationship Between Physical Activity and Psychological Health

We have seen that poor psychological health is associated with poor physical health. Is there proof for the converse association? Is a healthy and fit body positively associated with psychological health? Were the ancient Greeks right in their assertion that a physically fit and strong body would lead to a sound mind?

The part of the brain that enables us to exercise, the motor cortex, lies only a few millimeters away from the part of the brain that deals with thought and feeling. Might this proximity mean that when exercise stimulates the motor cortex, it has a parallel effect on cognition and emotion?

Since the beginning of time many have believed in the "cerebral satisfaction" of exercise. The Greeks maintained that exercise made the mind more lucid. Aristotle started his "Peripatetic School" in 335 B.C—so

named because of Aristotle's habit of walking up and down *(peripaton)* the paths of the Lyceum in Athens while thinking or lecturing to his students walking with him. Plato and Socrates had also practiced the art of peripatetics as did the Roman *Ordo Vagorum* or walking scholars. Centuries later, Oliver Wendell Holmes explained that "in walking the will and the muscles are so accustomed to working together and perform their task with so little expenditure of force that the intellect is left comparatively free."

John F. Kennedy, echoed the Greek ideal when he said:

> "Physical fitness is not only one of the most important keys to a healthy body, it is the basis of dynamic and creative intellectual activity. Intelligence and skill can only function at the peak of their capacity when the body is strong. Hardy spirits and tough minds usually inhabit sound bodies."

The highly acclaimed 1978 "Perrier Survey of Fitness in America," conducted by Louis Harris and Associates, showed that modern-day men and women strongly believe in the Greek concept of a "strong mind in a strong body." The survey found that those who have a deep commitment to exercise report feeling more relaxed, less tired, more disciplined, more attractive, more self-confident, more productive in work, and in general, more at one with themselves.[23]

The Canadian Fitness Survey (CFS) assessed reasons for being active during leisure time.[1] Health-related reasons dominated the responses, especially "to feel better mentally and physically" (62 percent of adults said it was "very important" to them). Other health-related reasons given for activity were to control weight or look better (42 percent) and to relax or reduce stress (36 percent).

Figures 13.2 and 13.3 show the results of a large study of 2,300 Los Angeles marathon (LAM) runners.[24] Runners used a four-point Likert scale in evaluating their energy and stress levels, and in reporting their quality of sleep and overall feelings since they had started running (compared to pre-running years). From this self-reported information, runners were categorized as being in the "perceived low stress" group if they described as "definitely better" their sleep, energy, and stress levels, and overall feelings since starting running. The majority of LAM runners reported much improved sleep, energy, and stress levels.

Many cross-sectional studies of endurance athletes have found them to have more favorable profiles of mood states than their sedentary counterparts.[25] Figure 13.4 presents the results of one study of nine marathon runners. The marathoners were found to have more

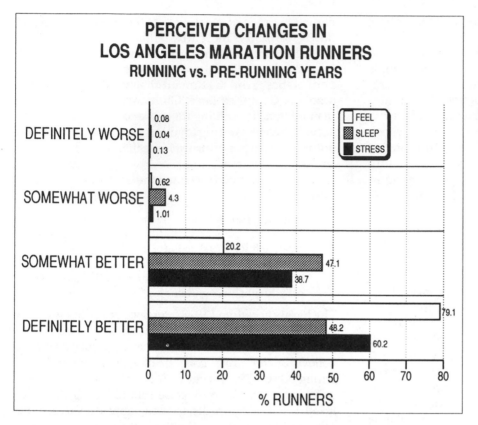

Figure 13.2 The majority of Los Angeles marathon runners studied reported that since starting regular running they felt and slept better, and were able to handle stress better. *Source:* Nieman DC, Johansen LM, Lee JW, Arabatzis K. Infectious Episodes in Runners Before and After the Los Angeles Marathon. J Sports Med (in press).

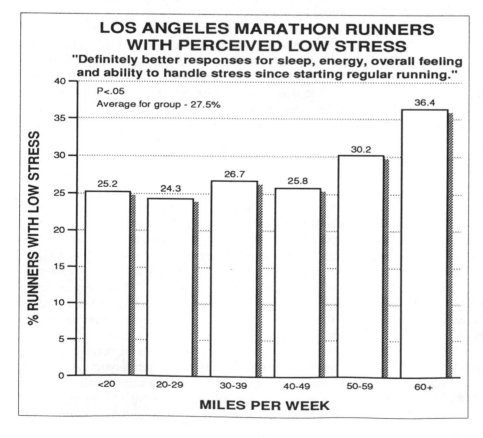

Figure 13.3 Quantity of running, correlated with the percentage of Los Angeles Marathon runners reporting their sleep, energy levels, overall feelings, and ability to handle stress ("perceived low stress") had been "definitely better" since they had started regular running. *Source:* Nieman DC, Johansen LM, Lee JW, Arabatzis K. Infectious Episodes in Runners Before and After the Los Angeles Marathon. J Sports Med (in press).

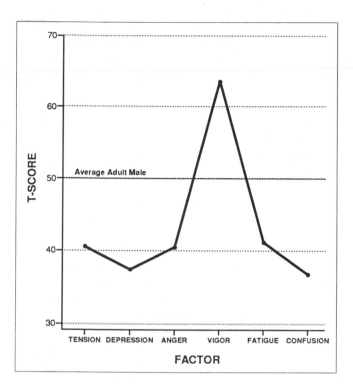

Figure 13.4 The Profile of Mood States inventory (POMS) is commonly used by researchers to determine levels of tension, depression, anger, vigor, fatigue, and confusion. In this study of nine male marathon runners, vigor was much higher, but all of the other mood states much lower than average. Interestingly, in this study, the higher the vigor rating, the longer it took for the runner to become exhausted (when running in a laboratory environment at 70 percent of $\dot{V}O_{2max}$). *Source:* Nieman DC, Carlson KA, Brandstater ME, Naegele RT, Blankenship JW. Running Endurance in 27-h-Fasted Humans. J Appl Physiol 63:2502–2509, 1987.

vigor, but less tension, depression, anger, fatigue, and confusion than the average adult male.

It has been common to find this "iceberg" pattern when comparing athletes with sedentary people. However, the possibility exists that heavy endurance training does not actually produce the mood state profile—that in fact people with such mood state profiles may choose to become endurance athletes. (In other words, a strong self-selection bias may be present when comparing athletes with the general population.)

Therefore, cross-sectional studies of the psychological profiles of athletes tell us little about whether or not sedentary people who choose to become active can expect to experience a comparable mood state. The best study design uses a controlled intervention format, in which a group of sedentary people are randomly divided into exercise and sedentary control groups, and

then followed for a number of weeks to measure any changes in psychological health.

Researchers have been very eager to study the common belief that physical activity improves psychological health. Well over 1,000 studies have now been conducted investigating whether or not exercise really results in measurable improvements in depression, anxiety, intelligence, self-concept, and other psychological parameters.[25] Unfortunately, in their eagerness to prove what so many already believe, most researchers have followed poor research designs. Only recently has some strong evidence emerged. Four studies have been particularly impressive.

General Well-Being in the Community

Previous studies provided little insight into the physical activity-mental health association for the general population. Recently, however, Dr. Tom Stephens directed a study of four independent national survey data bases, with analysis done by the Office of Analysis and Epidemiology, National Center for Health Statistics.[1] Each of the four data bases were derived from federal government surveys in the United States and Canada. Each was based on a sample of the national, non-institutionalized population; they were: the 1972–1973 National Health and Nutrition Examination Survey (NHANES I); the 1978–1979 Canada Health Survey (CHS); The 1979 National Survey of Personal Health Practices and Consequences (NSPHPC I); and the 1981 Canada Fitness Survey (CFS).

Six measures of psychological status were used, which have been shown to have good to excellent validity and reliability: General Well-Being (GWB), Blue-cheer index, Positive Affect Scale, Negative Affect Scale, CES-Depression (CES-D), and the Health Opinion Survey (HOS). The GWB consists of 18 items, covering such constructs as energy level, satisfaction, freedom from worry, and self-control. (See Physical Fitness Activity 13.1, end of this chapter.) A high score on the GWB represents an absence of bad feelings and an expression of positive feelings. The CES-D scale measures the frequency of 18 negative and two positive feelings (a low score represents an absence of depression). The Positive and Negative Affect Scales consist of five questions each on feelings. The HOS looks at the frequency of psychophysiological symptoms associated with anxiety and depression. The Blue-cheer index looks at the frequency of two positive and two negative self-descriptions (cheerful and lighthearted, downhearted and blue, happy all in all, and lonely). A high score represents a positive mood.

Results from these national surveys showed that higher scores for the GWB and Blue-cheer index (absence of bad feelings, and positive mood) were significantly associated with increased amounts of physical activity for older men, and for women in both younger and older groups.[1] For younger men, only the GWB was significantly related to physical activity. (See Figure 13.5.) Positive affect was significantly associated with amount of physical activity for all population groups measured. In general, depression and anxiety were lower for the physically active. (See Figure 13.6 for CES-D scores.)

The inescapable conclusion from these four national studies is that level of physical activity is positively associated with good mental health when mental health is defined as positive mood, general well-being, and relatively infrequent symptoms of anxiety and depression.[1] This relationship was found to be independent of education and physical health status. The physical activity-mental health relationship was found to be stronger for the older age group (+40 years of age) than for the younger, and stronger for women than for men.

These findings were supported recently by a representative sample of 400 adults in Illinois.[26] Icreased participation in exercise, sports, and physical activities was associated with improved psychological well-being.

Exercise was associated with decreased symptoms of depression, anxiety, and malaise. This was the first community survey using a large, representative sample to examine this relationship, supporting the findings from the larger national surveys.

Cardiovascular Reactivity to Mental Stress

A considerable amount of recent research has indicated that people with low levels of aerobic fitness experience greater cardiovascular and subjective responses to psychological stressors.[27-30] During stressful mental tasks, less-fit subjects have been found to have heart rates nearly 30 beats per minute higher than those of highly-fit subjects. Aerobic training programs for less-fit subjects has been found effective in reducing heart rate response to a psychological stressors.[27]

A recent analysis of 34 studies with 1,449 subjects showed comparable results—aerobically fit subjects had a significantly reduced psychosocial stress response to various stressors.[28] Exercise appears to act either as a coping strategy or an "inoculator" in response to psychosocial stressors.

Drs. Sinyor and Seraganian of Concordia University in Canada have shown that 10 weeks of aerobic exercise result in more effective coping with emotional

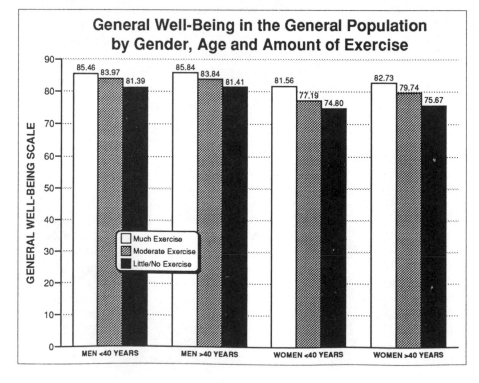

Figure 13.5 With increased exercise, scores from the General Well-Being test were higher for all age and gender subgroups measured. See the Physical Fitness Activity at the end of this chapter to see how you score. *Source:* Stephens T. Physical Activity and Mental Health in the United States and Canada: Evidence from Four Population Surveys. Prev Med 17:35–47, 1988.

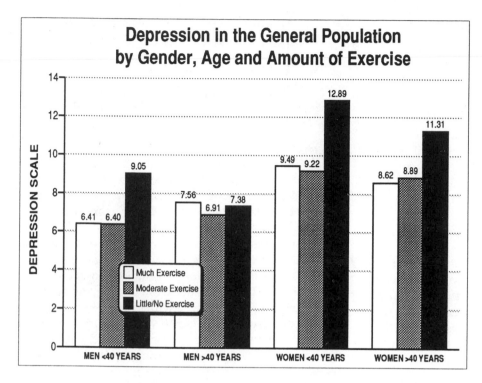

Depression in the General Population by Gender, Age and Amount of Exercise

Figure 13.6 Scores from the CES-Depression test tended to be lower (less depression) for people who reported being more physically active. *Source:* Stephens T. Physical Activity and Mental Health in the United States and Canada: Evidence from Four Population Surveys. Prev Med 17:35–47, 1988.

stress.[29] Subjects were randomly divided into a meditation group, a music appreciation class (the control groups), and an exercise group consisting of 30 minutes of calisthenics and jogging, four days per week for 10 weeks. In response to a battery of very stressful mental tasks, the exercise group at the end of 10 weeks demonstrated a faster recovery of the heart rate and autonomic system (skin electrical response) than the control groups did. Dr. Sinyor concluded that this faster recovery is very important in coping with stress. Since both exercise and mental stress increase the heart rate, blood pressure, adrenaline, and other biochemical measures, strengthening the body to adapt to exercise stress means better reactivity to mental stress.

Stressful Life Events and Somatic Illness

During the past 25 years, a very large number of studies have shown that life events of all types (marriage, divorce, buying a house, losing one's job, moving to a new location, surgery for health problems, etc.) are significant stressors, leading to predictable physical and psychological health problems. (For an example of the questionnaire, see: Holme TH. Life Situations, Emotions, and Disease. Psychosomatics 19:747–754, 1978). Several recent studies have shown, however, that such life stress has less impact on the health of physically active people.[31–33]

A 4-year longitudinal study of 278 managers from 12 corporations indicated that physical activity has a buffering effect on the relationship between life events and illness.[31]

A study of 112 students showed an association between a high level of life stress and poorer subsequent physical health for those with a low level of physical fitness, whereas students with a high level of physical fitness were "buffered" from the ill effects.[32] In a second study of college students who reported a high number of negative life events over the preceding year, experimental groups received either aerobic exercise training or relaxation training, and were compared to a no-treatment control group.[33] After 5 weeks, the exercise training had been more effective for reducing depression.

In summary, studies have found an association between stressful life change and subsequent physical and psychological health problems. Furthermore, there is evidence that regular aerobic exercise may help reduce the impact of stress on health.

Depression, Anxiety, and Mood Elevation

As discussed earlier in this chapter, depression and fatigue are very common complaints of Americans.[2, 34] National data have shown that adults who are physically inactive are at much higher risk for feeling fatigue and depression than those who are physically active.[1,35] Most individuals report that they "feel good" or "feel better" following vigorous aerobic exercise.[34] As the studies reviewed in this section will show, depression, anxiety, and mood state in general appear to be favorably affected by regular aerobic exercise.

A team of researchers at Duke University has shown the importance of exercise on various psychological traits such as depression, anxiety, and mood elevation.[45] In one study, 16 middle-aged men and women were matched with 16 controls. After ten weeks of walking and jogging 45 minutes, three times per week, the exercising adults showed decreased anxiety and depression, less fatigue and confusion, and elevated vigor.

In a study of 36 policemen and firemen, after 12 weeks of exercise, improvement in physical fitness was associated with decreased anxiety and depression.[46] Another study of depressed subjects compared the effects of a running program against those of psychotherapy. Running was found to be at least as effective as psychotherapy in alleviating moderate depression.[39, 44] Another study found that fourteen weeks of jogging about 8 miles per week significantly decreased anxiety.[47]

Running and walking are not the only aerobic exercises that are beneficial for the mind. A study comparing students in swimming classes with nonswimmers found the swimmers experienced less tension, depression, anger, and confusion, and more vigor.[48] Other studies have found that mixed aerobic programs of swimming, soccer, running, and aquatic and land calisthenics that are more moderate in intensity and more fun are helpful in reducing anxiety.[49] A study of 64 long-term unemployed women and men aged 25–45[50] showed that those exercising experienced a significant reduction in anxiety after three months of regular (2 hours per week) recreational (volleyball and badminton) and low-aerobic intensity activity (calisthenics and swimming).

A study of subjects with normal resting blood pressure compared the effectiveness of aerobic exercise versus quiet rest on state (short-term) anxiety and blood pressure.[51] Each subject on separate occasions either rested quietly in a sound chamber for 40 minutes or performed 40 minutes of self-selected aerobic exercise. Systolic blood pressure was reduced an average of 9 mm Hg in both conditions, but in the case of exercise, the reduction remained significant for 3 hours, whereas it returned to baseline within 20-minutes following quiet rest. State anxiety was reduced significantly following exercise, but not following rest.

Results from further study of 15 hypertensive subjects were similar. The researchers concluded that exercise and quiet rest have similar effects on state anxiety, and both conditions are followed by a transitory reduction in blood pressure. The anti-anxiety effects, however, are sustained for a longer period following exercise.[51]

Self-Concept

Exercise does more than decrease anxiety and depression and elevate mood. Self-concept is also improved and has been strongly correlated with exercise in many studies.[25] In a study of three groups of 40 college students, students were divided into a 10-week exercise group, a 10-week exercise group with supportive counseling, and a control group receiving no exercise or counseling.[52] The combination of running and supportive counseling helped those with low self-concept gain more positive views of themselves. In another study, a 10-week aerobic dancing course increased self-esteem and self-concept, especially for the subjects who were in the lowest fitness category to begin with.[53]

A study of women in a 12-week program of weight training showed an increase in both strength and self-concept.[54] So both aerobic and non-aerobic exercise may be helpful in improving self-concept.

Mental Cognition and Reaction Time

Results from some studies have suggested that short-term memory and intellectual function may be improved during or shortly after an exercise session, but much more study is needed in this area.[39, 55, 56]

The theory is of course consistent with that of the Greeks, who walked while they discussed topics of importance and were believers in the ability of exercise to improve mental function.

Mechanisms: How Physical Activity Helps Psychological Health

So far we've seen that mounting evidence backs up the Greek ideal of a "strong mind in a strong body." Regular exercise such as walking, jogging, and swimming is associated with decreased anxiety and depression, improved self concept, and an improvement in mood, with an increase in vigor and a decrease in fatigue. (See Figure 13.7.)

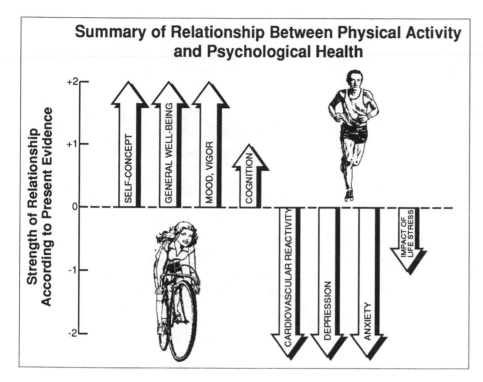

Figure 13.7 This figure summarizes the relationship between physical activity and psychological health using present evidence. The strength of the relationship is represented on the vertical axis, with "2" representing strong evidence in support and "1" representing preliminary supporting evidence, with more research needed to confirm the association.

The support for these assertions is growing fast. A state-of-the-art workshop dealing with exercise and mental health was sponsored by the National Institute of Mental Health during 1984.[34] A consensus statement was submitted, and included the following:

- Physical fitness is positively associated with mental health and well-being.
- Exercise is associated with the reduction of stress emotions such as state anxiety.
- Anxiety and depression are common symptoms of failure to cope with mental stress, and exercise has been associated with a decreased level of mild to moderate depression and anxiety.
- Long-term exercise is usually associated with reductions in traits such as neuroticism and anxiety.
- Appropriate exercise results in reductions in various stress indices such as neuromuscular tension, resting heart rate, and some stress hormones.
- Current clinical opinion holds that exercise has beneficial emotional effects across all ages and in both sexes.

Explaining how and why exercise improves psychological health is at this time still in the speculation stage. Some of the more tenable theories are discussed in this section.

Endogenous Opioids

The body has an amazing, recently discovered hormonal system of morphine-like chemicals called "endogenous opioids." These are of interest because their receptors are found in the hypothalamus and limbic systems of the brain, areas associated with emotion and behavior. Endogenous opioids like β-endorphin have been associated with decrease of pain, increase of memory, and regulation of appetite, sex, blood pressure, and ventilation.[34, 57-72]

During exercise, the pituitary increases its production of β-endorphin, causing its concentration to rise in the blood. Several laboratories, including our own here at Loma Linda University, have now measured this increase of β-endorphin with exercise.

As Figure 13.8 shows, β-endorphin is a late-rising hormone, rising sharply only during very intense exercise.[63-66] Most researchers have found that β-endorphin does not increase unless exercise intensity exceeds 80 to 90 percent $\dot{V}O_{2max}$.

In our research, the increase in β-endorphin did not differ significantly between athletes and nonathletes, peaked at about 3 to 3.5 times baseline levels, and fell to near baseline levels after 45 minutes of recovery from graded maximal treadmill exercise.

Although it is widely accepted by the exercising public that endorphins are responsible for exercise-

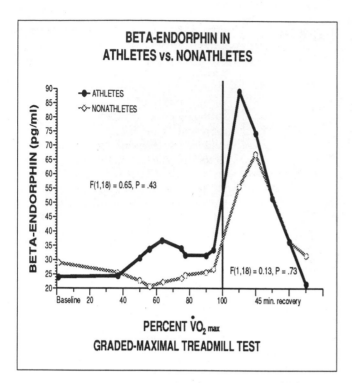

Figure 13.8 In this study, sedentary nonathletes and marathon athletes were exercised to exhaustion during a Balke treadmill, graded exercise test. The concentration of β-endorphin in the blood rose strongly during early recovery in response to near-maximal intensity exercise. *Source:* Nieman DC, Berk LS, Tan SA. Plasma β-endorphin During Graded Treadmill Exercise in Athletes and Non-Athletes. (Unpublished data.)

induced euphoria, compelling scientific evidence is largely absent.[67] Most researchers have found that despite significant decreases in tension during exercise, the increase in β-endorphin is unrelated to the improvement in the mood.[68–71]

Before any molecule from the blood can enter the brain cells, it must pass through what is called the blood-brain barrier, a highly selective barrier made up of special capillaries, connective tissue, and specialized brain cells called astrocytes. Most researchers have been unable to demonstrate that the endorphins secreted by the pituitary into the blood are able to gain entry into the brain. [62,60] (See Figure 13.9.) Unless they do, the decrease in pain, elevation in mood, and decrease in feelings of fatigue will not take place. In short, present research data do not support the belief that the elevation in mood and decrease in anxiety and depression that is associated with exercise is caused by exercise-related increases in blood concentrations of β-endorphin.

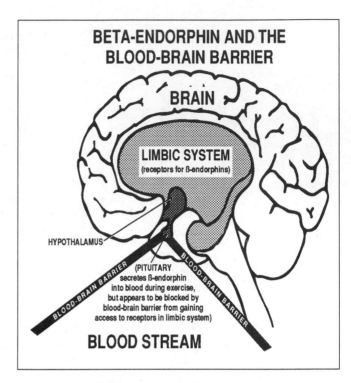

Figure 13.9 Although it is true that vigorous exercise increases the concentration of β-endorphin in the blood, this complex protein molecule is unable to cross the blood-brain barrier to gain access to the receptors located in the limbic system.

Alpha Brain Waves

Dr. James Wiese of Alberta Hospital and a research team at Arizona State University have both discovered that during exercise there is increased brain emission of alpha waves—brain waves associated with a relaxed, meditation-like state.[73, 74] These alpha waves appear approximately 20 minutes into a 30-minute jog, and are still measurable after the exercise is over. Researchers speculate that the increased alpha wave power could contribute to the psychological benefits of exercise, including reductions in anxiety and depression. Higher intensity exercise has been associated with higher alpha brain activity.[75] More research is needed.

Brain Neurotransmitters

Exercise may also enhance neurotransmitter activity in the brain. Although much more study is needed, it has been speculated that exercise may alter levels of norepinephrine, dopamine, and serotonin in the brain, decreasing depression.[76] There is evidence that neurotransmitters such as norepinephrine (NE) and serotonin

(5-HT) are involved in depression and schizophrenia.[34] Stress-induced depression is associated with a drop in NE in the brain stem of laboratory animals. Disturbance of NE or 5-HT takes place with human depression. Preliminary research shows that exercise training increases brain NE and 5-HT levels in rats. Thus, theoretically, the reduced depression observed with moderately depressed people following regular exercise may be due to increased levels of brain NE or 5-HT.[67]

Other Theories

Other researchers suggest that exercise decreases muscle electrical tension.[39] Some advance the idea that exercise increases oxygen transport to the brain. During exercise, deep body temperature is increased, and this increase is proportional to the intensity and duration of exercise. This temperature elevation has been found to decrease muscle tension, and may influence the release, synthesis, or uptake of certain brain neurotransmitters, inducing a slow wave sleep response.[67]

The possibility exists, of course, that psychological effects often attributed to exercise are actually caused by factors present with but separate from exercise.[67] An example would be the distraction hypothesis—based on the observation that resting quietly in an area free of distractions is associated with significant reductions in state anxiety and blood pressure. However, as discussed earlier in this chapter, aerobic exercise leads to reductions in blood pressure and anxiety that persist longer after exercise than they do following quiet rest.[51]

Whatever the real reasons for the positive impact of exercise on the brain—increase in β-endorphin, increase in brain alpha power, or enhanced brain neurotransmission—the evidence is very compelling, and more research is certainly warranted.

Precautions: Running Addiction, Mood Disturbance, and Sleep Disruption

Dr. Morgan from the Univeristy of Wisconsin has described individuals with "running addiction."[34,44] They are "addicted" to exercise, and have such a commitment that obligations to work, family, and interpersonal relationships, and ability to utilize medical advice suffer. Such people are also compulsive, use running for an escape, are overcompetitive, live in a state of chronic fatigue, are self-centered, and are preoccupied with

fitness, diet, and body image. Certainly this is taking exercise too far, negating any psychological benefit that more moderate exercise may bring.

Dr. Morgan has also reported that mood disturbance can increase when training loads are increased too greatly.[77] When swimmers increased their daily training distance from 4,000 to 9,000 meters per day during a 10-day period, there were significant increases in muscle soreness, depression, anger, fatigue, and overall mood disturbance, along with a decrease in general sense of well-being. Intense physical exercise such as a competitive marathon (26.2 miles) has been shown to disrupt both rapid eye movement (REM) sleep and total sleep time.[78]

Practical Implications

Although we are not sure why, the research presented in this chapter has shown that the same amount of exercise that helps the heart also helps the brain. The American College of Sports Medicine has established that three to five, 15-30 minute aerobic exercise sessions per week of moderate intensity, activities like jogging, swimming, bicycling, or brisk walking, are necessary to fully develop the heart-lung-blood vessel system. Most of the studies quoted in this article used these same exercise criteria, and thus showed that as the heart is strengthened, so is the brain.

We now can have confidence that in exercise we have a strong weapon to help counter the never-ending onslaught of stress, anxiety, and depression associated with our modern era. Exercise does help, acting as a buffer, decreasing the strain of stressful events. Exercise can help to fortify the brain, alleviating anxiety and depression while elevating mood.

Preliminary research is also indicating that the brain may function better cognitively during exercise. Though we need more research to evaluate the effect of regular exercise on overall mental function, there is evidence that it does more than just make people feel better. What this means for busy students and workers everywhere is that time spent in exercise may not be lost in terms of getting the job done. The half-hour exercise session may actually enhance mental functioning to the point of increasing overall time efficiency.

So the allocation of curricular time to physical education may not hamper academic achievement as some school boards have thought. And exercise breaks for normally sedentary office workers may actually enhance the productivity of a business. Research in the future should help to resolve some of these questions.

In essence, all of the evidence tends to support what we already strongly suspected and people like John and Donna at the beginning of the chapter have experienced. Exercise is good for both the body and the brain. Through regular, active use of the body, one can discover a greater sense of well-being, far greater vitality, and a calmer, more relaxed attitude toward daily pressures.

Sports Medicine Insight
Stress Management

Stress has been defined as any action or situation (stressor) that places special physical or psychological demands upon an individual; anything that unbalances one's equilibrium.[79, 80] Both good and bad stressors produce stress reactions in the body. A divorce is stressful—but so is getting married. Both upset an individual's equilibrium and require adjustment and adaptation.

Medical research on stress dates back to the 1920s, when Walter Cannon began experimenting with the physiological effect of stress on cats and dogs. Studying the animals' reactions to danger, the Harvard physiologist noted a regular and common pattern, now known as the fight-or-flight response.

Later, in the 1940s and 50s, Hans Selye, an endocrinologist at Montreal's Institute of Experimental Medicine and Surgery, extended Cannon's work and laid the foundation for much of today's work on stress. Experimenting with rats, he used various stressors, and found a regular pattern of responses, described by Selye as the General Adaptation Syndrome (alarm, resistance, exhaustion). Later researchers have focused on the effect of stressors on health and the complicated sequence of biochemical events that are put in motion by the perceived stressor and that lead to the stress response.[79]

The stressor itself does not create the response—it is the individual's reaction to the stressor. Therefore, individuals will have varying responses to the same stressor.

The body follows a typical physiological pattern (fight or flight response) when reacting to a stressor. The stress response appears to begin in the hypothalamus, which then affects the autonomic nervous system and the pituitary gland.

These two systems, acting in concert, alter the functioning of almost every part of the body. The muscles tense and tighten, the breathing becomes deeper and faster, the heart rate rises and blood vessels constrict (raising the blood pressure), the stomach and intestines temporarily halt digestion, perspiration increases, the secretion of saliva and mucus decreases, the sense organs sharpen perception, and the thyroid is stimulated. (See Figure 13.10.)

If the stressor is maintained for a prolonged period of time, Selye has shown that the body will go through what he has termed the "general adaptation syndrome."[81] After the alarm reaction (the fight or flight responses outlined above), there will be a stage in which resistance to stress rises and functions return to normal. Finally, there will be a stage of exhaustion in which the symptoms of the alarm reaction return. In animal experiments, the animals will die.

There can no longer be any doubt that a relationship exists between personality, stress, and disease. Numerous studies demonstrate the serious impact of stress on health and disease. Overall, it appears that chronic exposure to emotional stimuli leads to biochemical changes in the body, which may eventually predispose a person to illness and disease.

Stress may suppress the immune system, reducing resistance to viral or bacterial infections. For example, male college students who responded to a mental contest with extreme increases in heart rate and diastolic blood pressure were significantly more likely to have frequent minor illnesses than those responding with moderate or low increases. Marital discord has been associated with decreased immune function.[6, 7] High psychological and physiological stress responses before surgery have been associated with poorer outcomes and a depressed immune system.[82]

Clearly, it can be important to strengthen a patient's coping mechanism, potentially to alleviate illness and even to prevent death.

There are three basic strategies for managing stress:

1. **Environmental Engineering:** Manage stressors by controlling your pace of life and major life changes. Seek the social support of others. Don't crowd too much into the schedule. Adapt your environment (living arrangements, workload, transportation schedule, leisure plans, etc.) to your psychological makeup. Control your circumstances—don't let them control you.

2. **Mind Engineering:** Realize that when confronted by a stressor, your mind can choose your reaction. In other words, humans are largely responsible for creating their own emotional reactions and distress—and these can be controlled. So when an event takes place (e.g., a flat tire on your way to work), you can choose how you will react—you can let the stress response take over, with all of its health

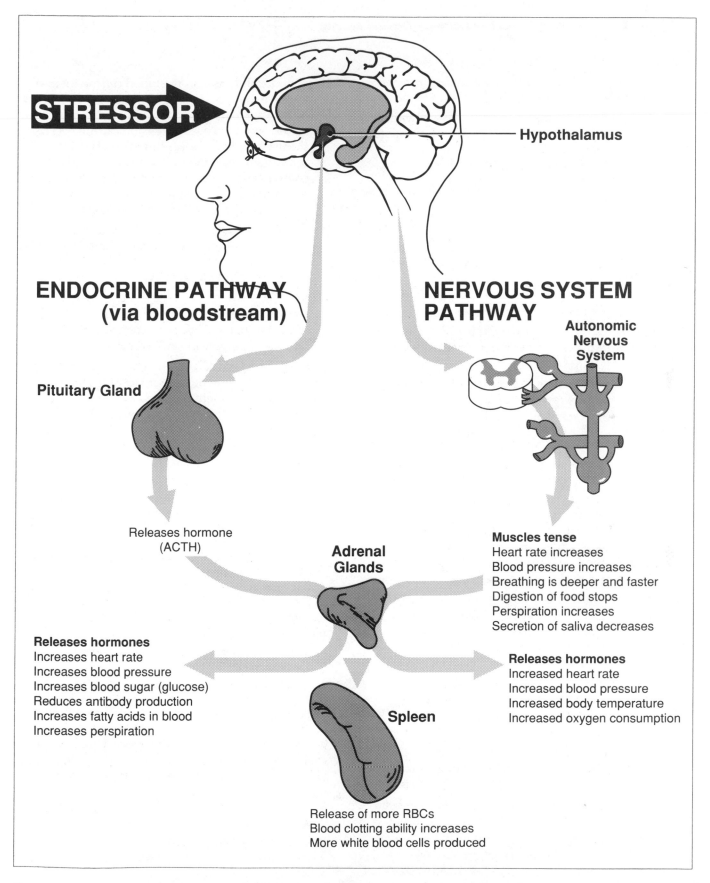

STRESSOR

Hypothalamus

ENDOCRINE PATHWAY
(via bloodstream)

NERVOUS SYSTEM
PATHWAY

Autonomic
Nervous
System

Pituitary Gland

Releases hormone
(ACTH)

Adrenal
Glands

Muscles tense
Heart rate increases
Blood pressure increases
Breathing is deeper and faster
Digestion of food stops
Perspiration increases
Secretion of saliva decreases

Releases hormones
Increases heart rate
Increases blood pressure
Increases blood sugar (glucose)
Reduces antibody production
Increases fatty acids in blood
Increases perspiration

Releases hormones
Increased heart rate
Increased blood pressure
Increased body temperature
Increased oxygen consumption

Spleen

Release of more RBCs
Blood clotting ability increases
More white blood cells produced

Figure 13.10 The stress response affects the entire body through both hormonal
and nerve pathways.

endangering effects, or you can choose a calmer, more reasoned, healthier reaction.

3. **Physical Engineering:** It is easier to deal with stress when your body is healthy from adequate exercise, sleep, food, fresh air and sunshine, water, and spiritual renewal. Take time to relax. It is a very important investment.

Summary

1. Nearly one out of five Americans is affected by one or more mental disorders, and one-half of U.S. adults experience at least a moderate amount of stress on a regular basis.

2. Many studies have shown that being chronically anxious, depressed, or emotionally distressed is associated with deterioration of health.

3. Studies of active people show them to have a better psychological profile than inactive people. However, a strong self-selection bias may be present when comparing active people with the general population. Controlled intervention studies are preferred when looking at the relationship between physical activity and psychological health.

4. A review of four national surveys has concluded that physical activity is positively associated with good mental health, defined as positive mood, general well-being, and relatively infrequent symptoms of anxiety and depression.

5. A considerable amount of research has indicated that less aerobically fit people show greater cardiovascular and subjective responses to psychological stressors than do those at high levels of aerobic fitness.

6. Stressful life events appear to cause fewer physical and psychological problems for physically active people than they do for inactive people.

7. Most studies support the proposition that depression, anxiety, and mood state in general are favorably affected by regular aerobic exercise.

8. Both aerobic and non-aerobic exercise have been shown to be helpful in improving self-concept.

9. Preliminary research suggests that short-term memory and intellectual function may be improved during or shortly after an exercise session. More research is needed to study the long-term effects.

10. β-endorphin rises in the blood during intense exercise, but not during low intensity exercise. Most researchers have found that despite significant decreases in tension during exercise, the increase in β-endorphin is unrelated to the improvement in mood. It appears that the complex β-endorphin protein molecule is unable to cross the blood-brain barrier to gain access to the receptors located in the limbic system.

11. During exercise, there is an increase in brain emission of alpha waves, brain waves associated with a relaxed, meditation-like state. These could contribute to the psychological benefits of exercise.

12. Exercise may enhance neurotransmitter activity in the brain, increasing the concentrations of brain norepinephrine and serotonin.

13. In the Sports Medicine Insight, the principles of stress management were reviewed. Three basic stress management methods were reviewed— environmental, mental, and physical engineering.

References

1. Stephens T. Physical Activity and Mental Health in the United States and Canada: Evidence from Four Population Surveys. Prev Med 17:35–47, 1988.

2. The Office of Disease Prevention and Health Promotion. U.S. Public Health Service. U.S. Department of Health and Human Services. Disease Prevention/ Health Promotion: The Facts. Palo Alto: Bull Publishing Company, 1988.

3. Regier DA, Boyd JH, Burke JD, et al. One-Month Prevalence of Mental Disorders in the United States. Arch Gen Psychiatry 45:977–986, 1988.

4. National Center for Health Statistics, C. A. Schoenborn. 1988. Health Promotion and Disease Prevention: United States, 1985. Vital and Health Statistics. Series 10, No. 163. DHHS Pub. No. (PHS) 88–1591. Public Health Service. Washington: U.S. Government Printing Office.

5. Girard DE. Psychosocial Events and Subsequent Illness—A Review. West J Med 142:358–363, 1985.

6. Kiecolt-Glaser JK, Fisher LD, Ogrocki P, et al. Marital Quality, Marital Disruption, and Immune Function. Psychosom Med 49:13, 1987.

7. Kiecolt-Glaser JK, Kennedy S, Malkoff S, et al. Marital Discord and Immunity in Males. Psychosom Med 50:213–229, 1988.

8. Venters M, Jacobs DR, Pirie P, et al. Marital Status and Cardiovascular Risk: The Minnesota Heart Survey and

the Minnesota Heart Health Program. Prev Med 15:591–605, 1986.

9. Kaplan GA, Salonen JT, Cohen RD, et al. Social Connections and Mortality From All Causes and From Cardiovascular Disease: Prospective Evidence From Eastern Finland. Am J Epidemiol 128:370–380, 1988.

10. Seeman TE, Kaplan GA, Knudsen L, et al. Social Network Ties and Mortality Among the Elderly in the Alameda County Study. Am J Epidemiol 126:714–723, 1987.

11. Kaprio J, Koskenvuo M, Rita H. Mortality After Bereavement: A Propsective Study of 95,647 Widowed Persons. Am J Public Health 77:283–287, 1987.

12. Ruberman W. Psychosocial Influences On Mortality After Myocardial Infarction. N Engl J Med 311:552–559, 1984.

13. Vaillant GE. Natural History of Male Psychologic Health. N Engl J Med 301:1249–1254, 1979.

14. Ragland DR, Brand RJ. Type A Behavior and Mortality From Coronary Heart Disease. N Engl J Med 318:65–69, 1988.

15. Kasl SV. Stress and Health. Annu Rev Public Health 5:319–341, 1984.

16. Dimsdale JE. A Perspective on Type A Behavior and Coronary Heart Disease. N Engl J Med 318:110–112, 1988.

17. Nunes EV, Frank KA, Kornfeld DS. Psychologic Treatment for the Type A Behavior Pattern and for Coronary Heart Disease: A Meta-Analysis of the Literature. Psychosom Med 48:159, 1987.

18. Siegel JM. Type A Behavior: Epidemiologic Foundations and Public Health Implications. Annu Rev Public Health 5:343–367, 1984.

19. Weidner G, Sexton G, McLellarn R, et al. The Role of Type A Behavior and Hostility in an Elevation of Plasma Lipids in Adult Women and Men. Psychosom Med 49:136, 1987.

20. Appels A, Mulder P, van 'T Hof M, et al. A Prospective Study of the Jenkins Activity Survey as a Risk Indicator for Coronary Heart Disease in the Netherlands. J Chron Dis 40:959–965, 1987.

21. Hecker MH, Chesney MA, Black GW, Frautschi N. Coronary–Prone Behaviors in the Western Collaborative Group Study. Psychosom Med 50:153–164, 1988.

22. Williams RB, Barefoot JC, Haney TL, et al. Type A Behavior and Angiographically Documented Coronary Atherosclerosis in a Sample of 2,289 Patients. Psychosom Med 50:139–152, 1988.

23. Stephens T. Secular Trends in Adult Physical Activity: Exercise Boom or Bust? Res Quart Exerc Sport 58:94–105, 1987.

24. Nieman DC, Johansen LM, Lee JW, Arabatzis K. Infectious Episodes in Runners Before and After the Los Angeles Marathon. J Sports Med (in press).

25. Hughes JR. Psychological Effects of Habitual Aerobic Exercise: A Critical Review. Prev Med 13:66–78, 1984.

26. Ross CE, Hayes D. Exercise and Psychologic Well–Being in the Community. Am J Epidemiol 127:762–771, 1988.

27. Holmes DS, McGilley BM. Influence of a Brief Aerobic Training Program on Heart Rate and Subjective Response to a Psychologic Stressor. Psychosom Med 49:366–374, 1987.

28. Crews DJ, Landers DM. A Meta-Analytic Review of Aerobic Fitness and Reactivity to Psychosocial Stressors. Med Sci Sports Exerc 19:S114–S120, 1987.

29. Sinyor D, Seraganian P. Aerobic Fitness Level and Reactivity to Psychosocial Stress: Physiological, Biochemical, and Subjective Measures. Psychosom Med 45:205–216, 1983.

30. Siconolfi SF. Exercise Training Attenuated the Blood Pressure Response to Mental Stress. Med Sci Sports Exerc 17:281, 1985.

31. Howard JH, Cunningham DA, Rechnitzer PA. Physical Activity As A Moderator of Life Events and Somatic Complaints: A Longitudinal Study. Can J Appl Sports Sci 9:194–200, 1984.

32. Roth DL, Holmes DS. Influence of Physical Fitness In Determining the Impact of Stressful Life Events on Physical and Psychologic Health. Psychosom Med 47:164–173, 1985.

33. Roth DL, Holmes DS. Influence of Aerobic Exercise Training and Relaxation Training on Physical and Psychologic Health Following Stressful Life Events. Psychosom Med 49:355–365, 1987.

34. Morgan WP. Affective Beneficence of Vigorous Physical Activity. Med Sci Sports Exerc 17:94–100, 1985.

35. Chen MK. The Epidemiology of Self-Perceived Fatigue Among Adults. Prev Med 15:74–81, 1986.

36. Eide R. The Relationship Between Body Image, Self-Image and Physical Activity. Scand J Soc Med, Suppl 29:109–112, 1982.

37. Eide R. The Effect of Physical Activity On Emotional Reactions, Stress Reactions and Related Physiological Reactions. Scand J Soc Med [Suppl].29:103–107, 1982.

38. Fasting K. Leisure Time, Physical Activity and Some Indices of Mental Health. Scand J Soc Med [Suppl] 29:113–119, 1982.

39. Folkins CH, Sime WE. Physical Fitness Training and Mental Health. Amer Psychol 36:373–389, 1981.

40. Lichtman S, Poser EG. The Effects of Exercise On Mood and Cognitive Functioning. J Psychosom Res 27:43–52, 1983.

41. Lobstein DD, Mosbacher BJ, Ismail AH. Depression As A Powerful Discriminator Between Physically Active and Sedentary Middle-Aged Men. J Psychosom Res 27:60–76, 1983.

42. Mellion MB. Exercise Therapy for Anxiety and Depression. Postgrad Med 77:59–66, 91–96, 1985.

43. Porter K. Psychological Characteristics of the Average Female Runner. Physician Sportsmed 13:171–175, 1985.

44. Taylor CB, Sallis JF, Needle R. The Relation of Physical Activity and Exercise to Mental Health. Public Health Rep 100:195–202, 1985.

45. Blumenthal JA, Williams RS, Needels TL, Wallace AG. Psychological Changes Accompany Aerobic Exercise in Healthy Middle-Aged Adults. Psychosom Med 44:529–536, 1982.

46. Folkins CH. Effects of Physical Training on Mood. J Clin Psychol 32:385–388, 1976.

47. McGlynn GH. The Effect of Aerobic Conditioning and Induced Stress on State-Trait Anxiety, Blood Pressure, and Muscle Tension. J Sports Med Phys Fitness 23:341–351, 1983.

48. Berger BG, Owen DR. Mood Alteration With Swimming—Swimmers Really Do "Feel Better". Psychosom Med 45:425–433, 1983.

49. Goldwater BC, Collis ML. Psychologic Effects of Cardiovascular Conditioning: A Controlled Experiment. Psychosom Med 47:174–181, 1985.

50. Fasting K, Gronningsaeter H. Unemployment, Trait Anxiety, and Physical Exercise. Scand J Sports Sci 8:99–103, 1986.

51. Raglin JS, Morgan WP. Influence of Exercise and Quiet Rest on State Anxiety and Blood Pressure. Med Sci Sports Exerc 19:456–463, 1987.

52. Hilyer JC, Mitchell W. Effect of Systematic Physical Fitness Training Combined With Counseling on the Self-Concept of College Students. J Counsel Psychol 26:427–436, 1979.

53. Eickhoff J, Thorland W, Ansorge C. Selected Physiological and Psychological Effects of Aerobic Dancing Among Young Adult Women. J Sports Med Phys Fitness 23:278, 1983.

54. Brown RD, Harrison JM. The Effects of a Strength Training Program on the Strength and Self-Concept of Two Female Age-Groups. Res Quart Exerc Sport 57:315–329, 1986.

55. Tomporowski PD, Eillis NR. Effects of Exercise on Cognitive Processes: A Review. Psychol Bul 99:338–346, 1986.

56. Hilmer W, Lehri S, Mohr W, Dorner H. Influence on Short-Term Memory by Standardized Ergometric Stress. Int J Sports Med 8:120, 1987 (abstract).

57. Appenzeller O. Opioids and Endurance Training; Longitudinal Study. Ann Sports Med 2:22–25, 1984.

58. De Meirleir K. Effects of Opiate Antagonism On Physiological and Hormonal Responses to Acute Dynamic Exercise. Med Sci Sports Exerc 17:235, 1985.

59. Grossman A, Bouloux P. The Role of Opioid Peptides in the Hormonal Responses to Acute Exercise in Man. Clin Sci 67:P483–491, 1984.

60. Grossman A. Endorphins: "Opiates for the Masses." Med Sci Sports Exerc 17:101–104, 1985.

61. Harber VJ, Sutton JR. Endorphins and Exercise. Sports Med 1:154–171, 1984.

62. Sutton JR. Endorphins in Exercise (Symposium). Med Sci Sports Exerc 17:73–92, 1985.

63. Langenfeld ME, Hart LS, Kao PC. Plasma ß-endorphin Responses to One-Hour Bicycling and Running At 60% VO2 max. Med Sci Sports Exerc 19:83–86, 1987.

64. Donevan RH, Andrew GM. Plasma ß–endorphin Immunoreactivity During Graded Cycle Ergometry. Med Sci Sports Exerc 19:229–233, 1987.

65. McMurray RG, Forsythe WA, Mar MH, Hardy CJ. Exercise Intensity-Related Responses of Beta-Endorphin and Catecholamines. Med Sci Sports Exerc 19:570–574, 1987.

66. Rahkila P, Hakala E, Salminen K, Laatikainen T. Response of Plasma Endorphins to Running Exercises in Male and Female Endurance Athletes. Med Sci Sports Exerc 19:451–455, 1987.

67. Morgan WP, O'Connor PJ. Exercise and Mental Health. In: Dishman RK (ed). Exercise Adherence. Champaign, Illinois: Human Kinetics Books, 1988.

68. Farrell PA, Gustafson AB, Garthwaite TL, et al. Influence of Endogenous Opioids on the Response of Selected Hormones to Exercise in Humans. J Appl Physiol 61:1051–1057, 1986.

69. Sforzo GA, Seeger TF, Pert CB, Pert A, Dotson CO. In Vivo Opioid Receptor Occupation in the Rat Brain Following Exercise. Med Sci Sports Exerc 18:380–384, 1986.

70. Goldfarb AH, Hatfield BD, Sforzo GA, et al. Serum ß-endorphin Levels During A Graded Exercise Test to Exhaustion. Med Sci Sports Exerc 19:78–82, 1987.

71. Farrell PA, Gustafson AB, Morgan WP, et al. Enkephalins, Catecholamines, and Psychological Mood Alterations: Effects of Prolonged Exercise. Med Sci Sports Exerc 19:347–353, 1987.

72. Allen ME, Coen D. Naloxone Blocking of Running-Induced Mood Changes. Ann Sports Med 3:190–195, 1987.

73. Fernhall B, Daniels FS. Electroencephalographic Changes After a Prolonged Running Period: Evidence for a Relaxation Response. Med Sci Sports Exerc 16:181, 1984.

74. Wiese J, Singh M, Yeudall L. Occipital and Parietal Alpha Power Before, During and After Exercise. Med Sci Sports Exerc 14:117, 1982.

75. Daugherty PL, Fernhall B, McCanne TR. The Effects of Three Exercise Intensities on the Alpha Brain Wave Activity of Adult Males. Med Sci Sports Exerc 19:S23, 1987.

76. Ransford CP. A Role for Amines in the Antidepressant Effect of Exercise: A Review. Med Sci Sports Exerc 14:1–10, 1982.

77. Morgan WP, Costill DL, Flynn MG, Raglin JS, O'Connor PJ. Mood Disturbance Following Increased Training in Swimmers. Med Sci Sports Exerc 20:408–414, 1988.

78. Montgomery I, Trinder J, Paxton S, Fraser G. Sleep Disruption Following a Marathon. J Sports Med 25:69–74, 1985.

79. McNeil C. Focus: The Dimensions of Stress. Perspect Prevent 2(2):6–8, 1988.

80. Kasl SV. Stress and Health. Annu Rev Public Health 5:319–341, 1984.

81. Selye H. Stress Without Distress. The New American Library Inc., 1974.

82. Linn BS, Linn MW, Klimas NG. Effects of Psychological Stress on Surgical Outcome. Psychosom Med 50:230–244, 1988.

Physical Fitness Activity 13.1— The General Well-Being Scale

As described earlier in this chapter, one measure of psychological status that has been used with good success in national surveys is the General Well-Being scale (GWB). The GWB was designed by the National Center for Health Statistics and consists of 18 items in six subscales covering such constructs as energy level, satisfaction, freedom from worry, and self-control. A high score on the GWB represents an absence of bad feelings and an expression of positive feelings. Results from national surveys have shown that higher scores for the GWB are significantly associated with increased amounts of physical activity for all age groups and for both men and women. (See: Stephens T. Physical Activity and Mental Health in the United States and Canada: Evidence from Four Population Surveys. Prev Med 17:35–47, 1988.)

In this physical fitness activity, the 18 questions of the GWB are listed, with an interpretation of results.

The General Well-Being Scale

Instructions:

The following questions ask how you feel and how things have been going for you *during the past month*. For each question, mark an "x" for the answer that most nearly applies to you. Since there are no right or wrong answers, it's best to answer each question quickly without pausing too long on any one of them.

1. How have you been feeling in general?
    - 5[ ] In excellent spirits
    - 4[ ] In very good spirits
    - 3[ ] In good spirits mostly
    - 2[ ] I've been up and down in spirits a lot
    - 1[ ] In low spirits mostly
    - 0[ ] In very low spirits

2. Have you been bothered by nervousness or your "nerves"?
    - 0[ ] Extremely so—to the point where I could not work or take care of things
    - 1[ ] Very much so
    - 2[ ] Quite a bit
    - 3[ ] Some-enough to bother me
    - 4[ ] A little
    - 5[ ] Not at all

3. Have you been in firm control of your behavior, thoughts, emotions or feelings?
    - 5[ ] Yes, definitely so
    - 4[ ] Yes, for the most part
    - 3[ ] Generally so
    - 2[ ] Not too well
    - 1[ ] No, and I am somewhat disturbed
    - 0[ ] No, and I am very disturbed

4. Have you felt so sad, discouraged, hopeless, or had so many problems that you wondered if anything was worthwhile?

    0[ ] Extremely so—to the point I have just about given up

    1[ ] Very much so

    2[ ] Quite a bit

    3[ ] Some—enough to bother me

    4[ ] A little bit

    5[ ] Not at all

5. Have you been under or felt you were under any strain, stress, or pressure?

    0[ ] Yes—almost more than I could bear

    1[ ] Yes—quite a bit of pressure

    2[ ] Yes—some, more than usual

    3[ ] Yes—some, but about usual

    4[ ] Yes—a little

    5[ ] Not at all

6. How happy, satisfied, or pleased have you been with your personal life?

    5[ ] Extremely happy—couldn't have been more satisfied or pleased

    4[ ] Very happy

    3[ ] Fairly happy

    2[ ] Satisfied—pleased

    1[ ] Somewhat dissatisfied

    0[ ] Very dissatisfied

7. Have you had reason to wonder if you were losing your mind, or losing control over the way you act, talk, think, feel, or of your memory?

    5[ ] Not at all

    4[ ] Only a little

    3[ ] Some, but not enough to be concerned

    2[ ] Some, and I've been a little concerned

    1[ ] Some, and I am quite concerned

    0[ ] Much, and I'm very concerned

8. Have you been anxious, worried, or upset?

    0[ ] Extremely so—to the point of being sick, or almost sick

    1[ ] Very much so

    2[ ] Quite a bit

    3[ ] Some—enough to bother me

    4[ ] A little bit

    5[ ] Not at all

9. Have you been waking up fresh and rested?

    5[ ] Every day

    4[ ] Most every day

    3[ ] Fairly often

    2[ ] Less than half the time

    1[ ] Rarely

    0[ ] None of the time

10. Have you been bothered by any illness, bodily disorder, pain, or fears about your health?

    0[ ] All the time

    1[ ] Most of the time

    2[ ] A good bit of the time

    3[ ] Some of the time

    4[ ] A little of the time

    5[ ] None of the time

11. Has your daily life been full of things that are interesting to you?

    5[ ] All the time

    4[ ] Most of the time

    3[ ] A good bit of the time

    2[ ] Some of the time

    1[ ] A little of the time

    0[ ] None of the time

12. Have you felt downhearted and blue?

    0[ ] All of the time

    1[ ] Most of the time

    2[ ] A good bit of the time

    3[ ] Some of the time

    4[ ] A little of the time

    5[ ] None of the time

13. Have you been feeling emotionally stable and sure of yourself?

    5[ ] All of the time

    4[ ] Most of the time

    3[ ] A good bit of the time

    2[ ] Some of the time

    1[ ] A little of the time

    0[ ] None of the time

14. Have you felt tired, worn out, used-up, or exhausted?

    0[ ] All of the time

    1[ ] Most of the time

    2[ ] A good bit of the time

    3[ ] Some of the time

    4[ ] A little of the time

    5[ ] None of the time

Note: For each of the four scales below, the words at each end describe opposite feelings. Circle any number along the bar that seems closest to how you have felt generally *during the past month.*

15. How concerned or worried about your health have you been?

Not						Very
concerned						concerned
at all						
	10	8	6	4	2	0

16. How relaxed or tense have you been?

Very						Very tense
relaxed						
	10	8	6	4	2	0

17. How much energy, pep, and vitality have you felt?

No energy						Very
at all,						energetic,
listless						dynamic
	0	2	4	6	8	10

18. How depressed or cheerful have you been?

Very						Very
depressed						cheerful
	0	2	4	6	8	10

Directions: Add up all the points from the boxes you have checked for each question. Compare your total score with the norms listed below.

National Norms for the General Well-Being Scale

Stress State	Total Stress Score	% Distribution U.S. Population
Positive well-being	81–110	55%
Low positive	76–80	10%
Marginal	71–75	9%
Indicates stress problem	56–70	16%
Indicates distress	41–55	7%
Serious	26–40	2%
Severe	0–25	<1%

Note: Figure 13.5 gives the scores for the U.S. population by age, gender, and amount of exercise. Notice that all subgroups reporting "much exercise" fell within the "positive well-being" range of 81–110.

Note: Software for analyzing the General Well-Being Scale is available from: Wellsource, 15431 S.E. 82nd Dr., Suite F, Clackamas, OR 97015.

Chapter 14

Additional Benefits of Physical Activity

"Diabetes is a major excuse to run. In that sense, diabetes supports my lifestyle, rather than vice versa."—Tom McManus, Jr., marathon runner[1]

Introduction

Many of the important benefits of regular physical activity have already been reviewed in Chapters 10 through 13. We've discussed the important relationships between physical activity and heart disease, obesity, aging, and psychological health. In Chapter 15, the risks of exercise will be reviewed, and then balanced with all of the benefits described in this book. Several special topics will also be addressed in Chapter 15, including the relationship between physical activity and the health of the immune system, asthma, and pregnancy, as well as other topics.

Recently, evidence has been reported by a growing number of researchers that physical activity may be meaningful to two other areas of common concern for Americans—diabetes mellitus and cancer. The relationship between physical activity and these two diseases will be discussed in this chapter.

Diabetes Mellitus

The concept that physical activity is beneficial for the diabetic is not new. It was promoted as a valuable adjunct to diabetic control in 600 A.D. by Chao Yuan-Fang, a prominent Chinese physician of the Sui Dynasty.[1] Researchers in this century have shown repeatedly that physical exercise can improve both the health and disease status of diabetics.

The Magnitude of Diabetes

Since 1932, diabetes has ranked among the 10 leading causes of death in the United States.[2] It is cause of about 36,000 deaths annually, and a contributing cause in an additional 95,000 deaths. It is the principal or secondary diagnosis in about 2.8 million hospitalizations each year, and is a major cause of blindness, renal failure, lower extremity amputations, and congenital malformations. The risk of dying from cardiovascular disease is two to three times greater among diabetics than among nondiabetics.[3]

Self-reported diabetes has increased from 0.9 percent in 1958 to 2.6 percent in 1985.[2] Only about half of diabetics, however, know that they are diabetic. Eleven percent of the U.S. population ages 20–74 (17 million) exhibit some degree of glucose intolerance (See Figure 14.1.)

Prevalence rises with age, and is higher among blacks than among whites. Gender differences are smaller. People who are 50 percent over desirable weight are five times as likely to be diabetic than those of

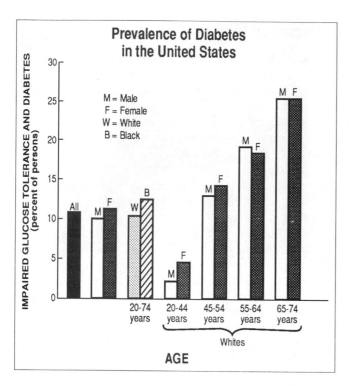

Figure 14.1 More than 11 percent of the U.S. population ages 20–74 are either diabetic or have impaired glucose tolerance. Prevalence rises with age, and is higher among blacks and females than whites and males. It afflicts more than 25 percent of the 65–74 age group. *Source:* see reference 2.

normal weight. The cost to society is $18 billion per year.[4]

Definitions and Classifications

Diabetes mellitus (commonly called diabetes) is the name given to a group of disorders characterized by metabolic abnormalities, of which the most evident is an elevated concentration of glucose in the blood.[5] Long-term complications involving the eyes, kidneys, nerves, and blood vessels result from a deficiency in the amount or effectiveness of the hormone insulin.[6] There are two major forms of diabetes mellitus: Type I, or *insulin-dependent* (IDDM), and Type II, or *noninsulin-dependent* (NIDDM).

IDDM can occur at any age, but especially in the young.[5-7] IDDM develops in 7 to 27 persons per 100,000 per year, depending on age. IDDM develops more frequently during puberty and after age 40. The risk of it is lowest in France and highest in Finland (the United States is third after Sweden). During the first 30 years of this century, the incidence of IDDM was fairly constant,

but the rate has nearly tripled during the past three decades, a trend seen in many other countries.[8]

IDDM is characterized by the abrupt onset of symptoms, resulting from a deficiency of insulin production by the pancreas, and dependence on injected insulin to sustain life.[5-7] (The beta-cells of the pancreas of IDDM patients, which normally produce and secrete insulin, are destroyed by the immune system.[8])

Only about 10 percent of all diabetics have IDDM. Classical first-appearance symptoms include excessive urination (*polyuria*), excessive thirst (*polydipsia*), unsatisfied hunger (*polyphagia*), weight loss, cessation of growth among the young, irritability, and drowsiness or coma. Glucose in the urine (*glycosuria*), excessive levels of glucose in the blood (*hyperglycemia*), and high levels of ketone bodies in the blood (*ketosis*) are associated with uncontrolled IDDM.

NIDDM accounts for approximately 90 percent of all cases, and affects at least 10 million Americans,[6] NIDDM usually occurs in people over age 40, and most frequently in the 55 and over group. Approximately 85 percent of patients with NIDDM are obese at the time of diagnosis.

The onset of the disease is gradual, and many patients have a long history of mild symptoms or display no symptoms at all. Often, the condition is first diagnosed without prior symptoms on the basis of elevated fasting blood glucose levels discovered during a routine physical examination. Symptoms may include fatigue, urination at night, constant thirst, and weight loss just before diagnosis. Genetic predisposition appears to play an important role in Type II as well as in Type I diabetes.

NIDDM patients may have normal pancreatic beta cells, and secrete insulin normally in response to carbohydrate ingestion. However, because the body cells are less able to use the insulin (insulin insensitivity), blood glucose levels are high. Patients with NIDDM are not dependent on insulin, and are not prone to ketosis. However, they may require insulin for correction of high blood glucose levels if dietary intervention and exercise, or oral agents (*sulfonylureas* or oral hypoglycemia agents) are not effective.

Recommended Procedures for the Diagnosis of Diabetes

Any one of the following are considered diagnostic of diabetes:[5]

- Presence of the classic symptoms of diabetes, such as polyuria, polydipsia, ketones in the urine, and rapid weight loss, together with elevation of plasma glucose.

- Elevated fasting glucose concentration on more than one occasion. Elevated serum glucose levels are defined as being greater than or equal to 140 mg/dl (7.8 mmol/L). Normal serum glucose levels are less than 115 mg/dl (6.4 mmol/L). Borderline or *impaired glucose tolerance* is between 115 and 140 mg/dl).

The oral glucose tolerance test (OGTT) is a 75-gram glucose solution given after an overnight fast of 10–16 hours. This test is usually given for people with borderline fasting serum glucose levels (115–140 mg/dl). (See Figure 14.2.) If the fasting glucose concentration is greater than 140 mg/dl, the OGTT is not needed.

Treatment of Diabetes

Treatment of diabetes centers around control of blood glucose levels, keeping them within the narrow limits maintained (by the pancreas) by healthy people. The three principal approaches to diabetes management are

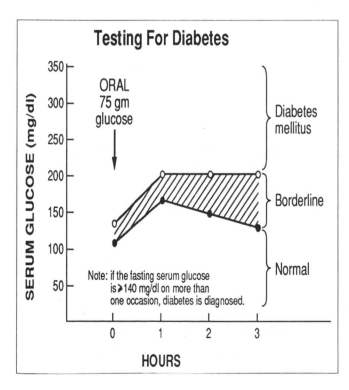

Figure 14.2 The oral glucose tolerance test is often given if the fasting glucose level is borderline (115–140 mg/dl). Diabetes is diagnosed if the serum glucose levels are 200 mg/dl or higher during and after 2 hours of follow-up after a 75-gram glucose meal. *Source:* see reference 5.

diet, exercise, and treatment with oral antidiabetic agents or insulin.[6]

Effective treatment of IDDM became possible when Banting and Best isolated and purified insulin in 1921. Commercial extraction and purification followed, leading quickly to widespread clinical use.

At first it was hoped that insulin would "cure" diabetes. Unfortunately, as patients began to survive for years, a host of disabling or lethal vascular, renal, ocular, and neurologic problems developed. It was natural to assume that these complications were caused by prolonged high serum glucose levels, and a belief arose that normalization of blood glucose concentrations would prevent or delay their occurrence. This assumption has been difficult to prove.[7]

About one-fourth of known diabetics in the United States are being treated with insulin, about half are receiving oral agents, and about one-fourth are not receiving any antidiabetic medication. Yet it is estimated that with optimum long-term diet and exercise therapy only about 25 percent would require any kind of medication.[8] Ninety percent of NIDDM is preventable with proper diet-exercise regimens.[1, 9]

There are several problems associated with insulin and oral agent treatment. Intensive conventional therapy with insulin requires that the patient measure his blood glucose level several times daily. The patient must be willing to take multiple injections every day. Insulin pump therapy is costly ($5 per day for supplies alone), and 10 percent of users become inflamed and infected where the needle is inserted.[7] Patients on insulin must keep meticulous records and be very regular and consistent about lifestyle habits such as eating times, amounts and types of foods, and activity.[9] For IDDMs, however, insulin injection is essential.

Oral hypoglycemic agents such as sulfonylureas (tolbutamide, tolazamide, acetohexamide, and chlorpropamide) can enhance the glucose utilization of NIDDM (but not of IDDM) patients who secrete reasonable amounts of insulin. The sulfonylureas stimulate the release of insulin from the beta cells of the pancreas.

Unfortunately, a long-term study by the University Group Diabetes Program in 12 university medical centers discovered that administration of oral hypoglycemic drugs is associated with increased cardiovascular mortality, compared treatment with diet alone or diet plus insulin. A new warning label that taking oral hypoglycemic drugs to treat NIDDM can increase the risk of death from cardiovascular disease will soon be required on these drugs.[10]

For these reasons and others, many researchers have been looking into the potential benefits of diet, exercise, and weight reduction in treating diabetes, especially for obese NIDDM patients.

Various researchers are beginning to suggest that a diet high in complex carbohydrates and fiber may actually be the safest, most effective, and least expensive treatment option for close to 90 percent of diabetics not totally dependent on insulin. Moreover, this diet may lessen the risk of long-term complications of diabetes (especially heart disease, the major cause of death for American diabetics).[11-16] (See the Sports Medicine Insight at end of this chapter.)

The single most important objective for the obese NIDDM is to achieve and maintain a desirable body weight. It has long been known that weight reduction by the obese reduces serum glucose and lipid levels, and also elevated blood pressure, factors associated with an increased risk for heart disease. With weight loss and successful maintenance of that weight loss, glucose levels in many NIDDM patients return to normal, requiring no further treatment with insulin or oral hypoglycemic agents.[5, 8, 13-16]

The Importance of Exercise for Diabetics

Although the concept that physical activity is beneficial for patients with diabetes mellitus is centuries old, there is considerable controversy regarding its value.[17-48] The issue requires an understanding of the effects of exercise on blood glucose levels.

During prolonged exercise, serum glucose levels stay remarkably stable for hours, despite the large use of serum glucose by the working muscles.[17] As depicted in Figure 14.3, the pancreas secretes two hormones, *insulin* and *glucagon*, to help maintain blood glucose levels. During rest, when blood glucose levels rise after a meal, insulin is secreted to help move the glucose into the body cells for formation of glycogen. Receptors on the body cells require that insulin be present before glucose can enter. On the other hand, when blood glucose levels drop, glucagon is secreted to increase blood glucose levels by stimulating the breakdown of liver glycogen and production of glucose by the liver.[48]

During prolonged aerobic exercise, blood insulin concentrations drop, while blood glucagon concentrations increase. These changes take place to counterbalance the "insulin-like" effect of muscle contraction.[29] As the muscles contract during exercise, they do not need the same amounts of insulin they needed during rest to transport glucose into muscle cells. This is because the movement of the muscle cells during exercise makes their membranes more permeable to glucose.[29] In addition, the receptors become more "sensitive" to the lower amount of insulin present during exercise.

There are four reasons why regular physical activity is promoted for diabetics of both types:

Improved Diabetic Control

It has been known for nearly 50 years that regular aerobic exercise will reduce the insulin requirements of well-controlled IDDM patients by 30–50 percent and requirements of those obese NIDDM patients by up to 100 percent (when combined with weight reduction).

One of the most consistent findings by researchers has been that with as little as one to three weeks of regular physical activity (20–30 minute sessions, three to five days a week), *insulin sensitivity* improves 20–50 percent.[19, 23, 24, 30, 31, 35, 36, 38, 42-46] This results in an improvement in blood glucose levels and cardiorespiratory fitness, even when accompanied by reductions in insulin dose by IDDM or drug use by NIDDM patients.[24] The rate of glucose uptake by the body cells is increased as a result of the increase in insulin sensitivity, lowering blood glucose levels.

Although regular exercise leads to reduced insulin requirements, recent studies have failed to show that long-term metabolic control is improved.[48] Although each exercise session has an acute glucose-lowering effect, fasting glucose levels remain unchanged.[32] Thus for the IDDM patient, regular exercise is important more for the cardiorespiratory and psychological benefits than for diabetic control.

The major aim of therapy for NIDDM patients is to improve insulin sensitivity through appropriate use of diet, exercise, and weight reduction.[48] The evidence from research with IDDM that exercise training reduces resistance to insulin has generated interest in the possibility that exercise may be useful in the treatment of mild NIDDM.

Recent studies are in fact showing that in contrast to results with IDDM patients, regular exercise by NIDDM patients does lead to improved long-term diabetic control. In one study, training for just seven days at an intensity of 60–68 percent VO_{2max} for 50–60 min each session led to strong improvements in the glucose tolerance if ten men with mild NIDDM.[36] The improvement in glucose tolerance, however, appeared to be a consequence of the last bout of exercise rather than of long-term adaptations to training.

This interpretation is supported by other studies that show that the increased insulin action found in people who exercise regularly is lost within a few days

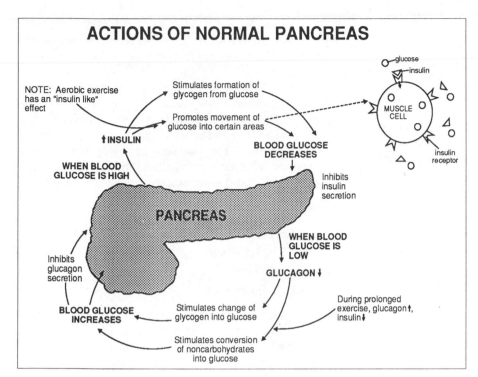

Figure 14.3 The pancreas secretes two hormones, insulin and glucagon, to control blood glucose levels. During exercise, glucagon rises while insulin falls to counterbalance the "insulin-like" effect of muscle contraction and the large glucose demands of the working muscle.

after exercise is stopped.[31] In a study in which those studied walked 20 to 40 minutes, blood glucose levels fell 6–16 mg/dl immediately after the bout.[37] They remained at the lower level during a 30-minute rest period, but returned to original levels when the next meal was consumed. It seems clear that NIDDM patients can improve diabetic control and insulin sensitivity only if they are regular in their exercise.

Several epidemiological research studies have found that the risk of developing diabetes is lower for active people.[20, 47] In one study, women who had been former college athletes had less than half the risk of nonathletic classmates of developing diabetes, despite similar family histories of diabetes.

For NIDDM patients, despite the important role of regular physical exercise in improving blood glucose levels, greater benefits can usually be achieved by weight loss.[13] Because many of the metabolic effects of exercise are short-lived, it is extremely important that NIDDM patients choose exercises that they are likely to continue over their lifetimes.

Correction or Prevention of Obesity

As stated previously, the vast majority of NIDDM diabetics are obese. In December of 1986, a Consensus Development Conference on Diet and Exercise in Non-Insulin-Dependent Diabetes Mellitus was sponsored by the National Institutes of Health. Important conclusions from this conference included the following:

- There is strong evidence that NIDDM is genetically determined, and that obesity and aging promote the development of the disease among those who are susceptible.

- Upper-body or android obesity appears to be more strongly associated with diabetes than lower-body or gynoid obesity.

- Obesity is characterized by insulin resistance, and when weight is lost the resistance is reduced. In addition, blood glucose levels usually return to normal with weight loss. Weight loss also improves hypertension and elevated blood lipids.

- For those with NIDDM, the primary dietary treatment is weight reduction through caloric restriction. Moderate caloric restriction 500 to 1,000 kcal below daily requirements may be optimal for producing gradual, sustained weight loss.

Thus weight reduction by obese NIDDM patients is of the utmost importance. (As reviewed in Chapter 11, the real power in weight loss is control of caloric intake, primarily dietary fat. Regular physical exercise is of secondary importance, but can help some people to cope better with their weight reduction diets.)

Reduced Risk of Coronary Heart Disease

Diabetics are at high risk for cardiovascular disease (CHD). Exercise, when combined with a high-carbohydrate, high-fiber reducing diet, leads to reduced blood pressure, total cholesterol, LDL-C, and triglycerides, and an increase in HDL-C. There is an inverse relationship between physical activity levels and incidence of coronary heart disease and associated mortality. (See Chapter 10.)

Psychosocial Benefits

As discussed in Chapter 13, regular physical activity results in a variety of psychological and social benefits that improve the quality of life. Improved feelings of well-being, health consciousness, self-confidence, self-control, self-esteem, and vigor are especially important for patients with a chronic disease like diabetes.[18]

Exercise Precautions and Guidelines for IDDM Patients

While non-diabetic people usually experience little change in blood glucose levels during exercise, IDDM patients may sustain either an increase or a decrease, depending on their initial serum glucose levels.[48]

IDDM patients who have blood glucose levels greater than 250 mg/dl with ketones in the urine or blood will experience a rapid rise in blood glucose levels upon starting exercise, and the development of ketosis.[48] When this happens, exercise should be postponed and supplemental insulin taken to reestablish proper blood glucose levels.

For the IDDM patient, the principal risk is insulin reaction or *hypoglycemia*.[17] If the blood glucose level of the IDDM sufferer is less than 100 mg/dl and insulin was injected within the past 60–90 minutes, carbohydrate should be consumed before and during exercise to avoid hypoglycemia.[21,48] In general, the diabetic should avoid strenuous exercise until reasonable diabetic control is established.

The phenomenon for IDDM patients of late-onset hypoglycemia after vigorous physical activity is not widely recognized among physicians.[25] In one study of 300 children and adolescents with IDDM, 16 percent experienced postexercise *late-onset (PEL) hypoglycemia*. Typically, PEL hypoglycemia happened during the night and occurred 6–15 hours after the completion of unusually strenuous exercise or play. In more than half the cases the hypoglycemia resulted in loss of conscious-

ness or seizures and necessitated treatment. Patients with tendencies toward PEL hypoglycemia should avoid exercise in the evening when hypoglycemia effects are most pronounced.[17]

Box 14.1 summarizes the important guidelines for IDDM patients to follow to avoid hypoglycemia during or after exercise.[17,48] A regular pattern of exercise and diet should be adopted to help monitor the effectiveness of the guidelines.[40] Exercise should be performed at the same convenient time every day at approximately the same intensity and duration. Morning appears to be

---

Box 14.1 Guidelines for IDDMs to Avoid Hyperglycemia or Hypoglycemia During and After Exercise

1. Consume carbohydrates (15-30 grams or 60-120 Calories for every 30 minutes of moderately intense exercise). A meal 1-3 hours before exercise is recommended.

2. Consume a snack of slowly absorbed carbohydrate (e.g., legumes, fructose, pasta, milk) following prolonged exercise sessions.

3. Reduce the insulin dose before exercise:

   a. Intermediate-acting insulin: reduce by 30-35 percent on the day of exercise.

   b. Intermediate- and short-acting insulin: omit dose of short-acting insulin that precedes exercise.

   c. Multiple doses of short-acting insulin: reduce the dose prior to exercise by 30-35 percent and supplement carbohydrates.

   d. Continuous subcutaneous infusion: eliminate mealtime bolus or increment that precedes or immediately follows exercise.

4. Avoid exercising the muscle area underlying injections of short-acting insulin for at least one hour.

5. Avoid late-evening exercise.

6. Monitor blood glucose before, during, and after exercise.

7. Learn individual glucose responses to different types of exercise.

Source: see reference 17, 48.

preferable to evening for most IDDM sufferers.[17] It is best that exercise not be performed at the time of peak insulin effect.

Because of the insulin-like effect of exercise, the IDDM patient initiating an exercise program will have to reduce insulin dosage or increase food intake. Insulin injections should not be at sites of the body that will be exercised (e.g., legs in running or cycling). During prolonged activities, a 15–30 gram carbohydrate snack is recommended for each 30 minutes of activity. Sugar cubes should be carried during exercise. Activities should be interrupted for a carbohydrate snack at initial warning symptoms of hypoglycemia. Adequate fluid replacement during and after exercise is important to avoid dehydration.

Diabetics should not exercise alone. Also, as with all at high-risk, it is good to have a careful medical examination before embarking on an exercise program. And gradual progression is advised.

Several of the long-term complications of diabetes may be worsened by exercise.[48] For example, because of the possible risks of retinal detachment and eye fluid hemorrhage, diabetic patients who have complications in their retinas should avoid exercise that requires straining and breath holding.[13] Because of the problems with peripheral blood circulation and nerve sensitivity, IDDM patients should be particularly careful to avoid cuts, blisters, and pounding exercises of the lower extremities. Good footware and careful foot hygiene is very important for IDDM patients. (As will be reviewed in Chapter 15, vigorous exercise may precipitate heart attack when there is underlying coronary artery disease.)

In general, with appropriate support and education, children, adolescents, and adults with IDDM can exercise and even perform athletically as well as their peers.[33,34] Much more care, precaution, and regularity is demanded, but the benefits appear to outweigh the potential risks.

A recently published retrospective study concluded that IDDM patients who had participated in team sports in high school or college were less likely than non-participants to have developed cardiovascular disease or diabetic complications, or to have died.[47] With proper instruction, careful monitoring, appropriate adjustments in insulin and food intake, and individual experience, many IDDM patients can learn to exercise safely, and many have achieved the status of world-class athletes.[48]

Box 14.2 summarizes the major benefits and potential risks of exercise for IDDM and NIDDM diabetics.[13, 21]

Box 14.2　Benefits and Risks Of Exercise for Individuals with Diabetes

Possible Benefits:

1. decreased blood glucose
2. increased insulin sensitivity
3. improved blood lipoprotein profile and lowered blood pressure
4. improved cardiorespiratory fitness
5. usefulness as adjunct to diet for weight reduction
6. increased sense of well-being and quality of life

Possible Risks:

1. hypoglycemia during or after exercise
2. increased blood glucose values among poorly-controlled patients
3. complications of atherosclerotic cardiovascular disease
4. degenerative joint disease
5. worsening of diabetic complications

Source: see references 13, 21.

Cancer

The Problem of Cancer in the United States

Cancer is a large group of diseases characterized by uncontrolled growth and spread of abnormal cells.[62, 63] About 75 million Americans now living (30 percent) will eventually have cancer. Of every 5 deaths in the United States, one is from cancer, making this disease the second leading cause of death. The number one cancer killer for men and women is lung cancer. The second leading cancer killer for men and third for women is colon cancer. The second leading cancer killer for women is breast cancer.

Relationship Between Cancer and Lifestyle

The National Cancer Institute (NCI) has set a goal of reducing the 1985 cancer mortality rate by 50 percent by the year 2000.[63] Research data support the estimate that lifestyle and environmental factors contribute to roughly 90 percent of cancer incidence.

There is a growing consensus among scientists that as much as 25 to 35 percent of cancer mortality is related to dietary factors.[63] A high intake of fat is associated with cancers of the breast, colon, rectum, uterus, prostate, and possibly several other sites.[62, 63] A high intake of dietary fiber, on the other hand, is associated with lower risk for colon and rectal cancers. These dietary relationships to cancer are reviewed in this chapter's Sports Medicine Insight.

Physical Activity and Cancer

Most of the studies examining the relationship between physical activity and cancer have concluded that there is a moderate protective effect, especially against colon and breast cancer.[49-61] However, these results are preliminary, and much more research is needed before firm conclusions can be drawn.[57]

Several researchers have reported that people holding sedentary jobs have a 30–100 percent greater risk of contracting colon cancer.[49, 50, 52, 53]

Some researchers theorize that exercise stimulates muscle movement (peristalsis) of the large intestine, thus shortening the time that the intestinal wall is in contact with any cancer producing chemical in the fecal matter.[51, 55, 64, 65] In addition, active people tend to be less obese than sedentary people (obesity is associated with increased risk of colon cancer). Active people may also eat differently than inactive people, but this has proven difficult to measure.

One study has suggested that active women may experience less breast and reproductive system cancers.[54] Women who were athletes in college were found to have significantly lower prevalence rates than nonathletes for cancers of the reproductive system and breast cancer. Risk of developing breast cancer was 86 percent lower and risk of reproductive cancers 162 percent lower among the former athletic women than the nonathletic women. Family histories for the two groups were comparable for these cancers.

A higher risk of cancer of the breast and of the uterus is associated with early menarche, later menopause, and obesity.[62, 66] Women who exercise vigorously from childhood tend to have later onset of menarche, earlier menopause, and are generally leaner. Thus active athletic women may be protected from breast and uterine cancer because of the indirect effects of exercise on puberty, menopause, and fatness. One recent study

has shown that risk of breast cancer is increased for women with fewer bowel movements (constipation).[67] By promoting more frequent bowel movements, regular physical activity may indirectly lower risk of breast cancer.

Animal studies generally support the beneficial effects of physical activity in reducing risk of cancer. For example, breast tumor growth has been reduced when rats exercise regularly.[68] This may be due to enhanced immune system function, but data are only suggestive at this time.[58] The animal study results are difficult to apply to humans.[56] Much more study is needed before more definite conclusions can be reached regarding the protective effect of exercise on cancer.

Sports Medicine Insight
Dietary Management for Diabetics and Prevention of Cancer

Treatment of diabetes and prevention of cancer are more strongly related to dietary than exercise habits. It is important that the sports medicine specialist understand these nutritional principles in order to give professional counseling and referral.

Nutritional Principles for the Diabetic

In 1986, the American Diabetes Association submitted their position statement entitled "Nutritional Recommendations and Principles for Individuals With Diabetes Mellitus."[69] A brief summary of these principles follows.

1. The caloric intake should be adjusted to achieve and maintain a desirable body weight.

2. The amount of carbohydrates should be liberalized, ideally up to 55–60 percent of total Calories, and individualized, with the amount dependent on the impact on blood glucose and lipid levels and individual eating patterns.

3. Whenever acceptable to the patient, foods containing unrefined carbohydrate with fiber should be substituted for highly refined carbohydrates, which are low in fiber. The goal is more than 40 grams of fiber per day (25 g/1000 kcal for people on low-Calorie diets).

4. For some people, modest amounts of sucrose and other refined sugars may be acceptable, contingent on metabolic control and body weight.

5. Americans in general consume too much protein. The RDA is 0.8 g/kg of body weight for adults.

6. Fat should comprise less than 30 percent of total Calories, and cholesterol intake should be less than 300 mg per day. Polyunsaturated fatty acids (mainly plant oils) should represent 6–8 percent of total Calories. Saturated fatty acids (primarily animal fats) should be less than 10 percent, with monounsaturated fatty acids (olives, nuts, fish) making up the balance.

7. The use of various nutritive and nonnutritive sweeteners (aspartame, saccharin) is acceptable in the management of diabetes.

8. The recommended sodium intake is 1000 mg/1000 Calories, not to exceed 3000 mg/day.

9. The same cautions regarding the use of alcohol that apply to the general public (moderation) apply to people with diabetes.

10. Vitamins and minerals should meet the recommended requirements for health. There is no evidence to warrant supplementation unless the patient is on a very-low-Calorie diet or other special circumstances warrant it.

Dietary goals for diabetic management include:

- Restore normal blood glucose and optimal lipid levels.
- Maintain normal growth rates and body weight.
- Stay consistent in the timing of meals and snacks (especially IDDM patients).
- Individualize the meal plan, based on lifestyle and diet history.
- Management of weight is very important for obese NIDDMs.
- Improve the overall health of diabetics through optimal nutrition.

The American Diabetes Association and American Dietetic Association have published the "Exchange Lists for Meal Planning."[70] The six exchange lists make meal planning easier for diabetics, helping the IDDM to be more consistent and helping the NIDDM patient to watch Calories more closely. The exchange lists make it easy to identify high fiber and high sodium foods.

Nutritional Guidelines for Prevention of Cancer

The American Cancer Society (ACS), together with several other organizations has submitted nutrition guidelines to help Americans prevent cancer. The ACS recommendations include the following:[62]

1. Avoid obesity: Those 40 percent or more overweight increase their risk of colon, breast, prostate, gallbladder, ovary, and uterine cancers. Women who are obese have a 55 percent greater risk, and obese men have a 33 percent greater risk of cancer than those of normal weight.

2. Cut down on total fat intake: A diet high in fat may be a factor in the development of certain cancers, particularly of the breast, colon, and prostate. In addition, by restricting fatty foods, people are better able to control body weight.

3. Eat more high-fiber foods such as whole grain cereals, fruits, and vegetables. Some studies suggest that diets high in fiber may help to reduce the risk of colon cancer. Americans now eat only about 12–18 grams of dietary fiber a day. Populations that consume diets containing twice this amount have lower rates of cancers of the colon and rectum. The data suggest that if dietary fiber of Americans is increased to a per capita figure of 20–30 grams per day, a 50 percent reduction in cancer of the colon and rectum is possible. In addition, foods high in fiber are a good substitute for foods high in fat.

4. Include foods rich in vitamins A and C in the daily diet: Vitamin A and its precursor, beta-carotene, appear to be particularly valuable in cancer prevention, and vitamins E and C may be protective to a lesser degree.

   About 20 studies in various parts of the world suggest an inverse association between eating foods containing vitamin A or beta-carotene and various types of human cancer, with risk reduced 30–50 percent.[63] These studies have shown that eating such foods (especially dark green and orange vegetables and various fruits) may lower the risk of cancers of the larynx, esophagus, and lung.

5. Include cruciferous vegetables in your diet: *Cruciferous vegetables* belong to the mustard family, whose plants have flowers with four leaves in the pattern of a cross. These include

cabbage, broccoli, brussels sprouts, kohlrabi, and cauliflower. Some studies have suggested that consumption of these vegetables may reduce the risk of cancer, particularly of the gastrointestinal and respiratory tracts.

6. Be moderate in consumption of alcoholic beverages: Heavy drinkers of alcohol, especially those who are also cigarette smokers, are at unusually high risk for cancers of the oral cavity, larynx, and esophagus.

7. Be moderate in consumption of salt-cured, smoked and nitrite-cured foods: Smoked foods such as hams, some varieties of sausages, fish, etc., absorb some of the tars that come from incomplete combustion. These tars contain cancer-causing chemicals, similar to those of cigarette smoke. Evidence shows that salt-cured or pickled foods may increase the risk of stomach and esophageal cancer. Nitrites are used with meats to help protect against food poisoning (botulism), and to improve color and flavor. These lead to the formation of nitrosamines, which are powerful cancer causing chemicals.

Summary

1. More than 11 percent of the U.S. population age 20–74 are diabetic or have impaired glucose tolerance. Diabetes is major medical disorder, and is related to a wide variety of health problems and early death.

2. Diabetes mellitus is characterized by metabolic abnormalities, the most evident being an elevated serum glucose. There are two major forms of diabetes mellitus: Type I, or insulin-dependent (IDDM), and Type II, or noninsulin-dependent (NIDDM).

3. IDDM can occur at any age, and is characterized by abrupt onset of symptoms, a deficiency of insulin production by the pancreas, and dependence on injected insulin to sustain life.

4. NIDDM is more common, and usually occurs in people over age 40. The onset of the disease is gradual. The vast majority of NIDDM patients are obese. NIDDM patients may have normal pancreatic beta cells, but because the body cells are less able to use the insulin, blood glucose levels are high.

5. The usual method for diagnosing diabetes is by measuring the fasting blood glucose level. When serum glucose is greater than or equal to 140 mg/dl on more than one occasion, diabetes is diagnosed.

6. Treatment of diabetes centers around control of blood glucose levels. The goal is to keep the blood glucose levels within the narrow limits of healthy people. The three principal approaches to diabetes management are diet, exercise, and treatment with oral antidiabetic agents or insulin.

7. The single most important objective for the obese NIDDM is to achieve and maintain a desirable body weight.

8. Although the concept that physical activity is beneficial for patients with diabetes mellitus is centuries old, there is considerable controversy regarding its value. In general, long- term diabetic control with physical activity has been shown effective for NIDDM patients but not IDDM patients.

9. One of the most consistent findings by researchers has been that with as little as one to three weeks of regular physical activity, insulin sensitivity improves 20–50 percent. However, improvement in glucose tolerance appears to be a consequence of the last bout of exercise rather than of long-term adaptations to training.

10. Physical activity by diabetics is important for other reasons, including management of obesity, reduced risk of coronary heart disease, and psychosocial benefits.

11. IDDM patients can experience hyperglycemia or hypoglycemia during and after exercise sessions, depending on initial blood glucose levels. The diabetic should avoid strenuous exercise until reasonable diabetic control is established. (Guidelines for preventing these problems were summarized in Box 14.1.)

12. Several of the long-term complications of diabetes may be worsened by exercise unless appropriate precautions are taken. With proper instruction, careful monitoring, appropriate adjustments in insulin and food intake, and individual experience, many IDDM patients can learn to exercise safely and many have achieved the status of world-class athletes.

13. Most of the studies examining the relationship between physical activity and cancer have concluded that there is a moderate protective effect, especially against colon and breast

cancer. However, these results are preliminary, with much more research needed before firm conclusions can be drawn.

References

1. Cantu RC. Diabetes and Exercise. Ithaca, New York: Mouvement Publications, 1982.

2. Kovar MG, Harris MI, Hadden WC. The Scope of Diabetes in the United States Population. Am J Public Health 77:1549–1550, 1987.

3. Kleinman JC, Donahue RP, Harris MI, et al. Mortality Among Diabetics in a National Sample. Am J Epidemiol 128:389–401, 1988.

4. The Carter Center of Emory University. Diabetes Care 8:391–406, 1985.

5. National Diabetes Data Group. Classification and Diagnosis of Diabetes Mellitus and Other Categories of Glucose Intolerance. Diabetes 28:1039–1057, 1979.

6. U.S. Department of Health and Human Services. The Surgeon General's Report on Nutrition and Health. DHHS (PHS) Publication No. 88–50211. U.S. Government Printing Office: Washington, D.C., 1988.

7. Loewenstein JE. Insulin Pumps and Other Recent Advances in the Outpatient Treatment of Diabetes. Arch Intern Med 144:755–758, 1984.

8. Krolewski AS, Warram JH, Rand LI, Kahn CR. Epidemiologic Approach to the Etiology of Type I Diabetes Mellitus and Its Complications. N Engl J Med 317:1390–1398, 1987.

9. Anderson JW. Diabetes: A Practical New Guide to Healthy Living. New York: Arco Publishing, Inc., 1982.

10. FDA Consumer, July–August, 1984.

11. Mann JI. Diet and Diabetes. Diabetologia 18:89–95, 1980.

12. Arky RA. Prevention and Therapy of Diabetes Mellitus. Nutr Rev 41:165–173, 1983.

13. National Institutes of Health. Consensus Development Conference on Diet and Exercise in Non-Insulin-Dependent Diabetes Mellitus. Diabetes Care 10:639–644, 1987.

14. American Diabetes Association. Position Statement: Nutritional Recommendations and Principles for Individuals With Diabetes Mellitus: 1986. Diabetes Care 10:126–132, 1987.

15. Vinik AI, Jenkins DJA. Dietary Fiber in Management of Diabetes. Diabetes Care 11(2):160–173, 1988.

16. Anderson JW, Gustafson NJ, Bryant CA, Tietyen-Clark J. Dietary Fiber and Diabetes: A Comprehensive Review and Practical Application. J Am Diet Assoc 87:1189–1197, 1987.

17. Vitug A, Schneider SH, Ruderman NB. Exercise and Type I Diabetes Mellitus. 16:285–304, 1988.

18. Leon AS. Diabetes. In: Skinner JS (ed). Exercise Testing and Exercise Prescription for Special Cases. Philadelphia: Lea & Febiger, 1987, pp. 115–134.

19. Jennings G, Nelson L, Nestel P, et al. The Effects of Changes in Physical Activity On Major Cardiovascular Risk Factors, Hemodynamics, Sympathetic Function, and Glucose Utilization In Man: A Controlled Study of Four Levels of Activity. Circulation 73:30–40, 1986.

20. Frisch RE, Wyshak G, Albright TE, Albright NL, Schiff I. Lower Prevalence of Diabetes in Female Former College Athletes Compared with Nonathletes. Diabetes 35:1101, 1986.

21. Franz MJ. Exercise and the Management of Diabetes Mellitus. J Am Diet Assoc 87:872–882, 1987.

22. Fremion AS, Marrero DG, Golden MP. Maximum Oxygen Uptake Determination in Insulin-Dependent Diabetes Mellitus. Physician Sportsmed 15(7):119–126, 1987.

23. Oshida Y, Yamanouchi K, Hayamizu S, Sato Y. Long–Term Mild Jogging Increases Insulin Action Despite No Influence on Body Mass Index or VO_{2max}. J Appl Physiol 66:2206–2210, 1989.

24. Stratton R, Wilson DP, Endres RK, Goldstein DE. Improved Glycemic Control After Supervised 8-wk Exercise Program in Insulin-Dependent Diabetic Adolescents. Diabetes Care 10:589–593, 1987.

25. MacDonald MJ. Postexercise Late-Onset Hypoglycemia in Insulin-Dependent Diabetic Patients. Diabetes Care 10:584–588, 1987.

26. Heath GW, Leonard BE, Wilson RH, et al. Community-Based Exercise Intervention: Zuni Diabetes Project. Diabetes Care 10:579–583, 1987.

27. Richter EA, Galbo H. Diabetes, Insulin and Exercise. Sports Med 3:275–288, 1986.

28. West MW. Diabetes Mellitus. In: Nutritional Support of Medical Practice (Schneider HA, Anderson CE, Coursin DB, eds). New York: Harper and Row, 1983.

29. Ivy JL. The Insulin-Like Effect of Muscle Contraction. Exerc Sport Sci Rev 15:29–54, 1987.

30. Holloszy JO, Schultz J, Kusnierkiewicz J, et al. Effects of Exercise on Glucose Tolerance and Insulin Resistance: Brief Review and Some Preliminary Results. Acta Med Scand (Suppl) 711:55–65, 1986.

31. King DS, Dalsky GP, Clutter WE, et al. Effects of Exercise and Lack of Exercise on Insulin Sensitivity and Responsiveness. J Appl Physiol 64:1942–1946, 1988.

32. Zinman B, Vranic M. Diabetes and Exercise. Med Clin North Am 69:145–157, 1985.

33. Blackett PR. Child and Adolescent Athletes With Diabetes. Physician Sportsmed 16(3):133–149, 1988.

34. Stratton R, Wilson DP, Endres RK. Acute Glycemic Effects of Exercise in Adolescents With Insulin Dependent Diabetes Mellitus. Physician Sportsmed 16(3):150–157, 1988.

35. Goodyear LJ, Hirshman MF, Knutson SM, Horton ED, Horton ES. Effect of Exercise Training on Glucose Homeostasis in Normal and Insulin-Deficient Diabetic Rats. J Appl Physiol 65:844–851, 1988.

36. Rogers MA, Yamamoto C, King DS, Hagberg JM, Ehsani AA, Holloszy JO. Improvement in Glucose Tolerance After 1 Wk of Exercise in Patients With Mild NIDDM. Diabetes Care 11:613–618, 1988.

37. Bayles-Paternostro M, Wing RR, Robertson RJ. Effect of Life-Style Activity of Varying Duration on Glycemic Control in Type II Diabetic Women. Diabetes Care 12:34–37, 1989.

38. Rauramaa R. Relationship of Physical Activity, Glucose Tolerance, and Weight Management. Prev Med 13:37–46, 1984.

39. Seals DR, et al. JAMA 252:645–649, 1984.

40. Kemmer FW, Berger M. Exercise In Therapy and the Life of Diabetic Patients. Clin Sci 67:279–283, 1984.

41. Nathan DM, et al. Programming Pre-Exercise Snacks to Prevent Post-Exercise Hypoglycemia in Intensively Treated Insulin-Dependent Diabetics. Ann Intern Med 102:483–486, 1985.

42. Rosenthal M, Haskell WL, et al. Demonstration of a Relationship Between Level of Physical Training and Insulin-stimulated Glucose Utilization in Normal Humans. Diabetes 32:408–411, 1983.

43. Bogardus C, et al. Effects of Physical Training and Diet Therapy On Carbohydrate Metabolism in Patients with Glucose Intolerance and Non-Insulin-depdendent Diabetes Mellitus. Diabetes 33:311–318, 1984.

44. Trovati M, Carta Q, et al. Influence of Physical Training on Blood Glucose Control, Glucose Tolerance, Insulin Secretion, and Insulin Action in Non-insulin-dependent Diabetic Patients. Diabetes Care 7:416–420, 1984.

45. Reitman JS, Vasquez B, et al. Improvement of Glucose Homeostasis After Exercise Training in Non-insulin-dependent Diabetes. Diabetes Care 7:434–441, 1984.

46. Landt KW, Campaigne BN, James FW, Sterling MA. Effects of Exercise Training on Insulin Sensitivity in Adolescents with Type I Diabetes. Diabetes Care 8:461–465, 1985.

47. LaPorte RE, Dorman JS, Tajima N, et al: Pittsburgh Insulin-Dependent Diabetes Mellitus Morbidity and Mortality Study: Physical Activity and Diabetic Complications. Pediatrics 78:1027–1033, 1986.

48. Horton ES. Role and Management of Exercise in Diabetes Mellitus. Diabetes Care 11(2):201–211, 1988.

49. Gerhardsson M, Norell SE, Kiviranta H, et al. Sedentary Job and Colon Cancer. Am J Epidemiol 123:775–780, 1986.

50. Garabrant DH, Peters JM, Mack TM, et al. Job Activity and Colon Cancer Risk. Am J Epidemiol 119:1005–1014, 1984.

51. Cordain L, Latin RW, Behnke JJ. The Effects of an Aerobic Running Program on Bowel Transit Time. J Sports Med 26:101–104, 1986.

52. Vena JE, Graham S, Zielezny M, et al. Lifetime Occupational Exercise and Colon Cancer. Am J Epidemiol 122:357–365, 1985.

53. Vena JE, Graham S, Zielezny M, Brasure J, Swanson MK. Occupational Exercise and Risk of Cancer. Am J Clin Nutr 45:318–327, 1987.

54. Frisch RE, Wyshak G, Albright NL, et al. Lower Lifetime Occurrence of Breast Cancer and Cancers of the Reproductive System Among Former College Athletes. Am J Clin Nutr 45:328–335, 1987.

55. Slattery ML, Schumacher MC, Smith KR, West DW, Abd-Elghany N. Physical Activity, Diet, and Risk of Colon Cancer in Utah. Am J Epidemiol 128:989–999, 1988.

56. Shephard RJ. Exercise and Malignancy. Sports Med 3:235–241, 1986.

57. Paffenbarger RS, Hyde RT, Wing AL. Physical Activity and Incidence of Cancer in Diverse Populations: A Preliminary Report. Am J Clin Nutr 45:312–317, 1987.

58. Eichner ER. Exercise, Lymphokines, Calories, and Cancer. Physician Sportsmed 15(6):109–116, 1987.

59. Kohl HW, LaPorte RE, Blair SN. Physical Activity and Cancer: An Epidemiological Perspective. Sports Med 6:222–237, 1988.

60. Frisch RE, Wyshak G. Albright NL, et al. Lower Prevalence of Non-Reproductive System Cancers Among Female Former College Athletes. Med Sci Sports Exerc 21:250–253, 1989.

61. Albanes D, Blair A, Taylor PR. Physical Activity and Risk of Cancer in the NHANESI Population. Am J Public Health 79:744–750, 1989.

62. American Cancer Society. Cancer Facts & Figures-1988. American Cancer Society, 90 Park Avenue, New York, NY 10016.

63. Greenwald P, Sondik E. Diet and Chemoprevention in NCI's Research Strategy to Achieve National Cancer Control Objectives. Ann Rev Public Health 7:267–291, 1986.

64. Keeling WF, Martin BJ. Gastrointestinal Transit During Mild Exercise. J Appl Physiol 63:978–981, 1987.

65. Gauthier MM. Can Exercise Reduce the Risk of Cancer? Physician Sportsmed 14(10):171–178, 1986.

66. Lane HW, Carpenter JT. Breast Cancer: Incidence, Nutritional Concerns, and Treatment Approaches. J Am Diet Assoc 87:765–769, 1987.

67. Micozzi MS, Carter CL, Albanes D, et al. Bowel Function and Breast Cancer in US Women. Am J Public Health 79:73–75, 1989.

68. Cohen LA, Choi K, Wnag CX. Influence of Dietary Fat, Caloric Restriction, and Voluntary Exercise in N-Nitro-

somethylurea-Induced Mammary Tumorgenesis in Rats. Cancer Res 48:4276–4283, 1988.

69. American Diabetes Association. Position Statement: Nutritional Recommendations and Principles for Individuals With Diabetes Mellitus: 1986. Diabetes Care 10:126–132, 1987.

70. American Diabetes Association and American Dietetic Association. Exchange Lists for Meal Planning, 1986. Diabetes Information Service Center, 1660 Duke Street, Alexandria, VA 22314.

Chapter 15

Precautions for Physical Activity

"The athlete's habit of body neither produces a good condition for the general purposes of civic life, nor does it encourage ordinary health and the procreation of children. Some amount of exertion is essential for the best habit, but it must be neither violent nor specialized, as is the case with the athlete. It should rather be a general exertion, directed to all the activities of a free man."—Aristotle

Introduction: The Harmful Effects of Too Much Exercise

The modern-day fitness movement is not yet 25 years old. It was given its first great impetus in 1968, when Dr. Kenneth Cooper, a medical doctor for the Air Force, published his book, *Aerobics*. In this book, Cooper challenged Americans to take personal charge of their lifestyles, and counter the "epidemics" of heart disease, obesity, and rising health care costs. Millions took up the "aerobic challenge" and began jogging, cycling, walking, and swimming their ways to better health—thus starting the new fitness revolution.

Americans are now exercising more than at any other time in our modern era. Exercise is suddenly prestigious. But with the prestige have come some real problems.

One product of the added prestige is "overzealousness." Excessive exercise appears to be America's newest elixir in that endless search for the "fountain of youth." Some people, allured by the media reports, and perhaps overreacting to health problems, job dissatisfaction, boredom, marital difficulties, and a fear of growing old, have seized on exercise as a panacea. Americans, who have a history of being a people of two-fold judgments (either all or none), have taken a good thing and once again carried it too far.

From Ironman Triathalons, to six-day running events, to transcontinental bicycle or foot races, we have it all today in the U.S.A. Most symbolic, however, of America's obsession with over-exercise is marathon running.

Runner's World magazine estimates that there are over 12 million runners in the United States, with one third of these considered to be in "serious" training.[1] And the goal of most, if they are serious runners, is the 26.2-mile marathon, an event highly glamorized by the media.

In 1984 when marathoning peaked, over 80,000 runners toed the line of 380 U.S. marathons.[2] Although the number is now coming down, the numbers are still large—the biggest marathons (like New York and Los Angeles) are attracting more than 20,000 runners each. More than 21,000 runners finished the 1988 New York Marathon (compared with only 55 in 1970).[3]

Marathoners try to run at least 40–60 miles per week, with some of the elite runners running 130 miles per week. As many recent articles in the medical literature have shown, such excessive training has brought a host of problems. The list is swelling as medical science discovers a wide array of harmful side-effects. This chapter will review the major risks, and in the Sports Medicine Insight, compare them with the benefits of exercise reviewed in Chapters 10 to 14.

Musculoskeletal Injuries

The muscles, joints, and supporting ligaments and tendons of the legs and feet respond very poorly to excessive exercise, especially activities that require running and jumping. (See Figure 15.1.)

Running Injuries

Many studies have explored the relationship between running and *musculoskeletal injuries*.[4-23] Several of the major studies are summarized below.

The Extent of the Problem

The Centers for Disease Control (CDC) in Atlanta evaluated the injury rates for 2,500 male and female runners for one year.[4-6] More than 35 percent developed orthopedic injuries serious enough to reduce weekly running

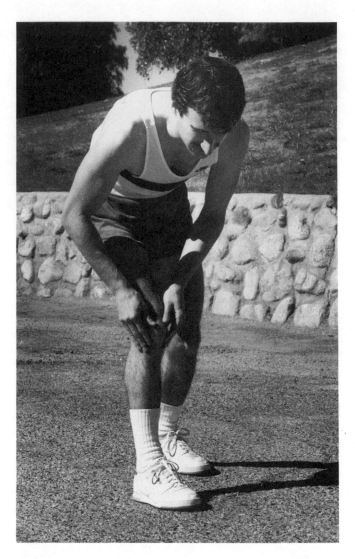

Figure 15.1 Activities that require running and jumping often cause trauma to the muscles, joints, and supporting ligaments and tendons of the legs and feet, especially when done to excess.

mileage. Of these, 40 percent sought medical consultation for their injuries. The risk of injury increased with weekly running mileage, with 53 percent injured when running 30–39 miles per week, and 65 percent injured when running more than 50 miles per week.

Sixty percent of the injuries involved the knee and foot areas. The researchers concluded that the average runner has a one-in-three chance of being injured within any given year, and a one-in-ten likelihood of incurring an injury that will require medical attention. A person running 15 miles a week can count on one injury every two years.

In the author's study of 2,307 runners about to participate in the 1987 Los Angeles Marathon, runners were asked to report any injury causing enough pain "so that your normal running program was interrupted (weekly mileage reduced)". Nearly one out of five runners (20.7 percent) reported at least one injury during the month prior to the race. Figure 15.2 shows that in common with other studies, most of the injured runners reported knee and foot injuries.

In one of the largest studies ever conducted on running injuries, a study of 4,358 male and 428 female joggers in Switzerland, researchers reported that 45.8 percent and 40 percent, respectively, had sustained a jogging injury during the preceding year.[7,8] Every fifth male runner was forced to fully interrupt his exercise routine. Because of the injuries, one out of every seven male joggers sought medical treatment, and one out of 40 missed work. Frequency of jogging injuries increased with increase in weekly distance jogged. (See Figure 15.3.)

In another study, the training habits and injury experience of 688 adult Canadian runners were assessed.[10] Injuries during the previous 12 months (serious enough to reduce running mileage, require medication, or cause a visit to a health professional) were reported by 57 percent. Professional assistance was sought by 52 percent. The knee was the most frequent site, followed by the foot, hip, heel, and ankle.

The knee is the most common site of injury for the runner.[17,20,21] In the CDC study, 38 percent of the injuries

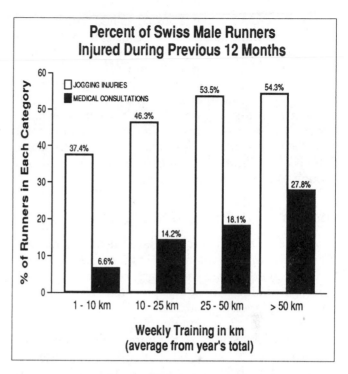

Figure 15.3 Frequency of jogging injuries and medical consultations as a result of jogging injuries, according to weekly training distance of Swiss male runners. *Source:* Marti B, Vader JP, Minder CE, Abelin T. On the Epidemiology of Running Injuries. Am J Sports Med 16:285–294, 1988.

Figure 15.2 Nearly a third of the injuries reported by runners preparing for the 1987 Los Angeles Marathon were to the knee. Foot and leg injuries were reported by one-fourth and one-fifth of the injured runners, respectively. *Source:* Nieman DC, Johanssen LM, Lee JW. Injuries to Runners Preparing for the Los Angeles Marathon. (Manuscript in progress.)

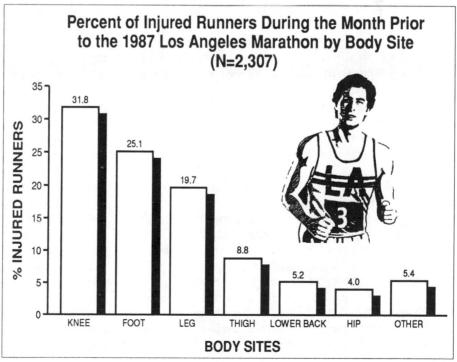

occurred there. Most knee pain associated with running occurs around the patella, and is caused by preexisting problems and overuse, especially from sudden changes in running mileage or intensity of workout.[18-23]

In summary, running is associated with a high rate of musculoskeletal injuries, with 35 to 60 percent of runners reporting injuries within a given year. And during just one month prior to a marathon, 21 percent reported injuries. Although most of the runners usually don't seek medical help, the pain is frequently serious enough to disrupt the running routine.

Factors Associated With Injuries

Researchers have tried to measure the factors responsible for the high prevalence of injuries among runners, and have three that are particularly common: improper training techniques, poor equipment, and biomechanical/anthropometric abnormalities.[15]

Running is a traumatic form of exercise for the musculoskeletal system of the human body. Studies of triathletes have found that relatively few of their injuries involve their bicycling and swimming—most are from running. In one study, 70 percent of the injuries sustained by 168 triathletes occurred during running practice sessions.[14]

The sudden impact of the foot with the running surface causes a force equal to 2.5 times one's body weight.[18] The human body appears to be able to handle moderate amounts of running, but when it is excessive or when distances are suddenly increased, injuries become common.

The injuries most frequently associated with running are those classified as *overuse syndromes*, especially common among runners who run excessive distances in their training.[6, 15] In one study of 60 runners, improper training techniques, especially excessive distance and sudden change in training routines, were responsible for 72 percent of reported injuries.[12] Malalignment of the legs and feet of the runners were involved in 40 percent of cases.

Overtraining creates an imbalance between training and recovery.[19] It can cause staleness as the physical and emotional stress of the exercise program exceeds the individual coping capacity (stress response). Clinical signs of overtraining include increased resting heart rate, inferior performance, reduced appetite, weight loss, retarded recovery after exercise, increased irritability and emotional lability, disturbed sleep, loss of training and competitive desire, increased resting blood pressure, *postural hypotension* (reduction in blood pressure when standing after sitting or lying down), in-

creased incidence of injuries, increased incidence of infections, and reduced maximal power output.[19] One of the most effective ways of avoiding overtraining is to follow a well-balanced, progressive training schedule. Sudden increases in training should be avoided. Some coaches follow the 10-percent rule, by which week-to-week training distances are never increased by more than 10 percent.

The running style (biomechanical factors) and anatomical structure of runners have both been associated with running injuries.[15] A high degree of motion in the foot or differences in leg length can be important factors. In one study, 48 trained runners with runner's knee were examined, treated, and followed for 8 months to identify the causes of this most prevalent of all running injuries and its response to treatment.[17] Most were found to have anatomic malalignment of the lower limb. Sixty-nine percent were also predisposed to runner's knee because of suddenly increased running distance, hill running, interval training, or racing too often.

One-third of the runners showed improvement with a change in shoes. In fact, one researcher has blamed the problem of running injuries on the thick soles of modern day running shoes.[18](In this report, the sensory insulation inherent in the modern running shoe was shown to be an important factor behind running injuries).

Factors not apparently associated with running injuries are age, stretching routines, type of running surface, type of terrain, and speed of training.[13] Although some exercise physiologists have theorized that muscle tightness (lack of flexibility) may be related to injuries, support for this theory is lacking.[16]

To determine what training factors are associated with running injuries, 451 randomly selected runners in a 10-km race completed a questionnaire about running habits, injuries sustained within the last two years, treatment, and demographic information. Of the 210 that reported having been injured within the past two years, mileage and number of days run per week were most highly associated with injury. (See Figure 15.4.)

Beginner runners are especially prone to musculoskeletal injury. A study of jail inmates found injury rates of 39 percent for those previously sedentary running 5 days per week, and only 12 percent for those running 3 days per week.[24, 25] Where they exercised for 45 minutes, the injury rates were 54 percent, against 22 percent with 15-minute work-outs. The conclusion was that running programs of 45-minutes in duration with five sessions per week are excessive for beginning joggers.

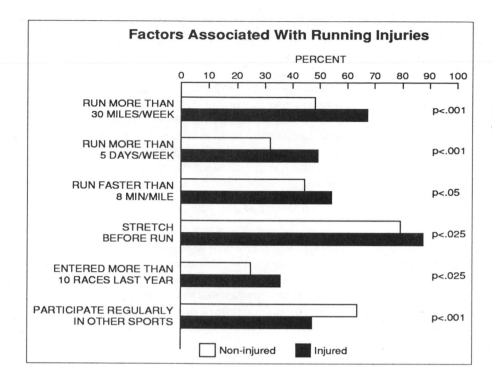

Figure 15.4 Training factors found to be significantly associated with injury incidence among 451 randomly selected runners over a two-year period. *Source:* Jacobs SJ, Berson BL. Injuries to Runners. A Study of Entrants to a 10,000 Meter Race. Am J Sports Med 14:151–155, 1986.

Aerobic Dance Injuries

Runners are not the only ones getting injured. Aerobic dancing, making exercise fun and socially-oriented, has attracted millions who might otherwise not have joined the fitness movement.[26] Unfortunately, there is increasing evidence that aerobic dance programs are associated with an alarming number of exercise injuries.[26-34]

Aerobic dance is probably the most popular organized fitness activity for women in the United States, with approximately 23 million participants.[27] Aerobic dance traces its origins to Jacki Sorenson, the wife of a naval pilot, who began conducting exercise classes at a U.S. Navy base in Puerto Rico in 1969. The growth of aerobic dance has been more recently stimulated by the production of videotaped dance exercise programs.

The original aerobic dance programs consisted of an eclectic combination of various dance forms, including ballet, modern jazz, disco, and folk, as well as calisthenic-type exercises. More recent innovations include water aerobics in a swimming pool, non-impact or low-impact aerobics (one foot on the ground at all times), specific dance aerobics, and "assisted" aerobics with weights worn on the wrists and/or ankles.

Concerns regarding the aerobic dance movement have been two-fold: (1) Do the programs promote cardiorespiratory endurance? (2) Are musculoskeletal injuries increased? Few researchers have examined the cardiorespiratory benefits of aerobic dance. In general,

however, when participants follow appropriate levels of intensity, frequency, and duration, there is a demonstrable training effect. (See Chapter 8.)

Exercise physiologists were concerned that the early dance aerobic programs were conceived by people with little or no background in medicine, kinesiology, or exercise physiology. In addition, some of the activities and positions utilized in the aerobic dance programs were potentially injurious.

The major studies examining the injury potential of aerobic dance have found that about 45 percent of students and 75 percent of instructors report injuries.[27-31, 34] Rates of injury for students are about one injury per 100 hours of dancing, and for instructors, about one per 400 hours. Most of these injuries, however, are mild, causing some pain and some disruption in participation, but generally not leading participants to stop dancing or to seek professional medical assistance. The lower extremities account for about 80 percent of all injuries.

What factors are associated with increased risk of aerobic dance injuries? In one study of 1,123 female and 164 male aerobics students, those who exercised more than three times per week, wore improper shoes, and exercised on non-resilient surfaces suffered the most injuries.[34] Apparently lower-leg injuries were the result of excessive physical trauma. Statistics like these support those who urge a substitution of low-impact aerobic routines for the high-impact (jumping and dancing on the balls of the feet) variety.[32, 33] In low-impact dance aerobics, the common denominator is that at least one foot is touching the floor throughout the aerobic portion of the workout. Movements are not ballistic, but focus on large-muscle upper body movements and arm movements above heart level, combined with leg kicks, high-powered steps, side-to-side movements, and lunges.

Research comparing injury rates is very limited, but because low-impact movements are often exaggerated, they can place unusual stress on the knees, ankles, and lower back.

Preliminary evidence shows that while high-impact routines give a more intense workout, low-impact aerobics meet the minimum exercise prescription criteria. (See Chapter 8.) Use of ankle and wrist weights can enhance the intensity, but may promote injury.

Bicycling Injuries

Bicyclers also suffer their share of injuries, but they are usually caused by accidents.[35-41] Bicycling injuries account for at least 1,000 deaths and 500,000 emergency

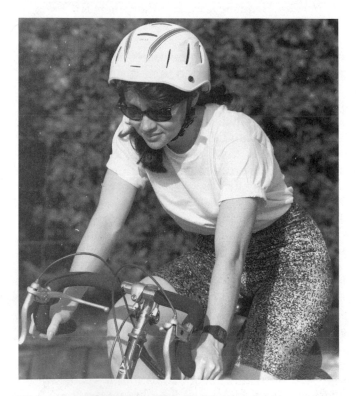

Figure 15.5 Nationwide, only 8 to 10 percent of bicyclers wear helmets. And yet, head injuries account for approximately 85 percent of bicycling deaths and two-thirds of bicycle-related hospital admissions.

room visits each year in the United States.[35] Head injuries account for approximately 85 percent of bicycling deaths and two-thirds of bicycle-related hospital admissions, yet nationwide, only 8 to 10 percent of bicyclists use helmets.[35, 37] Nearly half of the deaths are of children under the age of 14.[36] Among children less than 10 years old, more die from bike accidents than from firearm accidents, accidental poisonings, or falls.[38] College students have 510 accidents per million cycled miles, compared to 720 for children.[40]

Swimming Injuries

Competitive swimmers may swim 8,000 to 20,000 yards per day, 5 to 7 days each week (the latter being comparable to running 45 miles daily). Shoulder pain is the most common musculoskeletal complaint, usually resulting from supraspinatus or biceps tendonitis.[42] Symptoms include point tenderness on the anterior part of the tip of the shoulder. (It is painful to raise the bent arm overhead.)

In severe cases, total rest may be necessary to alleviate the pain. Physical therapy may be helpful.

Knee pain can occur among breaststroke swimmers (involving pain and tenderness in the medial aspect of the knee joint,[42] apparently related to the breaststroke "whip kick"). Leg strengthening and flexibility exercises may be helpful, and coaching on proper technique should be emphasized.

Osteoarthritis

Concerns have been raised that running may accelerate the development of *osteoarthritis* in weight-bearing joints—that runners may be sacrificing their joints to save their hearts.[43-45] Osteoarthritis is a chronic disease involving the joints, especially those bearing weight, characterized by destruction of articular cartilage, overgrowth of bone with lipping and spur formation, and impaired function.

The research to date indicates that many years of high-mileage running is not associated with premature degeneration of the joints or osteoarthritis.[43-45] One study of 50 to 72-year-old long-distance runners found they had less physical disability and greater functional capacity than average members of the community. The runners sought medical services less often (one-third of runner visits were for running-related injuries), weighed less, and experienced less musculoskeletal disability as they got older.[43]

Little is known about the effects of long distance running on the specialized growth cartilage in the extremity and spine bones of growing children,[46-48] although there are anecdotal data that repetitive microtrauma to these growth plates may lead to increased injury and perhaps disruption of growth. Until more is known, it is probably wise to limit children who have not yet completed growth to no more than 5 miles per day of training and no more than 10-km competitive distances.

Delayed Soreness and Muscle Cell Damage

There are two types of muscle soreness, acute and delayed. *Acute muscle soreness* occurs during and immediately following exercise. The muscular tension developed during the exercise reduces blood flow to the active muscles, causing lactic acid and potassium to build up, stimulating pain receptors.

Delayed soreness (often called *delayed-onset muscle soreness* or DOMS) occurs from 1 to 5 days following unaccustomed or severe exercise.[23, 49-55] DOMS is usually caused by structural damage to skeletal muscle after eccentric exercise, in which muscles produce force while lengthening, as in running downhill.[53] During the soreness, the muscles temporarily lose their usual capacity to produce force.

Injury to the membrane of the muscle (*sarcolemma*) is a normal consequence of extreme exertion. The risk is compounded if an untrained person performs eccentric exercise in a hot environment, or there is any preceding infectious disease, drug ingestion, or underlying metabolic disorder.[49] Once the membrane is injured, cell contents leak out and extracellular components leak in, resulting in muscle pain and weakness.

Intensive training for and competition in endurance events like the marathon are accompanied by injury to muscle cells. Evidence of injury shows up in the increase in intramuscular enzymes and myoglobin found in the blood following the exercise, and from direct microscopic examination of muscle samples.[50] Although training reduces the magnitude of the damage,[59-61] well-trained competitors in endurance events can experience chronic muscle injury because of increasing training intensities and challenges. [In one study of athletes who had completed Ironman distances—a 2.4-mile swim, 112-mile bicycling session, and 26.2-mile run—white blood cell counts tripled, and muscles enzymes such as *lactic dehydrogenase* (LDH) and *creatine phosphokinase* (CPK) rose dramatically in the blood, indicating considerable muscle cell damage.][56]

Endurance athletes, because of the continual damage to their muscle cells, often have different blood test profiles than nonathletes.[57, 58] The white blood cell count at rest will be higher than normal when the muscles are inflamed from overracing or overtraining, and may remain high for 2–3 weeks—a time to reduce training.

The blood levels of several enzymes reflect the degree of muscle tissue breakdown. The highest postexercise serum enzyme activities are found after very prolonged competitive exercise, such as ultradistance marathon running, or eccentric muscular activities (e.g., bench stepping and downhill running). World-class runners, particularly European athletes like Grete Waitz, undergo regular blood testing to monitor the levels of CPK and LDH enzymes. The higher the level of CPK in the blood, the greater the muscle damage and the greater the need for rest.

CPK values for runners may be two to three times those considered normal for short time periods, indicating that muscle fibers are in a state of flux as they react to the hard training. While this may be okay for a limited time, persistently elevated levels means the runners should back off from the hard training. LDH is another enzymatic marker for muscle cell damage, although not as sensitive as CPK. Interestingly, these enzymes (CPK, LDH) are also indicators of heart muscle damage to cardiac patients.[58]

R.I.C.E.—Treatment of Musculoskeletal Pain and Injury

Treatment of musculoskeletal pain and injury during the first 48 to 72 hours centers around rest, ice, compression, and elevation (*R.I.C.E.*)[62-65] Controlling the edema (accumulation of fluid) and swelling that accompany the injury is of the utmost importance. Control of edema brings about more rapid and complete healing, allowing more normal joint function and reducing pain and necrotic tissue buildup.

Compression of the area appears to be the most effective deterrent to swelling. Applying external compression inhibits the seepage of fluid into underlying tissue spaces and disperses excess fluid.

Initial rest for the injured area is also important. Movement that causes severe pain should be avoided (athletes who want to continue exercising should engage in some form of substitute activity that does not cause pain).

A new treatment called *cryokinetics* (alternating cold and exercise) is becoming a popular treatment for traumatic musculoskeletal injuries. Use of the affected muscles as soon as possible (guided by the pain response), promotes a return to full functional recovery.

Progressive resistance exercises are used to restore full muscle and joint function. The treatment involves 13 minutes of cold to anesthetize the injured area, followed by 3 minutes of exercise (like walking on a treadmill if the knee or ankle is involved), followed by 3 minutes of cold again. This is repeated for five cycles. (The danger of frostbite is virtually eliminated by wrapping the ice in cloth and limiting exposure to a maximum duration of 30 minutes).

If cryokinetics is initiated very early, grade-4 ankle sprains (unable to bear weight) can be brought to complete recovery in 13 days—compared with 30 days if cryotherapy is used too late, or 33 days if heat treatment is used.

Early heat treatment is discouraged, because it leads to an increase in blood flow to the injured area, increasing hemorrhage and exaggerating the acute inflammatory response.

Potential Problems of Excess Exercise for Women

Oligomenorrhea and Amenorrhea

There has been a rash of articles lately on the effects of hard exercise on the menstrual cycle.[66–90] Studies have shown that exercise increases the rate of *oligomenorrhea* (scanty or infrequent menstrual flow) and *amenorrhea* (absence of menstruation), effecting from about 5 percent of the sedentary population, to approximately 10–20 percent of women who exercise regularly and vigorously, and up to 50 percent of competitive athletes.[74–76]

The rates vary widely, however, depending on the type of athlete and the amount of training. Runners and ballet dancers, for example, have much higher rates than swimmers and cyclists. Nearly half of runners who train 80 miles per week or more are amenorrheic, compared to only about 10 percent of runners who run more moderate distances.

The author, in his study of 300 women runners preparing for the 1987 Los Angeles Marathon, found that approximately 10 percent of the women reported no more than three menstrual periods during the prior 12 months. (See Figure 15.6.) These oligoamenorrheic women tended to train more than women who reported more than three menstrual periods during the prior year. But in general, the prevalence of oligoamenorrhea was small among this group of women, who were not running excessively.

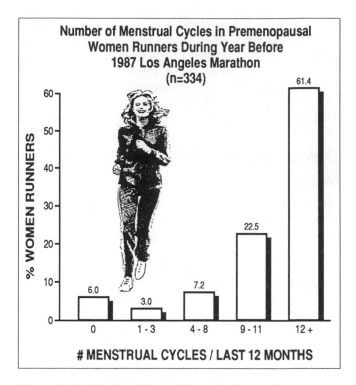

Figure 15.6 The prevalence of amenorrhea and oligomenorrhea (defined as 3 or less menstrual cycles per year) was relatively low in this group of 301 premenopausal women preparing for the 1987 Los Angeles Marathon. Most of the women did not train excessively.

Oligoamenorrhea is associated with increased risk of musculoskeletal problems. Many researchers have now reported that spinal bone mass is 20 to 30 percent lower for women with oligoamenorrhea, with the prevalence of stress fractures and musculoskeletal injuries higher.[75, 77–79, 84–86, 93] (See Figure 15.7.)

The causes of oligoamenorrhea and the associated loss in bone mineral mass are still hotly debated,[69, 71, 74, 81] but may include the direct effect of exercise itself on the sex hormones, or some indirect effect of exercise, such as psychological stress, decrease in body fat, or malnutrition. Chronic exercise appears to stimulate marked alterations in the human menstrual cycle, causing shortened luteal phases, delayed menses, abnormal bleeding, and loss of luteinizing hormone surge.[67] Research has shown that the hormones estrogen and parathyroid hormone (PTH) of oligoamenorrheic women are lower, while their cortisol is higher, which may be related to the loss of bone mineral mass.[75, 79, 84–86]

Although there is evidence that oligoamenorrheic women athletes have unusually low body fat levels,[88] body fat levels do not seem to be an important factor.[71, 82]

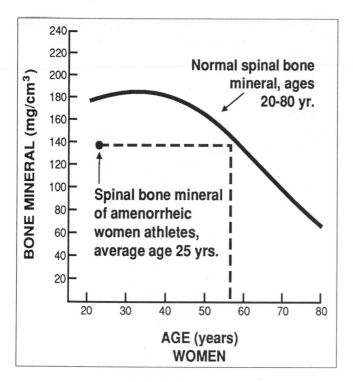

Figure 15.7 Several researchers have found that the spinal bone mineral mass of amenorrheic women athletes at age 25 is equal to that of women twice their age. (See references 75, 84–86, 93.)

Although anorexia nervosa and other eating disorders have been related to oligoamenorrhea among ballet dancers,[76] in general, the diets of oligoamenorrheic women athletes do not seem to be substantially different from those of women athletes in general.[80, 83, 84]

All women who stop menstruating or menstruate irregularly because of their exercise program should be examined by a physician.[81] Oligoamenorrhea appears to be rapidly reversible upon cessation of hard training.[68, 90–92] Even the loss of bone mineral mass has been found to be reversible when runners reduce their running distances, gain weight, and resume regular menses.[91]

Women are not alone in suffering disturbances in reproductive function with excessive exercise. Testosterone has been found unusually low among endurance trained male athletes,[94–97] apparently because their chronic endurance training has impaired testicular function.

Although sex drive appears to be decreased, most males in high-distance training appear to have normal sexual function. Interestingly, decreased bone mineral mass has been reported among males who exercise excessively while eating too little.[96]

Exercise and Pregnancy

Some women on regular exercise programs refuse to reduce their normal exercise when becoming pregnant. You probably have read some of the case stories. Ingride Kristiansen, the famous runner from Norway, for example, ran to the day of labor, and delivered a healthy baby (1983). Five months later she ran a 2:27 marathon, then a few months later, a 2:24, and in 1985 held the world records for the 5K, 10K, and marathon. These types of stories have been a cause of concern for many who provide reproductive health care to women.[98–123]

Exercise during pregnancy serves to increase the fitness of the mother, but we are not sure about the influence on fetal development. Theoretically, adverse effects to the fetus could occur from several exercise-induced changes, including decreased blood flow to the uterus (maternal muscles use more blood during exercise), leading to a temporary reduction in the oxygen supply to the fetus, reduced fetal heart rate, increased temperature in the uterus, and a diversion of the glucose supply from the fetus to the mother.

Most recent studies, however, show that moderate exercise during pregnancy appears to pose no harm to the fetus. Only when exercise becomes excessive does fetal development appear to be affected.

Several researchers using animal models have shown that hard exercise during gestation decrease the weight of the fetus.[107, 112] In one study with humans,[101] women who continued endurance exercise during pregnancy, gained on the average 10 pounds less, delivered 8 days earlier, and had offspring weighing 1.1 pounds less than those who stopped exercising prior to the 28th week.

Moderate exercise during pregnancy appears to benefit the mother, apparently without harm to the fetus.[110, 114–120] Submaximal exercise, such as walking, apparently does not reduce uterine blood flow,[118, 119] nor does it affect fetal heart rates.[113, 123] Moderate intensity exercise increases the mother's cardiorespiratory fitness,[115, 117, 120] and in one study led to a shortening of active labor.[114]

In 1985, the American College of Obstetricians and Gynecologists released their guidelines for exercise during pregnancy and postpartum.[111] They urged moderate exercise, aiming for limits of 140 beats per minute for heart rate, and 38°C for core body temperatures. Pregnant women were urged not to perform exercise in the supine position after the fourth month of gestation, (but recent research has shown that it is safe for pregnant women to engage in supine exercise for short durations of time).[122] Also discouraged were exercises of a competitive nature and those using ballistic movements or deep flexion or extension of joints.

Although these guidelines caused some outcry among exercise physiologists, who thought they were too cautious,[109] in general, they appear prudent in light of present knowledge. Box 15.2 summarizes these and other published exercise guidelines for pregnant women.[104, 106, 111]

So in summary, extremely strenuous exercise presents potential risks to the pregnant woman and her fetus. On the basis of present knowledge, it does appear prudent for women to reduce their exercise near the middle of the second trimester and to be very careful not too overexert. In moderation, exercise may provide both short-term and long-term benefits.

When counseling pregnant women, clinicians should use an individualized approach.[121] Exercise prescriptions should consider the woman's health, potential pregnancy complications, previous exercise history, and present exercise goals. There is general agreement that if a woman participated in an exercise program before pregnancy, she can continue it with some modification during pregnancy, erring on the side of moderation. (See Figure 15.8.)

Heat Injuries

During the 1984 Olympics, an event occurred that had a deep impact on Americans. Swiss marathoner Gabriella Anderson-Schiess, suffering from heat exhaustion, staggered incoherently through the last lap of the women's Olympic marathon. Before tens of thousands of horrified spectators and millions of television viewers, she finally collapsed into the arms of a race official after crossing the finish line.[124]

The American College of Sports Medicine has advised runners that heat exhaustion and heat strokes are their number one enemies.[125] When the temperature and humidity are high, runners have been warned to greatly reduce their exercise training and drink large amounts of water. Yet marathon competition can cause runners to ignore such precautions.

During the 1984 New York City Marathon, temperatures rose to 74°F in 94-percent humidity. Times were slow as runners struggled to finish, and 209 run-

---

BOX 15.2 Summary of Exercise Principles for Pregnant Women[104, 106, 111]

- Do not suddenly increase the amount of exercise undertaken.
- Do not exceed the amount of exercise normally undertaken before pregnancy.
- Eliminate sports in which the risk of injury is high (i.e., water skiing, contact sports, scuba diving).
- Late in pregnancy, avoid excessive aerobic exercise.
- Avoid exercises that require lying on the back for more than 5 minutes.
- Avoid exercises where balance is of major importance.
- In the latter part of pregnancy, avoid activities likely to cause joint strains.
- Avoid changing positions quickly (to avoid dizziness).
- Wear good supportive footwear and adequate breast support while exercising.

- Do not exercise to the point of exhaustion or severe breathlessness.
- Try not to sweat profusely during exercise or elevate body temperature too highly.
- Remember the importance of good nutrition.
- Monitor pulse rate and keep within the low end of the target heart rate range.
- Consult a health-care provider to discuss exercise plans.
- Consider reducing weight-bearing exercises like jogging and concentrating on non-weight-bearing exercises like swimming and cycling.
- Limit activity to shorter intervals than normal.
- Drink plenty of water.
- Stop exercising immediately if shortness of breath, dizziness, numbness, tingling, abdominal pain, or vaginal bleeding is experienced.

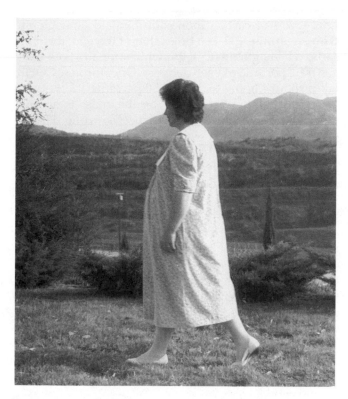

Figure 15.8 Regular brisk walking during pregnancy can improve the cardiorespiratory fitness level of the mother while posing no known harm to the fetus.

ners were treated at hospitals for dehydration, muscle spasms, cramps, and strains. This was but 2 months after Gabriella Anderson-Schiess had demonstrated to an onlooking world that hard exercise in the heat can be so very devastating. Obviously, the New York City marathoners chose to disregard this lesson.[126]

The problems of heat during exercise were discussed in Chapter 9. Hyperthermia and heat stroke are among the most serious complications associated with endurance exercise.[125] During heavy physical activity, especially on hot, humid days, large quantities of water can be lost through sweating. Early warning signals of possible heat injury include piloerection ("goosebumps") on the chest and upper arms, chilling, throbbing pressure in the head, unsteadiness, nausea, and dry skin. As body temperature rises, three major forms of heat injury become possibilities—heat cramps, heat exhaustion, and heat stroke.

Heat Cramps

Heat cramps involve muscular pains and spasms. First aid includes moving the victim to a cool place, having him lie down if he feels faint, and administering one or

two glasses of liquid with one-half teaspoon of salt added to each glass.

Heat Exhaustion

Heat exhaustion is characterized by fatigue, weakness, and collapse. There is profuse sweating, and the skin is often pale and clammy, while body temperature is usually close to normal. First aid includes moving the victim to the coolest possible place, removing clothing, and cooling (potentially with cold water applications, fans to create a draft, or ice packs). Care should be taken to avoid chilling the victim. He should be given saltwater (one teaspoon per glass), about half a glass every 15 minutes for one hour, and made to lie down and kept quiet.

Heat Stroke

Heat stroke is distinguished by extremely high body temperature and disturbance of the sweating mechanism. The skin is hot, red, and dry, the pulse is rapid and strong, and the victim may be unconscious. First aid includes moving the victim to a cool place, removing clothing, and cooling as fast as possible with all available means, including cold water, ice, fans, or rubbing alcohol. Speed is of the essence. Heat stroke is a life-threatening situation.

Measuring Temperature for Exercise Risk

The simplest measurement of environmental heat stress is the *wet bulb temperature* (WBT). It is obtained by putting a wick around the bulb of a thermometer, wetting it, and then blowing air by it with a fan to determine the effects of evaporation on the temperature reading. Since evaporation is effected by humidity, the WBT will help provide a guide to the degree of environmental stress. WBT of 78°F or higher require that exercise be postponed.

The *wet bulb globe temperature* (WGBT) consists of a dry bulb temperature reading, a wet bulb temperature reading, and a black globe temperature reading. The black globe, which is simply a thermometer placed with its bulb inside a copper toilet float painted black, measures the effect of radiant heat from the sun. All readings are taken in the open, allowing 30 minutes of exposure before readings are taken. To compute WBGT, the following formula is used:

$$WBGT\ (°F) = (0.7 \times wb) + (0.2 \times g) + (0.1 \times db)$$

wb = wet bulb temperature
g = globe temperature
db = dry bulb temperature (°F)

The following standards have been developed, designed primarily for mass participation runs:[125]

Below 64 WBGT—Low Risk
64–72 WBGT——Moderate Risk
73–82 WBGT——High Risk
+82 WBGT——Extremely High Risk

Environmental Pollution

Ozone

Air pollution adversely affects athletic performance.[127–137] During rest the average human ventilates only 6 liters of air per minute. During heavy exercise, women can ventilate 60 to 90 liters of air per minute, and males 100–130 liters of air per minute. Obviously, the dosage of air pollutants entering the body is increased, and exercise can exaggerate the normal pulmonary effects of air pollution.[133, 135]

There are two kinds of air pollutants—primary and secondary.[133] *Primary air pollutants* include carbon monoxide (CO), carbon dioxide (CO_2, sulfur dioxide (SO_2), nitrogen oxide (NO), and particulate material such as lead, graphite carbon, and fly ash. *Secondary air pollutants* are formed by the chemical action of the primary pollutants and the natural chemicals in the atmosphere. Examples include ozone (O_3), sulfuric acid (H_2SO_4), nitric acid (HNO_3), peroxyacetyl nitrate, and a host of other inorganic and organic compounds.

Ozone is produced by the photochemical reaction of sunlight and hydrocarbons and nitrogen dioxide from car exhaust.[136] Stage 1 alerts are called when ozone reaches 0.2 ppm, Stage 2 at 0.35 ppm. In the Los Angeles area, ozone levels reach 0.2 ppm levels for one hour or more on about 180 days per year.[135]

Ozone's toxicity is due to its action as an oxidant.[136] It is extremely reactive, affecting the pulmonary membranes. Ozone reacts rapidly and probably does not penetrate deeper than the mucosal surface. Symptoms include chest tightness, coughing, headache, dyspnea, nausea, throat irritation, and burning of the eyes.

Carbon monoxide is a tasteless, odorless, colorless gas, produced mainly during combustion of fossil fuels such as coal and gasoline. Cigarettes are also a source.

Low levels of carbon monoxide bind to hemoglobin with an affinity 100–200 times that of oxygen, forming carboxyhemoglobin (COHb), which impairs both oxygen transport and oxygen delivery. Once formed, COHb takes about 4 hours to decline 50 percent.

The pollutant regarded as the most toxic and detrimental to athletic performance is ozone. Heavy exercise in air polluted with ozone impairs the ability to exercise and reduces lung function, at least temporarily.[132, 134, 135] Statistically significant impairment of exercise performance can occur at 0.2 ppm. Individuals vary widely, however, in their response to ozone.[134] Reported subjective symptoms have included shortness of breath, coughing, excess sputum, raspy throat, and wheezing.

Interestingly, sensitivity to ozone has been found to diminish with repeated exposure.[127, 135, 137] Results show that by the end of four day periods of repeated exercise in polluted air, significant improvements are experienced in $\dot{V}O_{2max}$ and performance time, with decreased subjective symptoms.[137] Although habituation may benefit competitive performance, however, the long-term consequences of repeated exposures may be undesirable.

Other Pollutants

In one study, runners developed an average COHb level of five percent after only one-half hour of exercise in the heavy traffic of New York.[130] This is equivalent to the COHb that results from smoking one-half to one pack of cigarettes. Other studies have shown that maximal performance time is significantly reduced when the blood COHb level of nonsmokers exceeds 2.6 percent. $\dot{V}O_{2max}$ is affected at 4.3 percent, and is reduced linearly with increased levels of COHb from 5 percent to 35 percent.[129]

At rest, breathing air with 35 ppm CO for one hour is sufficient to produce a COHb of 1.5 percent; with 50 ppm CO, the COHb can rise to 5 percent in five hours. Those exercising heavily are at much greater risk. Levels of CO in traffic average about 37 ppm, but can rise to 54 ppm in heavy traffic and peak as high as 120 ppm at stop signals. These high levels may extend as far as 20 meters outward from the edge of the street. Joggers should avoid heavily traveled roadways, or stay at least 50–75 feet off to the side if possible.

Other air pollutants combined with ozone, such as nitrogen dioxide or sulphur dioxide, do not appear to reduce exercise performance. Peroxyacetyl nitrate, however, does appear to have an additive effect.[135]

Sudden Death from Heart Attack

Of all the potential problem areas associated with exercise, the one that has caused the most controversy is the effect on the heart.

The Saga of Jim Fixx

In northern Vermont, late on the afternoon of Friday, July 20, 1984, a passing motorcyclist discovered a man lying dead beside the road. He was clad only in shorts and running shoes. The man was Jim Fixx, author of *The Complete Book of Running*. This amazingly successful book had topped the bestseller lists for nearly two years, helping to accelerate the running boom of the late 1970s. Jim Fixx had become one of the leading spokesmen on the health benefits of running. Now he lay dead—with his running shoes on. And this is why so many Americans were disturbed. Jim Fixx died of cardiac arrest pounding the pavement to gain the fitness and health he advocated for all.[124, 138-140]

On autopsy, it was discovered that all of Jim Fixx's blood vessels were partially or nearly completely blocked from atherosclerotic plaque buildup. The left circumflex coronary artery was 98-percent occluded. How could a man in seemingly peak condition, having run 60–70 miles per week for over 12 years, be stricken by a disease most strongly associated with a sedentary life?

As a matter of fact, Jim Fixx, despite his running, was at extremely high risk for heart disease—yet he chose to ignore the warning signals. Jim's father had died of a heart attack at age 43. (Family history of heart disease, especially before the age of 55, is an extremely potent risk factor for it.) (See Chapter 10.)

Up to his mid-30s, Jim Fixx was smoking two packs of cigarettes per day, weighed 220 pounds, and had a high-stress, executive job. At age 35, he suddenly tried to turn his life around by running a lot of miles. He lost weight, and soon began racing marathons. He chose to continue his poor quality diet, however, and decided there was no need ever to see a doctor, even when experiencing heart disease warning signals such as throat and chest tightness. In addition, Jim Fixx was not handling at all well the strain, stress, and pressure of notoriety.

Seventeen years later Jim Fixx lay dead by the side of that Vermont back road, dead of a heart attack. Running may have lengthened his life a bit, but it probably ended up killing him as well.

The Magnitude of the Problem

Paralleling the boom in fitness activities has been an apparently disturbing number of sudden deaths (promptly reported by the media) during exercise.[141-148] (See Box 15.1.) The principal cause of death of adults during any form of exercise is coronary heart attack. In fact, however, these events are very rare.

Researchers have reported one death per 396,000 hours of jogging.[141, 147] A retrospective survey of the incidence of cardiovascular complications among participants at YMCA sports centers found one death per 2,897,057 person-hours and one nonfatal cardiac arrest per 2,253,267 person-hours.[141] For the cardiac patient population, the risk is higher, however. In surveys of cardiac rehabilitation programs, investigators have reported an average of one nonfatal and one fatal cardiovascular complication every 35,000–80,000 and 120,000–800,000 hours, respectively.[141]

Although sudden death during exercise is rare, exercise does increase the risk above normal. The risk of dying during exercise is seven times the risk for sedentary activities, and 17 times the risk of dying during the same time period by chance alone.[141, 142, 147]

However, most of the people who die during exercise (including young U.S. Air Force recruits, in one study) have some type of underlying heart disease.[142, 143, 145] In one study of 81 people who had died suddenly during exercise, 88 percent of them died because of underlying coronary artery disease.[147] Thirty-six cases of heart attack or sudden death in marathon runners have been reported in the world literature to date.[143] Seventy-one percent of them had had previous symptoms, but for the most part had ignored the symptoms and continued to train and race. Fifty percent of all cardiac events occurred either during or within 24 hours of competitive running events or long training runs.

Marathon runners, especially those with a family history of heart disease and/or other coronary risk factors, should not consider themselves immune to either sudden death or to coronary heart disease, but should seek medical advice immediately if they develop any symptoms suggestive of ischemic heart disease.

It has been found that unusual exercise (like shoveling snow after a storm) among those who were usually sedentary greatly increased their chances of dying of a sudden heart attack.[148] For those who were usually active, however, exercise proved in the study to be of more help than harm. Active people had a slightly elevated risk of sudden heart attack during any particular exercise session, but overall had a 60-percent reduced risk of fatal heart attack. (See Chapter 10.)

In other words, vigorous exercise is both a protector from and a provoker of sudden cardiac death. But any short-term risk of exercise is greatly outweighed by the long-term beneficial effects of exercise, especially for those who are habitually active. There remains, however, the important message that those at higher risk for heart disease need to be very careful.

Other Harmful Effects of Excessive Exercise

Sports Anemia

The problem of iron deficiency in athletes, especially runners, was fully discussed in Chapter 9. A substantial number of long distance runners have been found to have lower-than- optimal iron stores.[149-151] This may be due to increased loss of blood in the urine and stools, loss of iron in the sweat, decreased iron absorption in the intestinal tract, and/or the breakdown of red blood cells in the capillaries of the feet due to the pounding on hard surfaces. Some researchers feel that the flat, stale, leg-weary state that many competitive distance runners experience can be partially explained by low body iron stores.

Increased Risk of Infection

Much attention has been focused recently on stress, both physical and psychological, as a potent suppressor of the immune system.[152-180] Athletes training for long endurance events such as the marathon undergo repeated cycles of physical stress, sometimes accompanied by mental stress. Anecdotal information from coaches has reflected a concern about the risk of infection on the part of competitive endurance athletes.[163, 168, 175]

Research studies suggest that intense exertion, whether short-term and maximal[152-154, 156, 161-164, 169] or long-term and submaximal,[155, 158, 165, 166-168, 173, 176, 178, 179] may have harmful effects on the immune system and render athletes in hard training more susceptible to infections.[158, 166, 168] On the other hand, some researchers have suggested that moderate, submaximal exercise bouts[157, 159, 160, 163, 170] and long-term training[169, 170, 177] may enhance immunosurveillance, potentially decreasing the risk of infection.

A study of 2,300 Los Angeles Marathoners (Figure 15.9) showed that the odds of an upper respiratory tract infectious episode (cold, flu, sore throat) during the week following the race increased six-fold for those participating in the race.[166, 168] In another study, ten marathoners were exercised in a laboratory for 3 hours to exhaustion.[179] Cortisol, a known suppressant of the immune system, was elevated for about 1.5 hours following the run. During this time, natural killer cell activity was depressed, and many other immune system parameters demonstrated significant changes, lasting even to the next morning.

Exercise-Induced Bronchospasm

During and following strenuous exercise, 90–95 percent of asthmatics experience *exercise-induced bronchospasm* (EIB).[180-185] EIB is defined as a diffuse bronchospastic response in both large and small airways following

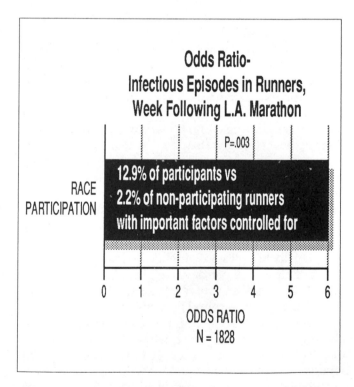

Figure 15.9 Participation in the Los Angeles marathon was associated with a six-fold increase in odds of an infectious episode, compared with similarly experienced runners who applied for but then did not run the race. *Source:* Nieman DC, Johansen LM, Lee JW. Cermak J, Arabatzis K: Infectious episodes in runners before and after the Los Angeles Marathon. Med Sci Sports Exerc 20:S42, 1988.

heavy exercise. Post-exercise symptoms include difficulty in breathing, coughing, shortness of breath, and wheezing. In the laboratory, EIB is often induced by exercising at 85 percent $\dot{V}O_{2max}$ for 5 to 8 minutes. It usually lasts 5 to 15 minutes, with a spontaneous resolution by 45–60 minutes post-exercise. A few asthmatics will have a late response 4–6 hours later, but this is uncommon.[183]

Asthma is a relatively common problem, affecting 5 to 10 percent of the adult population.[184] Although asthmatics are most susceptible to EIB, 30–35 percent of all other athletes with allergies are also prone to EIB symptoms.[182, 185]

The causes are still hotly debated.[180,181,184] In recent years, the humidity and temperature of air in the respiratory tract have become the focus of inquiry into the causes of EIB.[182, 185] Exercise, cold air, and fog may precipitate bronchospasms among those susceptible. The EIB response may be due to a cooling and drying of the mast cells in the air passageways, causing a release of chemicals that cause the bronchospasms.[180]

EIB can be controlled. A survey by the U.S. Olympic Committee and the American Academy of Allergy and Immunology found that 67 of 597 U.S. athletes in the 1984 summer games, or 11.2 percent, suffered from EIB.[182, 185] These athletes won 41 medals. EIB can be controlled by exercising in a warm, humid environment, exercising in repeated spurts of less than five minutes each, less than 40 minutes apart, breathing slowly through the nose, exercising at intensities below 85 percent $\dot{V}O_{2max}$, and using appropriate medications. Table 15.1 summarizes the medications that have been approved by the International Olympic Committee for managing EIB.[182]

Gastrointestinal Problems

Gastrointestinal (GI) symptoms are very common among athletes; they are bothersome, but usually not serious.[186–189] Precipitating or aggravating factors include intensity of exercise, anxiety, recentness of meals, and the ingestion of specific foods or drinks such as high-fiber foods, coffee, and orange juice. Women have reported an increased risk of abdominal cramps when exercising during their menses. Swimming and cycling have been reported to caused remarkably few GI symptoms compared to running.

Recent reports have shown that blood can appear in the urine and stool following intense exercise.[187–190] The source of the blood is not yet known, but may include bleeding from the kidney or bladder, and bleeding from the stomach or GI tract walls from GI tract wall infections, the use of aspirin or other drugs, or the stress of exercise, especially running. More research is needed to establish the reasons for the bleeding. Eating a precompetition meal low in dietary fiber 3 to 4 hours prior to the event may help avoid some of the GI tract problems.[186]

Exercise Principles to Lessen Risks

The saga of Jim Fixx points out two crucial lessons for the rest of us. First of all, running is not a panacea.

Table 15.1 Medications That Have Been Approved by the International Olympic Committee for Managing EIB

Medication	When to Take Before Exercise	Duration of Effect
Inhaled beta-adrenergic agents (not oral) such as Albuterol	10–20 min before	4–6 hr
Terbutaline, metaproterenol	5–10 min before	2–4 hr
Cromolyn sodium	20 min before	1–2 hr
Theophylline		
(Short-acting)	30 min before	2–4 hr
(Long-acting)	1-2 hr before	4–6 hr

Medications not allowed by the IOC for EIB are: inhaled epinephrine (Primatene Mist), isoproterenol, isoetharine, and decongestants (eg, ephedrine, pseudoephedrine, phenylephrine, phenylpropanolamine). *Source:* Katz RM. Coping With Exercise-Induced Asthma In Sports. Physician Sportsmed 15(7):101-108, 1987.

Running or any type of exercise cannot in isolation produce good health. Exercise is only one factor of many conducive to wellness, and must be combined with others, including stress management, a low-fat, high complex-carbohydrate diet, regular medical check-ups, and the avoidance of smoking.

Secondly, while no worthwhile human endeavor is totally free of risks, they can be minimized. In regard to exercise, this means seeing a doctor, and having a treadmill-EKG test before starting a vigorous exercise program, especially when one is at high risk. (See Chapter 3.) The typical risk factors include smoking, hypertension, high blood cholesterol, obesity, stress, family history, diabetes, and age.

Another key exercise safety principle is to start at a low-intensity level and progress gradually. For most, this means a walking program. An exercise rule-of-thumb is that one should not even think of jogging until three miles can be walked in under 45 minutes.

The common exercise termination signals should be respected. These include feeling abnormal heart beats (irregular fluttering), pain or pressure in the center of the chest, dizziness, lightheadedness, nausea or vomiting during or after exercise, extreme breathlessness continuing after exercise, musculoskeletal pains, or prolonged fatigue and insomnia.

The prevention of musculoskeletal injuries revolves around several principles:

- Stretching the major joints after every exercise session.

- Engaging in muscle strengthening exercises in combination with aerobic exercise to keep all muscles in balance. (Investigations to date suggest that weight training can aid in injury prevention.)[191]

- Warming-up and warming-down with slow aerobics before and after each hard aerobic session.

- Using proper equipment. Most important are shoes. The runner should pay $30–$50 for a good pair of shoes from a sports store that has qualified personnel to help individualize the shoe selection. Aerobic dancers can now purchase shoes especially made for the demands of that sport, with more ball-of-the-foot cushioning, and more leather in the uppers for side-to-side support.[192] Aerobic dancers should avoid concrete floors that are not well padded and carpeted, or seek out facilities with suspended wood floors.

- Gradual progression and moderation are essential. As discussed previously, one of the most important causes of musculoskeletal injuries is over-use, especially from sudden increases in mileage or exercise intensity and time.[193] Beginning exercisers should always err on the side of too little exercise rather than too much. Aerobic dance instructors are often overzealous. Seek out instructors with proper certification and an ability to adapt for slower members of the group.

- Obtain proper rest along with the exercise. Exercise plus rest equals fitness. Exercise tends to tear down, rest builds up.

- Exercise technique is important. When running, the body should be in an upright position, the arms at a 90-degree angle, swinging from the shoulder. The feet should land almost flatfooted with the weight well back toward the heel. (Do not run on the ball of the foot.) Breathing should be through the mouth and nose in a regular fashion. Overall, the body should be loose, natural, and poised. During aerobic dancing, try to avoid too much jumping up and down on the ball of the foot until your musculoskeletal system has strengthened. Substitute walking in place for jumping in place whenever possible.

All of the exercise risks, however, must be put into their proper perspective. Not exercising at all is worse than too much exercise, while moderate exercise is a virtue. The well-documented benefits of moderate exercise are too valuable to be neglected. (See Sports Medicine Insight.)

Figure 15.10 attempts to summarize the risks vs. the benefits of exercise.[5] The greatest gain in the risk-benefit relationship occurs at the lower end of the activity spectrum. In other words, the greatest benefits of exercise are gained by previously sedentary people just beginning moderate exercise programs. Risks are low at the lower levels of activity, but become increasingly more frequent and severe at higher levels. Thus such activities as brisk walking are highly recommended, producing many benefits with few risks.

Sports Medicine Insight
Risks Versus Benefits— A Summary

Broad claims have been made regarding the health benefits of physical activity—but claiming too much can ruin the message.[194] Many of the benefit claims are not supported by all researchers. In addition, benefits must be balanced against the risks, which rise exponentially with excessive exercise.

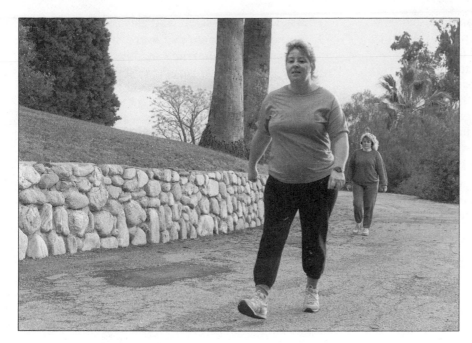

Figure 15.10 The increase in benefits from regular exercise are greatest at low levels and diminish with increasing activity. Risks, on the other hand, are less at lower levels, and become increasingly more frequent and severe at higher levels. *Source:* Powell KE, Paffenbarger RS. Workshop on Epidemiologic and Public Health Aspects of Physical Activity: A Summary. Public Health Rep 100:118–126, 1985.

Table 15.2 is a summary of the major benefits of exercise described in Chapters 10 through 14, balanced against the potential risks outlined in this chapter. The summary represents the author's evaluation of present evidence and published data. The "surety rating" is an estimate of the strength of the data, using the following point rating system:

> 0 = data do not support this viewpoint
> 1+ = most data are supportive, but many reports do not support the claim
> 2+ = established consensus with little or no conflicting data

Summary

1. This chapter surveyed some of the risks involved with exercise, especially when performed excessively. These include musculoskeletal injuries, disruption of normal reproductive function of women, possible problems for women who are pregnant, heat injury, effects of air pollution on performance, sudden death from heart attack, sports anemia, increased risk of infectious episodes, exercise-induced bronchospasm, and gastrointestinal problems.

2. The musculoskeletal injury potential was reviewed for running, aerobic dance, bicycling, and swimming. Most of the injuries are related to overtraining and accidents. The muscles,

joints, and supporting ligaments and tendons of the legs and feet respond very poorly to excessive exercise, especially activities that require running and jumping.

3. Running is associated with a high rate of musculoskeletal injuries, with 35 to 60 percent of runners reporting injuries within a given year. Although most of the runners usually don't seek medical help, the pain is frequently serious enough to disrupt the running routine.

4. Researchers have tried to measure the factors responsible for the high prevalence of injuries among runners. Three important factors are improper training techniques, poor equipment, and biomechanical/anthropometric abnormalities.

5. The major studies examining the injury potential of aerobic dance have found that about 45 percent of students and 75 percent of instructors report injuries. Most of these injuries, however, are mild, causing some pain and some disruption in participation, but generally falling short of leading participants to cease aerobic dance activities or seek professional medical assistance.

6. Evidence to date indicates that many years of high mileage running are not associated with premature degeneration of the joints or osteoarthritis

7. There are two types of muscle soreness, acute and delayed. Acute soreness occurs during and immediately following exercise. Delayed soreness (DOMS) occurs from 1 to 5 days following unaccustomed or severe exercise. DOMS is most likely caused by structural damage to skeletal muscle after eccentric exercise. Once the membrane is injured, cell contents leak out and extracellular components leak in. Muscle pain and weakness ensue.

8. Treatment of musculoskeletal pain and injury during the first 48 to 72 hours centers around rest, ice, compression, and elevation (R.I.C.E.).

9. Studies have shown that exercise increases the rates of oligomenorrhea and amenorrhea; they vary widely, however, depending on the type of athlete and the amount of training. The causes are still hotly debated. Loss of bone mineral mass is a problem for oligoamenorrheic athletes.

10. Exercise during pregnancy serves to increase the fitness of the mother, but its influence on fetal development is uncertain. Pregnant women should err on the side of moderation until more is known.

Table 15.2 Health Benefits and Risk of Aerobic Physical Activity

Benefit	Surety Rating	Risk	Surety Rating
Cardiorespiratory System			
Improved functional capacity ($\dot{V}O_{2max}$), ventilation, cardiac output, etc.)	2+		
Heart Disease and Risk Factors			
Control of BP in hypertensives	2+	Cardiac arrest for those at high risk	2+
Prevention of hypertension	1+		
Improved lipoprotein profile	2+		
Smoking cessation/prevention	1+		
Prevention of heart disease	2+		
Cardiac rehab—improved life quality	2+		
Obesity			
Prevention of obesity	1+	Musculoskeletal injury	1+
Treatment of obesity	1+		
Increase in BMR after fitness session	1+		
Decrease in appetite, short term only	1+		
Increase in TEF with exercise prior to or after meal	1+		
Psychological			
Elevation in mood	2+	Exercise addiction	1+
Decrease in anxiety	2+	Mood disturbance with excessive increases in training	1+
Decrease in depression	2+		
Increase in self-concept	2+		
Improved mental cognition, short-term	1+		
Improved sleep	0		
Decrease in substance abuse (OH, drugs)	0		
Musculoskeletal			
Prevention of bone mineral loss	1+	Injury with overuse	2+
Treatment of osteoporosis	1+	Osteopenia among women, oligoamenorrhea	2+
		Increased osteoarthritis with long years of training	0

0 = data do not support this viewpoint; 1+ = most data are supportive, but many reports do not support the claim; 2+ = established consensus with little or no conflicting data

(Continued)

Table 15.2 Health Benefits and Risk of Aerobic Physical Activity (Continued)

Benefit	Surety Rating	Risk	Surety Rating
Nutrition			
Improves quality of diet	0	Vitamin/mineral deficiency	0
		Iron deficiency with excessive exercise	1+
Diabetes			
Improved glycemic control Type I + II	2+	Hypoglycemia in uncontrolled Type I	2+
Prevention of Type II	0		
Cancer			
Prevention of bowel cancer	1+		
Increased colonic motility	1+		
Immune System			
Moderate exercise improves immune function	1+	Excessive exercise depresses immune function	1+
		Excessive exercise increases risk of infectious episode	1+
Hormonal Reproduction			
Moderate exercise, increased libido	0	Excessive exercise, decreased libido	1+
Healthier baby from pregnant women who exercise regularly during gestation	0	Exessive exercise, oligoamenorrhea	2+
Increased cardiorespiratory fitness of pregnant women who train during gestation	2+	Risk to fetus of pregnant woman who trains heavily	1+
Environment			
Heat acclimatization	2+	Heat injury in hot, humid weather	2+
		Decreased performance with ozone 0.20 ppm	2+
Aging			
Improved functional capacity of elderly	2+		
Lengthens life expectancy by reducing risk of chronic disease	2+		
Lengthens life-span	0		

0 = data do not support this viewpoint; 1+ = most data are supportive, but many reports do not support the claim; 2+ = established consensus with little or no conflicting data

11. The American College of Sports Medicine has advised athletes that the risk of heat exhaustion and heat stroke during high temperature and humidity is greatly increased. Heat injury is a major cause of death among exercising athletes, and appropriate measures should be taken, including postponing the exercise.

12. The air pollutant regarded as the most detrimental to athletic performance is ozone. Heavy exercise in air polluted with ozone has been shown to impair the ability to exercise and decrease lung function at least temporarily. Other air pollutants appear to have little relative effect.

13. The principal cause of death among adults during exercise is coronary heart attack. It happens rarely however, and more often to those with underlying heart disease.

14. Excessive exercise has been associated with increased risk of infectious health problems. Moderate exercise may be protective, but little research has been conducted so far to verify this.

15. During and following strenuous exercise, the majority of asthmatics experience exercise-induced bronchospasm (EIB). EIB can be controlled with appropriate medications and exercise techniques.

16. Gastrointestinal symptoms among athletes, especially runners, are very common and bothersome, but are usually not serious.

17. Important principles for minimizing exercise associated risks include undergoing proper screening procedures, progressing gradually, obeying exercise termination signals, and following prevention principles.

18. The risks of exercise must be balanced with all of its documented benefits. The greatest gain in the risk-benefit relationship occurs at the lower end of the activity spectrum.

References

1. Runner's World. Who Is The American Runner. Runner's World, August, 1984.

2. Stephens T. Secular Trends in Adult Physical Activity: Exercise Boom or Bust? Res Quart Exerc Sport 58:94–105, 1987.

3. New York by Numbers. Runner's World, November, 1988, p 58.

4. Koplan JP, et al. An Epidemiologic Study of the Benefits and Risks of Running. JAMA 248:3118–3121, 1982.

5. Koplan JP, et al. The Risks of Exercise: A Public Health View of Injuries and Hazards. Public Health Rep 100:189–195, 1985.

6. Powell KE, Kohl HW, Caspersen CJ, Blair SN. An Epidemiological Perspective on the Causes of Running Injuries. Physician Sportsmed 14(6):100–114, 1986.

7. Marti B, Vader JP, Minder CE, Abelin T. On the Epidemiology of Running Injuries. Am J Sports Med 16:285–294, 1988.

8. Marti B. Benefits and Risks of Running Among Women: An Epidemiologic Study. Int J Sports Med 9:92–98, 1988.

9. Jacobs SJ, Berson BL. Injuries to Runners. A Study of Entrants to a 10,000 Meter Race. Am J Sports Med 14:151–155, 1986.

10. Walter SD, Hart LE, Sutton JR, et al. Training Habits and Injury Experience in Distance Runners: Age-and Sex-Related Factors. Physician Sportsmed 16(6):101–113, 1988.

11. Pagliano JW, Jackson DW. A Clinical Study of 3,000 Long-Distance Runners. Ann Sports Med 3:88–91, 1987.

12. Lysholm J, Wiklander J. Injuries in Runners. Am J Sports Med 15:168–168, 1987.

13. Blair SN, Kohl HW, Goodyear NN. Rates and Risks for Running and Exercise Injuries: Studies in Three Populations. Res Quart Exerc Sport 58:221–228, 1987.

14. Ireland ML, Micheli LJ. Triathletes: Biographic Data, Training, and Injury Patterns. Ann Sports Med 3:117–120, 1987.

15. Messier SP, Pittala KA. Etiologic Factors Associated with Selected Running Injuries. Med Sci Sports Exerc 20:501–505, 1988.

16. Ekstrand J, Gillquist J. The Frequency of Muscle Tightness and Injuries in Soccer Players. Am J Sports Med 10:75–78, 1982.

17. Pretorius DM, Noakes TD, Irving G, Allerton K. Runner's Knee: What Is It and How Effective Is Conservative Management? Physician Sportsmed 14(12):71–81, 1986.

18. Robbins SE, Hanna AM. Running-Related Injury Prevention Through Barefoot Adaptations. Med Sci Sports Exerc 19:148–156, 1987.

19. Kuipers H, Keizer HA. Overtraining in Elite Athletes: Review and Directions for the Future. Sports Med 6:79–92, 1988.

20. Newell SG, Bramwell ST. Overuse Injuries to the Knee in Runners. Physician Sportsmed 12:79–92, 1984.

21. Percy EC, Strother RT. Patellalgia. Physician Sportsmed 13:43–58, 1985.

22. Grana WA, Coniglione TC. Knee Disorders in Runners. Physician Sportsmed 13:127–133, 1985.

23. Tidus PM, Ianuzzo CD. Effects of Intensity and Duration of Muscular Exercise On Delayed Soreness and Serum Enzyme Activities. Med Sci Sports Exerc 15:461–465, 1983.

24. Pollock ML. How Much Exercise Is Enough? Physician Sportsmed 6: 1978.

25. Pollock ML, et al. Effects of Frequency and Duration of Training On Attrition and Incidence of Injury. Med Sci Sports Exerc 9:31–36, 1977.

26. Wolfe MD. Avoiding Aerobics Injuries. Athletic Business, March 1985, pp. 10–16.

27. Garrick JG, Requa RK. Aerobic Dance: A Review. Sports Med 6:169–179, 1988.

28. Garrick JG, Gillien DM. A Prospective Study of Aerobic Dance Injuries. Corporate Fitness and Recreation, June 1986, pp 29–32.

29. Garrick JG, Gillien DM, Whiteside P: The Epidemic of Aerobic Dance Injuries. Am J Sports Med 14:67–72, 1986.

30. Rothenberger LA, Chang JI, Cable TA. Prevalence and Types of Injuries in Aerobic Dancers. Am J Sports Med 16:403–407, 1988.

31. Mutoh Y, Sawai S, Takanashi Y, Skurko L. Aerobic Dance Injuries Among Instructors and Students. Physician Sportsmed 16:81–88, 1988.

32. Priest NN, Priest PW. Low-Impact Aerobics. Corporate Fitness and Recreation, June-July 1986, pp. 19–21.

33. Koszuta LE. Low-Impact Aerobics: Better Than Traditional Aerobic Dance? Physician Sportsmed 14(7):156–161, 1986.

34. Richie DH, Kelso SF, Bellucci PA. Aerobic Dance Injuries: A Retrospective Study of Instructors and Participants. Physician Sportsmed 13:130–140, 1985.

35. Wasserman RC, Waller JA, Monty MJ, Emergy AB, Robinson DR. Bicyclists, Helmets and Head Injuries: A Rider-Based Study of Helmet Use and Effectiveness. Am J Public Health 78:1220–1221, 1988.

36. Weiss BD, Duncan B. Bicycle Helmet Use by Children: Knowledge and Behavior of Physicians. Am J Public Health 76:1022–1023, 1986.

37. Kraus JF, Fife D, Conroy C. Incidence, Severity, and Outcomes of Brain Injuries Involving Bicycles. Am J Public Health 77:76–78, 1987.

38. Ward A. Improving Bicycle Safety for Children. Physician Sportsmed 15(6):203–208, 1987.

39. Watts CK, Jones D, Crouch D, et al. Survey of Bicycling Accidents in Boulder, Colorado. Physician Sportsmed 14(3):99–104, 1986.

40. Kiburz D, Jacobs R, Reckling F, Mason J. Bicycle Accidents and Injuries Among Adult Cyclists. Am J Sports Med 14:416, 1986.

41. Selbst SM, Alexander D, Ruddy R. Bicycle-Related Injuries. Am J Dis Child 141:140–144, 1987.

42. Johnson JE, Sim FH, Scott SG. Musculoskeletal Injuries in Competitive Swimmers. Mayo Clin Proc 62:289–304, 1987.

43. Lane NE, Bloch DA, Wood PD, Fries JF. Aging, Long-Distance Running, and the Development of Musculoskeletal Disability. Am J Med 82:772–780, 1987.

44. Lane NE, Block DA, Jones HH, et al. Long-Distance Running, Bone Density, and Osteoarthritis. JAMA 255:1147–1151, 1986.

45. Panush RS, Schmidt C, Caldwell JP, et al. Is Running Associated With Degenerative Joint Disease? JAMA 255:1152–1154, 1986.

46. Rowland TW, Walsh CA. Characteristics of Child Distance Runners. Physician Sportsmed 13:45–53, 1985.

47. Micheli LJ, Micheli ER. Children's Running: Special Risks? Ann Sports Med 2:61–63, 1985.

48. Caine DJ, Lindner KJ. Overuse Injuries of Growing Bones: The Young Female Gymnast at Risk? Physician Sportsmed 13:51–64, 1985.

49. Milne CJ. Rhabdomyolysis, Myoglobinuria and Exercise. Sports Med 6:93–106, 1988.

50. Armstrong RB. Muscle Damage and Endurance Events. Sports Med 3:370–381, 1986.

51. Armstrong RB. Mechanisms of Exercise-Induced Delayed Onset Muscular Soreness: A Brief Review. Med Sci Sports Exerc 16:529–538, 1984.

52. Schwane JA, et al. Delayed-Onset Muscular Soreness and Plasma CPK and LDH Activities From Downhill Running. Med Sci Sports Exerc 15:51–56, 1983.

53. Evans WJ. Exercise-Induced Skeletal Muscle Damage. Physician Sportsmed 15(1):89–100, 1987.

54. Hagerman FC, et al. Muscle Damage in Marathon Runners. Physician Sportsmed 12:39–48, 1984.

55. Dressendorfer RH, Wade CE. The Muscular Overuse Syndrome in Long-Distance Runners. Physician Sportsmed 11:116–126, 1983.

56. Farber H, Arbetter J, Schaefer E, et al. Acute Metabolic Effects of An Endurance Triathlon. Ann Sports Med 3:131–138, 1987.

57. Eichner R. A Little Drop Will Do You. Runner's World, August 1987, pp 43–47.

58. Noakes TD. Effect of Exercise on Serum Enzyme Activities in Humans. Sports Med 4:245–267, 1987.

59. Schwane JA, Williams JS, Sloan JH. Effects of Training on Delayed Muscle Soreness and Serum Creatine Kinase Activity After Running. Med Sci Sports Exerc 19:584–590, 1987.

60. Stauber WT, Fritz VK, Vogelbach DW, Dahlmann B. Characterization of Muscles Injured by Forced Lengthening. I. Cellular Infiltrates. Med Sci Sports Exerc 20:345–353, 1988.

61. Clarkson PM, Tremblay I. Exercise-Induced Muscle Damage, Repair, and Adaptation in Humans. J Appl Physiol 65:1–6, 1988.

62. Knight KL, Londeree BR. Comparison of Blood Flow in the Ankle of Uninjured Subjects During Therapeutic Applications of Heat, Cold, and Exercise. Med Sci Sports Exerc 12:76–80, 1980.

63. Wilkerson GB. External Compression for Controlling Traumatic Edema. Physician Sportsmed 13:97–106, 1985.

64. Kellett J. Acute Soft Tissue Injuries—A Review of the Literature. Med Sci Sports Exerc 18:489–500, 1986.

65. Meeusen R, Lievens P. The Use of Cryotherapy in Sports Injuries. Sports Med 3:398–414, 1986.

66. Bonen A, Keizer HA. Athletic Menstrual Cycle Irregularity: Endocrine Response to Exercise and Training. Physician Sportsmed 12:78–94, 1984.

67. Bullen BA, et al. Induction of Menstrual Disorders By Strenuous Exercise In Untrained Women. N Eng J Med 312:1349–53, 1985.

68. Calabrese LH, et al. Menstrual Abnormalities, Nutritional Patterns, and Body Composition in Female Classical Ballet Dancers. Physician Sportsmed 11:86–98, 1983.

69. Highet R. Athletic Amenorrhea. Sports Med 7:82–108, 1989.

70. Lutter JM, Cushman S. Menstrual Patterns in Female Runners. Physician Sportsmed 10:60–72, 1982.

71. Loucks AB, Horvath SM. Athletic Amenorrhea: A Review. Med Sci Sports Exerc 17:56–72, 1985.

72. Prior JC, Vigna Y. The Short Luteal Phase: A Cycle in Transition. Contemporary OB/GYN: The Active Woman. May 1985, pp. 167–177.

73. Stager JM, et al. Delayed Menarche in Swimmers in Relation to Age at Onset of Training and Athletic Performance. Med Sci Sports Exerc 16:550–555, 1984.

74. Shangold MM. Cause, Evaluation, and Management of Athletic Oligo-/Amenorrhea. Med Clinics N Amer 69:83–95, 1985.

75. Lloyd T, Triantafyllou SJ, Baker ER, et al. Women Athletes With Menstrual Irregularity Have Increased Musculoskeletal Injuries. Med Sci Sports Exerc 18:374–379, 1986.

76. Brooks-Gunn J, Warren WP, Hamilton LH. The Relation of Eating Problems and Amenorrhea in Ballet Dancers. Med Sci Sports Exerc 19:41–44, 1987.

77. Barrow GW, Saha S. Menstrual Irregularity and Stress Fractures in Collegiate Female Distance Runners. Am J Sports Med 16:209–216, 1988.

78. Stager JM, Hatler LK. Menarche in Athletes: The Influence of Genetics and Prepubertal Training. Med Sci Sports Exerc 20:369–373, 1988.

79. Nelson ME, Fisher EC, Catsos PD, et al. Diet and Bone Status in Amenorrheic Runners. Am J Clin Nutr 43:910–916, 1986.

80. Deuster PA, Kyle SB, Moser PB, et al. Nutritional Intakes and Status of Highly Trained Amenorrheic and Eumenorrheic Women Runners. Fertil Steril 46:636–643, 1986.

81. Shangold MM. How I Manage Exercise-Related Menstrual Disturbances. Physician Sportsmed 14(3):113–120, 1986.

82. Sanborn CF, Albrecht BH, Wagner WW. Athletic Amenorrhea: Lack of Association With Body Fat. Med Sci Sports Exerc 19:207–212, 1987.

83. Weight LM, Noakes TD. Is Running an Analog of Anorexia?: A Survey of the Incidence of Eating Disorders in Female Distance Runners. Med Sci Sports Exerc 19:213–217, 1987.

84. Cook SD, Harding AF, Thomas KA, et al. Trabecular Bone Density and Menstrual Function in Women Runners. Am J Sports Med 15:503–507, 1987.

85. Lloyd T, Buchanan JR, Bitzer S, et al. Interrelationships of Diet, Athletic Activity, Menstrual Status, and Bone Density in Collegiate Women. Am J Clin Nutr 46:681–684, 1987.

86. Ding J, Sheckter CB, Drinkwater BL, et al. High Serum Cortisol Levels in Exercise-Associated Amenorrhea. Ann Int Med 108:530–534, 1988.

87. Hohtari H, Elovainio R, Salminen K, Laatikainen T. Plasma Corticotropin-Releasing Hormone, Corticotropin, and Endorphins at Rest and During Exercise in Eumenorrheic and Amenorrheic Athletes. Fertil Steril 50:233–238, 1988.

88. Toriola AL. Survey of Menstrual Function in Young Nigerian Athletes. Int J Sports Med 9:29–34, 1988.

89. Loucks AB; Horvath SM. Exercise-Induced Stress Responses of Amenorrheic and Eumenorrheic Runners. J Clin Endocrinol Metab 59:1109–1120, 1984.

90. Stager JM. Amenorrhea in Athletes. Sports Med 1:337–340, 1984.

91. Lindberg JS, Powell MR, Hunt MM, et al. Increased Vertebral Bone Mineral in Response to Reduced Exercise in Amenorrheic Runners. West J Med 146:39–42, 1987.

92. Drinkwater BL, Nilson K, Ott S, Chesnut CH. Bone Mineral Density After Resumption of Menses in Amenorrheic Athletes. JAMA 256:380–382, 1986.

93. Drinkwater BL, et al. Bone Mineral Content of Amenorrheic and Eumenorrheic Athletes. N Eng J Med 311:277–281, 1984.

94. Cumming DC, Wheeler GD, McColl EM. The Effects of Exercise on Reproductive Function in Men. Sports Med 7:1–17, 1989.

95. Hackney AC, Sinning WE, Bruot BC. Reproductive Hormonal Profiles of Endurance-Trained and Untrained Males. Med Sci Sports Exerc 20:60–65, 1988.

96. Rigotti NA, Neer RM, Jameson L. Osteopenia and Bone Fractures in a Man With Anorexia Nervosa and Hypogonadism. JAMA 256:385–388, 1986.

97. Wheeler GD, et al. Reduced Serum Testosterone and Prolactin Levels in Male Distance Runners. JAMA 252:514–516, 1984.

98. Artal R, et al. Fetal Bradycardia Induced By Maternal Exercise. Lancet, August 4, 1984, pp. 258–260.

99. Barman MR. Readers' Advice to Their Patients. Contemporary OB/GYN: Active Woman. May 1985, pp. 27–31.

100. Botti JJ, Jones RL. Aerobic Conditioning, Nutrition, and Pregnancy. ClinNutr 4:14–17, 1985.

101. Clapp JF, Dickstein S. Endurance Exercise and Pregnancy Outcome. Med Sci Sports Exerc 16:556–562, 1984.

102. Jopke T. Pregnancy: A Time to Exercise Judgment. Physician Sportsmed 11:139–148, 1983.

103. Jovanovic L, et al. Human Maternal and Fetal Response to Graded Exercise. J Appl Physiol 58:1719–1722, 1985.

104. Maeder EC. Effects of Sports and Exercise In Pregnancy. Postgrad Med 77:112–114, 1985.

105. Massey JB. Reproductive Effects of Aerobic Exercise In Women. J Med Assoc Georgia 73:457–459, 1984.

106. Paolone AM, Worthington S. Cautions and Advice On Exercise During Pregnancy. Contemporary OB/GYN: Active Woman. May 1985, pp. 150–164.

107. Treadway J, Dover EV, Morse W, et al. Influence of Exercise Training on Maternal and Fetal Morphological Characteristics in the Rat. J Appl Physiol 60:1700–1703, 1986.

108. Morton MJ, Paul MS, Metcalfe J. Exercise During Pregnancy. Med Clin North Am 69:97–107, 1985.

109. Gauthier MM. Guidelines for Exercise During Pregnancy: Too Little or Too Much? Physician Sportsmed 14(4):162–169, 1986.

110. Artal R, Wiswell RA. Exercise in Pregnancy. Los Angeles: Williams & Wilkins, 1986.

111. American College of Obstetricians and Gynecologists. Exercise During Pregnancy and the Postnatal Period (ACOG Home Exercise Programs). Washington, D.C.: ACOG, 1985.

112. Garris DR, Kasperek GJ, Overton SV, Alligood GR. Effects of Exercise on Fetal-Placental Growth and Uteroplacental Blood Flow in the Rat. Biol Neonate 47:223–229, 1985.

113. Carpenter MW, Sady SP, Hoegsberg B, Sady MA, et al. Fetal Heart Rate Response to Maternal Exertion. JAMA 259:3006–3009, 1988.

114. Wong SC, McKenzie DC. Cardiorespiratory Fitness During Pregnancy and Its Effect on Outcome. Int J Sports Med 8:79–83, 1987.

115. Kulpa PJ, White BM, Visscher R. Aerobic Exercise in Pregnancy. Am J Obstet Gynecol 156:1395–1403, 1987.

116. Rauramo I, Forss M. Effect of Exercise on Maternal Hemodynamics and Placental Blood Flow in Healthy Women. Acta Obstet Gynecol Scand 67:21–25, 1988.

117. Yates CY, Boylan LM, Lewis RD, Driskell JA. Maternal Aerobic Exercise and Vitamin B-6 Status. Am J Clin Nutr 48:117–121, 1988.

118. Moore DH, Jarrett JC, Bendick PJ. Exercise-Induced Changes in Uterine Artery Blood Flow, As Measured by Doppler Ultrasound, In Pregnant Subjects. Am J Perinatol 5:94–97, 1988.

119. Steegers EA, Buunk G, Binkhorst RA, Jongsma HW, et al. The Influence of Maternal Exercise on the Uteroplacental Vascular Bed Resistance and the Fetal Heart Rate During Normal Pregnancy. Eur J Obstet Gynecol Reprod Biol 27(1):21–26, 1988.

120. South-Paul JE, Rajagopal KR, Tenholder MF. The Effect of Participation in a Regular Exercise Program Upon Aerobic Capacity During Pregnancy. Obstet Gynecol 71(2):175–179, 1988.

121. Wallace AM, Engstrom JL. The Effects of Aerobic Exercise on the Pregnant Woman, Fetus, and Pregnancy Outcome. J Nurse-Midwifery 32(5):277–290, 1987.

122. Nesler CL, Hassett SL, Cary S, Brooke J. Effects of Supine Exercise on Fetal Heart Rate in the Second and Third Trimesters. Am J Perinatol 5:159–163, 1988.

123. Paolone AM, Shangold M, Paul D, et al. Fetal Heart Rate Measurement During Maternal Exercise—Avoidance of Artifact. Med Sci Sports Exerc 19:605–609, 1987.

124. Maranto G. Exercise: How Much Is Too Much? Discover, October, 1984.

125. American College of Sports Medicine. Position Stand on Prevention of Thermal Injuries During Distance Running. Med Sci Sports Exerc 16: 1984.

126. Ryan AJ. NYC Marathon: Should It Have Been Stopped? Physician Sportsmed 12:23, 1984.

127. Goldstein E. Photochemical Air Pollution, Part II. West J Med 142:523–531, 1985.

128. Hage P. Air Pollution: Adverse Effects On Athletic Performance. Physician Sportsmed 10:126–132, 1982.

129. Klausen K, Anderson C, Nandrup. Acute Effects of Cigarette Smoking and Inhalation of Carbon Monoxide During Maximal Exercise. Eur J Appl Physiol 51:371–379, 1983.

130. Nicholson JP, Case DB. Carboxyhemoglobin Levels in New York City Runners. Physician Sportsmed 11:135–138, 1983.

131. Rogers CC. The Los Angeles Olympic Games: Effects of Pollution Unclear. Physician Sportsmed 12:172–183, 1984.

132. Folinsbee LJ, et al. Pulmonary Function Changes After 1 H Continuous Heavy Exercise in 0.21 PPM Ozone. J Appl Physiol 57:984–988, 1984.

133. Pierson WE, Covert DS, Koenig JQ, et al. Implications of Air Pollution Effects on Athletic Performance. Med Sci Sports Exerc 18:322–327, 1986.

134. Schelegle ES, Adams WC. Reduced Exercise Time in Competitive Simulations Consequent to Low Level Ozone Exposure. Med Sci Sports Exerc 18:408–414, 1986.

135. Adams WC. Effects of Ozone Exposure at Ambient Air Pollution Episode Levels on Exercise Performance. Sports Med 4:395–424, 1987.

136. Lippmann M. Effects of Ozone on Respiratory Function and Structure. Annu Rev Public Health 10:49–67, 1989.

137. Foxcroft WJ, Adams WC. Effects of Ozone Exposure On Four Consecutive Days On Work Performance and VO_2 max. J Appl Physiol 61:960–966, 1986.

138. Higdon H. Jim Fixx: How He Lived, Why He Died. The Runner, November, 1984.

139. Van Camp, SP. The Fixx Tragedy: A Cardiologist's Perspective. Physician Sportsmed 12:153–155, 1984.

140. Cooper KH. Running Without Fear. New York: Bantam Books, 1985.

141. Franklin BA. Safety of Outpatient Cardiac Exercise Therapy: Reducing the Incidence of Complications. Physician Sportsmed 14(9):235–248, 1986.

142. Phillips M, Robinowitz M, Higgins JR, et al. Sudden Cardiac Death in Air Force Recruits. JAMA 256:2696–2699, 1986.

143. Noakes TD. Heart Disease in Marathon Runners: A Review. Med Sci Sports Exerc 19:187–194, 1987.

144. Kark JA, Posey DM, Schumacher HR, et al. Sickle Cell Trait as a Risk Factor for Sudden Death in Physical Training. N Engl J Med 317:781–787, 1987.

145. Van Camp SP. Exercise-Related Sudden Death: Risks and Causes. Physician Sportsmed 16(5):97–112, 1988.

146. Nortcote RJ, Ballantyne D. Sudden Death and Sport. Sports Med 1:181–186, 1984.

147. Ragosta M, et al. Death During Recreational Exercise In the State of Rhode Island. Med Sci Sports Exerc 16:339–342, 1984.

148. Siscovick DS, et al. The Incidence of Primary Cardiac Arrest During Vigorous Exercise. N Eng J Med 311:874–877, 1984.

149. Falsetti HL, et al. Hematological Variations After Endurance Running With Hard- and Soft-Soled Running Shoes. Physician Sportsmed 11:118–124, 1983.

150. Potera C. GI Bleeding Found In Long-Distance Runners. Physician Sportsmed 12:29, 1984.

151. Spitler DL, et al. Haptoglobin and Serum Enzymatic Response to Maximal Exercise In Relation to Physical Fitness. Med Sci Sports Exerc 16:366–370, 1984.

152. Berk LS, Nieman DC, Tan SA, Nehlsen-Cannarella S, Kramer J, Eby WC, Owens M. Lymphocyte Subset Changes During Acute Maximal Exercise. Med Sci Sports Exerc 18:706, 1986 (abstract).

153. Berk LS. Tan SA, Nieman DC, Eby W. Stress from Maximal Exercise Modifies T-Helper and T-Suppressor Lymphocyte Subpopulations and Their Ratio in Man. In: Dotson CO, Humphrey JH (eds.) Exercise Physiology: Current Selected Research. New York: AMS Press, Inc. 3:1–11, 1988.

154. Brahmi Z, Thomas JE, Park M, Park M, Dowdeswell IAG: The Effect of Acute Exercise on Natural Killer-Cell Activity of Trained and Sedentary Human Subjects. J Clin Immunol 5:321–328, 1985.

155. Davidson RJL, Robertson JD, Galea G, Maughan RJ. Hematological Changes Associated With Marathon Running. Int J Sports Med 8:19–25, 1987.

156. Deuster PA, Curiale AM, Cowan ML, Finkelman FD. Exercise-Induced Changes in Populations of Peripheral Blood Mononuclear Cells. Med Sci Sports Exerc 20:276–280, 1986.

157. Edwards AJ, Bacon TH, Elms CA, Verardi R, Felder M, Knight SC:.Changes in the Populations of Lymphoid Cells in Human Peripheral Blood Following Physical Exercise. Clin Exp Immunol 58:420–427, 1984.

158. Eskola J, Ruuskanen O, Soppi E, Viljanen MK, Järvinen M, Toivonen H, Kouvalainen K. Effect of Sport Stress on Lymphocyte Transformation and Antibody Formation. Clin Exp Immunol 32:339–345, 1978.

159. Hedfors E, Holm G, Ivansen M, Wahren J. Physiological Variation of Blood Lymphocyte Reactivity: T-cell Subsets, Immunoglobulin Production, and Mixed-Lymphocyte Reactivity. Clin Immunol Immunopath 27:9–14, 1983.

160. Hedfors E, Holm G, Ohnell B. Variations of Blood Lymphocytes During Work Studied by Cell Surface Markers, DNA Synthesis and Cytotoxicity. Clin Exp Immunol 24:328–335, 1976.

161. Landmann RMA, Müller FB, Perini CH, Wesp M, Erne P, Bühler FR. Changes of Immunoregulatory Cells Induced by Psychological and Physical Stress: Relationship to Plasma Catecholamines. Clin Exp Immunol 58:127–135, 1984.

162. Lewicki R. Tchórzewski H, Majewska E, Nowak Z, Baj Z. Effect of Maximal Physical Exercise On T-lymphocyte Subpopulations and On Interleukin 1 (IL 1) and Interleukin 2 (IL 2) Production in Vitro. Int J Sports Med 9:114–117, 1988.

163. MacKinnon LT, Tomasi TB. Immunology of Exercise. Ann Sports Med 3:1–4, 1986.

164. Masuhara M, Kami K, Umebayasi K, Tatsumi N. Influences of Exercise on Leukocyte Count and Size. J Sports Med Phys Fit 27:285–290, 1987.

165. Moorthy AV, Zimmerman SW. Human Leukocyte Response to an Endurance Race. Eur J Appl Physiol 38:271–276, 1978.

166. Nieman DC, Johansen LM, Lee JW, Cermak J, Arabatzis K. Infectious Episodes in Runners Before and After the Los Angeles Marathon. Med Sci Sports Exerc 20:S42, 1988.

167. Oshida Y, Yamanouchi K, Hayamizu S, Sato Y. Effect of Acute Physical Exercise on Lymphocyte Subpopulations in Trained and Untrained Subjects. Int J Sports Med 9:137–140, 1988.

168. Peters EM, Bateman ED. Respiratory Tract Infections: An Epidemiological Survey. S Afr Med J 64:582–584, 1983.

169. Roberston AJ, Ramesar KCRB, Potts RC, Gibbs JH, Browning MCK, Borwn RA, Hayes PC, Beck JS. The Effect of Strenuous Physical Exercise On Circulating Blood Lymphocytes and Serum Cortisol Levels. Clin Lab Immunol 5:53–57, 1981.

170. Soppi E, Varjo P, Eskola J, Laitinen LA. Effect of Strenuous Physical Stress On Circulating Lymphocyte Number and Function Before and After Training. J Clin Lab Immunol 8:43–46, 1982.

171. Steel CM. Evans J, Smith MA. Physiological Variation in Circulating B cell:T cell Ratio in Man. Nature 247:387–388, 1974.

172. Stephenson LA, Kolka MA, Wilerson JE. Effect of Exercise and Passive Heat Exposure On Immunoglobulin and Leukocyte Concentrations. In: Dotson CO, Humphrey JH (eds): Exercise Physiology: Current Select Research, Volume 1. New York, AMS Press, Inc., 1985, p 145.

173. Wells CL, Stern JR, Hecht LH. Hematological Changes Following a Marathon Race in Male and Female Runners. Eur J Appl Physiol 48: 41–49, 1982.

174. Yu DTY. Clements PJ, Pearson CM. Effect of Corticosteroids On Exercise-induced Lymphocytosis. Clin Exp Immunol 28:326–331, 1977.

175. Simon HB. The Immunology of Exercise. JAMA 252:2735–2738, 1984.

176. Tomasi TB, Trudeau FB, Czerwinski D, et al. Immune Parameters in Athletes Before and After Strenuous Exercise. J Clin Immunol 2: 173–178, 1982.

177. Watson RR, Moriguchi S, Jackson JC, et al. Modification of Cellular Immune Functions in Humans by Endurance Exercise Training During Beta-adrenergic Blockade With Atenolol or Propranolol. Med Sci Sports Exerc 18:95–100, 1986.

178. Nieman DC, Tan SA, Lee JW, Berk LS. Complement and Immunoglobulin Levels in Athletes and Sedentary Controls. Int J Sports Med 10:124–128, 1989.

179. Nieman DC, Berk LS, Simpson-Westerberg M, Arabatzis K, Youngberg WS, Tan SA, Lee JW, Eby WC. The Effects of Long Endurance Running on Immune System Parameters and Lymphocyte Function in Experienced Marathoners. Int J Sports Med 10:317–323, 1989.

180. Sly MR. History of Exercise-Induced Asthma. Med Sci Sports Exerc 18:314–317, 1986.

181. Eggleston PA. Pathophysiology of Exercise-Induced Asthma. Med Sci Sports Exerc 18:318–321, 1986.

182. Katz RM. Coping With Exercise-Induced Asthma In Sports. Physician Sportsmed 15(7):101–108, 1987.

183. Rubinstein I, Levison H, Slutsky AS, et al. Immediate and Delayed Bronchoconstriction After Exercise in Patients With Asthma. N Engl J Med 317:482–485, 1987.

184. Roberts JA. Exercise-Induced Asthma in Athletes. Sports Med 6:193–196, 1988.

185. Katz RM. Prevention With and Without the Use of Medications for Exercise-Induced Asthma. Med Sci Sports Exerc 18:331–333, 1986.

186. Larsen DC, Fisher R. Management of Exercise-Induced Gastrointestinal Problems. Physician Sportsmed 15(9):112–126, 1987.

187. Robertson JD, Maugham RJ, Davidson RJL. Fecal Blood Loss in Response to Exercise. Br Med J 295:303–305, 1987.

188. Schoch DR, Sullivan AL, Grand RJ, Eagan WF. Gastrointestinal Bleeding in an Adolescent Runner. J Pediatr 111:302–304, 1987.

189. Sullivan SN. Exercise-Associated Symptoms in Triathletes. Physician Sportsmed 15(9):105–109, 1987.

190. Alvarez C, Mir J, Obaya S, Fragoso M. Hematuria and Microalbuminuria After a 100. Kilometer Race. Am J Sports Med 15:609–611, 1987.

191. Fleck SJ, Falkel JE. Value of Resistance Training for the Reduction of Sports Injuries. Sports Med 3:61–68, 1986.

192. Wolfe MD. Avoiding Aerobics Injuries. Athletic Business, March 1985, pp. 10–16.

193. Renstrom P, Johnson RJ. Overuse Injuries In Sports: A Review. Sports Medicine 2:316–333, 1985.

194. Phelps JR. Physical Activity and Health Maintenance— Exactly What is Known? West J Med 146:200–206, 1987.

Physical Fitness Activity 15.1— Benefits and Risks of Exercise: A Personal Assessment

Review the Sports Medicine Insight. List below seven benefits that *you personally* feel are most important. In other words, drawing on your own experience, what benefits are most valuable to you. List the benefit, and then explain why you chose it. Assign priorities to the listing of benefits. In your description, be sure to explain any discrepancy with the surety rating given in the Sports Medicine Insight.

1. _____
   _____

2. _____
   _____

3. _____
   _____

4. _____
   _____

5. _____
   _____

6. _____
   _____

7. _____
   _____

Review the Sports Medicine Insight again. List below three risks that *you personally* feel have been most bothersome in your own experience. In other words, drawing on your own experience, what risks have caused you the most pain and grief. List the risk, and then explain why you chose it. Assign priorities to the listing of risks. In your description, be sure to explain any discrepancy with the surety rating given.

1. _____
   _____

2. _____
   _____

3. _____
   _____

Questionnaires

Employee Wellness Questionnaire

**Loma Linda University Medical Center,
Center for Health Promotion**

Prepared by Dr. David Abbey, Research Director

Testing Date: _____

Name: _____

Home Address: _____

_____

City: _____ State: _____ Zip: _____

Home Phone: _____ SS#: _____

Employee #: _____ Company: _____

Work Department: _____

Work Phone Number: _____

Questions regarding health practices related to risk of certain diseases and past history of disease will be asked. Please answer every question so that an accurate assessment can be made. Your response will be treated in a confidential manner.

Center for Health Promotion

Employee Wellness Questionnaire

Please answer every question. No analysis can be done if data is missing. Thank you.

Physical Activity

1. How would you rate your physical activity level? *Note:* Physical activity includes work and leisure activities that require sustained physical exertion such as walking briskly, running, lifting and carrying.

   1 [ ] Level 1—Little or no physical activity

   2 [ ] Level 2—Occasional physical activity

   3 [ ] Level 3—Regular physical activity at least 3 times per week.

2. Does your work or daily activity primarily involve: (Check only one.)

   1 [ ] Sitting

   2 [ ] Standing

   3 [ ] Walking or other active exercise

   4 [ ] Heavy labor (such as lifting heavy objects)

   5 [ ] Other (please specify): _____

   _____

3. Outside of your normal work or daily responsibilities, how often do you engage in *vigorous* exercise which markedly increases your breathing such as: vigorous walking, cycling, running, swimming, etc.?

   1 [ ] Seldom or never

   2 [ ] Less than 1 time per week

   3 [ ] 1–2 times per week

   4 [ ] 3–5 times per week

   5 [ ] 6 or more times per week

4. When you do vigorous exercise, how long do you spend at each session?

   1 [ ] 0–14 minutes

   2 [ ] 15–29 minutes

   3 [ ] 30–44 minutes

   4 [ ] 45–59 minutes

   5 [ ] 60 or more minutes

5. On the average, how many times per day do you lift objects which weigh 25 pounds or more?

   1 [ ] Rarely or Never

   2 [ ] 1–4 times

   3 [ ] 5–14 times

   4 [ ] 15–24 times

   5 [ ] 25 times or more

6. Does your work involve moving or lifting heavy objects (50 pounds or more) on a daily basis?

    1 [ ] Yes

    2 [ ] No

7. How many times in the last year have you experienced back or neck pain?

    1 [ ] None

    2 [ ] Once or twice

    3 [ ] 3–6 times

    4 [ ] 7 or more times

8. Have you ever experienced back or neck pain which was severe enough to interfere with your normal activities for more than 3 days?

    1 [ ] Yes—How many times? _____

    2 [ ] No

Lifestyle

Please check how often you use each of the following on a WEEKLY basis. Please mark a box for every food item according to your usual intake. If you eat some foods only rarely or occasionally, mark the "less than 1" category.

	Times Per Week				
	None	<1	1–3	4–7	>7
9. a. Cheeses (cream, cottage, cheddar, swiss, etc.)	1 [ ]	2 [ ]	3 [ ]	4 [ ]	5 [ ]
b. Eggs (eaten as egg dish or in cooking)	1 [ ]	2 [ ]	3 [ ]	4 [ ]	5 [ ]
c. Fried foods (potato chips, french fries, fried meat, eggs, etc.)	1 [ ]	2 [ ]	3 [ ]	4 [ ]	5 [ ]
10. Fish other than shellfish	1 [ ]	2 [ ]	3 [ ]	4 [ ]	5 [ ]
11. Shellfish or organ meats (liver, kidney, giblets, etc.)	1 [ ]	2 [ ]	3 [ ]	4 [ ]	5 [ ]
12. Beef, pork, veal, or lamb	1 [ ]	2 [ ]	3 [ ]	4 [ ]	5 [ ]
13. Poultry (chicken, turkey, etc.)	1 [ ]	2 [ ]	3 [ ]	4 [ ]	5 [ ]
14. Drugs or medication (prescription or other)	1 [ ]	2 [ ]	3 [ ]	4 [ ]	5 [ ]
a. For headaches	1 [ ]	2 [ ]	3 [ ]	4 [ ]	5 [ ]
b. To help you sleep	1 [ ]	2 [ ]	3 [ ]	4 [ ]	5 [ ]
c. Which affect your mood or help you relax	1 [ ]	2 [ ]	3 [ ]	4 [ ]	5 [ ]
d. To help you make it through the day	1 [ ]	2 [ ]	3 [ ]	4 [ ]	5 [ ]
e. For recreational use	1 [ ]	2 [ ]	3 [ ]	4 [ ]	5 [ ]

15. How often do you use whole milk or cream products (whipped cream, sour cream, half and half, evaporated milk, butter, etc.)

    1 [ ] Rarely

    2 [ ] Less than once per day

    3 [ ] 1–2 times per day

    4 [ ] 3–5 times per day

    5 [ ] More than 5 times per day

16. Have you ever used alcoholic beverages? (Please check the category below which best describes you.)

    1 [ ] Non-drinker or less than 1 drink per week (*Skip* to #21)

    2 [ ] Ex-drinker (*Skip* to #21)

    3 [ ] Presently use alcoholic beverages

If you presently use alcoholic beverages, please enter the average number of drinks per week you use of each of the following: (Be sure to put 0 in the blank if you do not use that type of drink.)

    _____ Bottles or 8 oz. cans of beer per week

    _____ Glasses of wine per week

    _____ Mixed drinks or shots of liquor per week

17. Have you ever felt you ought to cut down on your drinking?

    1 [ ] Yes

    2 [ ] No

18. Have people annoyed you by criticizing your drinking?

    1 [ ] Yes

    2 [ ] No

19. Have you ever felt bad or guilty about your drinking?

    1 [ ] Yes

    2 [ ] No

20. Have you ever had a drink first thing in the morning to steady your nerves or get rid of a hangover?

    1[ ] Yes

    2[ ] No

21. Do you now or have you ever used tobacco in any form?

    1 [ ] Yes, currently use tobacco (*Skip* to #23)

    2 [ ] Have in the past but not now (*Continue* with #22 and #23 recording past tobacco use in #23)

    3 [ ] Have never used tobacco (*Skip* to #24)

22. _____ How many years has it been since you stopped using tobacco? (Put 1 if it has been less than 1 year.)

23. Please enter the average amount of tobacco used per *day* in the last 5 years. (Ex-users should use the last 5 years before quitting.)

Cigarettes	1 [ ]_____	(Number per *day*)
Pipes/cigars (smoke inhaled)	2 [ ]_____	(Number per *day*)
Pipes/cigars (smoke not inhaled)	3 [ ]_____	(Number per *day*)
Other forms of tobacco	4 [ ]_____	(Number per *day*)

Habit Patterns

24. How many of the following things do you usually do?

- Hitchhike or pick up hitchhikers
- Criticize or argue with strangers
- Carry a gun or knife for protection
- Live or work at night in a high-crime area
- Keep a gun at home for protection
- Seek entertainment at night in high-crime areas or bars

  1 [ ] 3 or more

  2 [ ] 1 or 2

  3 [ ] None

25. _____ Miles per year as a driver or passenger of an automobile (Average = 10,000).

26. _____ What percent of the time do you use seat belts? (Put 0 if never use).

Social Networks

27. How many friends and relatives (including your husband/wife) do you feel close to? (People that you feel at ease with, can talk to about private matters, and can call on for help.)

  1 [ ] None

  2 [ ] One or two

  3 [ ] Three to five

  4 [ ] Six to nine

  5 [ ] Ten or more

28. In general how strong are your social ties with your family and friends?

  1 [ ] Very strong

  2 [ ] About average

  3 [ ] Weaker than average

Mental/Social/Spiritual Well-Being

29. In general how satisfied are you with your life?

  1 [ ] Mostly satisfied

  2 [ ] Partly satisfied

  3 [ ] Mostly disappointed

30. How often do you get insufficient rest so that you are unable to function efficiently?

    1 [   ] Less than weekly

    2 [   ] Usually one night per week

    3 [   ] 2 or 3 nights per week

    4 [   ] 4 or more nights per week

31. How often does your day include planned periods of relaxation?

    1 [   ] Never

    2 [   ] Rarely

    3 [   ] Sometimes

    4 [   ] Usually

    5 [   ] Always

32. How would you describe the emotional stress you experience:

On the Job

    1 [   ] Experience much stress and often feel unable to cope with it

    2 [   ] Experience much stress but am able to cope with it

    3 [   ] Experience average or low levels of stress

At Home

    1 [   ] Experience much stress and often feel unable to cope with it

    2 [   ] Experience much stress but am able to cope with it

    3 [   ] Experience average or low levels of stress

33. How often do you feel worried, tense or upset about something?

    1 [   ] Several times per day

    2 [   ] A few times per day

    3 [   ] Several times per week

    4 [   ] A few times per week

    5 [   ] A few times per month

    6 [   ] Rarely or never

34. Have you suffered a serious personal loss or misfortune in the past year? (For example, a job loss, disability, divorce, separation, jail term, or death of a close person)

    1 [   ] Yes, two or more serious losses

    2 [   ] Yes, one serious loss

    3 [   ] No

35. How often in the past year did you witness or become involved in a violent or potentially violent argument?

    1 [   ] 4 or more times

    2 [   ] 2 to 3 times

    3 [   ] Once or never

36. Do you have a religious preference?

    1 [ ] No

    2 [ ] Yes (Please specify) _____

    _____

Medical History

37. Considering your age, how would you describe your overall physical health?

    1 [ ] Excellent

    2 [ ] Good

    3 [ ] Fair

    4 [ ] Poor

38. When did you have your last medical examination?

    1 [ ] Within the last year

    2 [ ] 1–2 years ago

    3 [ ] 3 or more years ago

39. Do you have an annual rectal exam?

    1 [ ] Yes

    2 [ ] No

40. Did either of your parents die of a heart attack before age 60?

    1 [ ] Yes, one of them

    2 [ ] Yes, both of them

    3 [ ] No

    4 [ ] Not sure

41. Did your mother, father, sister, or brother have diabetes?

    1 [ ] Yes

    2 [ ] No

    3 [ ] Not sure

42. Do you have diabetes?

    1 [ ] Yes, not controlled

    2 [ ] Yes, controlled

    3 [ ] No

    4 [ ] Not sure

43. Please check which of the following conditions you have had or now have: (Check as many as apply.)

Have Had	Now Have	
[ ]	[ ]	Arthritis
[ ]	[ ]	Gout
[ ]	[ ]	Heart attack/coronary

Have Had	Now Have	
[ ]	[ ]	Other heart problems (rheumatic fever, etc. Please specify) _____ _____
[ ]	[ ]	High blood pressure
[ ]	[ ]	Lung/breathing problem (pneumonia/emphysema/asthma/chronic bronchitis/etc.)
[ ]	[ ]	Stomach/duodenal ulcer
[ ]	[ ]	Stroke
[ ]	[ ]	Diabetes
[ ]	[ ]	Thyroid problems
[ ]	[ ]	Varicose veins, etc.
[ ]	[ ]	Rectal growth
[ ]	[ ]	Rectal bleeding
[ ]	[ ]	Cancer
[ ]	[ ]	Allergies
[ ]	[ ]	Depression/nervousness
[ ]	[ ]	Any other health problems (Please specify) _____ _____

44. Please check any of the following medications you currently take regularly:

    [ ] Heart medicine

    [ ] Blood pressure medicine

    [ ] Hormones/birth control pills

    [ ] Medicine for your breathing or lungs

    [ ] Insulin

    [ ] Arthritis medicine

45. Sex

    [ ] Male (*Skip* to #51)

    [ ] Female (*Continue* with #46)

Women Only

46. Have you had a hysterectomy?

    1 [ ] Yes

    2 [ ] No

47. How often do you have a Pap Smear?

    1 [   ] At least once per year

    2 [   ] At least once every 3 years

    3 [   ] More than 3 years apart

    4 [   ] Have never had one

    5 [   ] Not applicable

48. Was your last Pap Smear normal?

    1 [   ] Yes

    2 [   ] No

    3 [   ] Not sure

    4 [   ] Not applicable

49. Did your mother, sister, or daughter have breast cancer?

    1 [   ] Yes

    2 [   ] No

    3 [   ] Not sure

50. How often do you examine your breasts for lumps?

    1 [   ] Monthly

    2 [   ] Once every few months

    3 [   ] Rarely or never

    4 [   ] Not applicable

Dental Care

51. How often do you visit your dentist?

    1 [   ] At least once every 6 months

    2 [   ] At least once a year

    3 [   ] Less than yearly

    4 [   ] Only when I have pain or other problems

52. How often do you brush your teeth/dentures?

    1 [   ] 2 or 3 times a day

    2 [   ] Once a day

    3 [   ] Less than once a day

53. Do you have dentures?

    1 [   ] No

    2 [   ] Yes, partial

    3 [   ] Yes, complete upper and lower (*Skip* to #55)

54. How often do you floss your teeth?

    1 [   ] One or more times a day

    2 [   ] Less than once a day

    3 [   ] Never

55. Since your last dental visit, have you ever experienced: (Check YES or NO for each.)

Yes	No	
[ ]	[ ]	A toothache
[ ]	[ ]	New sensitivity to sweets, hot, or cold
[ ]	[ ]	Dark spots or holes in teeth
[ ]	[ ]	Stains or calculus (tartar) on teeth
[ ]	[ ]	Swollen, red, or bleeding gums
[ ]	[ ]	Bad breath or bad taste in mouth
[ ]	[ ]	Loose or drifting teeth
[ ]	[ ]	Pain, grating, or clicking in jaw joints
[ ]	[ ]	Loose dentures or sore spots under dentures

Demographics

56. _____ Age

57. Race/Origin:

1 [ ] White (Non-Hispanic origin)

2 [ ] Black (Non-Hispanic origin)

3 [ ] Hispanic

4 [ ] Asian/Pacific Islander

5 [ ] American Indian/Alaskan Native

6 [ ] Other

58. What is your marital status?

1 [ ] Single (Never married)

2 [ ] Married

3 [ ] Separated

4 [ ] Widowed

5 [ ] Divorced

6 [ ] Other

59. What is the highest level of education you have completed? (Please check only one)

1 [ ] Did not graduate from high school

2 [ ] High School

3 [ ] Some college/trade or business school

4 [ ] College/Professional degree

60. Which of the following best describes your present employment status? (Please check only one)

1 [ ] Employed full-time

2 [ ] Employed part-time

3 [ ] Unemployed

4 [ ] Homemaker/Volunteer/Student

5 [ ] Retired/Other

61. What is your occupation?

_____

(Write in occupation on line above, then circle appropriate occupational category)

  1. Student (not working full-time)
  2. Homemaker (not employed outside the home)
  3. Laborer or farm worker
  4. Owner or manager of small business, agency, or farm which sells produce (insurance agent, contractor, etc.)
  5. Owner or executive of large business or high level government agency
  6. Operator (truck driver, factory machine operator, etc.)
  7. Service worker (fireman, police, orderly, LPN, postman, maid, janitor, barber, etc.)
  8. Skilled craftsman or foreman (carpenter, plumber, mechanic, factory foreman, painter, electrician, etc.)
  9. Clerical/sales (bookkeeper, secretary, typist, salesclerk, salesman, etc.)
  10. Health professional (physician, nurse, dentist, etc.)
  11. Other professional (teacher, minister, etc.)
  12. None of the above categories fit

Occupational Health

62. Please describe your main job duties. _____

_____

63. How long have you been working in your current job position?
  _____ yrs. _____ mo.

64. After a day's work do you often have pain or stiffness which lasts for more than 3 hours?

  1 [ ] Yes (Please describe what joints or muscles are involved)

_____

  2 [ ] No

	All of the time	Most of the time	Some of the time	Rarely or never	N/A
65. How often are there high noise levels on the job so that you have to raise your voice to be heard?	1 [ ]	2 [ ]	3 [ ]	4 [ ]	5 [ ]
66. How often do you wear hearing protective devices when there are high noise levels on the job?	1 [ ]	2 [ ]	3 [ ]	4 [ ]	5 [ ]
67. How often do you handle chemicals other than medicine on the job which could come in contact with your skin?	1 [ ]	2 [ ]	3 [ ]	4 [ ]	5 [ ]
68. How often do you have itching skin or rashes from things you handle at work?	1 [ ]	2 [ ]	3 [ ]	4 [ ]	5 [ ]

	All of the time	Most of the time	Some of the time	Rarely or never	N/A
69. When you handle such substances or other chemicals at work, how often do you use protective devices (such as face mask, gloves, work coat, work boots)?	1 [ ]	2 [ ]	3 [ ]	4 [ ]	5 [ ]
70. How often are there chemical fumes on the job which cause nose or eye irritation?	1 [ ]	2 [ ]	3 [ ]	4 [ ]	5 [ ]
71. How often does the air you breathe at work contain dust or chemical fumes (such as insecticides, paint fumes, etc.)?	1 [ ]	2 [ ]	3 [ ]	4 [ ]	5 [ ]
72. How often do you wear a breathing filter when the air at work contains a lot of dust or chemical fumes?	1 [ ]	2 [ ]	3 [ ]	4 [ ]	5 [ ]
73. How often do you work with grinding wheels, drills, welding torches, or other devices which cause sparks or flying particles?	1 [ ]	2 [ ]	3 [ ]	4 [ ]	5 [ ]
74. How often do you wear goggles or a face shield when working with such devices?	1 [ ]	2 [ ]	3 [ ]	4 [ ]	5 [ ]
75. How often do you work in situations where you could fall more than 10 feet?	1 [ ]	2 [ ]	3 [ ]	4 [ ]	5 [ ]
76. How often do you find it difficult to concentrate on your tasks while at work?	1 [ ]	2 [ ]	3 [ ]	4 [ ]	5 [ ]

77. Do you operate machinery at work which could cause you physical injury?

    1 [ ] Yes

    2 [ ] No

78. On your present job, have you ever experienced an accident related to your work which resulted in loss of work for two days or more?

    1 [ ] Yes—How many times?_____

    2 [ ] No

Consent to Graded Exercise Testing and Other Physical Fitness Tests

Testing Objectives: I understand that the tests that are about to be administered to me are for the purpose of determining my physical fitness status, including heart, lung, and blood vessel capacities for whole body activity, body composition (ratio of body fat to muscle, bone, and water), muscular endurance and strength, and joint flexibility.

Explanation of Procedures: I understand that the tests which I will undergo will be performed on a treadmill, bicycle, or steps. The tests are designed to increase the demands on the heart, lung, and blood vessel system. This increase in effort will continue until exhaustion or other symptoms prohibit further exercise. During the test, heart rate, blood pressure, and electrocardiographic data will be periodically measured. Body composition will be determined through use of skinfolds or underwater weighing to determine levels of body fat versus fat-free weight. Muscular endurance and strength will be determined through use of body calisthenics and/or equipment. The sit-and-reach test will be used to determine the flexibility of the hip joint.

Description of Potential Risks: I understand that there exists the possibility that certain abnormal changes may occur during the testing. These changes could include abnormal heart beats, abnormal blood pressure response, various muscle and joint strains or injuries, and in rare instances, heart attack. Professional care throughout the entire testing process should provide appropriate precaution against such problems.

Benefits to be Expected: I understand that the results of these tests will aid in determining my physical fitness status, and in determining potential health hazards. These results will facilitate a better individualized exercise prescription.

I have read the foregoing information and understand it. Questions concerning these procedures have been answered to my satisfaction. I also understand that I am free to deny answering any questions during the evaluation process, or to withdraw consent and discontinue participating in any procedures. I have also been informed that the information derived from these tests is confidential and will not be disclosed to anyone other than my physician or others who are involved in my care or exercise prescription without my permission. However, I am in agreement that information from these tests not identifiable to me can be used for research purposes.

Participant's Signature _____ Date _____

Witness Signature _____ Date _____

Consent for Physical Fitness Programs

General Statement of Program Objectives and Procedures: I understand that this physical fitness program may include exercises to build the cardiorespiratory system (heart and lungs), the musculoskeletal system (muscle endurance and strength, and flexibility), and to improve body composition (decrease of body fat in individuals needing to lose fat, with an increase in weight of muscle and bone). Exercises may include aerobic activities (treadmill walking/running, bicycle riding, rowing machine exercise, group aerobic activity, swimming, and other such activities), calisthenics, and weight lifting to improve muscular strength and endurance, and flexibility exercises to improve joint range of motion.

Description of Potential Risks: I understand that the reaction of the heart, lung, and blood vessel system to such exercise cannot always be predicted with accuracy. I know there is a risk of certain abnormal changes occurring during or following exercise which may include abnormalities of blood pressure or heart rate, ineffective functioning of the heart, and in rare instances, heart attacks. Use of the weight lifting equipment, and engaging in heavy body calisthenics, can lead to musculoskeletal strains, pain, and injury if adequate warm-up, gradual progression, and safety procedures are not followed. Safety procedures are listed on the wall of the fitness facility. In addition, trained staff members will be supervising during all times to help ensure that these risks are minimized. The staff are trained in CPR and first aid, and regularly practice emergency procedures. Equipment is inspected and maintained on a regular basis.

Description of Potential Benefits: I understand that a program of regular exercise for the heart and lungs, muscles and joints, has many associated benefits. These may include a decrease in body fat, improvement in blood fats and blood pressure, improvement in psychological function, and a decrease in risk of heart disease.

I have read the foregoing information and understand it. Any questions which may have occurred to me have been answered to my satisfaction. I understand that I am free to withdraw from this program without prejudice at any time I desire. I am also free to decline answering specific items or questions during interviews or when filling out questionnaires. The information which is obtained will be treated as privileged and confidential and will not be released or revealed to any person other than my physician without my expressed written consent. The information obtained, however, may be used for a statistical or scientific purpose with my right of privacy retained.

Signature of Participant _____ Date _____

Signature of Witness _____ Date _____

Survey of Health/Fitness Club/Spa

NAME _____ DATE _____

Class Assignment: Visit a local fitness club and fill in the following:

Name of Fitness Club _____

Address _____

1. Number of paid members? _____

2. What type of screening do applicants go through to become members?

   A. [ ] None—all are allowed to become members by simply paying

   B. [ ] Applicants fill out a simple questionnaire (or index card) which is not used seriously

   C. [ ] Apparently healthy/high-risk determination is calculated from an in-depth questionnaire and interview process. High-risk applicants are advised to receive further testing by a physician.

   D. [ ] The club conducts its own physical fitness testing under the supervision of a medical director for high-risk applicants (and/or apparently healthy individuals who desire it).

   E. [ ] Other: explain below

   _____

   _____

3. What qualifications does the club director have?

   A. [ ] No formal training in exercise (less than a college degree in physical education or exercise physiology). Experience only.

   B. [ ] No formal college training in exercise, but is certified by the American College of Sports Medicine.

   C. [ ] Both formal college training or advanced degree, and certification by the American College of Sports Medicine.

   D. [ ] Is a medical doctor with expertise in exercise and fitness.

   E. [ ] Other: explain below

   _____

   _____

4. What qualifications do staff members have?

   A. [ ] Good looking bodies, but no certification or formal training.

   B. [ ] No certification, formal training, but do have CPR.

   C. [ ] American College of Sports Medicine certification.

   D. [ ] ACSM certification and formal college or higher education

   E. [ ] Other: explain below

   _____

   _____

5. Do staff members provide individualized exercise prescriptions for each member?

[ ] Yes [ ] No

Explain _____

_____

6. Does the club organize periodic retesting of its members to monitor progress towards individualized goals?

[ ] Yes [ ] No

Explain _____

_____

7. Does the club have adequate cardiorespiratory fitness equipment?

[ ] Yes [ ] No

If yes, check types of cardiorespiratory equipment available:

		Brand Name
A. [ ] Treadmills		_____
B. [ ] Stationary bicycles		_____
C. [ ] Rowing machines		_____
D. [ ] Cross-country ski simulators		_____
E. [ ] Stair-climbers		_____
F. [ ] Other: list		_____

_____

8. Are members trained and supervised to measure their intensity of exercise with either the Borg RPE scale or heart rate (percent of max HR or Karvonen formula)?

[ ] Yes [ ] No

Explain:_____

_____

9. Does the club urge that members practice both warm-up and flexibility exercises?

[ ] Yes [ ] No

Explain: _____

_____

10. What type of equipment does the club have for developing muscle strength and endurance?

A. [ ] Weight stacks

B. [ ] Free weights

C. [ ] Nautilus

D. [ ] Hydra-fitness

E. [ ] Other: list:_____

_____

11. Are members supervised at all times during their exercise (in all rooms)?

    [   ] Yes   [   ] No

    Explain _____

    _____

12. Does the club have a governing body/advisory committee composed of appropriate professionals?

    [   ] Yes   [   ] No

    Explain _____

    _____

13. Does the club have specific written policies for the protection of the rights and safety of the members?

    [   ] Yes   [   ] No

    Explain _____

    _____

14. Does the club conduct regular in-service training for its staff?

    [   ] Yes   [   ] No

    Explain _____

    _____

15. Does the club have liability insurance?

    [   ] Yes   [   ] No

    Explain _____

    _____

16. Are the locker rooms and restrooms well ventilated, easily accessible, secure, and supervised?

    [   ] Yes   [   ] No

    Explain _____

    _____

17. How extensively does the club market its services to the community?

    _____

    _____

18. Does the club use an award or incentive system to encourage members to stick with their exercise programs?

    [   ] Yes   [   ] No

    Explain _____

    _____

19. What type of payment schedule does the club follow? Are members allowed a 3-month trial period? Are large sums of money encouraged in advance for long time periods? Does the club try to sign up more members than it can handle, worrying little of membership retention?

    Explain _____

    _____

20. Summary: summarize your survey of this club

_____

_____

_____

_____

_____

_____

_____

_____

Physical Fitness Test Norms

Physical Fitness Test Norms for Children, Adolescents and College Students

National Children and Youth Fitness Study I (NCYFS I)

In 1984, the Public Health Service (Office of Disease Prevention and Health Promotion, U.S. Department of Health and Human Services), in response to the landmark government report, *Promoting Health/Preventing Disease: Objectives for the Nation,* launched the National Children and Youth Fitness Study to determine how fit and how active 1st through 12th-grade students actually are. Data on 10 to 18-year-olds were collected from a random sample of 10,275 students from 140 public and private schools in 19 States between February and May 1984. The NCYFS I was the first nationwide assessment of the physical fitness of American young people in nearly a decade, and the most rigorous study of fitness among our youth ever conducted in the U.S.

Test items of the NCYFS I include:

- Triceps and subscapular skinfolds for body composition.
- One-mile walk/run for cardiorespiratory endurance
- Sit-and-reach test for lower back/hamstring flexibility
- Pull-up for upper body muscular strength and endurance
- One minute bent-knee sit-ups for abdominal strength/endurance

(*Note:* see description of methods in Chapters 4 to 6).
Source: Public Health Service. Summary of Findings from National Children and Youth Fitness Study. JOPHER/January 1985, pp. 44–90.

Interpretations of Norms:
<25% = Unacceptable or Poor
25–50% = Minimal or Fair
50–75% = Acceptable or Good
>75% = Optimal or Excellent

Table 1   Sum of Triceps and Subscapular Skinfolds—Boys (total mm)

Age	10	11	12	13	14	15	16	17	18
%									
99	9	9	9	9	9	10	10	10	11
90	12	12	12	11	12	12	12	13	13
80	13	13	13	13	13	13	13	14	14
75	14	14	14	13	13	14	14	14	15
70	15	15	15	14	14	14	14	15	15
60	16	16	16	15	15	15	15	16	17
50	17	18	17	17	17	17	17	17	18
40	20	20	20	19	18	18	18	19	19
30	22	23	22	21	21	20	20	21	22
25	24	25	24	23	22	22	22	22	24
20	25	26	28	25	25	24	23	24	25
10	35	36	38	34	33	32	30	30	30

Table 2   Sum of Triceps and Subscapular Skinfolds—Girls (total mm)

Age	10	11	12	13	14	15	16	17	18
%									
99	10	11	11	12	12	13	13	16	14
90	13	14	15	15	17	19	19	20	19
80	15	16	17	18	19	21	21	22	21
75	16	17	18	19	20	23	22	23	22
70	17	18	18	20	21	24	23	24	23
60	18	19	21	22	24	26	24	26	25
50	20	21	22	24	26	28	26	28	27
40	22	24	24	26	28	30	28	31	28
30	25	28	27	29	31	33	32	34	32
25	27	30	29	31	33	34	33	36	34
20	29	33	31	34	35	37	35	37	36
10	36	40	40	43	40	43	12	42	42

Table 3   Chin-Ups—Boys (hands in underhand position, palms toward subject)

Age	10	11	12	13	14	15	16	17	18
%									
99	13	12	13	17	18	18	20	20	21
90	8	8	8	10	12	14	14	15	16
80	5	5	6	8	9	11	12	13	14
75	4	5	5	7	8	10	12	12	13
70	4	4	5	7	8	10	11	12	12
60	2	3	4	5	6	8	10	10	11
50	1	2	3	4	5	7	9	9	0
40	1	1	2	3	4	6	8	8	9
30	0	0	1	1	3	5	6	6	7
25	0	0	0	1	2	4	6	5	6
20	0	0	0	0	1	3	5	4	5
10	0	0	0	0	0	1	2	2	3

Table 4   Chin-Ups for Girls (hands in underhand position, palms toward subject)

Age	10	11	12	13	14	15	16	17	18
%									
99	8	8	8	5	8	6	8	7	6
90	3	3	2	2	2	2	2	2	2
80	2	1	1	1	1	1	1	1	1
75	1	1	1	1	1	1	1	1	1
70	1	1	1	0	1	1	1	1	1
60	0	0	0	0	0	0	0	0	0
50	0	0	0	0	0	0	0	0	0
40	0	0	0	0	0	0	0	0	0
30	0	0	0	0	0	0	0	0	0
20	0	0	0	0	0	0	0	0	0
10	0	0	0	0	0	0	0	0	0

Table 5 Bent-Knee Sit-Ups—Boys (number in one minute) (arms crossed on chest)

Age	10	11	12	13	14	15	16	17	18
%									
99	60	60	61	62	64	65	65	68	67
90	47	48	50	52	52	53	55	56	54
80	43	43	46	48	49	50	51	51	50
75	40	41	44	46	47	48	49	50	50
70	38	40	43	45	45	46	48	49	48
60	36	38	40	41	43	44	45	46	44
50	34	36	38	40	41	42	43	43	43
40	32	34	35	37	39	40	41	41	40
30	30	31	33	34	37	37	39	39	38
25	28	30	32	32	35	36	38	37	36
20	26	28	30	31	34	35	36	35	35
10	22	22	25	28	30	31	32	31	31

Table 6 Bent-Knee Sit-Ups—Girls (number in one minute) (arms crossed on chest)

Age	10	11	12	13	14	15	16	17	18
%									
99	50	53	66	58	57	56	59	60	65
90	43	42	46	46	47	45	49	47	47
80	39	39	41	41	42	42	42	41	42
75	37	37	40	40	41	40	40	40	40
70	36	36	39	39	40	39	39	39	40
60	33	34	36	35	37	36	37	37	38
50	31	32	33	33	35	35	35	36	35
40	30	30	31	31	32	32	33	33	33
30	27	28	30	28	30	30	30	31	30
25	25	26	28	27	29	30	30	30	30
20	24	24	27	25	27	28	28	29	28
10	20	20	21	21	23	24	23	24	24

Table 7   Sit-and-Reach, Flexibility Test—Boys (Footline set at 0; measurement in inches, plus or minus)

Age	10	11	12	13	14	15	16	17	18
%									
99	6	6.5	6.5	7.5	8	9.5	10	9.5	10
90	4	4.5	4	4.5	5.5	6	7	7.5	7.5
80	3	3.5	3	3	4	5	6	6	6
75	2.5	3	3	3	3.5	4.5	5	5.5	5.5
70	2.5	2.5	2.5	2.5	3	4	5	5	5
60	2	2	1.5	1.5	2	3	4	4	4
50	1.5	1	1	1	1.5	2	3	3.5	3
40	0.5	1.5	0	0.5	1	1.5	2	2.5	2.5
30	0	0	−.5	0	0	0.5	1.5	1.5	1.5
25	−0.5	−0.5	−1	−1	−1	0	1	1	1
20	−1	−1	−1.5	−1.5	−1	−0.5	0	−0.5	−0.5
10	−2	−2.5	−3.5	−3	−3	−2.5	−2	−1.5	−2

Table 8   Sit-and-Reach Flexibility Text—Girls (Footline set at 0; measurement in inches, plus or minus)

Age	10	11	12	13	14	15	16	17	18
%									
99	8.5	8.5	9	10	10	11	11	11	10.5
90	5.5	6	7	8	7.5	8	8.5	8.5	8.5
80	4.5	5	6	7	7	7	7.5	7.5	7.5
75	4.5	4.5	5	6	6.5	7	7	7	7
70	4	4.5	5	5.5	6	6.5	7	7	6.5
60	3	3.5	4	5	5.5	6	6	6	6
50	2.5	3	3.5	4	5	5	5.5	6	5.5
40	2	2	3	3.5	4	5	5	5	5
30	1	1.5	2.5	2.5	3	4	4.5	4	4
25	1	1	2	2	3	3.5	4	3.5	3.5
20	0	1	1.5	1.5	2	3	3.5	3	3
10	−1.5	−0.5	0	0	0.5	1.5	2	1.5	1

Table 9   One Mile Run—Boys (min:sec)

Age	10	11	12	13	14	15	16	17	18
%									
99	6:55	6:21	6:21	5:59	5:43	5:40	5:31	5:14	5:33
90	8:13	7:25	7:13	6:48	6:27	6:23	6:13	6:08	6:10
80	8:35	7:52	7:41	7:07	6:58	6:43	6:31	6:31	6:33
75	8:48	8:02	7:53	7:14	7:08	6:52	6:39	6:40	6:42
70	9:02	8:12	8:03	7:24	7:18	7:00	6:50	6:46	6:57
60	9:26	8:38	8:23	6:46	7:34	7:13	7:07	7:10	7:15
50	9:52	9:03	8:48	8:04	7:51	7:30	7:27	7:31	7:35
40	10:15	9:25	9:17	8:26	8:14	7:50	7:48	7:59	7:53
30	10:44	10:17	9:57	8:54	8:46	8:18	8:04	8:24	8:12
20	11:25	10:55	10:38	9:20	9:28	8:50	8:34	8:55	9:10
10	12:27	12:07	11:48	10:38	10:34	10:13	9:36	10:43	10:50

Table 10   One Mile Run—Girls (min:sec)

Age	10	11	12	13	14	15	16	17	18
%									
99	7:55	7:14	7:20	7:08	7:01	6:59	7:03	6:52	6:58
90	9:09	8:45	8:34	8:27	8:11	8:23	8:28	8:20	8:22
80	9:56	9:52	9:30	9:13	8:49	9:04	9:06	9:10	9:27
75	10:09	9:56	9:52	9:30	9:16	9:28	9:25	9:26	9:31
70	10:27	10:10	10:05	9:48	9:31	9:49	9:41	9:41	9:36
60	10:51	10:35	10:32	10:22	10:04	10;20	10:15	10:16	10:08
50	11:14	11:15	10:58	10:52	10:32	10:46	10:34	10:34	10:51
40	11:54	11:46	11:26	11:22	10:58	11:20	11:08	10:59	11:27
30	12:27	12:33	12:03	11:55	11:35	11:53	11:49	11:43	11:58
25	12:52	12:54	12:33	12:17	11:49	12:18	12:10	12:03	12:14
20	13:12	13:17	12:53	12:43	12:10	12:48	12:32	12:30	12:37
10	14:20	14:35	14:07	13:45	13:13	14:07	13:42	13:46	15:18

National Children and Youth Fitness Study II

As described in chapter 1, the second National Children and Youth Fitness Study (NCYFS II) was launched to study the physical fitness and physical activity habits of 4,678 children ages six to nine. The study was the first to assess the fitness and activity patterns of six- to nine-year-olds.

Test items of the NCYFS II include:

- Triceps, subscapular, and medial calf skinfolds for body composition.
- One-mile (age 8 or 9) or half-mile (age 6 or 7) walk/run for cardiorespiratory endurance
- Sit-and-reach test for lower back/hamstring flexibility
- Modified pull-up for upper body muscular strength and endurance
- One minute bent-knee sit-ups for abdominal strength/endurance

Interpretations of Norms: <25% = Unacceptable or Poor; 25–50% = Minimal or Fair; 50–75% = Acceptable or Good; >75% = Optimal or Excellent

(*Note:* see description of methods in Chapters 4 to 6).

Source: Ross JG, Pate RR, Delpy LA, Gold RS, Svilar M. New Health-Related Fitness Norms. JOPERD/November-December, 1987, pp. 66–70.

Table 11   Triceps Skinfold (in millimeters)

| | Age | | | | | | | |
| | Boys | | | | Girls | | | |
Percentile	6	7	8	9	6	7	8	9
99	5	5	5	5	5	6	6	6
95	6	5	6	6	7	7	7	7
90	6	6	6	6	8	7	8	8
85	7	7	7	7	8	8	8	9
80	7	7	7	7	9	8	9	10
75	7	7	7	8	9	9	9	10
70	7	7	8	8	9	9	10	11
65	8	8	8	9	10	10	10	11
60	8	8	8	10	10	10	11	12
55	8	8	9	10	11	11	12	12
50	8	9	9	10	11	11	12	13
45	9	9	10	11	12	12	13	14
40	9	10	10	12	12	12	14	14
35	10	10	11	13	13	13	15	15
30	10	11	12	14	13	13	16	16
25	10	11	13	15	14	14	17	18
20	11	12	14	16	14	15	18	19
15	12	14	15	18	15	17	19	21
10	13	16	19	21	17	19	21	22
5	16	20	23	23	20	22	25	25

Table 12   Subscapular Skinfold (in millimeters)

| | Age | | | | | | | |
| | Boys | | | | Girls | | | |
Percentile	6	7	8	9	6	7	8	9
99	4	4	4	4	4	4	4	4
95	4	4	4	4	4	4	5	5
90	4	4	4	5	5	5	5	5
85	4	5	5	5	5	5	5	5
80	5	5	5	5	5	5	5	6
75	5	5	5	5	5	5	6	6
70	5	5	5	5	5	5	6	6
65	5	5	5	6	6	6	6	6
60	5	5	5	6	6	6	6	7
55	5	5	6	6	6	6	7	7
50	5	5	6	6	6	6	7	8
45	5	6	6	7	6	7	7	8
40	6	6	6	7	7	7	8	9
35	6	6	6	7	7	7	8	9
30	6	6	7	8	7	8	9	10
25	6	7	7	9	8	9	10	12
20	7	7	8	10	8	10	12	15
15	7	8	10	12	10	11	15	17
10	8	10	14	15	12	13	17	21
5	12	16	19	20	16	19	21	25

Table 13 Sum of Triceps and Medial Calf Skinfolds (in millimeters)

| | Age | | | | | | | |
| | Boys | | | | Girls | | | |
Percentile	6	7	8	9	6	7	8	9
99	9	9	9	9	11	11	11	12
95	11	11	11	11	13	13	14	14
90	12	12	12	12	15	15	15	16
85	12	13	13	13	16	16	16	18
80	13	13	13	14	17	17	18	19
75	14	14	14	15	18	18	19	20
70	14	14	15	16	18	18	20	21
65	15	16	17	18	20	20	22	23
60	15	16	17	18	20	20	22	23
55	16	16	17	19	21	21	23	25
50	16	17	18	21	21	22	24	26
45	17	18	19	22	22	23	26	27
40	17	19	20	23	23	24	27	29
35	18	20	21	25	24	25	29	30
30	20	21	23	27	25	26	31	32
25	20	22	24	29	27	28	33	35
20	22	24	27	31	28	31	35	37
15	23	27	31	35	30	33	38	41
10	27	32	37	40	33	37	43	45
5	33	39	44	47	38	43	49	52

Table 14 Modified Pull-Ups (number completed)

| | Age | | | | | | | |
| | Boys | | | | Girls | | | |
Percentile	6	7	8	9	6	7	8	9
99	25	27	38	35	24	27	25	30
95	18	20	21	25	17	20	20	20
90	15	19	20	20	13	16	17	17
85	12	15	17	20	11	14	14	15
80	11	13	15	17	10	12	12	13
75	10	13	14	15	9	11	11	12
70	9	12	13	14	9	10	11	11
65	8	11	12	13	7	9	10	10
60	7	10	11	12	7	8	9	10
55	7	9	10	11	6	8	9	9
50	6	8	10	10	6	7	8	9
45	6	8	9	10	5	7	7	8
40	5	7	8	9	5	6	6	7
30	4	5	7	7	4	4	5	5
35	5	6	8	7	4	4	5	5
25	3	4	6	6	3	4	4	4
20	3	4	5	5	2	3	4	4
15	2	3	4	4	1	2	3	2
10	1	1	3	3	0	1	1	1
5	0	0	1	2	0	0	0	0

The child is positioned on his back with the shoulders directly below a bar that is set at a height one or two inches beyond the child's reach. An elastic band is suspended across the uprights parallel to and about seven to eight inches below the bar. In the start position, the child's buttocks are off the floor, the arms and legs are straight, and only the heels are in contact with the floor. An overhand grip (palm away from the body) is used and thumbs are placed around the bar. A pull-up is completed when the chin is hooked over the elastic band. The movement should be accomplished using only the arms and the body must be kept rigid and straight. (See Chapter 6).

Table 15 Timed Bent-Knee Sit-Ups (number in 60 seconds)

Percentile	Age							
	Boys				**Girls**			
	6	7	8	9	6	7	8	9
99	36	42	43	48	36	40	44	43
95	31	35	38	42	31	35	37	39
90	28	32	35	39	28	33	34	36
85	26	30	33	36	26	30	32	34
80	25	29	32	35	24	28	30	32
75	24	28	30	33	23	27	29	31
70	22	27	29	32	22	26	28	30
65	21	26	28	31	21	24	27	29
60	20	25	27	30	20	23	26	28
55	19	24	26	29	19	22	25	26
50	19	23	26	28	18	21	25	26
45	17	21	24	26	17	20	23	24
40	17	21	24	26	17	20	23	24
35	16	20	23	24	15	17	20	22
30	15	19	21	24	15	17	20	22
25	14	18	20	23	14	16	19	21
20	12	16	19	22	12	15	17	19
15	11	14	17	19	10	13	16	17
10	9	12	15	16	6	11	13	15
5	4	7	11	13	1	7	9	10

See Chapter 6 for details on methods.

Table 16   Sit-and-Reach Flexibility Test (in inches) (footline set at zero)

Percentile	Age							
	Boys				Girls			
	6	7	8	9	6	7	8	9
99	5.5	6.0	6.0	5.5	6.5	6.0	7.0	7.0
95	4.5	4.5	4.5	4.0	5.5	5.5	5.5	6.0
90	4.0	4.0	4.0	3.5	4.5	5.0	5.0	5.0
85	3.5	4.0	3.5	3.0	4.0	4.5	4.5	4.5
80	3.0	3.5	3.0	2.5	4.0	4.0	4.0	4.0
75	3.0	3.0	2.5	2.5	3.5	4.0	4.0	4.0
70	2.5	2.5	2.5	2.0	3.0	3.0	3.0	3.0
65	2.0	2.0	2.0	2.0	3.0	3.0	3.0	3.0
60	2.0	2.0	2.0	1.5	3.0	3.0	3.0	3.0
55	1.5	1.5	1.5	1.0	2.5	3.0	2.5	2.5
50	1.5	1.5	1.5	1.0	2.0	2.5	2.0	2.0
45	1.0	1.0	1.0	0.5	2.0	2.5	2.0	2.0
40	0.5	0.5	0.5	0	2.0	2.0	1.5	2.0
35	0.5	0.5	0.5	0	1.5	2.0	1.5	1.5
30	0	0	0	−0.5	1.0	1.5	1.0	1.0
25	0	−0.5	−0.5	−1.0	0.5	1.0	0.5	0.5
20	−0.5	−0.5	−1.0	−1.5	0	0.5	0	0
15	−1.0	−1.0	−1.5	−2.0	0	0	−0.5	−0.5
10	−1.5	−2.0	−2.5	−2.5	−0.5	−0.5	−1.0	−1.0
5	−2.0	−3.0	−3.5	−4.0	−1.5	−1.5	−2.0	−3.0

Table 17 Distance Walk/Run (Mile walk/run for children age 8 and over; half mile walk/run for children under age 8) (in minutes and seconds)

	Age							
	Boys				Girls			
	Half Mile		Mile		Half Mile		Mile	
Percentile	6	7	8	9	6	7	8	9
99	3:53	3:34	7:42	7:31	4:05	4:03	8:18	8:06
95	4:15	3:56	8:18	7:54	4:29	4:18	9:14	8:41
90	4:27	4:11	8:46	8:10	4:46	4:32	9:39	9:08
85	4:35	4:22	9:02	8:33	4:57	4:38	9:55	9:26
80	4:45	4:28	9:19	8:48	5:07	4:46	10:08	9:40
75	4:52	4:33	9:29	9:00	5:13	4:54	10:23	9:50
70	4:59	4:40	9:40	9:13	5:20	5:00	10:35	10:15
65	5:04	4:46	9:52	9:29	5:25	5:06	10:46	10:31
60	5:10	4:50	10:04	9:44	5:31	5:11	10:59	10:41
55	5:17	4:54	10:16	9:58	5:39	5:18	11:14	10:56
50	5:23	5:00	10:39	10:10	5:44	5:25	11:32	11:13
45	5:28	5:05	11:00	10:27	5:49	5:32	11:46	11:30
40	5:33	5:11	11:14	10:41	5:55	5:39	12:03	11:46
35	5:41	5:17	11:30	10:59	6:00	5:46	12:14	12:09
30	5:50	5:28	11:51	11:16	6:07	5:55	12:37	12:26
25	5:58	5:35	12:14	11:44	6:14	6:01	12:59	12:45
20	6:09	5:46	12:39	12:02	6:27	6:10	13:26	13:13
15	6:21	6:06	13:16	12:46	6:39	6:20	14:18	13:44
10	6:40	6:20	14:05	13:37	6:51	6:38	14:48	14:31
5	7:15	6:50	15:24	15:15	7:16	7:09	16:35	15:40

1985 SCHOOL POPULATION FITNESS SURVEY
President's Council on Physical Fitness and Sports

As described in chapter 1, in 1985, the President's Council on Physical Fitness and Sports School Population Fitness Survey was conducted. Data were collected to assess the physical fitness status of American public school children ages 6–17. A four stage probability sample was designed to select approximately 19,200 boys and girls from 57 school districts and 187 schools.

The test was not designed to measure all of the health-related fitness components (body composition was not assessed). In addition, several skill-related tests were included. Nine test items were selected for both boys and girls. Norms are given for boys and girls aged 6–17.

- Pull-ups
- Flexed-arm hang
- Curl-ups
- One-mile run/walk
- V-sit reach
- Shuttle run
- Two-mile walk
- 50-yard dash
- Standing long jump

Source: Youth Physical Fitness in 1985. The President's Council on Physical Fitness and Sports School Population Fitness Survey. President's Council on Physical Fitness and Sports. 450 Fifth St NW, Suite 7103, Washington, DC 20001.

Suggested interpretation of norms:
90–100% Excellent
75–85% Very good
60–70% Good
45–55% Average
30–40% Fair
15–25% Poor
0–10% Very poor

Table 18 Pull-Up for Boys (Overhand Grasp—Palms Facing Away)—1985 School Population Fitness Survey—Norms for boys aged 6–17

Per-centile	Age												Per-centile
	6–	7	8	9	10	11	12	13	14	15	16	17	
100	11	14	15	21	22	25	21	20	23	29	26	26	100
95	5	6	8	8	9	10	10	11	13	14	15	17	95
90	3	5	6	6	7	7	8	9	11	12	12	15	90
85	2	4	5	5	6	6	7	7	10	11	11	13	85
80	1	4	4	5	5	5	6	7	9	10	10	12	80
75	1	3	4	4	4	4	5	6	8	10	10	11	75
70	1	2	3	4	4	4	5	5	7	9	9	10	70
65	0	2	3	3	3	3	4	5	6	8	8	10	65
60	0	2	2	3	3	3	3	4	6	7	8	10	60
55	0	1	2	2	2	2	3	4	5	7	7	9	55
50	0	1	1	2	2	2	2	3	5	6	7	8	50
45	0	1	1	1	2	1	2	2	4	5	7	7	45
40	0	1	1	1	1	1	1	2	4	5	6	7	40
35	0	0	0	1	1	1	1	1	3	4	5	6	35
30	0	0	0	0	1	0	1	1	3	4	5	5	30
25	0	0	0	0	0	0	0	1	2	3	4	5	25
20	0	0	0	0	0	0	0	0	1	2	4	4	20
15	0	0	0	0	0	0	0	0	1	2	3	3	15
10	0	0	0	0	0	0	0	0	0	1	2	2	10
5	0	0	0	0	0	0	0	0	0	0	0	1	5
0	0	0	0	0	0	0	0	0	0	0	0	0	0

Table 19 Flexed-Arm Hang for Boys (Seconds)—1985 School Population Fitness Survey—Norms for boys aged 6–17

Per-centile	Age												Per-centile
	6–	7	8	9	10	11	12	13	14	15	16	17	
100	55	95	63	101	120	101	111	127	117	130	125	116	100
95	23	60	34	40	48	52	47	48	68	79	71	64	95
90	16	23	28	28	38	37	36	37	61	62	61	56	90
85	14	20	23	24	31	31	30	33	47	58	51	49	85
80	12	17	18	20	25	26	25	29	40	49	46	45	80
75	10	15	17	18	22	22	21	25	35	44	42	41	75
70	9	13	15	16	20	19	19	22	31	40	39	39	70
65	9	11	14	14	17	17	16	20	28	37	36	37	65
60	8	10	12	12	15	15	15	18	25	35	33	35	60
55	7	9	11	11	14	13	13	16	22	33	30	33	55
50	6	8	10	10	12	11	12	14	20	30	28	30	50
45	5	7	9	8	10	10	10	12	17	28	25	29	45
40	5	6	8	8	8	9	9	10	15	25	22	26	40
35	4	5	6	7	7	7	8	9	13	22	20	23	35
30	3	4	5	5	6	6	6	8	11	20	18	20	30
25	2	4	4	5	5	5	5	6	10	18	15	17	25
20	2	3	3	3	3	4	4	5	8	14	12	15	20
15	1	2	2	3	2	3	2	4	5	10	10	11	15
10	1	1	1	2	1	1	1	2	3	8	7	8	10
5	0	0	0	0	0	0	0	0	1	3	3	5	5
0	0	0	0	0	0	0	0	0	0	0	0	0	0

The height of the bar should be adjusted so it is approximately equal to or slightly higher than the subject's standing height. The subject should use an overhand grasp (palms facing away). With the assistance of two spotters who may help subject get to starting position, one in front and one in back of pupil, the subject raises her body off the floor to a position where the chin is above the bar without touching bar, the elbows are flexed, and the chest is close to the bar. The subject holds this position as long as possible. The stopwatch is started as soon as the subject takes the hanging position with no assistance. The watch is stopped when (a) subject's chin touches the bar, (b) subject's head tilts backward to keep chin above the bar, (c) subject's chin falls below the level of the bar.

**Table 20   Curl-Up for Boys (Flexed Leg) (Number in One Minute)—
1985 School Population Fitness Survey—Norms for boys aged 6–17**

Per-centile	Age												Per-centile
	6–	7	8	9	10	11	12	13	14	15	16	17	
100	53	56	58	60	64	68	67	76	79	81	77	73	100
95	40	42	47	48	51	51	57	59	62	62	62	61	95
90	37	38	42	44	48	49	53	55	58	59	58	57	90
85	33	36	40	41	45	47	50	53	56	57	56	55	85
80	31	34	38	40	43	45	48	51	54	55	53	53	80
75	28	33	37	38	41	43	47	50	52	53	51	51	75
70	26	31	36	37	40	42	45	48	51	51	50	50	70
65	25	31	35	35	40	40	44	46	49	50	48	48	65
60	24	30	34	34	38	39	43	45	48	49	48	46	60
55	23	29	32	33	36	38	42	43	47	47	46	45	55
50	22	28	31	32	35	37	40	42	45	45	45	44	50
45	21	26	30	31	34	36	39	41	44	44	44	43	45
40	20	25	29	30	33	35	38	40	42	43	42	41	40
35	19	24	28	29	32	34	37	39	41	41	40	40	35
30	17	22	26	27	30	32	35	38	40	40	40	40	30
25	16	21	25	26	30	31	34	36	39	38	38	38	25
20	14	20	23	24	28	29	32	34	37	36	37	36	20
15	13	18	20	22	25	27	30	32	35	35	35	35	15
10	10	15	18	20	23	25	27	30	33	32	31	32	10
5	7	12	14	16	19	20	25	26	28	29	27	27	5
0	0	1	0	1	4	0	7	0	0	0	6	1	0

The subject lies on the floor with knees bent, feet on floor, heels not more than 12 inches from the buttocks, and the back flat on the floor. The angle at the knees should be less than 90 degrees. The subject crosses the arms and places the fingers on the opposite shoulder. The arms are held in contact with the chest at all times. Subject's feet are held on the surface by a partner. The subject raises the head, shoulders and trunk, curling upward so that the elbows touch the thighs. This constitutes one curl-up. The subject lowers the back to the surface so that the scapula touches the floor before starting another curl-up. The timer calls out the signal, "Ready—Go!", and the curl-up performance is started on the word "go." Performance is stopped on the word "stop." The number of correctly executed curl-ups completed in 60 seconds is the score.

Table 21   1-Mile Run for Boys (Minutes and Seconds)—1985 School Population Fitness Survey—Norms for boys aged 6–17

Per-centile	Age 6–	7	8	9	10	11	12	13	14	15	16	17	Per-centile
100	6'18"	7'41"	6'30"	6'50"	6'24"	6'29"	6'03"	5'40"	4'30"	4'42"	4'49"	4'46"	100
95	8'54"	8'31"	8'00"	7'48"	7'10"	6'56"	6'43"	6'25"	6'01"	5'50"	5'40"	5'35"	95
90	9'41"	8'56"	8'28"	8'14"	7'39"	7'17"	6'57"	6'39"	6'13"	6'07"	5'56"	5'57"	90
85	10'15"	9'22"	8'48"	8'31"	7'57"	7'32"	7'11"	6'50"	6'26"	6'20"	6'08"	6'06"	85
80	10'32"	9'43"	9'00"	8'47"	8'08"	7'45"	7'25"	7'00"	6'33"	6"29"	6'18"	6'14"	80
75	10'53"	10'02"	9'23"	9'04"	8'19"	8'00"	7'41"	7'11"	6'45"	6'38"	6'25"	6'23"	75
70	11'17"	10'20"	9'38"	9'12"	8'37"	8'14"	7'56"	7'20"	6'59"	6'48"	6'33"	6'32"	70
65	11'41"	10'34"	9'56"	9'30"	8'59"	8'27"	8'05"	7'29"	7'09"	6'57"	6'44"	6'40"	65
60	12'00"	10'55"	10'15"	9'47"	9'11"	8'45"	8'14"	7'41"	7'19"	7'06"	6'50"	6'50"	60
55	12'20"	11'19"	10'39"	10'07"	9'29"	.9'01"	8'25"	7'55"	7'29"	7'16"	6'58"	6'57"	55
50	12'36"	11'40"	11'05"	10'30"	9'48"	9'20"	8'40"	8'06"	7'44"	7'30"	7'10"	7'04"	50
45	13'00"	11'56"	11'27"	10'46"	10'10"	9'46"	8'58"	8'17"	7'59"	7'39"	7'20"	7'14"	45
40	13'39"	12'17"	11'55"	11'03"	10'32"	10'07"	9'11"	8'35"	8'13"	7'52"	7'35"	7'24"	40
35	14'11"	12'50"	12'08"	11'20"	10'58"	10'25"	9'40"	8'54"	8'30"	8'08"	7'53"	7'35"	35
30	14'48"	13'23"	12'30"	11'44"	11'14"	10'54"	10'00"	9'10"	8'48"	8'29"	8'09"	7'52"	30
25	15'12"	13'49"	12'54"	12'08"	11'40"	11'25"	10'22"	9'35"	9'10"	8'49"	8'37"	8'06"	25
20	15'34"	14'16"	13'23"	12'33"	12'15"	12'00"	10'52"	10'02"	9'35"	9'05"	8'56"	8'25"	20
15	16'30"	15'00"	14'10"	12'59"	13'07"	12'29"	11'30"	10'39"	10'18"	9'34"	9'22"	8'56"	15
10	17'25"	16'12"	14'57"	13'52"	13'50"	13'08"	12'11"	11'43"	11'22"	10'10"	10'17"	9'23"	10
5	18'12"	17'43"	16'08"	15'01"	14'47"	14'35"	13'14"	12'47"	12'11"	11'25"	11'49"	10'15"	5
0	22'05"	21'20"	22'40"	19'40"	23'00"	23'32"	23'05"	24'12"	18'10"	21'44"	20'15"	16'49"	0

The subject is to run one mile as fast as possible. Walking is permitted, but the object is to cover the distance in the shortest possible time. Record in minutes and seconds.

**Table 22 V-Sit Reach for Boys (Inches)—
1985 School Population Fitness Survey—Norms for boys aged 6–17**

| Per-centile | Age | | | | | | | | | | | | Per-centile |
	6–	7	8	9	10	11	12	13	14	15	16	17	
100	7.0	9.0	7.0	13.0	14.5	14.5	13.5	11.0	12.0	12.0	13.0	12.5	100
95	5.0	5.0	4.0	5.0	7.0	6.5	5.5	5.0	6.5	7.0	8.0	8.5	95
90	4.0	4.0	3.5	4.0	5.0	5.0	5.0	4.0	5.0	6.0	7.0	8.0	90
85	3.5	3.5	3.0	3.0	4.0	4.0	4.0	3.5	4.5	5.0	6.0	7.0	85
80	3.0	3.0	2.5	3.0	3.0	4.0	3.0	3.0	4.0	5.0	5.5	6.0	80
75	2.0	2.0	2.0	2.0	3.0	3.0	3.0	2.5	3.5	4.0	5.0	5.5	75
70	2.0	2.0	2.0	2.0	2.0	2.5	2.0	2.0	3.0	4.0	4.5	5.0	70
65	1.5	2.0	1.0	1.5	2.0	2.0	2.0	1.5	2.5	3.0	4.0	4.5	65
60	1.0	1.5	1.0	1.0	1.5	2.0	1.5	1.0	2.0	3.0	3.5	4.0	60
55	1.0	1.0	1.0	1.0	1.0	1.0	1.0	1.0	2.0	2.5	3.0	3.5	55
50	1.0	1.0	0.5	1.0	1.0	1.0	1.0	0.5	1.0	2.0	3.0	3.0	50
45	0.5	0.5	0.0	0.0	0.5	1.0	0.0	0.0	1.0	2.0	2.0	3.0	45
40	0.0	0.0	0.0	0.0	0.0	0.0	0.0	0.0	1.0	1.0	2.0	2.0	40
35	0.0	0.0	–1.0	–0.5	0.0	0.0	–0.5	–1.0	0.0	1.0	1.5	1.5	35
30	0.0	–0.5	–1.0	–1.0	0.0	–1.0	–1.0	–1.0	0.0	0.0	1.0	1.0	30
25	–1.0	–1.0	–1.5	–1.5	–1.0	–1.0	–2.0	–2.0	–1.0	0.0	0.5	1.0	25
20	–1.5	–1.0	–2.0	–2.0	–2.0	–2.0	–2.0	–2.5	–2.0	–1.0	0.0	0.0	20
5	–2.0	–2.0	–3.0	–2.5	–2.5	–3.0	–3.0	–3.0	–2.0	–2.0	–1.0	–1.0	15
0	–3.0	–3.0	–3.0	–3.0	–3.5	–3.5	–4.5	–4.0	–4.0	–3.0	–3.0	–2.0	10
5	–4.5	–4.0	–4.0	–5.0	–5.0	–5.0	–6.0	–6.0	–5.0	–5.0	–4.0	–4.0	5
0	–10.0	–9.0	–10.0	–3.0	–12.0	–10.0	–12.0	–12.5	–12.0	–10.0	–12.0	–10.0	0

A straight line two feet long is marked on the floor. This is the baseline. At the midpoint of the baseline draw a line that is perpendicular to the baseline that extends two feet on each side of the baseline. This is the measuring line. Place "one inch" and "one-half inch" marks along the measuring line on each side of the baseline. The "0" point is where the baseline and measuring line intersect. A yardstick or measuring tape can be used to determine the plus or minus distance from the zero point. Subject removes shoes and sits on the floor so that the measuring line is between the legs, and the soles of the feet are placed immediately behind the baseline. The feet should be 8–12 inches apart. The subject clasps thumbs so that the hands are together, palms down, and placed on the floor between the lower legs. While the legs are held flat on the floor by a partner, subject keeps soles of feet perpendicular to the floor, and slowly reaches forward along the measuring line as far as possible, keeping the fingers in contact with the floor and both hands held down. Three practice extensions are given. On the fourth extension the subject holds the farthest point for a count of three seconds while that distance is recorded.

**Table 23 Shuttle Run for Boys (Seconds)—
1985 School Population Fitness Survey—Norms for boys aged 6–17**

Per-centile	Age												Per-centile
	6–	7	8	9	10	11	12	13	14	15	16	17	
100	11.0	8.3	8.0	8.1	7.4	7.0	7.5	8.0	6.6	6.3	6.5	6.9	100
95	11.7	10.8	10.4	10.4	9.8	9.5	9.4	9.0	8.8	8.5	8.4	8.5	95
90	12.0	11.2	10.9	10.6	10.0	9.9	9.6	9.3	9.0	8.8	8.6	8.6	90
85	12.1	11.5	11.1	10.9	10.3	10.0	9.8	9.5	9.1	9.0	8.7	8.7	85
80	12.3	11.7	11.2	11.0	10.5	10.2	9.9	9.6	9.3	9.1	8.9	8.9	80
75	12.4	12.0	11.4	11.1	10.7	10.4	10.0	9.8	9.4	9.2	8.9	8.9	75
70	12.5	12.2	11.5	11.3	10.8	10.5	10.1	9.9	9.5	9.3	9.0	9.0	70
65	12.8	12.4	11.8	11.5	11.0	10.6	10.3	10.0	9.6	9.4	9.1	9.1	65
60	13.0	12.5	11.9	11.6	11.2	10.8	10.4	10.1	9.7	9.5	9.2	9.2	60
55	13.1	12.7	12.0	11.8	11.3	11.0	10.5	10.1	9.8	9.5	9.3	9.3	55
50	13.3	12.8	12.2	11.9	11.5	11.1	10.6	10.2	9.9	9.7	9.4	9.4	50
45	13.5	13.0	12.3	12.0	11.6	11.2	10.7	10.3	10.0	9.8	9.5	9.5	45
40	13.7	13.2	12.5	12.2	11.8	11.4	10.8	10.4	10.1	9.9	9.6	9.6	40
35	13.8	13.3	12.7	12.5	12.0	11.5	11.0	10.6	10.2	10.0	9.7	9.6	35
30	14.0	13.5	13.0	12.8	12.2	11.7	11.1	10.7	10.3	10.1	9.8	9.8	30
25	14.3	13.8	13.3	13.0	12.4	12.0	11.2	10.8	10.5	10.2	10.0	9.9	25
20	14.5	14.0	13.6	13.3	12.7	12.2	11.4	11.0	10.7	10.4	10.1	10.1	20
15	14.8	14.5	13.8	13.6	13.1	12.6	11.6	11.1	11.0	10.7	10.3	10.3	15
10	15.2	14.9	14.2	14.1	13.6	13.0	12.0	11.4	11.3	11.0	10.6	10.6	10
5	16.0	15.4	15.0	14.5	14.5	13.5	12.4	12.0	12.0	11.8	11.1	11.1	5
0	19.5	25.0	18.0	18.8	16.9	16.8	16.1	16.4	19.9	19.8	23.0	23.0	0

Two parallel lines are marked on the floor 30 feet apart. The width of a regulation volleyball court is a suitable area. Place the blocks of wood behind one of the lines. The subject starts from behind the other line. On the signal "Ready? Go!" the subject runs to the blocks, picks one up, runs back to the starting line, places the block behind the line, subject then runs back and picks up the second block, and carries it back across the starting line. If the scorer has two stopwatches or one with a split-second timer, it is preferable to have two subjects running at the same time. To eliminate the necessity of returning the blocks after each race, start the races alternately, first from behind one line and then from behind the other. Allow two trials with some rest between. Record the time of the better of the two trials to the nearest tenth of a second.

**Table 24 2-Mile Walk/Boys (Minutes and Seconds)—
1985 School Population Fitness Survey—Norms for boys aged 6–17**

Per-centile	6–	7	8	9	10	11	12	13	14	15	16	17	Per-centile
100	24'01"	24'00"	24'13"	24'06"	24'00"	24'05"	24'00"	24'00"	24'00"	24'00"	24'00"	24'00"	100
95	25'59"	25'43"	25'19"	25'06"	24'36"	24'30"	24'30"	24'14"	24'10"	24'24"	24'20"	24'32"	95
90	27'23"	27'24"	26'12"	25'55"	25'12"	24'57"	24'55"	24'40"	24'30"	24'45"	24'50"	24'57"	90
85	28'05"	28'18"	27'20"	26'44"	25'42"	25'25"	25'07"	25'01"	24'50"	25'08"	25'16"	25'20"	85
80	28'49"	28'50"	28'01"	27'37"	26'25"	25'50"	25'29"	25'30"	25'06"	25'30"	25'34"	25'37"	80
75	29'20"	29'25"	28'43"	28'07"	27'00"	26'37"	25'58"	26'07"	25'20"	25'50"	25'48"	26'00"	75
70	30'28"	30'16"	29'23"	28'38"	27'30"	27'00"	26'18"	26'24"	25'40"	26'29"	26'13"	26'30"	70
65	31'21"	30'46"	30'00"	28'59"	28'00"	27'30"	26'43"	26'55"	26'16"	27'00"	26'35"	26'53"	65
60	31'48"	31'20"	30'29"	29'27"	28'35"	27'44"	27'04"	27'18"	26'44"	27'15"	27'10"	27'16"	60
55	33'01"	31'57"	31'27"	30'39"	29'03"	28'06"	27'31"	27'48"	27'25"	27'34"	27'30"	27'40"	55
50	34'07"	32'40"	32'10"	31'14"	29'56"	28'52"	28'03"	28'14"	28'02"	27'57"	27'55"	28'06"	50
45	34'36"	33'36"	32'50"	31'45"	30'34"	29'41"	28'31"	28'29"	28'21"	28'27"	28'10"	28'33"	45
40	35'15"	34'40"	33'26"	32'30"	31'29"	30'25"	28'51"	29'00"	28'57"	29'08"	28'59"	29'15"	40
35	35'44"	35'36"	34'22"	33'02"	32'03"	31'31"	29'05"	29'13"	29'27"	29'53"	29'44"	29'34"	35
30	36'35"	36'20"	35'00"	33'45"	32'43"	32'25"	30'00"	30'01"	30'10"	30'22"	30'30"	29'55"	30
25	37'08"	37'04"	35'44"	34'24"	33'26"	32'59"	31'01"	30'50"	30'54"	31'10"	31'00"	30'30"	25
20	38'50"	38'16"	37'13"	35'31"	34'20"	33'26"	31'48"	31'40"	31'53"	31'43"	31'48"	31'07"	20
15	40'20"	40'00"	38'37"	36'57"	35'29"	35'00"	33'10"	33'18"	32'44"	32'40"	32'40"	32'13"	15
10	41'10"	40'48"	39'56"	38'19"	37'30"	36'06"	34'14"	34'34"	34'30"	34'23"	33'47"	33'32"	10
5	43'35"	44'45"	41'55"	40'45"	38'53"	38'16"	36'00"	36'34"	36'02"	35'59"	35'15"	35'10"	5
0	49'37"	57'33"	56'30"	58'23"	62'01"	47'55"	42'02"	40'30"	50'23"	44'18"	45'30"	42'00"	0

Subjects are instructed to walk the distance as fast as possible. One foot must contact the ground at all times or the subject is running. Scoring is to the nearest second.

Table 25 50-Yard Dash for Boys (Minutes and Seconds)—
1985 School Population Fitness Survey—Norms for boys aged 6–17

Per-centile	Age												Per-centile
	6–	7	8	9	10	11	12	13	14	15	16	17	
100	7.4	7.0	7.0	6.5	6.0	6.1	5.4	5.6	5.1	5.0	5.0	5.1	100
95	8.1	8.0	7.8	7.6	7.3	7.1	6.7	6.4	6.1	6.1	5.9	6.0	95
90	8.5	8.5	8.0	7.9	7.5	7.3	6.9	6.6	6.3	6.2	6.0	6.0	90
85	9.0	8.8	8.2	8.0	7.7	7.4	7.0	6.8	6.5	6.3	6.2	6.1	85
80	9.2	9.0	8.4	8.1	7.8	7.5	7.1	6.9	6.6	6.4	6.3	6.2	80
75	9.4	9.1	8.5	8.2	8.0	7.6	7.3	7.0	6.7	6.5	6.3	6.3	75
70	9.5	9.3	8.6	8.3	8.1	7.8	7.3	7.1	6.8	6.6	6.4	6.4	70
65	9.6	9.4	8.8	8.4	8.2	7.9	7.5	7.1	6.9	6.6	6.5	6.4	65
60	9.8	9.5	8.9	8.5	8.3	8.0	7.5	7.2	7.0	6.7	6.6	6.5	60
55	10.0	9.6	9.0	8.6	8.3	8.1	7.7	7.3	7.0	6.8	6.6	6.6	55
50	10.1	9.8	9.1	8.7	8.4	8.1	7.8	7.4	7.1	6.9	6.7	6.6	50
45	10.3	9.9	9.2	8.8	8.5	8.3	7.8	7.5	7.2	6.9	6.7	6.7	45
40	10.5	10.0	9.4	8.9	8.7	8.4	8.0	7.6	7.3	7.0	6.8	6.8	40
35	10.8	10.0	9.5	9.0	8.8	8.5	8.0	7.7	7.4	7.1	6.8	6.9	35
30	10.9	10.1	9.8	9.1	8.9	8.7	8.2	7.9	7.5	7.1	6.9	6.9	30
25	11.0	10.3	10.0	9.2	9.0	8.9	8.3	8.0	7.6	7.2	7.0	7.0	25
20	11.3	10.7	10.1	9.4	9.2	9.0	8.4	8.1	7.8	7.4	7.1	7.1	20
15	11.5	11.0	10.3	9.6	9.5	9.2	8.7	8.3	7.9	7.5	7.3	7.3	15
10	11.8	11.3	10.6	9.9	9.8	9.5	8.9	8.5	8.2	7.7	7.5	7.5	10
5	12.5	12.0	11.1	10.4	10.2	10.1	9.4	9.0	8.8	8.2	8.1	7.8	5
0	14.8	13.9	13.8	13.6	14.8	13.0	13.0	12.9	14.5	13.9	14.0	14.6	0

It is preferable to administer this test to two pupils at a time. Have both take positions behind the starting line. The starter will use the commands "Are you ready?" and "Go!" The latter will be accompanied by a downward sweep of the starter's arm to give a visual signal to the timer who stands at the finish line. The score is the amount of time between the starter's signal and the instant the pupil crosses the finish line. Record in seconds to the nearest tenth of a second.

Table 26 Standing Long Jump for Boys (Feet and Inches)—1985 School Population Fitness Survey—Norms for boys aged 6–17

Per-centile	Age 6–	7	8	9	10	11	12	13	14	15	16	17	Per-centile
100	8'0"	5'7"	7'6"	6'4"	8'8"	8'7"	9'6"	9'9"	9'6"	9'0"	10'1"	9'10"	100
95	4'8"	4'11"	5'4"	5'9"	6'2"	6'5"	6'8"	7'3"	7'11"	8'0"	8'4"	8'6"	95
90	4'6"	4'9"	5'2"	5'6"	5'10"	6'2"	6'4"	6'11"	7'6"	7'10"	8'0"	8'4"	90
85	4'4"	4'7"	5'0"	5'4"	5'9"	6'0"	6'3"	6'9"	7'4"	7'8"	7'10"	8'1"	85
80	4'3"	4'6"	4'10"	5'2"	5'7"	5'11"	6'1"	6'7"	7'2"	7'6"	7'8"	8'0"	80
75	4'1"	4'5"	4'9"	5'1"	5'6"	5'9"	6'0"	6'6"	7'0"	7'4"	7'7"	7'10"	75
70	4'0"	4'4"	4'8"	5'0"	5'4"	5'8"	5'10"	6'4"	6'10"	7'3"	7'6"	7'9"	70
65	3'11"	4'3"	4'7"	4'11"	5'3"	5'7"	5'9"	6'3"	6'9"	7'11"	7'4"	7'8"	65
60	3'10"	4'2"	4'6"	4'10"	5'2"	5'6"	5'8"	6'2"	6'7"	7'0"	7'3"	7'6"	60
55	3'9"	4'1"	4'5"	4'9"	5'0"	5'5"	5'7"	6'1"	6'6"	6'11"	7'2"	7'5"	55
50	3'8"	4'0"	4'4"	4'7"	4'11"	5'3"	5'5"	6'0"	6'4"	6'9"	7'1"	7'4"	50
45	3'7"	3'11"	4'3"	4'6"	4'10"	5'2"	5'4"	5'10"	6'3"	6'8"	7'0"	7'3"	45
40	3'6"	3'10"	4'2"	4'5"	4'9"	5'1"	5'3"	5'9"	6'2"	6'7"	6'10"	7'1"	40
35	3'5"	3'9"	4'1"	4'4"	4'8"	5'0"	5'2"	5'8"	6'0"	6'5"	6'9"	7'0"	35
30	3'4"	3'7"	4'0"	4'3"	4'6	4'11"	5'1"	5'6"	5'11"	6'4"	6'7"	6'11"	30
25	3'3"	3'6"	3'11"	4'2"	4'5"	4'9"	5'0"	5'4"	5'9"	6'1"	6'6"	6'10"	25
20	3'2"	3'5"	3'9"	4'0"	4'3"	4'7"	4'10"	5'2"	5'7"	6'0"	6'3"	6'8"	20
15	3'1"	3'3"	3'8"	3'11"	4'1"	4'5"	4'8"	5'1"	5'5"	5'10"	6'0"	6'5"	15
10	2'11"	3'1"	3'6"	3'8"	4'0"	4'2"	4'6"	4'10"	5'2"	5'7"	5'9"	6'1"	10
5	2'8"	2'10"	3'3"	3'7"	3'9"	3'11"	4'2"	4'6"	4'9"	5'2"	5'4"	5'8"	5
0	1'8"	2'0"	2'1"	2'2"	2'9"	2'0"	3'2"	2'6"	3'4"	3'0"	3'6"	4'4"	0

Pupil stands with the feet several inches apart and the toes just behind the takeoff line. Preparatory to jumping, the pupil swings the arms backward and bends the knees. The jump is accomplished by simultaneously extending the knees and swinging forward the arms. Allow three trials. Measure from the takeoff line to the heel or other part of the body that touches the floor nearest the takeoff line. When the test is given indoors, it is convenient to tape the tape measure to the floor at right angles to the takeoff line and have the pupils jump along the tape. The scorer stands to the side and observes the mark to the nearest inch. Record the best of the three trials in feet and inches to the nearest inch.

Table 27   Pull-Up for Girls—1985 School Population Fitness Survey Norms for girls aged 6–17

Per-centile	Age												Per-centile
	6–	7	8	9	10	11	12	13	14	15	16	17	
100	8	8	14	11	9	24	22	18	44	14	10	31	100
95	4	4	5	4	5	5	5	5	4	3	4	4	95
90	3	3	3	3	3	3	3	2	3	2	2	2	90
85	2	2	2	2	3	3	2	2	2	2	1	1	85
80	1	1	2	2	2	2	2	1	1	1	1	1	80
75	1	1	1	1	2	2	1	1	1	1	1	1	75
70	1	1	1	1	1	1	1	0	1	1	1	1	70
65	0	0	1	1	1	1	0	0	1	0	0	1	65
60	0	0	0	0	1	0	0	0	0	0	0	0	60
55	0	0	0	0	0	0	0	0	0	0	0	0	55
50	0	0	0	0	0	0	0	0	0	0	0	0	50
45	0	0	0	0	0	0	0	0	0	0	0	0	45
40	0	0	0	0	0	0	0	0	0	0	0	0	40
35	0	0	0	0	0	0	0	0	0	0	0	0	35
30	0	0	0	0	0	0	0	0	0	0	0	0	30
25	0	0	0	0	0	0	0	0	0	0	0	0	25
20	0	0	0	0	0	0	0	0	0	0	0	0	20
15	0	0	0	0	0	0	0	0	0	0	0	0	15
10	0	0	0	0	0	0	0	0	0	0	0	0	10
5	0	0	0	0	0	0	0	0	0	0	0	0	5
0	0	0	0	0	0	0	0	0	0	0	0	0	0

**Table 28   Flexed Arm Hang for Girls (Seconds)—
1985 School Population Fitness Survey—Norms for girls aged 6–17**

Per-centile	Age												Per-centile
	6–	7	8	9	10	11	12	13	14	15	16	17	
100	55	72	97	78	152	150	99	68	100	125	131	127	100
95	22	29	26	35	38	33	37	35	38	41	40	37	95
90	15	21	21	23	29	25	27	28	31	34	30	29	90
85	13	17	17	20	22	10	21	21	25	28	24	24	85
80	11	14	15	16	19	16	16	19	21	23	21	20	80
75	10	12	13	14	16	14	14	16	18	18	18	18	75
70	9	11	11	12	14	13	13	14	16	15	16	15	70
65	8	9	10	11	12	11	11	12	13	12	13	12	65
60	6	8	10	10	11	9	10	10	11	10	10	11	60
55	6	7	9	9	9	8	8	9	10	9	9	10	55
50	5	6	8	8	8	7	7	8	9	7	7	7	50
45	5	5	7	7	7	6	6	6	7	6	6	6	45
40	4	5	6	6	6	5	5	5	6	5	5	5	40
35	3	5	5	5	5	4	4	5	5	4	4	5	35
30	3	4	4	4	4	4	3	4	4	4	3	4	30
25	2	3	3	3	3	3	2	3	3	3	2	2	25
20	1	2	3	2	2	2	1	1	2	2	2	2	20
15	1	1	1	1	1	1	1	1	1	1	1	1	15
10	0	0	0	0	0	0	0	0	0	1	0	1	10
5	0	0	0	0	0	0	0	0	0	0	0	0	5
0	0	0	0	0	0	0	0	0	0	0	0	0	0

Table 29 Curl-Up for Girls (Flexed Leg) (Number in One Minute)— 1985 School Population Fitness Survey—Norms for girls aged 6–17

Per-centile	Age												Per-centile
	6–	7	8	9	10	11	12	13	14	15	16	17	
100	55	55	59	62	61	67	62	72	72	74	77	67	100
95	36	42	43	45	45	48	50	52	53	55	53	53	95
90	33	36	40	41	42	44	47	50	49	51	49	47	90
85	32	34	38	39	40	42	45	46	47	48	45	44	85
80	31	32	36	38	38	40	43	44	45	46	43	41	80
75	30	31	35	36	37	39	41	42	43	44	41	40	75
70	28	30	33	35	35	37	40	42	42	41	40	38	70
65	27	29	31	34	34	35	39	40	41	40	38	37	65
60	25	27	30	32	32	35	38	40	40	39	37	36	60
55	24	26	30	31	32	33	36	38	39	37	36	35	55
50	23	25	29	30	30	32	35	37	37	36	35	34	50
45	21	24	28	30	29	31	34	36	36	35	34	33	45
40	20	23	27	29	28	30	32	35	35	34	33	31	40
35	20	22	25	27	27	29	31	33	34	32	32	30	35
30	19	21	24	26	26	28	30	31	32	31	30	30	30
25	17	20	23	25	25	27	29	30	31	30	30	28	25
20	16	19	22	23	23	25	27	28	30	28	27	25	20
15	14	17	20	20	21	24	5	26	28	26	25	25	15
10	11	15	18	19	19	20	23	23	25	23	23	22	10
5	7	10	12	13	14	16	20	19	20	20	19	19	5
0	0	0	0	0	0	2	0	0	0	0	0	0	0

**Table 30 1-Mile Run for Girls (Minutes and Seconds)—
1985 School Population Fitness Survey—Norms for girls aged 6–17**

Per-centile	Age												Per-centile
	6–	7	8	9	10	11	12	13	14	15	16	17	
100	8'36"	8'04"	8'00"	6'11"	6'26"	7'07"	6'22"	5'42"	5'00"	5'51"	5'58"	6'20"	100
95	10'06"	9'30"	9'10"	8'21"	8'07"	8'06"	7'35"	7'21"	7'20"	7'25"	7'26"	7'22"	95
90	10'29"	10'05"	9'45"	9'07"	8'49"	8'40"	8'00"	7'49"	7'43"	7'52"	7'55"	7'58"	90
85	11'20"	10'36"	10'02"	9'30"	9'19"	9'02"	8'23"	8'13"	7'59"	8'08"	8'23"	8'15"	85
80	11'37"	10'55"	10'20"	10'03"	9'38"	9'22"	8'52"	8'29"	8'20"	8'24"	8'39"	8'34"	80
75	12'00"	11'17"	10'55"	10'22"	10'08"	9'44"	9'15"	8'49"	8'36"	8'40"	8'50"	8'52"	75
70	12'12"	11'25"	11'20"	10'45"	10'19"	10'04"	9'36"	9'09"	8'50"	8'55"	9'11"	9'15"	70
65	12'20"	11'45"	11'38"	10'58"	10'42"	10'24"	10'05"	9'30"	9'09"	9'09"	9'25"	9'33"	65
60	12'31"	12'20"	11'53"	11'13"	10'52"	10'42"	10'26"	9'50"	9'27"	9'23"	9'48"	9'51"	60
55	12'45"	12'39"	12'10"	11'32"	11'00"	11'00"	10'44"	10'07"	9'51"	9'37"	10'09"	10'08'	55
50	13'12"	12'56"	12'30"	11'52"	11'22"	11'17"	11'05"	10'23"	10'06"	9'58"	10'31"	10'22"	50
45	13'56"	13'21"	12'46"	12'13"	11'40"	11'36"	11'23"	10'57"	10'25"	10'18"	10'58"	10'48"	45
40	14'14"	13'44"	13'07"	12'24"	11'58"	12'00"	11'47"	11'20"	10'51"	10'40"	11'15"	11'05"	40
35	14'45"	14'04"	13'31"	12'48"	12'08"	12'21"	12'01"	11'40"	11'10"	11'00"	11'44"	11'20"	35
30	15'09"	14'32"	13'56"	13'19"	12'30"	12'42"	12'24"	12'00"	11'36"	11'20"	12'08"	12'00"	30
25	15'27"	14'55"	14'21"	13'44"	13'00"	13'09"	12'46"	12'29"	11'52"	11'48"	12'42"	12'11"	25
20	16'10"	15'12"	14'53"	14'07"	13'29"	13'44"	13'35"	13'01"	12'18"	12'19"	13'23"	12'40"	20
15	16'45"	16'00"	15'19"	14'57"	14'00"	14'16"	14'12"	14'10"	12'56"	13'33"	14'16"	13'03"	15
10	17'36"	16'35"	15'45"	15'40"	14'30"	14'44"	14'39"	14'49"	14'10"	14'13"	16'03"	14'01"	10
5	19'00"	17'27"	16'55"	16'58"	15'43"	16'07"	16'00"	16'10"	15'44"	15'17"	18'00"	15'14"	5
0	21'40"	22'19"	20'40"	24'00"	24'00"	21'02"	24'54"	20'45"	20'04"	24'07"	21'00"	28'50"	0

Table 31 V-Sit Reach for Girls (Inches)—1985 School Population Fitness Survey— Norms for girls aged 6–17

Per-centile	Age												Per-centile
	6-	7	8	9	10	11	12	13	14	15	16	17	
100	9.5	9.0	12.0	14.0	13.0	15.0	14.5	14.5	14.0	15.0	15.0	15.0	100
95	7.0	6.5	6.0	8.0	8.0	10.0	9.0	9.0	10.0	10.0	10.5	10.5	95
90	6.0	5.5	5.0	6.0	7.0	8.0	8.0	8.0	8.5	9.0	9.5	9.0	90
85	5.5	5.0	4.5	5.5	6.0	6.5	7.0	7.0	8.0	8.0	9.0	8.0	85
80	5.0	4.5	4.0	5.0	5.0	6.0	6.0	6.0	7.0	7.5	8.0	7.5	80
75	5.0	4.0	4.0	4.0	5.0	5.0	6.0	6.0	6.5	7.0	8.0	7.0	75
70	4.0	4.0	3.5	4.0	4.0	5.0	5.0	5.0	6.0	6.5	7.0	6.0	70
65	3.5	3.0	3.0	3.5	4.0	4.5	5.0	5.0	6.0	6.0	7.0	6.0	65
60	3.0	3.0	3.0	3.0	3.0	4.0	4.5	4.5	5.0	6.0	6.0	5.5	60
55	3.0	3.0	2.5	3.0	3.0	4.0	4.0	4.0	5.0	5.0	6.0	5.0	55
50	2.5	2.0	2.0	2.0	3.0	3.0	3.5	3.5	4.5	5.0	5.5	4.5	50
45	2.0	2.0	2.0	2.0	2.5	3.0	3.0	3.0	4.0	4.5	5.0	4.0	45
40	1.5	2.0	1.5	2.0	2.0	2.5	3.0	3.0	4.0	4.0	4.5	4.0	40
35	1.0	1.5	1.0	1.0	2.0	2.0	2.5	2.5	3.5	3.5	4.0	3.5	35
30	1.0	1.0	1.0	1.0	1.0	1.5	2.0	2.0	3.0	3.0	4.0	3.0	30
25	1.0	1.0	0.5	0.0	1.0	1.0	2.0	2.0	2.5	2.0	3.0	2.5	25
20	0.0	0.0	0.0	0.0	0.5	1.0	1.0	1.0	2.0	2.0	2.5	2.0	20
15	0.0	0.0	0.0	−0.5	0.0	0.0	0.5	0.5	1.0	1.0	2.0	1.5	15
10	−1.0	−1.0	−1.0	−1.0	−1.0	−0.5	0.0	0.0	0.0	0.5	1.0	1.0	10
5	−2.5	−3.0	−2.5	−3.0	−2.5	−3.0	−2.5	−2.5	−1.5	−1.0	−0.5	−1.0	5
0	−9.0	−9.0	−6.0	−11.0	−17.0	−11.0	−11.0	−11.0	−10.0	−10.0	−6.0	−12.0	0

Table 32   Shuttle Run for Girls (Seconds)—1985 School Population Fitness Survey—Norms for girls aged 6–17

Per-centile	Age												Per-centile
	6–	7	8	9	10	11	12	13	14	15	16	17	
100	9.1	9.5	8.3	8.3	7.2	7.1	7.7	9.0	8.0	8.3	6.4	7.6	100
95	12.0	11.5	11.2	10.4	10.1	10.0	10.0	9.8	9.6	9.5	9.6	9.5	95
90	12.2	11.9	11.5	10.8	10.6	10.3	10.2	10.0	9.9	9.8	10.0	9.9	90
85	12.4	12.1	11.8	11.1	10.8	10.5	10.4	10.2	10.1	10.0	10.1	10.0	85
80	12.7	12.3	12.0	11.3	11.1	10.6	10.5	10.4	10.3	10.1	10.2	10.2	80
75	13.0	12.5	12.1	11.5	11.3	10.8	10.7	10.5	10.5	10.3	10.4	10.3	75
70	13.0	12.6	12.2	11.7	11.4	11.0	10.8	10.6	10.6	10.4	10.5	10.4	70
65	13.3	12.8	12.4	11.9	11.6	11.1	10.9	10.8	10.8	10.6	10.6	10.6	65
60	13.4	13.0	12.6	12.1	11.8	11.2	11.0	10.9	10.9	10.7	10.7	10.7	60
55	13.6	13.1	12.8	12.2	11.9	11.4	11.2	11.0	11.0	10.8	10.8	10.9	55
50	13.8	13.2	12.9	12.5	12.1	11.5	11.3	11.1	11.2	11.0	10.9	11.0	50
45	14.0	13.5	13.0	12.7	12.2	11.7	11.4	11.2	11.3	11.1	11.0	11.1	45
40	14.1	13.6	13.3	12.9	12.4	11.9	11.5	11.4	11.4	11.2	11.2	11.2	40
35	14.5	13.9	13.5	13.0	12.6	12.1	11.7	11.5	11.6	11.4	11.4	11.3	35
30	14.7	14.0	13.7	13.2	12.8	12.2	11.9	11.6	11.7	11.5	11.5	11.5	30
25	14.8	14.3	13.9	13.4	13.1	12.5	12.1	11.8	11.9	11.7	11.7	11.7	25
20	15.0	14.5	14.3	13.7	13.3	12.8	12.3	12.0	12.1	11.9	11.9	11.9	20
15	15.3	14.9	14.8	14.0	13.7	13.0	12.5	12.4	12.5	12.2	12.2	12.1	15
10	15.5	15.4	15.2	14.6	14.2	13.4	12.9	12.8	12.9	12.6	12.6	12.7	10
5	16.1	16.4	16.2	15.6	15.0	14.0	13.4	13.4	14.0	13.2	13.2	13.2	5
0	19.8	29.1	20.5	20.5	17.8	20.6	16.1	19.8	21.4	16.6	15.4	19.8	0

Table 33   2-Mile Walk for Girls (Minutes and Seconds)—
1985 School Population Fitness Survey—Norms for girls aged 6–17

Per-centile	6–	7	8	9	10	11	12	13	14	15	16	17	Per-centile
100	24'00"	24'08"	24'00"	24'00"	24'04"	24'23"	24'01"	24'02"	24'00"	24'05"	24'00"	24'03"	100
95	25'30"	26'53"	26'20"	25'56"	25'00"	25'30"	25'09"	24'49"	25'17"	25'30"	25'43"	25'20"	95
90	27'11"	28'20"	27'37"	27'06"	26'20"	26'35"	25'46"	25'54"	25'53"	26'30"	26'27"	26'30"	90
85	28'09"	29'57"	29'19"	28'04"	26'46"	27'11"	26'20"	26'24"	26'32"	27'09"	27'20"	26'59"	85
80	28'54"	30'46"	30'09"	28'53"	27'02"	27'43"	26'55"	27'00"	26'53"	27'46"	28'06"	27'24"	80
75	31'00"	31'36"	30'46"	29'09"	27'35"	28'23"	27'17"	27'11"	27'23"	28'09"	28'36"	27'58"	75
70	31'30"	32'30"	31'19"	29'56"	28'03"	28'50"	27'33"	27'39"	27'54"	28'30"	29'11"	28'22"	70
65	32'30"	33'13"	32'00"	30'35"	28'30"	29'34"	28'03"	28'08"	28'17"	28'49"	29'30"	28'48"	65
60	32'50"	33'41"	32'35"	31'15"	29'10"	30'06"	28'28"	28'27"	28'39"	29'10"	29'50"	29'17"	60
55	33'50"	34'10"	33'07"	31'45"	29'49"	30'37"	28'48"	28'47"	29'07"	29'42"	30'10"	29'40"	55
50	35'16"	35'10"	33'51"	32'45"	30'28"	31'15"	29'15"	29'01"	29'34"	30'06"	30'30"	30'10"	50
45	36'00"	35'52"	34'52"	33'30"	31'35"	31'35"	29'50"	29'30"	30'01"	30'30"	30'50"	30'20"	45
40	36'20"	36'15"	35'40"	33'57"	32'25"	32'35"	30'02"	29'58"	30'33"	30'50"	31'00"	30'49"	40
35	37'42"	37'09"	36'20"	34'36"	33'02"	32'55"	30'41"	30'32"	31'00"	31'10"	31'33"	31'03"	35
30	38'53"	38'19"	37'07"	35'06"	34'04"	34'00"	31'25"	30'57"	31'46"	31'40"	31'53"	31'37"	30
25	39'42"	40'18"	37'40"	35'36"	35'00"	34'55"	32'45"	31'47"	32'26"	32'17"	32'26"	32'01"	25
20	41'25"	41'20"	39'00"	37'05"	36'18"	36'00"	33'49"	32'40"	33'12"	33'00"	33'04"	32'24"	20
15	40'21"	42'00"	40'02"	39'00"	37'47"	37'24"	34'23"	33'56"	34'07"	33'38"	34'05"	32'40"	15
10	42'42"	43'00"	41'28"	40'38"	39'50"	39'00"	35'50"	34'55"	35'15"	34'45"	34'45"	33'42"	10
5	48'12"	46'30"	43'26"	42'36"	43'00"	42'50"	38'50"	37'00"	36'50"	36'36"	36'27"	34'50"	5
0	52'00"	55'47"	60'00"	49'20"	50'36"	51'55"	67'25"	67'25"	44'00"	44'00"	42'31"	45'32"	0

Table 34 50-Yard Dash for Girls (Seconds)—1985 School Population Fitness Survey Norms for girls aged 6–17

Per-centile	Age												Per-centile
	6–	7	8	9	10	11	12	13	14	15	16	17	
100	7.2	7.0	6.8	6.4	6.7	6.5	6.5	6.4	6.3	5.8	6.0	6.1	100
95	8.1	8.4	7.9	7.8	7.6	7.3	7.0	6.9	6.8	6.8	6.9	6.8	95
90	8.9	8.7	8.2	8.0	7.9	7.5	7.3	7.1	7.0	7.0	7.1	7.1	90
85	9.3	9.0	8.6	8.1	8.0	7.7	7.4	7.2	7.2	7.2	7.3	7.2	85
80	9.6	9.2	8.7	8.3	8.1	7.8	7.5	7.3	7.3	7.3	7.4	7.4	80
75	9.8	9.4	9.9	8.5	8.2	8.0	7.6	7.4	7.4	7.4	7.5	7.5	75
70	10.0	9.5	9.1	8.6	8.4	8.0	7.8	7.5	7.5	7.5	7.6	7.7	70
65	10.1	9.7	9.2	8.8	8.5	8.1	7.9	7.6	7.7	7.6	7.7	7.8	65
60	10.2	9.8	9.3	8.9	8.6	8.2	8.0	7.7	7.8	7.7	7.9	7.9	60
55	10.4	10.0	9.5	9.0	8.7	8.4	8.1	7.8	7.9	7.8	7.9	8.1	55
50	10.8	10.1	9.6	9.1	8.8	8.5	8.2	7.9	8.0	7.9	8.0	8.2	50
45	10.9	10.2	9.8	9.2	8.9	8.6	8.3	8.0	8.0	8.0	8.1	8.3	45
40	11.0	10.4	9.9	9.3	9.0	8.7	8.5	8.1	8.2	8.1	8.2	8.4	40
35	11.1	10.5	10.0	9.4	9.1	8.8	8.6	8.3	8.3	8.2	8.3	8.5	35
30	11.2	10.7	10.2	9.6	9.3	8.9	8.7	8.4	8.4	8.4	8.4	8.6	30
25	11.4	10.8	10.4	9.7	9.4	9.1	8.9	8.5	8.5	8.5	8.6	8.7	25
20	11.8	11.0	10.5	9.9	9.6	9.3	9.0	8.7	8.7	8.6	8.8	8.9	20
15	12.0	11.4	10.9	10.1	9.9	9.6	9.2	8.9	8.9	8.8	9.1	9.1	15
10	12.5	11.7	11.2	10.4	10.2	9.9	9.7	9.3	9.2	9.1	9.3	9.3	10
5	13.5	12.2	11.9	11.0	10.8	10.3	10.4	10.0	9.7	9.8	10.0	10.0	5
0	15.0	17.0	15.8	15.0	13.7	15.0	13.8	15.8	12.9	12.9	12.4	13.6	0

Table 35   Standing Long Jump for Girls (Feet and Inches)—
1985 School Population Fitness SurveyNorms for girls aged 6–17

| Per-centile | Age | | | | | | | | | | | | Per-centile |
	6–	7	8	9	10	11	12	13	14	15	16	17	
100	5'11	5'10	6'9"	6'1	7'0	7'3"	7'1"	7'4"	9'4"	8'7"	8'2"	7'7"	100
95	4'3"	4'8"	5'0"	5'5"	5'8"	6'0"	6'4"	6'6"	6'8"	6'7"	6'8"	6'9"	95
90	4'1"	4'6"	4'8"	5'1"	5'5"	5'9"	6'1"	6'2"	6'3"	6'4"	6'4"	6'5"	90
85	4'0"	4'3"	4'7"	4'11"	5'3"	5'6"	5'10"	6'0"	6'2"	6'2"	6'2"	6'2"	85
80	3'10"	4'2"	4'5"	4'9"	5'1"	5'5"	5'8"	5'11"	6'0"	6'0"	6'0"	6'1"	80
75	3'9"	4'0"	4'4"	4'7"	5'0"	5'4"	5'7"	5'9"	5'10"	5'11"	5'11"	6'0"	75
70	3'8"	3'11"	4'3"	4'6"	4'10"	5'3"	5'5"	5'8"	5'8"	5'9"	5'9"	5'11"	70
65	3'7"	3'10"	4'2"	4'5"	4'9"	5'1"	5'5"	5'7"	5'7"	5'8"	5'8"	5'9"	65
60	3'6"	3'9"	4'2"	4'4"	4'8"	5'0"	5'4"	5'5"	5'6"	5'6"	5'6"	5'8"	60
55	3'5"	3'8"	4'1"	4'3"	4'7"	4'11"	5'3"	5'4"	5'5"	5'4"	5'6"	5'6"	55
50	3'4"	3'7"	4'0"	4'2"	4'6"	4'9"	5'1"	5'3"	5'3"	5'3"	5'4"	5'5"	50
45	3'3"	3'6"	3'11"	4'1"	4'5"	4'8"	5'0"	5'1"	5'2"	5'2"	5'2"	5'4"	45
40	3'3"	3'5"	3'10"	4'0"	4'4"	4'7"	4'11"	5'0"	5'1"	5'1"	5'1"	5'3"	40
35	3'2"	3'4"	3'9"	3'10"	4'3"	4'6"	4'10"	4'11"	5'0"	5'0"	5'0"	5'1"	35
30	3'1"	3'3"	3'7"	3'9"	4'2"	4'5"	4'9"	4'9"	4'11"	4'11"	4'11"	5'0"	30
25	3'0"	3'2"	3'6"	3'8"	4'1"	4'4"	4'7"	4'8"	4'9"	4'9"	4'10"	4'10"	25
20	2'11"	3'1"	3'5"	3'7"	3'11"	4'2"	4'5"	4'6"	4'8"	4'7"	4'8"	4'8"	20
15	2'10"	3'0"	3'3"	3'6"	3'9"	4'0"	4'3"	4'5"	4'6"	4'5"	4'6"	4'5"	15
10	2'9"	2'11"	3'2"	3'4"	3'8"	3'10"	4'0"	4'2"	4'3"	4'3"	4'3"	4'2"	10
5	2'5"	2'8"	3'0"	3'2"	3'4"	3'7"	3'9"	3'11"	4'0"	4'0"	3'11"	4'0"	5
0	0'8"	1'10"	2'1"	2'1"	2'5"	2'4"	2'8"	2'8"	1'7"	2'5"	3'2"	2'3"	0

AAHPERD Norms for College-Aged Students

The American Association of Health, Physical Education, Recreation, and Dance (AAHPERD) released the results of their new testing program for college students in 1985. The study population consisted of 5,158 young adults in colleges from all geographic regions of the United States. The data for the study were collected under the supervision of twenty-four coinvestigators. The test items in order are as follows:

- Two-site skinfold test (triceps and subscapular)
- Mile run or nine-minute run for cardiorespiratory endurance
- Sit-and-reach test for flexibility
- One-minute timed sit-ups for abdominal muscular endurance

AAHPERD allows authors to publish only a limited part of the norms. The reader is urged to purchase the book from AAHPERD listed below.

Table 36   Health Related Physical Fitness Test Items—Males

%	Mile Run	Sit-Ups	Sit + Reach	Sum of Skinfold	% Body Fat
99	5:06	68	26	10	2.9
75	6:12	50	16	16	6.6
50	6:49	44	11	21	9.4
25	7:32	38	6	26	13.1
5	9:47	30	–4	40	20.4

Table 37   Health Related Physical Fitness Test Items—Females

%	Mile Run	Sit-Ups	Sit + Reach	Sum of Skinfold	% Body Fat
99	6:04	61	28	11	7.9
75	8:15	42	18	24	19.0
50	9:22	35	14	30	22.8
25	10:41	0	9	37	27.1
5	12:43	21	1	51	33.7

Mile run: Run one mile in the fastest possible time.
Sit-ups: As many correctly executed sit-ups as possible in 60 seconds.
Sit-and-reach: Footline is set at 0 cm. Score is cm beyond feet when legs are straight.
Sum of skinfolds: Triceps plus subscapular skinfolds.
See chapter 4 through 6 for details on how to administer tests.

Source: AAHPERD. Norms for College Students: Health Related Physical Fitness Test. 1985. Reprinted by permission of the American Alliance for Health, Physical Education, Recreation and Dance, 1900 Association Drive, Reston, Virginia 22091.

Cardiorespiratory Test Norms for Adults

(See Chapter 4 for instructions).

Table 38 YMCA Norms for Resting Heart Rate (beats/min)

Age (yrs.)	18–25		26–35		36–45		46–55		56–65		>65	
Gender	M	F	M	F	M	F	M	F	M	F	M	F
Excellent	49–55	54–60	49–54	54–59	50–56	54–59	50–57	54–60	51–56	54–59	50–55	54–59
Good	57–61	61–65	57–61	60–64	60–62	62–64	59–63	61–65	59–61	61–64	58–61	60–64
Above Average	63–65	66–69	62–65	66–68	64–66	66–69	64–67	66–69	64–67	67–69	62–65	66–68
Average	67–69	70–73	66–70	69–71	68–70	70–72	68–71	70–73	68–71	71–73	66–69	70–72
Below Average	71–73	74–78	72–74	72–76	73–76	74–78	73–76	74–77	72–75	75–77	70–73	73–76
Poor	76–81	80–84	77–81	78–82	77–82	79–82	79–83	78–84	76–81	79–81	75–79	79–84
Very Poor	84–95	86–100	84–94	84–94	86–96	84–92	85–97	85–96	84–94	85–96	83–98	88–96

Source: Adapted from: YMCA. Y'S Way to Fitness. 3rd edition. Champaign, Illinois: Human Kinetics Publishers, Inc., 1989. Reprinted with permission from the YMCA of the USA. Copies of the book may be purchased from the YMCA Program Store, Box 5077, Champaign, IL 61820, (217) 351–5077. See Chapter 4 for a description of this test.

Table 39 Resting Blood Pressure Standards

BP Range, mm Hg	Category
Diastolic Blood Pressure	
<85	Normal
85–89	High-normal
90–104	Mild hypertension
105–114	Moderate hypertension
≥115	Severe hypertension
Systolic Blood Pressure When Diastolic Blood Pressure is <90 mm Hg	
<140	Normal
140–159	Borderline isolated systolic hypertension
≥160	Isolated systolic hypertension

Note: Classification is based on the average of two or more readings on two or more occasions.

Source: 1988 Joint National Committee. The 1988 Report of the Joint National Committee on Detection, Evaluation, and Treatment of High Blood Pressure. Arch Intern Med 148:1023–1038, 1988.

Table 40 $\dot{V}O_{2max}$ Estimation from Running Tests

Estimation of $\dot{V}O_{2max}$ from Average Running Speed During Racing

Racing Distance	Equation to calculate $\dot{V}O_{2max}$	Correlation
1.5 km	METS = 2.4388 + (0.8343 x kmh)	0.95
1.6093 km (1 mile)	METS = 2.5043 + (0.8400 x kmh)	0.95
3 km	METS = 2.9226 + (0.8900 x kmh)	0.98
5 km	METS = 3.1747 + (0.9139 x kmh)	0.98
10 km	METS = 4.7226 + (0.8698 x kmh)	0.88
42.195 km (marathon)	METS = 6.9021 + (0.8246 x kmh)	0.85

Note: kmh = average racing speed in competition in kilometers per hour.

Note: 1 MET = 3.5 ml · kg^{-1}· min^{-1}. To calculate total oxygen power, multiply number of METS times 3.5 ml · kg^{-1}· min^{-1}. For example, if you can run a 5 km race in 18:30 (which is 16.2 kmh, calculated by multiplying the number of kilometers in the race by 60, and then dividing by the race time in decimal form $(5 \times 60)/18.5 = 16.2$ kmh), using the equation above, $\dot{V}O_{2max}$ in METS is equal to:

METS = 3.1747 + (0.9139 × 16.2) = 18 METS

$\dot{V}O_{2max}$ in ml · kg^{-1}· min^{-1} = 18 METS × 3.5 ml · kg^{-1}· min^{-1} = 63 ml · kg^{-1}· min^{-1}.

Equivalent Performances for Various Distances

$\dot{V}O_{2max}$ Performance Time for Various Distances (hours:minutes:seconds)

(ml · kg^{-1}· min^{-1})	1.5 km	Mile	5 km	10 km	42.2 km
28	13:30	14:46	56:49	2:39:14	31:41:25
31.5	11:27	12:29	47:04	2:02:00	16:35:05
35	9:56	10:49	40:10	1:38:53	11:13:52
38.5	8:46	9:33	35:02	1:23:08	8:29:26
42	7:51	8:33	31:04	1:11:43	6:49:30
45.5	7:07	7:44	27:54	1:03:03	5:42:21
49	6:30	7:03	25:20	0:56:15	4:54:07
52.5	5:59	6:29	23:11	0:50:47	4:17:48
56	5:32	6:01	21:23	0:46:17	3:49:28
59.5	5:09	5:36	19:50	0:42:30	3:26:44
63	4:50	5:14	18:30	0:39:33	3:08:06
66.5	4:32	4:55	17:20	0:36:33	2:52:34
70	4:17	4:38	16:18	0:34:10	2:39:23
73.5	4:03	4:23	15:23	0:32:12	2:28:05
77	3:50	4:09	14:34	0:30:12	2:18:16
80.5	3:39	3:57	13:50	0:28:33	2:09:41
84	3:29	3:46	13:10	0:27:04	2:02:06
87.5	3:20	3:36	12:34	0:25:44	1:55:21
See* $\dot{V}O_2$	3.2%	2.3%	2.3%	4.8%	5.6%

Source: Tokmakidis SP, Léer L, Mercier D, P´ronnet F, Thibault G. New Approaches to Predict $\dot{V}O_{2max}$ and Endurance from Running Performance. J Sports Med 27:401–409, 1987. *SEE = standard error of estimate

Table 41   YMCA 3-Minute Step Test   Post Exercise 1-Minute Heart Rate (beats/min)

Age (yrs.)	18–25		26–35		36–45		46–55		56–65		>65	
Gender	M	F	M	F	M	F	M	F	M	F	M	F
Excellent	70–78	72–83	73–79	72–86	72–81	74–87	78–84	76–93	72–82	74–92	72–86	73–86
Good	82–88	88–97	83–88	91–97	86–94	93–101	89–96	96–102	89–97	97–103	89–95	93–100
Above average	91–97	100–106	91–97	103–110	98–102	104–109	99–103	106–113	98–101	106–111	97–102	104–114
Average	101–104	110–116	101–106	112–118	105–111	111–117	109–115	117–120	105–111	113–117	104–113	117–121
Below average	107–114	118–124	109–116	121–127	113–118	120–127	118–121	121–126	113–118	119–127	114–119	123–127
Poor	118–126	128–137	119–126	129–135	120–128	130–138	124–130	127–133	122–128	129–136	122–128	129–134
Very poor	131–164	141–155	130–164	141–154	132–168	143–152	135–158	138–152	131–150	142–151	133–152	135–151

Source: Adapted from: YMCA. Y'S Way to Fitness. 3rd edition. Champaign, Illinois: Human Kinetics Publishers, Inc., 1989. Reprinted with permission from the YMCA of the USA. Copies of the book may be purchased from the YMCA Program Store, Box 5077, Champaign, IL 61820, (217) 351–5077. See Chapter 4 for a description of this test.
Note: See Chapter 4 tor instructions. Pulse is to be counted for one full minute following 3 minutes of stepping at 24 steps/min on a 12 inch bench.

Table 42   YMCA Physical Working Capacity Bicycle Test   (milliters of oxygen per minute arranged in order of high to low in each category)

Age (yrs.)	18–25		26–35		36–45		46–55		56–65		>65	
Gender	M	F	M	F	M	F	M	F	M	F	M	F
Excellent	2350–2065	1830–1440	2300–1950	1800–1330	2250–1815	1780–1215	2150–1645	1700–1130	2100–1485	1650–1015	1940–1235	1190–820
Good	1905–1705	1320–1175	1820–1665	1245–1115	1725–1565	1135–1035	1520–1385	1045–930	1400–1240	970–840	1175–1045	725–640
Above average	1630–1515	1120–1030	1600–1485	1065–985	1500–1375	980–880	1335–1240	885–815	1195–1100	790–720	1015–945	610–560
Average	1455–1350	990–915	1430–1325	955–885	1325–1235	835–765	1205–1130	790–730	1055–965	690–635	900–840	540–510
Below average	1305–1195	880–810	1270–1180	840–765	1190–1090	745–695	1090–1020	700–640	925–860	605–550	805–725	495–470
Poor	1135–1050	775–705	1135–1020	730–655	1045–945	670–575	950–885	610–545	830–740	530–475	695–610	460–395
Very poor	975–850	640–500	960–780	600–490	860–700	530–470	830–700	495–400	680–590	420–340	555–490	370–320

Source: Adapted from: YMCA. Y'S Way to Fitness. 3rd edition. Champaign, Illinois: Human Kinetics Publishers, Inc., 1989. Reprinted with permission from the YMCA of the USA. Copies of the book may be purchased from the YMCA Program Store, Box 5077, Champaign, IL 61820, (217) 351–5077. See instructions, Chapter 4.

Table 43 $\dot{V}O_{2max}$ Estimation from Treadmill Test
From length of time on treadmill until exhaustion

$\dot{V}O_2$ Max	METS	Bruce	Balke
(ml · kg⁻¹· min⁻¹)		(min:sec)	(min:sec)
14.0	4.0	2:30	2:00
15.7	4.5	4:00	3:00
20.2	5.8	6:00	6:00
24.2	6.9	7:20	8:00
27.7	7.9	8:20	9:45
31.1	8.9	9:15	12:00
34.8	9.9	10:10	14:30
38.2	10.9	11:00	17:00
42.5	12.1	12:00	19:00
45.7	13.1	12:45	21:30
49.6	14.2	13:40	24:15
53.0	15.2	14:30	26:15
56.1	16.0	15:15	27:45
59.7	17.1	16:10	29:00
62.7	17.9	17:00	30:00
66.1	18.9	18:00	31:15
70.0	20.0	19:20	32:00
73.6	21.0	21:00	33:45
75.4	21.5	22:30	35:45

Source: Estimated $\dot{V}O_{2max}$ for Bruce's treadmill protocol based on the equation:
$\dot{V}O_{2max}$ ml · kg⁻¹· min⁻¹ = 14.8 − 1.379(TIME) + 0.451(TIME²) − 0.012(TIME³)

Note: TIME = total time to exhaustion during the Bruce maximal graded treadmill exercise test. Foster C, Jackson AS, Pollock ML, et al. Generalized Equations for Predicting Functional Capacity From Treadmill Performance. Am Heart J 108:1229–1234, 1984.

Estimated $\dot{V}O_{2max}$ for Balke protocol taken from table adapted from Pollock ML, Wilmore JH, and Fox SM: Health and Fitness Through Physical Activity. New York: Macmillan, 1978. Reprinted with permission of the publisher.

Note: $\dot{V}O_{2max}$ is in mililiters of oxygen per kilogram of body weight per minute. One met = 3.5 ml/kg/min. See Chapter 4 for description of Bruce and Balke protocols on treadmill. Note that as a rough rule of thumb, the number of minutes a person exercises in the Bruce's protocol is nearly equal to the number of mets.

Table 44 $\dot{V}O_{2max}$ Norms

Women	Low	Fair	Avg	Good	High	Athletic	Olympic
20–29	<28	29–34	35–43	44–48	49–53	54–59	60+
30–39	<27	28–33	34–41	42–47	48–52	53–58	59+
40–49	<25	26–31	32–40	41–45	46–50	51–56	57+
50–65	<21	22–28	29–36	37–41	42–45	46–49	50+
Men							
20–29	<38	39–43	44–51	52–56	57–62	63–69	70+
30–39	<34	35–39	40–47	48–51	52–57	58–64	65+
40–49	<30	31–35	36–43	44–47	48–53	54–60	61+
50–59	<25	26–31	32–39	40–43	44–48	49–55	56+
60–69	<21	22–26	27–35	36–39	40–44	45–49	50+

Source: Adapted from Astrand: ACTA Physiol Scand 49 (Suppl):169,1960.
Reprinted with permission from Blackwell Scientific Publications LTD.

Note: $\dot{V}O_{2max}$ is expressed in tables as milliliters of oxygen per kilogram of body weight per minute.

Body Composition Test Norms for Adults

Table 45   1959 Metropolitan Height-Weight Tables
(In pounds by height and frame, in indoor clothing)

Men (In shoes, 1-inch heels)				Women (In shoes, 2-inch heels)			
Height (inches)	Frame small	medium	large	Height (inches)	Frame small	medium	large
62	112–120	118–129	126–141	58	92–98	96–107	104–119
63	115–123	121–133	129–144	59	94–101	98–110	106–122
64	118–126	124–136	132–148	60	96–104	101–113	109–125
65	121–129	127–139	135–152	61	99–107	104–116	112–128
66	124–133	130–143	138–156	62	102–110	107–119	115–131
67	128–137	134–147	142–161	63	105–113	110–122	118–134
68	132–141	138–152	147–166	64	108–116	113–126	121–138
69	136–145	142–156	151–170	65	111–119	116–130	125–142
70	140–150	146–160	155–174	66	114–123	120–135	129–146
71	144–154	150–165	159–179	67	118–127	124–139	133–150
72	148–158	154–170	164–184	68	122–131	128–143	137–154
73	152–162	158–175	168–189	69	126–135	132–147	141–158
74	156–167	162–180	173–194	70	130–140	136–151	145–163
75	160–171	167–185	178–199	71	134–144	140–155	149–168
76	164–175	172–190	182–204	72	138–148	144–159	153–173

Source: New Weight Standards for Men and Women. Stat Bull Metropol Life Insur Co. 40:1, 1959. Courtesy of the Metropolitan Life Insurance Company.

Table 46 1973 Fogarty Height-Weight Table
(Height without shoes; weight without clothing).

Height	Weight	
(inches)	Men	Women
58		92–121
59		95–124
60		98–127
61	105–134	101–130
62	108–137	104–134
63	111–141	107–138
64	114–145	110–142
65	117–149	114–146
66	121–154	118–150
67	125–159	122–154
68	129–163	126–159
69	133–167	130–164
70	137–172	134–169
71	141–177	
72	145–182	
73	149–187	
74	153–192	
75	157–197	

Source: Adapted from: New Weight Standards for Men and Women. Stat Bull Metropol Life Insur Co. 40:1, 1959. Courtesy of the Metropolitan Life Insurance Company.

Table 47 1983 Metropolitan height-Weight Tables (In pounds by height and frame, in indoor clothing, men 5 lbs, 1-inch heel; women 3 lbs, 1-inch heel).

Men Height (inches)	Frame small	medium	large	Women Height (inches)	Frame small	medium	large
62	128–134	131–141	138–150	58	102–111	109–121	118–131
63	130–136	133–143	140–153	59	103–113	111–123	120–134
64	132–138	135–145	142–156	60	104–115	113–126	122–137
65	134–140	137–148	144–160	61	106–118	115–129	125–140
66	136–142	139–151	146–164	62	108–121	118–132	128–143
67	138–145	142–154	149–168	63	111–124	121–135	131–147
68	140–148	145–157	152–172	64	114–127	124–138	134–151
69	142–151	148–160	155–176	65	117–130	127–141	137–155
70	144–154	151–163	158–180	66	120–133	130–144	140–159
71	146–157	154–166	161–184	67	123–136	133–147	143–163
72	149–160	157–170	164–188	68	126–139	136–150	146–167
73	152–164	160–174	168–192	69	129–142	139–153	149–170
74	155–168	164–178	172–197	70	132–145	142–156	152–173
75	158–172	167–182	176–202	71	135–148	145–159	155–176
76	162–176	171–187	181–207	72	138–151	148–162	158–179

Source: Reprinted with permission from the Metropolitan Life Insurance Company, New York.

Table 48 1985 NIH Consensus Panel Weight Table (Height without shoes; weight without clothing).

Height (inches)	Weight Men	Women
58		100–131
59		101–134
60		103–137
61	123–145	105–140
62	125–148	108–144
63	127–151	111–148
64	129–155	114–152
65	131–159	117–156
66	133–163	120–160
67	135–167	123–164
68	137–171	123–167
69	139–175	129–170
70	141–179	132–176
71	144–183	135–176
72	147–187	
73	150–192	
74	153–197	
75	157–202	

Source: Adapted from the 1983 Height-Weight Tables, Metropolitan. Courtesy of the Metropolitan Life Insurance Company.

Table 49   Body Mass Index Standards

The most commonly used body mass index is the quetelet index or kg/m² (body weight in kilograms divided by height in meters squared). Researchers from The Panel on Energy, Obesity, and Body Weight Standards have recommended that the following table be used when using the Quetelet index for obesity classification:

- 20–25 kg/m²—desirable range for adult men and women
- 25–29.9 kg/m²—Grade I obesity
- 30–40 kg/m²—Grade II obesity
- >40 kg/m²—Grade III obesity (morbidy obesity)

Source: Jéquier E. Energy, Obesity, and Body Weight Standards. Am J Clin Nutr 45:1035–1047, 1987.

The following table was developed by the Nutrition/Metabolism Laboratory, Cancer Research Institute, Boston MA, and represents another way of using the body mass index for medical classification of obesity.

Percent of desirable wt	Definition	Grade of Obesity	BMI (kg/m²)
225	Super morbid obesity	6	>50
200	Morbid obesity	5	45
180	Super obesity	4	40
160	Medically significant	3	35
135	Obesity	2	30
110	Overweight	1	25
100	Desirable weight	0	22
70	Medically significant starvation	–3	15

Source: Blackburn G, Kanders B. Evaluation and Treatment of the Medically Obese Patient with Cardiovascular Disease. Am J Cardiology 60:11, 1987.

Table 50   Triceps Skinfold Norms
Percentiles of Triceps Skinfold Thickness (mm) by Age Group & Sex

Males	—Lean—	—Good—	—Plump—	—Fat—	
Percentiles	5	15	50	85	95
Age group					
18–24	4	5	8	13	16
25–34	4	6	10	15	17
35–44	5	6	11	15	18
45–54	5	7	10	15	18
55–64	5	7	10	15	17
65–74	4	6	10	14	16
Females					
Percentiles	5	15	50	85	95
Age group					
18–24	9	11	17	23	26
25–34	10	13	20	26	29
35–44	12	15	22	29	32
45–54	12	16	24	31	33
55–64	12	16	24	31	33
65–74	11	15	22	29	31

Of the various skinfold sites, the triceps skinfold has been used most often in large population group studies. The data were derived from the first and second National Health and Examination Surveys (NHANES I and II) for 1971–1974 and 1976–1980. These surveys involved a multistage, stratified sampling of the noninstitutionalized civilians of the United States. Excluded in the development of the triceps skinfold norms were all individuals whose triceps skinfolds were above the 85th age- and sex-specific percentile. This resulted in the exclusion of 6,088 fat individuals and left a total sample of 23,120 nonfat subjects. Thus the triceps skinfold norms present reference percentile values based upon a sample that is not obese. Optimal values are thus at the 50th percentile.

Care should be taken when using just one skinfold site such as the triceps skinfold in classifying individuals as to their degree of obesity. No equations for body fat estimation have been developed using the triceps skinfold, and individuals must therefore compare their values to tables developed from national norms. Some individuals have more of their body fat distributed on the backs of their upper arms than others, which could lead to an overestimation of the degree of obesity (and vice versa). The single-site skinfold test should only be used as a rough approximation of the degree of obesity.

Source: Adapted from Frisancho AR, Frameter (1985). Health Products, 2126 Ridge, Ann Arbor, Michigan, 48104. Used with permission. (See Chapter 5).

Table 51   Percent Body Fat Classifications

Classification	Male	Female
Lean	<8	<13
Optimal	8–15	13–20
Slightly overfat	16–20	21–25
Fat	21–24	26–32
Obese (overfat)	≥25	≥32
Long distance runners	4–9	6–15
Wrestlers	4–10	—
Gymnasts	4–10	10–17
Body builders (elite)	6–10	10–17
Swimmers	5–11	14–24
Basketball athletes	7–11	18–27
Canoers/kayakers	11–15	18–24
Tennis players	14–17	19–22

Source: Adapted from: Lohman TG. The Use of Skinfold to Estimate Body Fatness on Children and Youth. JOPERD November-December, 1987, pp. 98–102. Fleck SJ. Body Composition of Elite American Athletes. Am J Sports Med 11:398, 1983. Wilmore JH. The Physiological Basis of the Conditioning Process. Boston: Allyn and Bacon, Inc., 1982.

Musculoskeletal Test Norms for Adults

See descriptions given with each test. Also review Chapter 6.

Table 52   One-Minute Timed, Bent-Knee Sit-Ups   Norms and Percentiles by Age Groups and Gender for Sit-Ups (number in 60 seconds)

Age(years)	15–19		20–29		30–39		40–49		50–59		60–69	
Gender	M	F	M	F	M	F	M	F	M	F	M	F
Excellent	≥48	≥42	≥43	≥36	≥36	≥29	≥31	≥25	≥26	≥19	≥23	≥16
Above Average	42–47	36–41	37–42	31–35	31–35	24–28	26–30	20–24	22–25	12–18	17–22	12–15
Average	38–41	32–35	33–36	25–30	27–30	20–23	22–25	15–19	18–21	5–11	12–16	4–11
Below Average	33–37	27–31	29–32	21–24	22–26	15–19	17–21	7–14	13–17	3–4	7–11	2–3
Poor	≤32	≤26	≤28	≤20	≤21	≤14	≤16	≤6	≤12	≤2	≤6	≤1

Procedures: Subject lies in a supine position, knees bent at a right angle, and feet shoulder-width apart. The hands are placed at the side of the head with the fingers over the ears. The elbows are pointed towards the knees. The hands and elbows must be maintained in these positions for the entire duration of the test. Also, the ankles of the participant must be held throughout the test by the appraiser to ensure that the heels are in constant contact with the mat. The participant is required to sit up, touch the knees with the elbows and return to the starting position (shoulders touch the floor). The participant performs as many sit-ups as possible within one minute. A rocking or bouncing movement is not permitted. The buttocks must remain in contact with the mat at all times.

Source: Fitness Canada. CSTF Operations Manual (Third Edition). Ottawa. Fitness and Amateur Sport, 1986. The Canadian Standardized Test of Fitness was developed by, and is reproduced with the permission of, Fitness Canada, Government of Canada.

Table 53   Push-Ups   Norms and Percentiles by Age Groups and Gender for Push-Ups

Age (years)	15–19		20–29		30–39		40–49		50–59		60–69	
Gender	M	F	M	F	M	F	M	F	M	F	M	F
Excellent	≥39	≥33	≥36	≥30	≥30	≥27	≥22	≥24	≥21	≥21	≥18	≥17
Above Average	29–38	25–32	29–35	21–29	22–29	20–26	17–21	15–23	13–20	11–20	11–17	12–16
Average	23–28	18–24	22–28	15–20	17–21	13–19	13–16	11–14	10–12	7–10	8–10	5–11
Below Average	18–22	12–17	17–21	10–14	12–16	8–12	10–12	5–10	7–9	2–6	5–7	1–4
Poor	≤17	≤11	≤16	≤9	≤11	≤7	≤9	≤4	≤6	≤1	≤4	≤1

Procedures: *Males*—The participant lies on his stomach, legs together. His hands, pointing forward, are positioned under the shoulders. The participant pushes up from the mat by fully straightening the elbows and using the toes as the pivotal point. The upper body must be kept in a straight line. The participant returns to the starting position, chin to the mat. Neither the stomach nor thighs should touch the mat. *Females:* Same as for males, except the knees are the pivotal point. The lower legs remain in contact with the mat, ankles plantar-flexed.

Source: Fitness Canada. CSTF Operations Manual (Third Edition). Ottawa. Fitness and Amateur Sport, 1986. The Canadian Standardized Test of Fitness was developed by, and is reproduced with the permission of, Fitness Canada, Government of Canada.

Table 54 Grip Strength Norms and Percentiles by Age Groups and Gender for Combined Right and Left Hand Grip Strength (kg)

Age (years)	5–19		20–29		30–39		40–49		50–59		60–69	
Gender	M	F	M	F	M	F	M	F	M	F	M	F
Excellent	≥113	≥71	≥124	≥71	≥123	≥73	≥119	≥73	≥110	≥65	≥102	≥60
Above Average	103–112	64–70	113–123	65–70	113–122	66–72	110–118	65–72	102–109	59–64	98–101	54–59
Average	95–102	59–63	106–112	61–64	105–112	61–65	102–109	59–64	96–101	55–58	86–92	51–53
Below Average	84–94	54–58	97–105	55–60	97–104	56–60	94–101	55–58	87–95	51–54	79–85	48–50
Poor	≤83	≤53	≤96	≤54	≤96	≤55	≤93	≤54	≤86	≤50	≤78	≤47

Procedures: Have the participant grasp the dynamometer in the right hand first. Adjust the grip of the dynamometer so the second joint of the fingers fits snugly under the handle. The participant holds the dynamometer in line with the forearm at the level of the thigh. The dynamometer is then squeezed vigorously so as to exert maximum force. During the test, neither the hand nor the dynamometer should touch the body or any other object. Measure both hands alternatively allowing two trials per hand. Record the scores for each hand to the nearest kilogram. Combine the maximum score for each hand.

Source: Fitness Canada. CSTF Operations Manual (Third Edition). Ottawa. Fitness and Amateur Sport, 1986. The Canadian Standardized Text of Fitness was developed by, and is reproduced with the permission of, Fitness Canada, Government of Canada.

Table 55 Sit and Reach Test for Low Back-Hamstring Flexibility Norms and Percentiles by Age Groups and Gender for Trunk Forward Flexion (cm)

Note: footline is set at 26 cm.

Age (years)	15–19		20–29		30–39		40–49		50–59		60–69	
Gender	M	F	M	F	M	F	M	F	M	F	M	F
Excellent	≥39	≥43	≥40	≥41	≥38	≥41	≥35	≥38	≥35	≥39	≥33	≥35
Above Average	34–38	38–42	34–39	37–40	33–37	36–40	29–34	34–37	28–34	33–38	25–32	31–34
Average	29–33	34–37	30–33	33–36	28–32	32–35	24–28	30–33	24–27	30–32	20–24	27–30
Below Average	24–28	29–33	25–29	28–32	23–27	27–31	18–23	25–29	16–23	25–29	15–19	23–26
Poor	≤23	≤28	≤24	≤27	≤22	≤26	≤17	≤24	≤15	≤24	≤14	≤23

Procedures: Have the participant warm-up for this test by performing slow aerobic activities and then stretching movements. The participant, barefoot, sits with legs fully extended with the soles of the feet placed flat against the flexibility box. (See Chapter 6). Keeping knees fully extended, arms evenly stretched, palms down, the participant bends and reaches forward without jerking, pushing the sliding marker along the scale with the fingertips as far as possible. The position of maximum flexion must be held for approximately two seconds. The test is repeated twice. The footline is set at 26 cm.

Source: Fitness Canada. CSTF Operations Manual (Third Edition). Ottawa. Fitness and Amateur Sport, 1986. The Canadian Standardized Text of Fitness was developed by, and is reproduced with the permission of, Fitness Canada, Government of Canada.

Note: There is some feeling that flexibility should not decrease with age if regular range of motion exercise is engaged in. The following norms are proposed:

Classification	Sit and Reach (inches) (footline at 0)
Excellent	≥+7
Good	+4–6.75
Average	+0–3.75
Fair	–3–0.25
Poor	<–3

Table 56   YMCA Endurance Bench Press Test—Total lifts
(Arranged in order of high to low in each category)

Age (yrs.)	18–25		26–35		36–45		46–55		56–65		>65	
Gender	M	F	M	F	M	F	M	F	M	F	M	F
Excellent	45–38	50–36	43–34	48–33	40–30	46–28	35–24	42–26	32–22	34–22	30–18	26–18
Good	34–30	32–28	30–26	29–25	28–24	25–21	22–20	22–20	20–14	20–16	14–10	14–12
Above average	28–25	25–22	25–22	22–20	22–20	20–17	17–14	17–13	14–10	15–12	10–8	11–9
Average	22–21	21–18	21–18	18–16	18–16	14–12	13–10	12–10	10–8	10–8	8–6	8–5
Below average	20–16	16–13	17–13	14–12	14–12	11–9	10–8	9–6	6–4	7–4	4	4–2
Poor	13–9	12–8	12–9	9–5	10–8	8–4	6–4	5–2	4–2	3–1	2	2–0
Very poor	8–0	5–1	5–0	2–0	5–0	2–0	2–0	1–0	0	0	0	0

Source: Adapted from: YMCA. Y'S Way to Fitness. 3rd edition. Champaign, Illinois: Human Kinetics Publishers, Inc., 1989. Reprinted with permission from the YMCA of the USA. Copies of the book may be purchased from the YMCA Program Store, Box 5077, Champaign, IL 61820, (217) 351–5077.
Note: See Chapter 6 for instructions. Women use a 35 pound bar; men, 85 lbs. Max repetitions in time to metronome at 30 lifts per minute.

Table 57   1-RM Bench Press Test

Men	Classification	Women
+1.2	Excellent	+48
0.99–1.19	Good	0.41–0.47
0.79–0.98	Average	0.30–0.40
0.69–0.78	Fair	0.21–0.29
0.00–0.68	Poor	0.00–0.20

Source: Johnson BL, Nelson JK. Practical Measurement for Evaluation in Physical Education. Minneapolis; Burgess Publishing Co., 1979. Reprinted with permission from Burgess Publishing, 7110 Ohms Lane, Edina, MN 55435.
Note: See Chapter 6 for instructions. The amount of pounds lifted in an all-out effort is divided by the body weight, and then compared with these norms.

Table 58   Pull-Ups

Classification	Number of pull-ups
Excellent	15+
Good	12–14
Average	8–11
Fair	5–7
Poor	0–4

Source: Johnson BL, Nelson JK. Practical Measurement for Evaluation in Physical Education. Minneapolis: Burgess Publishing Co., 1979. Reprinted with permission.
Note: See Chapter 6 for instructions. Norms are for college men.

Table 59   Parallel Bar Dips

Classification	Number of Bar Dips
Excellent	25+
Good	18–24
Average	9–17
Fair	4–8
Poor	0–3

Source: Same as above.
Note: See Chapter 6 for instructions.

Serum Cholesterol and LCL-C Levels in Americans

Total Cholesterol and LDL-Cholesterol Distribution(s) in the U.S. Population by Age and Sex NHANES Data (Serum)

Table 60 Mean Serum Cholesterol Levels of Men

Mean serum cholesterol levels of *men*, standard errors of the mean, age-adjusted values, selected percentiles, number of examined persons, and estimated population, by race and age: United States, 1976–80

Race and Age	Examined Persons	Estimated Population	Mean	SEM†	5th	10th	15th	25th	50th	75th	85th	90th	95th
All Races	Number	Number in Thousands			Serum Cholesterol in Milligrams Per Deciliter								
20–74 years	5,604	63,611	211	1.2	144	156	165	179	206	239	258	271	291
20–24 years	676	9,331	180	1.7	129	136	145	155	176	202	215	227	246
25–34 years	1,067	15,895	199	1.5	141	152	159	172	194	220	240	254	275
35–44 years	745	11,367	217	2.0	153	166	173	187	215	244	262	275	293
45–54 years	690	11,114	227	1.8	159	176	182	197	223	255	271	283	303
55–64 years	1,227	9,607	229	1.8	164	176	184	198	225	254	277	288	307
65–74 years	1,199	6,297	221	1.8	153	167	175	191	217	249	265	279	301
White													
20–74 years	4,883	55,808	211	1.2	145	157	166	179	207	239	258	271	291
20–24 years	581	8,052	180	1.8	131	138	146	155	176	202	216	229	244
25–34 years	901	13,864	199	1.7	144	153	161	172	194	220	239	254	273
35–44 years	653	9,808	217	1.8	153	166	173	187	214	244	260	272	291
45–54 years	617	9,865	227	1.8	160	177	181	198	222	254	271	283	303
55–64 years	1,086	8,642	230	2.0	164	178	185	199	225	255	278	289	307
65–74 years	1,045	5,576	222	2.0	153	167	175	191	217	250	266	281	301
Black													
20–74 years	607	6,102	208	2.5	133	146	156	171	200	238	260	273	301
20–24 years	79	1,043	171	*3.7	*	128	134	149	170	193	210	211	*
25–34 years	139	1,546	199	*4.1	129	136	144	163	192	226	248	259	301
35–44 years	70	1,112	218	*8.3	*	156	168	176	202	238	275	283	*
45–54 years	62	1,044	229	*7.1	*	174	184	195	232	261	268	279	*
55–64 years	129	801	223	*4.8	157	168	172	183	218	254	271	299	312
65–74 years	128	555	217	4.2	149	163	173	183	216	244	261	277	299

†SEM = Standard Error of the Mean.

Source: National Center for Health Statistics; Fulwood, R.; Kalsbeck, W.; Rifkind, B.; Russell-Briefel, R.; Muesing, R.; LaRosa, J.; Lippel, K. Total serum cholesterol levels of adults 20–74 years of age: United States, 1976–80. Vital and Health Statistics, Ser. II, No. 236. DHHS Pub. No. (PHS) 86–1686. Public Health Service. Washington, DC: US Government Printing Office, May 1986.

Table 61   Mean Serum Cholesterol Levels of Women

Mean serum cholesterol levels of *women*, standard errors of the mean, age-adjusted values, selected percentiles, number of examined persons, and estimated population, by race and age: United States, 1976–80

Race and Age	Examined Persons	Estimated Population	Mean	SEM†	Percentile 5th	10th	15th	25th	50th	75th	85th	90th	95th
All Races	Number	Number in Thousands			Serum Cholesterol in Milligrams Per Deciliter								
20–74 years	6,260	69,994	215	1.2	143	156	166	179	210	245	266	282	305
20–24 years	738	9,994	184	1.9	132	140	145	157	180	204	216	230	250
25–34 years	1,170	16,856	192	1.4	135	145	154	164	188	215	233	243	263
35–44 years	844	12,284	207	1.8	147	158	164	177	202	231	248	260	276
45–54 years	763	11,918	232	2.2	164	178	188	199	228	257	275	290	306
55–64 years	1,329	10,743	249	2.0	180	193	203	215	242	277	299	314	336
65–74 years	1,416	8,198	246	1.6	173	189	198	214	241	274	295	309	327
White													
20–74 years	5,418	60,785	216	1.3	143	156	166	179	210	246	267	282	305
20–24 years	624	8,408	184	2.1	133	140	147	159	181	204	215	230	249
25–34 years	1,000	14,494	192	1.5	135	145	153	164	188	215	235	244	261
35–44 years	726	10,584	207	1.9	147	157	164	177	203	231	248	250	277
45–54 years	647	10,369	232	2.6	166	179	188	199	228	257	274	290	308
55–64 years	1,176	9,601	249	1.7	180	193	203	215	244	277	298	312	330
65–74 years	1,245	7,329	246	1.7	174	190	199	214	242	275	296	309	328
Black													
20–74 years	729	7,579	212	3.1	140	154	166	176	205	237	263	279	308
20–24 years	94	1,304	185	*4.9	*	136	144	156	178	204	220	237	*
25–34 years	145	1,953	191	*4.1	129	144	156	167	190	212	226	235	267
35–44 years	103	1,415	206	*4.5	143	158	170	175	194	233	254	274	279
45–54 years	100	1,215	230	*7.2	150	172	181	200	226	263	277	291	306
55–64 years	135	959	251	*8.0	178	185	198	211	233	280	318	336	345
65–74 years	152	733	243	4.2	173	189	198	211	237	269	290	308	323

SEM† = Standard Error of the Mean.

Source: National Center for Health Statistics; Fulwood, R.; Kalsbeck, W.; Rifkind, B.; Russell-Briefel, R.; Muesing, R.; LaRosa, J.; Lippel, K. Total serum cholesterol levels of adults 20–74 years of age: United States, 1976–80. Vital and Health Statistics, Ser. II, No. 236. DHHS Pub. No. (PHS) 86–1686. Public Health Service. Washington, DC: US Government Printing Office, May 1986.

Table 62   Serum Low Density Lipoprotein Cholesterol

Calculated levels of *serum low density lipoprotein cholesterol*** for persons, ages 20–74 years fasting 12 hours or more by sex and age: means and selected percentile: United States, 1976–80.

Race and Age	Examined Persons	Estimated Population	Mean	SEM†	Percentile 5th	10th	15th	25th	50th	75th	85th	90th	95th
	Number	Number in Thousands			Serum LDL-Cholesterol in Milligrams Per Deciliter								
Male													
20–74 years	1,037	21,262	140	39	80	92	100	113	136	164	181	194	208
20–24 years	72	1,852	109	36	*	70	74	88	104	129	149	154	*
25–34 years	174	5,186	128	33	76	87	94	108	128	148	161	171	189
35–44 years	130	3,866	145	40	81	96	105	116	138	176	192	203	206
45–54 years	106	3,543	150	36	99	103	112	119	146	171	189	195	211
55–64 years	267	3,943	148	39	84	101	108	118	147	171	191	206	217
65–74 years	288	2,872	149	40	87	105	109	120	144	174	188	199	217
Female													
20–74 years	1,246	27,102	141	43	81	91	98	110	136	164	186	199	220
20–24 years	105	3,325	114	33	69	74	83	94	106	136	149	155	179
25–34 years	194	5,517	121	33	72	83	90	98	116	139	154	166	187
35–44 years	166	4,800	129	34	78	90	97	107	126	150	163	171	191
45–54 years	168	5,155	157	45	94	104	116	125	156	184	200	213	226
55–64 years	282	4,644	159	42	101	113	118	129	150	188	205	219	237
65–74 years	331	3,661	162	44	98	109	122	135	158	186	207	226	245

†SEM = Standard Error of the Mean.

** Serum LDL-Cholesterol = [Serum Total Cholesterol—(HDL-C + (Triglycerides/5))]. Equation from Friedewald, W.T. et al. Clin Chem 1972; 18:499–502. Persons with a serum triglyceride value greater than 400 mg/dl were excluded.

* Sample size insufficient to produce statistically reliable results.

Source: National Center for Health Statistics: Division of Health Examination Statistics, unpublished data from the second National Health and Nutrition Examination Survey, 1976–80.

Addresses of Professional Organizations and Equipment Suppliers

Addresses of Professional Organizations

Major organizations with an emphasis in sports medicine include:

Amateur Athletic Union of the United States (AAU)
AAU House, Box 68207, Indianapolis, IN 46268
(317) 872-2900
Publication: InfoAAU.

American Alliance for Health, Physical Education, Recreation and Dance (AAHPERD)
1900 Association Dr., Reston, VA 22091
(703) 476-3400
Publications include: Research Quarterly; Health Education; Journal of Physical Education, Recreation and Dance.

American College of Sports Medicine (ACSM)
Box 1440, Indianapolis, IN 46206-1440
(317) 637-9200
Publications include: Medicine and Science in Sports and Exercise; Sports Medicine Bulletin; Exercise and Sport Sciences Reviews. Certification program available.

American Dietetic Association (ADA)
Practice Group of Sports and Cardiovascular Nutritionists (SCAN)
216 W. Jackson Blvd., Chicago, IL 60606-6995
(312) 899-0040
Publication: SCAN Pulse.

American Medical Athletic Association (AMAA)
Box 4704, North Hollywood, CA 91607
(818) 989-3432
Publications include: Annals of Sports Medicine, AMAA/AMJA Newsletter.

American Orthopaedic Society for Sports Medicine (AOSSM)
70 W Hubbard, Suite 202, Chicago, IL 60610
(312) 644-2623
Publication: The American Journal of Sports Medicine.

Association for Fitness in Business (AFB)
965 Hope St., Stamford, CT 06907
(203) 359-2188
Publications include: AFB Action, Fitness in Business.

International Dance-Exercise Association (IDEA)
2431 Morena Blvd, Suite 2-D, San Diego, CA 92110
(619) 275-2450
Publication: Dance-Exercise Today. Certification program available.

Institute for Aerobics Research (IAR)
12330 Preston Rd, Dallas, TX 75230
(214) 701-8001
Publication: The Aerobics News. Certification program available.

President's Council on Physical Fitness and Sports (PCPFS)
450 Fifth St NW, Suite 7103, Washington, DC 20001
(202) 272-3421
Publication: PCPFS Newsletter.

Source: Anonymous. Sports Medicine Groups 1987. Physician Sportsmed 15(12):155-161, 1987.

Note: Each year, the Physician and Sportsmedicine journal publishes a "Sports Medicine Directory." Contact: The Physician and Sportsmedicine, Centers Project, 4530 W 77th St, Minneapolis, 55435, for information.

Other professional organizations include:

Aerobics and Fitness Association of America
15250 Ventura Blvd., Suite 310
Sherman Oaks, CA 91403
(800) 905-0040

American Academy of Orthopaedic Surgeons
222 S. Prospect Ave. Park Ridge, IL 60068
(312) 823-7186

American Academy of Podiatric Sports Medicine
1729 Glastonberry Rd., Potomac, MD 20845
(301) 424-7440

American Academy of Physical Medicine and Rehabilitation
122 S. Michigan Ave., Suite 1300, Chicago, IL 60603
(312) 922-9366

American Academy of Physical Education
Texas Women's University
Box 24142, Denton, TX 76204
(817) 383-2415

American Academy of Podiatric Sports Medicine
P.O. Box 31331, San Francisco, CA 94131

American Aerobics Association
P.O. Box 401, Durango, CO 81302
(303) 247-4109

American Association for Leisure and Recreation
1900 Association Drive, Reston, VA 22124
(703) 476-3471

American Association of Cardiovascular and Pulmonary Rehabilitation
53 Park Place, New York, NY 10007
(212) 575-6200

American Athletic Association of the Deaf
3916 Lantern Drive, Silver Spring, MD 20902

American Athletic Trainers Association and Certification Board
660 W. Duarte Road, Arcadia, CA 91006
(818) 445-1983

American Cancer Society
777 Third Ave., New York, NY 10017
(212) 586-8700

American College of Obstetricians and Gynecologists
600 Maryland Ave. S.W., Suite 300
Washington, DC 20024
(202) 638-5577

American Council on International Sports
817 23rd St. N.W., Washington, DC 20052
(202) 676-7246

American Dietetic Association
430 N. Michigan Ave., Chicago, IL 60611
(312) 899-0040

American Federation of Women Bodybuilders
31345 Tamarack #2213, Wixom, MI 48096

American Heart Association
7320 Greenville Ave. , Dallas, TX 75231
(214) 373-6300

American Lung Association
7400 Augusta St., River Forest, IL 60305
(312) 243-2000

American Massage Therapy Association
P.O. Box 1270, Kingsport, TN 37662
(615) 245-8071

American Medical Director Association
1200 15th St. N.W., Washington, DC 20005
(202) 659-3148

American Orthopaedic Society for Sports Medicine
70 West Hubbard St., Chicago, IL 60610
(312) 644-2623

American Osteopathic Academy of Sports Medicine
P.O. Box 623, Madison, WI 53562
(608) 831-4400

American Physical Fitness Research Institute Inc.
654 N. Sepulveda Blvd., Los Angeles, CA 90049
(213) 476-6241

American Physical Therapy Association
111 N. Fairfax St., Alexandria, VA 22314
(703) 684-2782

American Public Health Association
1015 15th St. N.W., Washington, DC 20005
(202) 789-5600

American Running and Fitness Association
2420 K St., N.W., Washington, DC 20037
(202) 667-4150

American Society of Biomechanics
Orthopaedic Research, University of California
Davis, CA 95616
(916) 752-3333

Association for the Advancement of Health Education
1900 Association Drive, Reston, VA 22091
(703) 476-3450

Athletic Training Council
c/o NAGWS
1900 Association Drive, Reston, VA 22091
(703) 476-3450

Athletics Congress of the USA
200 South Capitol Ave., Suite 140
Indianapolis, IN 46225
(317) 638-9155

Centers for Disease Control
1600 Clifton Road N.E., Atlanta, GA 30333
(404) 329-2888

Club Managers Association of America
7615 Winterberry Place, P.O. Box 34482
Bethesda, MD 20817
(301) 229-3600

International College of Applied Kinesiology
P.O. Box 25276, Shawnee Mission, KS 66212
(916) 648-2828

International Council for Health, Physical Education and Recreation
1900 Association Drive, Reston, VA 22091
(703) 476-3462

International Dance-Exercise Association
2431 Morena Blvd., Suite 2-D, San Diego, CA 92110
(619) 275-2450

Manager's Network
13670 N.W. Laidlaw Road, Portland, OR 97229
(503) 645-6543

National Athletic Trainers Association
1001 East 4th St., Greenville, NC 27834
(919) 752-1725

National Board YWCA
726 Broadway, New York, NY 10003
(212) 475-5990

National Council Against Health Fraud
Loma Linda University
Evans Hall, Loma Linda, CA 92350
(714) 796-3067

National Council of Better Business Bureaus
1515 Wilson Blvd., Arlington, VA 22209
(703) 276-0100

National Dance-Exercise Instructor's Training Association
1503 Washington Ave. So., Suite 208
Minneapolis, MN 55454
(612) 340-1306

National Health Information Clearing House
1555 Wilson Blvd., Rosslyn, VA 22209

National Institute for Occupational Safety and Health
944 Chestnut Ridge Road, Morgantown, WV 26505

National Recreation and Park Association
3101 Park Center Drive, Alexandria, VA 22302
(703) 820-4940

National Safety Council
444 No. Michigan Ave., Chicago, IL 60611

National Senior Sports Association
317 Cameron St., Alexandria, VA 22314
(703) 549-6711

National Sporting Goods Association
1699 Wall St., Mt. Prospect, IL 60056
(312) 439-4000

National Strength and Conditioning Association
P.O. Box 81410, Lincoln, N.E. 68501
(402) 472-3000

National Wellness Association
South Hall, University of Wisconsin
Stevens Point, WI 54481
(715) 346-2172

Sports and Cardiovascular Nutritionists
12450 N. Washington St., Thornton, CO 80241

U.S. Gymnastics Federation
200 S. Capitol Ave., Suite 110, Indianapolis, IN 46225
(317) 237-5050

U.S. Olympic Committee
1750 E. Boulder St., Colorado Springs, CO 80909
(303) 632-5551

U.S. Squash Racquets Association
211 Ford Road, Bala-Cynwyd, PA 19004
(215) 667-4006

U.S. Weightlifting Federation
1750 E. Boulder St., Colorado Springs, CO 80909
(303) 578-4508

Wellness Councils of America (WELCOA)
1301 Harney, Omaha, NE 68102
(402) 346-8962

Women's Sports Foundation
195 Moulton St., San Francisco, CA 94123

YMCA of the USA
101 North Wacker Drive, Chicago, IL 60606
(312) 269-0520

Addresses of Equipment Suppliers

Aerobics, Inc.
30 Colfax Ave., Clifton, NJ 07013
(201) 773-4143
Pace Master treadmills.

AMF American
200 American Ave., Jefferson, IA 50129
(800) 247-3978
Recumbent bike, Rower.

Avita Health and Fitness Products, Inc.
7140 180th Ave., Redmond, WA 98052
(800) 222-9995
Avita treadmills, bikes, rowers.

Bally Fitness Products Corp.
10 Thomas Rd., Irvine, CA 92718
(800) 543-2925
Lifecycle, Liferower.

Bow-Flex of America, Inc.
1153 Triton Dr., Suite D, Foster City, CA 94404
(800) 654-3539; in Calif. (415) 572-1123
Bow-Flex multigym, which can be used for rowing or
bicycling.

Cambridge Scientific Indus.
Moose Lodge Rd., P.O. Box 265, Cambridge, MD
21613
(800) 638-9566
Skinfold Calipers.

Chatillon and Sons
83-30 Kew Gardens Road, Kew Gardens, NY 11415
scales for hydrostatic weighing.

Concept II
RR 1, Box 1100, Morrisville, VT 05661
(802) 888-7971
Concept II rower.

Continental Scale Corporation
7400 West 100th Place, Bridgeview, IL 60455
(312) 598-9100
weighing scales.

County Technology, Inc.
P.O. Box 87, Gays Mills, WI 54631
(608) 735-4718
Gulick anthropometric measuring tape.

Creative Health Products
5148 Saddle Ridge Rd., Plymouth, MI 48170
(800) 742-4478
skinfold calipers, measuring tapes, fitness measuring
equipment.

Cybex
2100 Smithtown, Ronkonkoma, NY 11779-0903
(516) 585-9000
Fitron bikes.

Excel the Exercise Co.
9935 Beverly Blvd., Pico Rivera, CA 90660
(800) 347-2258
bikes, rowers.

Excelsior Fitness Equipment Co.
615 Landwehr Rd., Northbrook, IL 60062
(312) 291-9100
Schwinn Air-Dyne bike.

Exercycle Corp.
PO Box 1349, Woonsocket, RI 02895
(401) 769-7160
treadmills, bikes.

Fitness Master, Inc.
1260 Park Rd., Chanhassen, MN 55317
(800) 328-8995
Fitness Master ski simulator.

Fitness Systems
900 Wilshire Blvd, Suite 1500, Los Angeles, CA 90017
(800) 537-5512
treadmills.

Fit-Trail by SouthWood Corp.
P.O. Box 240457, Charlotte, NC 28224
(800) 438-6302
outside fitness trail.

Fuji America
118 Bauer Dr., Oakland, NJ 07436
(800) 631-8474
bicycles.

Genesis, Inc.
7920 Silverton Ave.
San Diego, CA 92126
(619) 586-1288
treadmills.

Heart Mate
260 W. Beach Ave., Inglewood, CA 90302
(213) 677-8131
Heart Mate bikes, rowers.

Heart Rate, Inc.
3188 Airway Ave., #E, Costa Mesa, CA 92626
(714) 850-9716
Versa-Climber stair climber.

Hydra-Fitness Indus.
P.O. Box 599, Belton, TX 76513-0599
(800) 433-3111
weight lifting equipment.

J. Oglaend, Inc.
40 Radio Cir., Mt. Kisco, NY 10549
(800) 828-1186
Bodyguard, Landice treadmills, bikes, rowers.

Lafayette Instrument Co.
P.O. Box 5729, Lafayette, IN 47903
(317) 423-1505
skinfold calipers, fitness measuring equipment.

Maclevy Health and Fitness Products
1 Lefrak City Plaza, Elmhurst, NY 11368
(800) MAC-LEVY
treadmills, bikes, rowers.

Marcy Fitness Products
1900 S. Burgundy Pl., Ontario, CA 91761
(800) 34M-MARCY
treadmills, bikes, rowers.

Nautilus Equipment
PO Box Drawer 809014, Dallas, TX 75380-9014
(800) 874-8941
weight systems.

NordicTrack
141 Jonathon Blvd. N, Chaska, MN 55318
(800) 328-5888
NordicTrack ski simulator.

Pacer Industries
1121 Crowley Rd., Carrollton, TX 75006
(800) 873-9090
treadmills.

Paramount Fitness Equipment Corp
6450 E. Bandini Blvd.
Los Angeles, CA 90040
(800) 421-6242
weight training equipment, exercise bicycles and treadmills.

Performance USA
106 Regal Row, Dallas, TX 75247
(800) 292-5866
Monark, Walton bikes, rowers; Coursesetter treadmills.

Pfister Import-Export, Inc.
450 Barell Avenue, Carlstadt, NJ 07072
(201) 939-4606
stadiometers, scales, skinfold calipers.

Precor Co.
P.O. Box 3004, Bothell, WA 98041
(800) 662-0606
treadmills, bikes, rowers, ski simulator.

Pro-Tec Sports, Inc.
5181 Argosy Dr., Huntington Beach, CA 92649
(800) 423-6382
PTS-TURBO 1000 recumbent bike.

Quinton Instrument Co.
2121 Terry Ave., Seattle, WA 98121-2791
(800) 426-0347
treadmills, bicycles, testing equipment, metabolic cart.

Ross Laboratories
625 Cleveland Avenue, Columbus, OH 43216
anthropometric tapes.

Spectrum Films, Inc., Div. The Altschul Group
930 Pitner Ave., Evanston, IL 60202;
(800) 421-2363
fitness films.

StairMaster Sports/Medical Products
259 Rt. 17K, Newburgh, NY 12550
(800) 772-0089
stair climbing machines.

Trackmaster Treadmills
P.O. Box 12445, Pensacola, FL 32582
(800) 225-2655
treadmills.

Trotter Treadmills, Inc.
1073 Main St., Millis, MA 02054
(800) 227-1632
treadmills.

Tunturi, Inc.
1776 136th Pl. NE, Bellevue, WA 98005
(800) 426-0858
Tunturi treadmills, bikes, rowers.

Universal Fitness Products, Universal Gym
Equipment
PO Box 1270, Cedar Rapids, IA 52406
(800) 553-7901
Tredex treadmills, Aerobicycle, weight lifting
equipment.

Vitamaster, Inc.
PO Box 778, Lincolnton, NC 28092
(800) 632-8800
Vitamaster treadmills, bikes.

Wellsource, Inc.
15431 S.E. 82nd Dr., Suite D, P.O. Box 569
Clackamas, OR 97015
(800) 533-9355
computer software.

Weslo, Inc.
875 S. Main St., Logan, UT 84321
(801) 750-5000
treadmills, rowers.

West Bend Co.
400 Washington St., West Bend, WI 53095
(800) 438-5326
treadmills, bikes, rowers.

Source: Fitness Management 5(4), 1989. A complete source book for
products and services can be obtained by writing to:

Fitness Management
3923 West 6th Street
Los Angeles, CA 90020
(213) 385-3926

Calisthenics for Development of Flexibility and Muscular Strength and Endurance

Flexibility Exercises

The key to developing good flexibility is to hold each of the following positions just short of pain for 15 to 20 seconds. *Relax* totally, letting your muscles slowly go limp as the tension of the stretched muscle area slowly subsides. After the tension has subsided, it is a good idea to stretch just a bit farther to better develop your flexibility (hold this "developmental stretch" also for 15 to 30 seconds). Be sure that you do not stretch to the point of pain for flexibility cannot be developed while the stretched muscle is in pain.

Flexibility exercises should be conducted *following* the aerobic phase. Research has shown that stretching is safer and more effective when done with warm muscles and joints. You can stretch farther without injury more often following stimulating aerobics than before.

Do not be worried if you seem "tighter" than other people in many of the following stretches. Flexibility is an individual matter, and each person should "make the most" of what they have, realizing there are genetic differences.

Flexibility #1

Lower Back, Hamstring Stretch (with Rope)

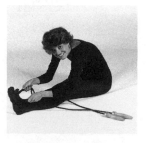

Start by sitting on the floor, one leg straight, the other relaxed off to the side (some people like the other leg bent at a 90° angle, foot against the other leg, some like it straight off to the side a bit, others slightly bent and loose). The rope should be doubled over the heel. (This exercise can also be done with both legs at one time.)

Stretch by reaching down the rope toward your foot with both hands until you feel a good tension in the back of your leg (some feel tension in the lower back also). Relax, breathe easily, letting the tension slowly subside, then reach a bit farther, holding this for 15 to 30 seconds also. Repeat with the other leg.

Benefits: This is perhaps the best stretch for the lower back and hamstrings (muscles on the back of your thigh). Your goal is to slowly work toward your foot as the weeks pass until you can at least hold on to your foot with one hand.

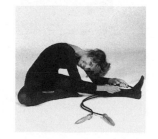

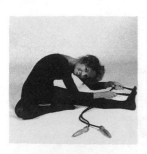
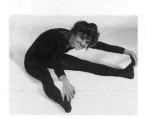

Flexibility #2

Calf Rope Stretch

Start just the same as the lower back, hamstring rope stretch, but put the rope on the ball of your foot.

Stretch by pulling your upper foot (easy does it) toward your body until you feel a good tension in the top of your calf muscle. Relax and hold this position for 15 to 30 seconds, then reach a bit farther down the rope for a second 15- to 30-second stretch. Repeat with the other leg.

Benefits: Stretches the calf muscle.

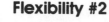

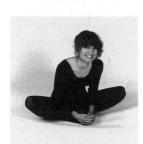

Flexibility #3

Groin Stretch

Start by sitting on the floor with the soles of your feet together, legs bent, knees up and out.

Stretch by pulling your feet with your hands to within a few inches of your crotch. Hold this position as you lean forward from the waist, keeping your chin up, and knees down as far as possible. Feel a good tension in the groin area and hold.

Benefits: Stretches the muscles in the groin area. Be careful that you do not overstretch.

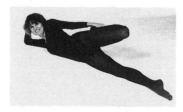

Flexibility #4

Quad Stretch

Start by lying on your right side, right hand supporting your head.

Stretch by bending your left leg, pulling the heel to your seat with the left hand grasping the ankle. Slowly move the entire left leg somewhat behind you until there is a good tension in front of the thigh, and hold. Repeat with the other leg.

Benefits: The muscles of the front of the thigh (quadriceps) are stretched in this exercise.

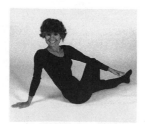

Flexibility #5

Spinal Twist

Start by sitting with your left leg straight out in front of you, your right leg bent, right foot crossed over the left knee.

Stretch by placing your left elbow on the outside of your right knee, pushing the right knee inward. At the same time, place your right hand on the ground behind you, and twist looking over your right shoulder. Keep pushing with your left elbow and twisting with your head over your right shoulder until you feel a good tension along your spine and hip, and hold for 15 to 30 seconds. Repeat on the other side.

Benefits: Stretches the muscles along the spine and side of the hips. Some people find this a hard stretch to coordinate. You may have to practice carefully with the pictures until you get used to all the important details.

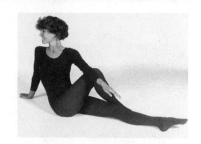

Flexibility #6

Downward Dog

Start by getting on all fours.

Stretch by humping your seat straight up, with legs straight. Walk in with your hands toward your feet until you are about 3 feet from your feet. Then try to keep your heels on the ground as you lean somewhat backward, keeping your legs straight, hands on the floor, and head down. You should feel a good tension all along your posterior leg. Hold for 15 to 30 seconds until the tension slowly subsides.

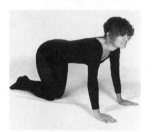

Benefits: This is an excellent stretch for the hamstrings and calves of your legs as well as the lower back. Running tends to tighten the posterior leg muscles, and this exercise helps to counter this. The key is to keep the heels on the ground, but be careful not to hold a painful position as this could injure your legs.

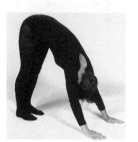

Flexibility #7

Upper Body Stretch

Start by grasping a rope or towel with your hands 2 to 4 feet apart.

Stretch by keeping your arms perfectly straight, and slowly circling them up and behind you. Move slowly, feeling the tension in the front of your chest and shoulders. If you cannot keep your arms straight, or if the pain is too intense, put your hands farther apart. Repeat several times.

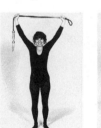
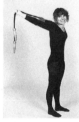

Benefits: Running tends to tighten the muscles in the front of the chest. This exercise helps to stretch those muscles, improving your posture.

Flexibility #8

Standing Side Stretch

Start by standing with your feet 3 feet apart, hands on your hips.

Stretch by raising your right hand up and over your head as you lean way over to the left side. Keep your legs straight and lean straight to the side. Hold the position, feeling the stretch along your right side and inner left thigh. Repeat with the other side.

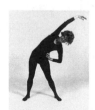
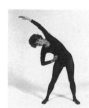

Benefits: This exercise stretches the muscles along both sides and inner thighs. If you do not feel a stretch in your thighs, put your feet farther apart.

Muscle Endurance and Strength Exercises

The following exercises localize movement to specific muscle groups, developing the strength and muscle endurance in each of these areas. Do 5 to 15 reps of each (remembering that a rep = one-one, two, three, two-one, two, three, etc.).

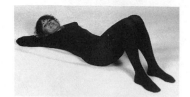

Abdomen #1

Bent Knee Sit-Ups

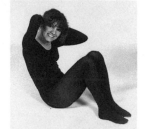

Start by lying on the ground, knees bent at a 90° angle. Most people need to tuck their feet under either another person or an object. If you are in good shape, you can put your hands behind your head. If your abdominal muscles are not in good shape, you can put your arms straight out in front of you (and even pull on your knees if you need to).

> 1—Sit up by flexing your abdominal muscles, and touch your elbows to your knees. If you need to, keep your arms out in front of you.
>
> 2—Lie back down, keeping your knees bent.
>
> 3 & 4—Repeat.

Continue for 5 to 10 counts (10 to 20 total sit-ups, or two every full repetition).
Benefits: The bent knee sit-up is an excellent exercise for toning up the abdominal muscles. The knees are bent so that the strong hip flexors will have minimal action, allowing the abdominal muscles to act.

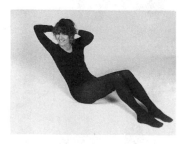

Abdomen #2

Ab-Curl Twisters

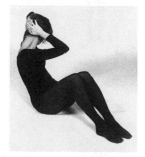

Start in the same basic position as the sit-up, except that you should have your torso two-thirds the way up toward your knees.

> 1—Keeping your body in a two-thirds sit-up position, twist to your left.
>
> 2—Next twist to your right.
>
> 3 & 4—Keep twisting back and forth, right and left, while leaning back, feeling a good tension in your abdominal area. If the movement becomes too hard, move closer to your knees.

Continue for 5 to 10 full repetitions.
Benefits: The sides of the abdomen are given a great workout as well as the middle abdominal muscles.

Abdomen #3

Straight Leg Ab-Twisters

Start by sitting with your legs together, straight out in front of you, arms crossed over your chest.

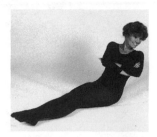

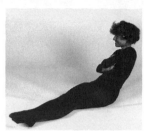

> 1—Lean back at least one-third of the way to the floor, hold this position throughout, and twist to the left, looking to the ground on the left side.
>
> 2—Next do the same to the right side.
>
> 3 & 4—Repeat, twisting left and right while leaning back, legs straight.

Continue for 5 to 10 repetitions.
> *Benefits:* This exercise also gives the sides of the abdomen a good workout while developing the muscle endurance of the middle abdominals as well.

Abdomen #4

Steam Engine

Start by lying on your back, hands behind the head. Then lift the head off the ground and touch your left elbow to your right knee. The right leg is bent, foot off the ground, while the left leg is straight, off the ground as well.

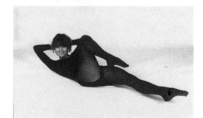

> 1—While maintaining the basic starting position, twist your torso to the left while bending the left leg and straightening the right leg. Touch in one smooth movement your right elbow to your left knee.
>
> 2—Return to the starting position, twisting your torso to the right.
>
> 3 & 4—Repeat, twisting right and left, touching the elbow on each side to the knee of the opposite bent leg. The alternating leg should be straight and off the ground.

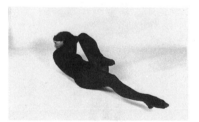

Continue for 5 to 20 repetitions.
> *Benefits*: This is probably the best abdominal exercise because the entire abdominal area is given a great workout. The abdominal muscles are best developed when the trunk is curled and twisted, as in the steam engine exercise.

Abdomen #5

Wringer

Start by lying on the ground, legs straight and together, but arms straight and out to the sides.

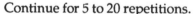

> 1—Lift your leg up and over to your outstretched right hand. Try to keep your leg straight, plus keep your left shoulder as close to the ground as possible.
>
> 2—Return your left leg to the starting position.

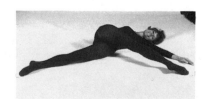

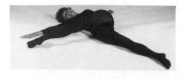

3—Repeat with your right leg, once again lifting it up and over to your left hand which is straight out perpendicular from your body.

4—Return your right leg to the starting position.

Continue for 10 to 15 full repetitions.

Benefits: This exercise will not only develop the muscular endurance of the hip flexors and abdominal muscles, but also stretch the muscles along the sides of the body.

Abdomen #6

Gut Tucks

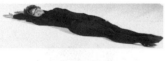

Start by sitting in a tuck position, with your legs drawn up close to your body, and hands on the floor slightly behind you for balance and support.

1—Lift your feet several inches off the ground as you straighten your legs halfway. It is important not to straighten the legs all the way because this places too great a strain on the lower back.

2—Return your legs to the tuck position, with your legs drawn up close to your body, and hands on the floor slightly behind you for balance and support.

3 & 4—Repeat, half straightening your legs and then tucking them back in, keeping the feet off the ground as you support yourself with your hands, leaning back slightly.

Continue for 5 to 10 repetitions.

Benefits: This is an excellent abdominal exercise, firming up the muscles in the lower abdominal area especially.

Abdomen #7

Half Pike Sit-Ups

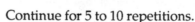
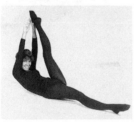

Start by lying on the ground on your back, body fully stretched out, legs together, and arms together over your head.

1—Lift your right leg up straight off the floor while lifting your arms, head, and shoulders up until you can touch your hands to your ankle or foot.

2—Return to the starting position.

3 & 4—Repeat with your left leg.

Continue for 10 repetitions.

Benefits: The hip flexors are given a good workout, while the abdominals are developed to a lesser extent because there is little abdominal curling going on.

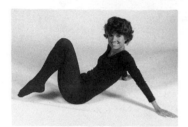
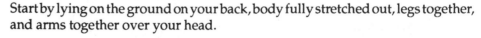

Abdomen #8

Single Leg Lifts

Start by supporting yourself on your elbows and seat, with your left leg bent, right leg straight.

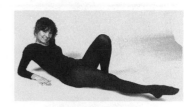

> 1—Lift your right leg, keeping it straight, up off the ground as high as you can.
>
> 2—Return your right leg to the starting position, but keep it several inches off the ground.
>
> 3 & 4—Repeat for 5 to 10 repetitions, then do the same with your left leg.

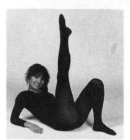

Continue lifting the straight leg up and down while keeping the other leg bent, supporting yourself with your elbows. It is important to stay in this position to prevent lower back strain from lifting the straight leg.

> *Benefits:* This exercise is especially good for the hip flexors, and secondarily for lower abdominal muscles.

Abdomen #9

Extended Leg Sit-Ups

Start by lying on your back, legs straight up in a "pike" position, with your hands joined together behind your head, elbows out.

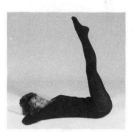

> 1—Lift your head, arms and shoulders up as high as you can off the ground, making sure to keep the elbows out.
>
> 2—Return to the starting position.
>
> 3 & 4—Repeat, curling your upper body up and then down while keeping the legs straight up off the ground.

Continue for 5 to 10 repetitions.

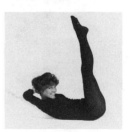

> *Benefits:* This is one of the best abdominal exercises you can do to develop a "flat tummy." The hip flexors are not involved because of the straight-leg-pike position which forces the abdominal muscles to curl your head and shoulders up.

Abdomen #10

Rowing

Start by lying on your back, arms and legs fully stretched and together.

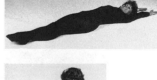

> 1—Draw your legs up to your body in a tuck position as you lift your upper body forward, reaching past your bent knees with your straight arms.
>
> 2—Return to the starting position.
>
> 3 & 4—Repeat, tucking your body into a tight ball, then returning to the starting position .

Continue for 5 to 10 repetitions.

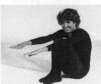

> *Benefits:* This is another excellent exercise for the abdominals and hip flexors. The tighter the ball you draw yourself into, the better.

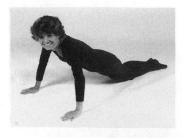

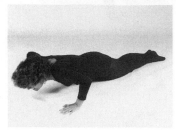

Arms-Shoulders #1

Push-Ups

Start by supporting yourself on your knees and hands. It is important that your back be straight, seat not humped up. Your shoulders should be over your hands, arms straight. You should feel that you are supporting a good part of your weight on your hands. *Note:* If you are strong enough, support yourself between your feet and hands, keeping the trunk of your body perfectly straight and rigid. This can strain the lower back, so be certain that you possess sufficient strength.

1—Lower yourself down to within a few inches off the ground, keeping your back rigid and straight, weight equally distributed between knees and hands.

2—Straighten your arms up, once again keeping the back rigid and straight. Avoid sagging or humping.

3 & 4—Repeat, lowering your body down and then pushing up, while the trunk is straight, and weight well felt on your arms and hands.

Continue for 5 to 15 repetitions (10 to 30 single push-ups).
Benefits: This exercise develops muscular strength and endurance of the muscles of the front of the chest (pectorals) and back of the upper arm (triceps). The muscles of the trunk are also developed as the body is kept in a straight and rigid position throughout the exercise.

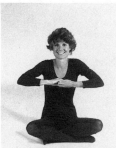

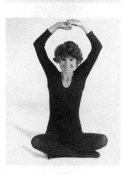

Arms-Shoulders #2

Sitting Hand Pull Raises

Start by sitting with your legs crossed, hands clasped together in the "Indian grip" (fingers hooked, hands opposite). Elbows should be out.

1—Pull hands apart, keeping them together with hooked fingers as you lift your hands and arms above your head. Keep pulling the hands hard the entire time.

2—Return the hands and arms to the starting position, still pulling hard.

3 & 4—Repeat, lifting the hands up and down as you try to pull them apart.

Continue for 5 to 10 repetitions.
Benefits: This calisthenic especially develops the muscles between the shoulder blades, the rhomboids. The muscles of the upper back and neck, the trapezius in particular, are also developed. The overall benefit is to improve back posture.

Arms-Shoulders #3

Isometric Rope Curls

Start by sitting with legs crossed. Sit on top of your jumping rope and grasp the rope with both hands, palms up, arms at a 90° angle.

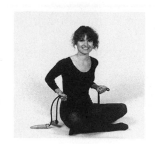

    1—Forcefully lift up, contracting your arm muscles as tightly as possible. Hold for 5 seconds and then relax. Isometric means that there is muscle contraction without movement.

Repeat 3 to 5 times, contracting as forcefully as you can each time.
    Benefits: This develops the biceps, the muscles on the front of your upper arms, plus other muscles of the forearm. This simple exercise has been scientifically proven to increase the strength of your arms.

Hips-Thighs-Lower Back #1

Bear Hugs

Start by standing in a normal position, feet together.

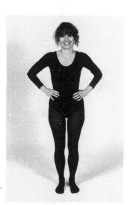

    1—Keeping your left foot in the same spot, step out straight to your right side, pointing your right foot in that direction. Reach out far enough so that your left leg remains straight, but your right leg is well bent. Wrap your arms around your right thigh as you finish stepping out to the right.

    2—Return to the starting position.

    3 & 4—Repeat with the left side. Continue stepping out to each side, hugging your thigh, and then returning back to the starting position.

Continue for 5 to 10 repetitions.
    Benefits: The hamstrings and gluteus maximus (back of upper thigh and buttock muscles) are well developed in this exercise. Be careful not to overdo the first several times, for several people experience quite a bit of soreness. This exercise also develops the quadricep muscles in the front of your thigh.

Hips-Thighs-Lower Back #2

Lateral Leg Raises

Start by lying on your right side, your head held propped up with your right hand, your left leg lying on top of your right leg.

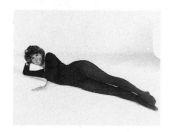

    1—Lift your left leg up as high as you can. Keep the leg straight.

    2—Return the leg to the down position.

    3 & 4—Repeat. Keep lifting the leg up, then down, concentrating on a full range of motion. Repeat with the other leg.

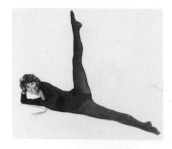

Continue for 5 to 10 repetitions.

Benefits: Develops the muscles on the side of your hip, the "abductors." As the muscles here are developed, you will lose inches from your hip measurement.

Hips-Thighs-Lower Back #3

Ballet Squats

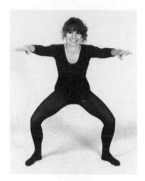

Start by standing with your feet three feet apart, toes pointing out at a 45° angle. The arms should be straight, parallel to the ground, and out to the sides or angled forward.

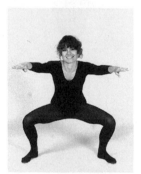

1—Squat down until the thighs are parallel to the ground.

2—Straighten your legs only halfway. Do not stand all the way up, but keep the knees well bent.

3 & 4—Repeat, moving up and down between a half squat and three-quarters squat position. The arms should be straight the entire time. The movement should be quick and almost bouncy.

Continue for 5 to 10 repetitions.

Benefits: The quadriceps, the muscles on the front of the thigh, are highly developed in this exercise. The buttock muscles also get a good workout.

Hips-Thighs-Lower Back #4

Kneeling Leg Raises

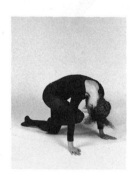

Start by kneeling down on all fours.

1—Lift your right leg slightly up and move it forward as you curl your head down, ending up with one-half of your body curled up. Your right knee should be close to your head.

2—Next lift your head up high as you also straighten and lift your right leg up high, arching your back.

3 & 4—Repeat, alternating curling and arching on one side of your body and then the other.

Continue for 5 to 10 repetitions.

Benefits: The major benefit is to the muscles of your back, especially near the neck and hip areas. Be careful not to strain your lower back by lifting your leg too high.

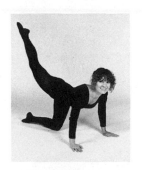

Hips-Thighs-Lower Back #5

Kneeling Leg Swings

Start by kneeling on all fours.

1—Straighten your leg and swing it out to the right side. Keep your leg straight, about 6 to 12 inches off the ground. Move your head and look right.

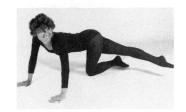

2—Next swing your leg behind you and cross over to the left side as far as you can while looking left. Your right leg should still be straight and off the ground 6 to 12 inches.

3 & 4—Repeat, swinging the leg back and forth, far to the right, and then crossing behind, while moving your head right, then left. Repeat with the other leg.

Continue for 5 to 10 repetitions.

Benefits: This is an excellent exercise for developing the muscles along the sides of the abdomen and in the lower back. In addition, the muscles along the sides of the trunk are given a good stretch each time the head and leg curl to the opposite side.

Hips-Thighs-Lower Back #6

Leg Pumps

Start by supporting yourself on your right side, right elbow, right hand, and bent right leg. Also put your left hand on the ground in front of you for support and balance. Your left leg should be straight, on top of the right.

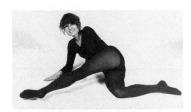

1—Forcefully swing your straight left leg forward, keeping it several inches off the ground.

2—Next swing your leg way back behind you (keep it straight off the ground several inches).

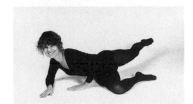

3 & 4—Repeat, swinging your leg forward and back over your bent right leg. Keep the top leg straight. Repeat with the other leg.

Continue for 5 to 10 repetitions.

Benefits: This calisthenic develops the muscles on the side of the hip, the "abductors" which will help to reduce the measurement of the hips. The muscles of the abdomen and lower back are also developed.

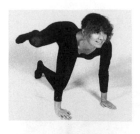

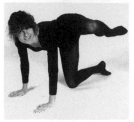

Hips-Thighs-Lower Back #7

Kneeling Bent Leg Raises

Start by supporting yourself on all fours.

>1—Lift your right leg, keeping it bent at a 90° angle, straight up to your side until it is parallel to the ground. Look at your leg with your head turned to the right side.
>
>2—Return to the starting position.
>
>3 & 4—Repeat, raising the bent leg up while looking right, and then returning to the starting position. Do the same on the other side.

Continue for 5 repetitions on each leg.
>*Benefits:* The muscles on the sides of the hips, the "abductors" are developed in this exercise.

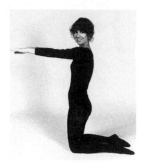

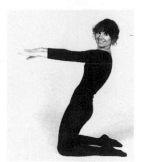

Hips-Thighs-Lower Back #8

Knee Leans

Start by kneeling, keeping your upper body straight, arms straight and reaching forward.

>1—Keeping your body rigid and straight, lean back over your heels.
>
>2—Return to the starting position.
>
>3 & 4—Repeat, leaning back and then going forward, keeping the trunk rigid. To get the full effect, it is important that you do not bend at the waist.

Continue for 5 to 10 repetitions.
>*Benefits:* This is an excellent exercise for developing the quadricep muscles, the big muscles on the front of your thighs. Be careful that you do not overdo the first several times, for these muscles can get very sore with this movement.

Hips-Thighs-Lower Back #9

Bent Over Squats

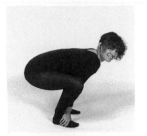

Start by squatting down, hands holding your feet (or if you are a stiff person, your ankles).

> 1—While holding your feet or ankles, straighten your legs so that your seat humps up above you. You should feel a good stretch as you straighten your legs.
>
> 2—Return to the starting position.
>
> 3 & 4—Repeat, straightening and bending the legs as you keep gripping your feet or ankles.

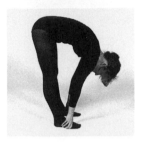

Continue for 5 to 10 repetitions.

> *Benefits:* This exercise does two things well—it develops the muscle endurance and strength of the quadricep muscles (front of the thigh), plus helps to stretch the muscles in the lower back and posterior leg. Be careful that you do not overstretch. The movement should be slow and methodical.

Major Bones, Muscles, and Arteries of the Human Body

Major Bones of Skeleton

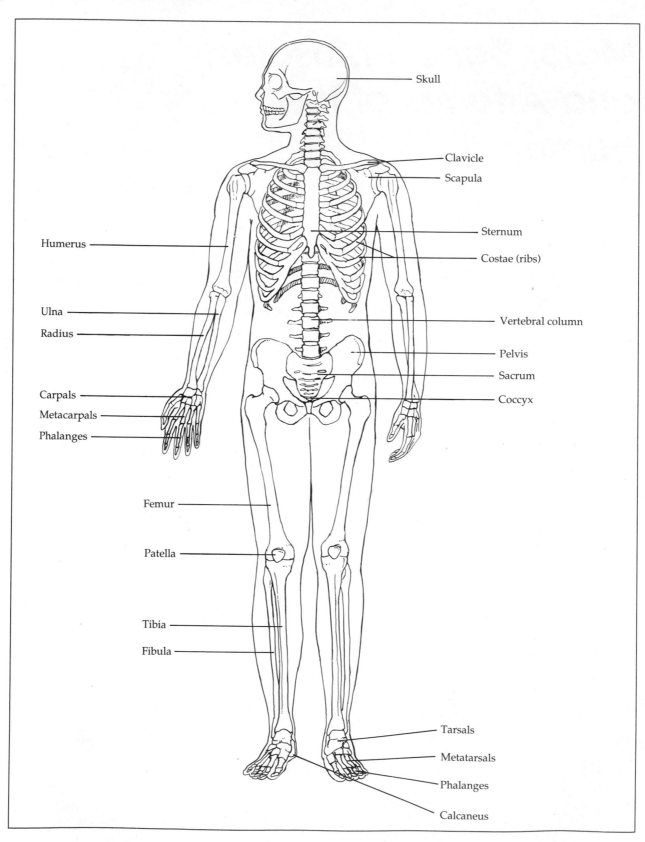

Skull

Clavicle

Scapula

Sternum

Costae (ribs)

Humerus

Ulna

Radius

Vertebral column

Pelvis

Sacrum

Carpals

Coccyx

Metacarpals

Phalanges

Femur

Patella

Tibia

Fibula

Tarsals

Metatarsals

Phalanges

Calcaneus

Major Muscles of Body *(Anterior)*

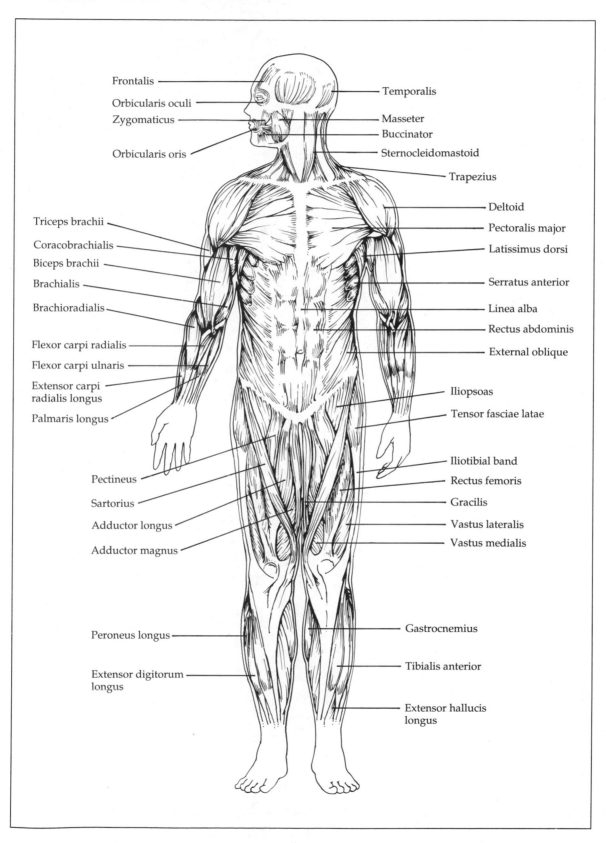

Frontalis

Orbicularis oculi

Zygomaticus

Orbicularis oris

Triceps brachii

Coracobrachialis

Biceps brachii

Brachialis

Brachioradialis

Flexor carpi radialis

Flexor carpi ulnaris

Extensor carpi
radialis longus

Palmaris longus

Pectineus

Sartorius

Adductor longus

Adductor magnus

Peroneus longus

Extensor digitorum
longus

Temporalis

Masseter

Buccinator

Sternocleidomastoid

Trapezius

Deltoid

Pectoralis major

Latissimus dorsi

Serratus anterior

Linea alba

Rectus abdominis

External oblique

Iliopsoas

Tensor fasciae latae

Iliotibial band

Rectus femoris

Gracilis

Vastus lateralis

Vastus medialis

Gastrocnemius

Tibialis anterior

Extensor hallucis
longus

Major Muscles of Body *(Posterior)*

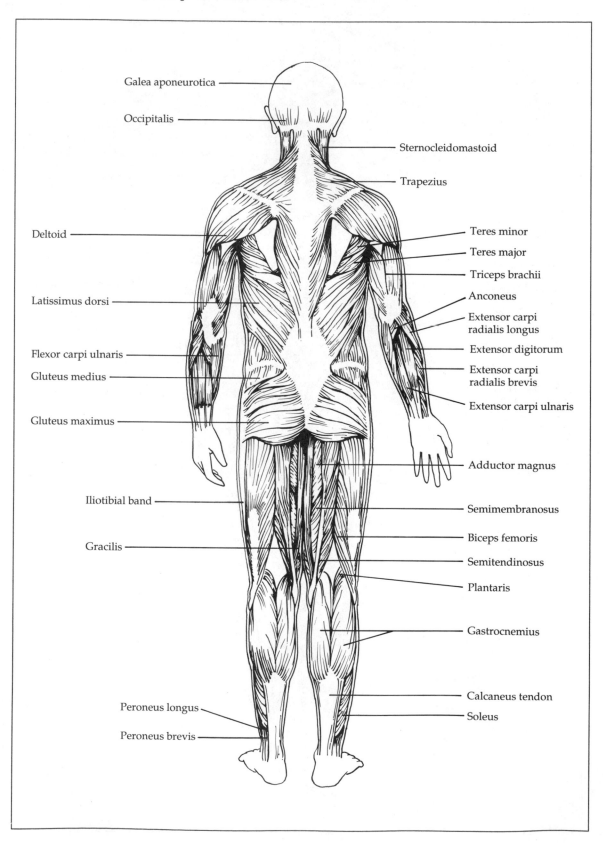

Galea aponeurotica

Occipitalis

Sternocleidomastoid

Trapezius

Deltoid

Teres minor

Teres major

Triceps brachii

Anconeus

Latissimus dorsi

Extensor carpi
radialis longus

Extensor digitorum

Flexor carpi ulnaris

Extensor carpi
radialis brevis

Gluteus medius

Extensor carpi ulnaris

Gluteus maximus

Adductor magnus

Iliotibial band

Semimembranosus

Biceps femoris

Gracilis

Semitendinosus

Plantaris

Gastrocnemius

Calcaneus tendon

Peroneus longus

Soleus

Peroneus brevis

Major Arteries of Circulatory System

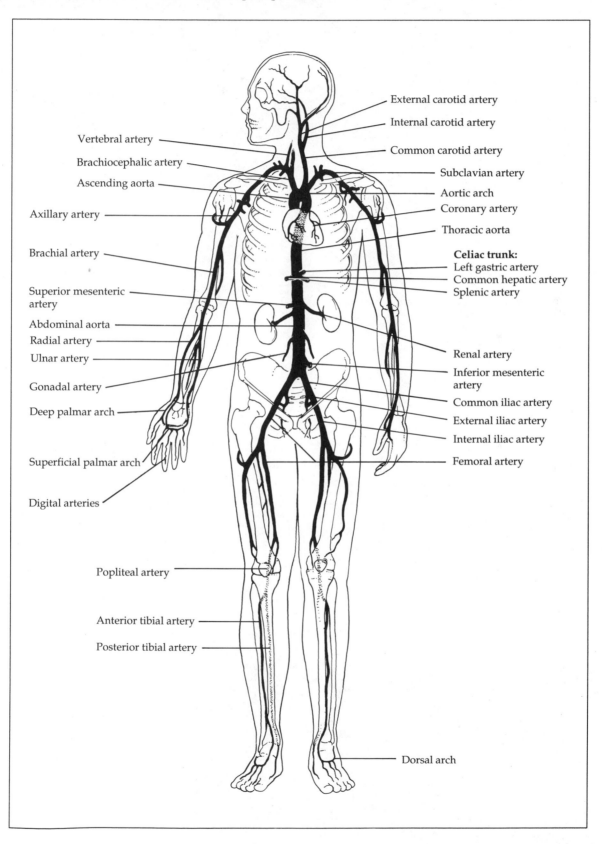

Vertebral artery

Brachiocephalic artery

Ascending aorta

Axillary artery

Brachial artery

Superior mesenteric artery

Abdominal aorta

Radial artery

Ulnar artery

Gonadal artery

Deep palmar arch

Superficial palmar arch

Digital arteries

Popliteal artery

Anterior tibial artery

Posterior tibial artery

External carotid artery

Internal carotid artery

Common carotid artery

Subclavian artery

Aortic arch

Coronary artery

Thoracic aorta

Celiac trunk:
Left gastric artery
Common hepatic artery
Splenic artery

Renal artery

Inferior mesenteric artery

Common iliac artery

External iliac artery

Internal iliac artery

Femoral artery

Dorsal arch

Glossary of Terms

Acclimatization The body's gradual adaptation to a changed environment, such as higher temperatures.

Acromegaly A chronic disease caused by excess production of growth hormone leading to elongation and enlargement of bones of the extremities and certain head bones.

Acute Sudden, short-term.

Acute muscle soreness Occurs during and immediately following the exercise. The muscular tension developed during the exercise reduces blood flow to the active muscles, causing lactic acid and potassium to build up, stimulating pain receptors.

Adenosine triphosphate (ATP) Energy released from the separation of high energy phosphate bonds from is the immediate energy source for muscular contraction

Adherence Sticking to something. Used to describe a person's continuation in an exercise program.

Adipose tissue Fat tissue.

Aerobic Using oxygen.

Aerobic activities Activities using large muscle groups at moderate intensities that permit the body to use oxygen to supply energy and to maintain a steady state for more than a few minutes.

Aerobic dance The original aerobic dance programs consisted of an eclectic combination of various dance forms including ballet, modern jazz, disco, and folk, as well as calisthenic-type exercises. More recent innovations include water aerobics (done in a swimming pool), non-impact or low-impact aerobics (one foot on the ground at all times), specific dance aerobics, and "assisted" aerobics whereby weights are worn on the wrists and/or ankles.

Aerobic power See maximal oxygen uptake.

Agility Relates to the ability to rapidly change the position of the entire body in space, with speed and accuracy.

Aging Refers to the normal yet irreversible biological changes that occur during the total years that a person lives.

Alcohol dependent Dependency on alcohol that leads to negative consequences such as arrest, accident, or impairment of health or job performance.

Alcoholism Alcoholism is a chronic, progressive, and potentially fatal disease. It is characterized by tolerance (brain adaptation to the presence of alcohol) and physical dependency (withdrawal symptoms occur when consumption of alcohol is decreased). Alcohol-related problems may include symptoms of alcohol dependence such as memory loss, inability to stop drinking until intoxicated, inability to cut down on drinking, binge drinking, and withdrawal symptoms.

Alveoli Air sacs of the lung.

Alzheimer's disease This disease progresses from short-term memory loss to a final stage requiring total care. It is a form of senile dementia, associated with atrophy of parts of the brain.

Amino acid An organic compound that makes up protein. Twenty amino acids are necessary for metabolism and growth, but only 11 are "essential" in that they must be provided from the food eaten. Some proteins contain all safe and adequate dietary intake is 0.05-0.20 mg per day. Peanuts, prunes, oils, various vegetables, whole wheat bread, and chicken are good sources of chromium.

Amenorrhea Absence of menstruation.

Anabolic The building up of a body substance.

Anabolic steroids A group of synthetic, testosterone-like hormones that promote anabolism, including muscle hypertrophy. Their use in athletics is considered unethical and carries numerous serious health risks.

Anaerobic Not using oxygen.

Anaerobic activities Activities using muscle groups at high intensities that exceed the body's capacity to use oxygen to supply energy and which create an oxygen debt by using energy produced without oxygen. See oxygen debt.

Anaerobic threshold The point at which blood lactate concentrations start to rise above resting values. The anaerobic threshold can be expressed as a percent of $\dot{V}O_{2max}$.

Androgenic Causing masculinization.

Android A type of obesity is characterized by the predominance of body fat in the upper half of the body.

Anemia Low hemoglobin concentration in the blood.

Aneurysm Localized abnormal dilatation of a blood vessel due to weakness of the wall.

Angina A gripping, choking or suffocating pain in the chest (angina pectoris) caused most often by insufficient flow of oxygen to the heart muscle during exercise or excitement.

Anorexia Lack of appetite. Anorexia nervosa is a psychological and physiological condition characterized by inability or refusal to eat, leading to severe weight loss, malnutrition, hormone imbalances and other potentially life-threatening biological changes.

Anthropometry The science dealing with the measurement (size, weight, proportions) of the human body.

Anticipatory response Prior to exercise, heart rates can rise due to anticipation of the exercise bout.

Apoprotein The protein part of the lipoprotein. They are important in activating or inhibiting certain enzymes involved in the metabolism of fats.

Aquasize Aerobic dance in the water.

Arrhythmia Any abnormal rate or rhythm of the heart beat.

Arteriosclerosis Commonly called hardening of the arteries, this includes a variety of conditions that cause the artery walls to thicken and lose elasticity.

Arteriovenous oxygen difference ($\bar{a}$ - $\bar{v}O_2$ difference) The difference between the oxygen content of arterial and venous blood.

Artery Vessel which carries blood away from the heart to the tissues of the body

Asthma A disease characterized by wheezing caused by a spasm of the bronchial tubes or by swelling of their mucous membranes.

Atherosclerosis A very common form of arteriosclerosis, in which the arteries are narrowed by deposits of cholesterol and other material in the inner walls of the artery.

Atrioventricular (AV) Node A small mass of specialized conducting tissue at the bottom of the right atrium through which the electrical impulse stimulating the heart to contract must pass to reach the ventricles.

Auscultation Process of listening for sounds within the body with the stethoscope.

Balance Relates to the maintenance of equilibrium while stationary or moving.

Ballistic movement An flexibility exercise movement in which a part of the body is sharply moved against the resistance of antagonist muscles or against the limits of a joint.

Basal metabolic rate The minimum energy required to maintain the body's life functions at rest. Usually expressed in calories per day.

Bee pollen A substance gleaned from honey that is claimed by some to have unusual nutritional qualities enhancing performance. Double blind placebo studies do not support this claim.

Behavior modification Behavior modification considers in great detail the eating behavior to be changed, events which trigger the eating, and its consequences.

Binge eating The consumption of large quantities of rich foods within short periods of time.

Blood doping An ergogenic procedure wherein an athlete's own blood or transfusion of type matched donor's blood is infused to enhance endurance performance.

Blood pressure The pressure exerted by the blood on the wall of the arteries. Measures are in millimeters of mercury (as 120/80 mm Hg).

Bodybuilding A unique activity in which competitors work to develop the mass, definition, and symmetry of their muscles, rather than the strength, skill, or endurance required for more common athletic events.

Body composition The proportions of fat, muscle and bone making up the body. Usually expressed as percent of body fat and percent of lean body mass.

Body density The specific gravity of the body, which can be tested by underwater weighing. Compares the weight of the body to the weight of the same volume of water. Result can be used to estimate the percentage of body fat.

Body mass index (BMI) Body weight and height indices for determining degree of obesity.

Bradycardia Slow heart beat of less than 60 beats per minute at rest.

Branched chain amino acids Valine, isoleucine, leucine.

BTPS The volume of air at the temperature and pressure of the body, and 100 percent saturated with water vapor.

Bundle of His A bundle of fibers of the impulse-conducting system of the heart. From its origin in the A-V node it enters the interventricular septum where it divides into two branches (bundle branches) whose fibers pass to the right and left ventricles, becoming continuous with the Purkinje fibers of the ventricles.

Caffeine A methylxanthine found in many plants. Caffeine has unpredictable effects on endurance performance, but may increase muscle utilization of free fatty acids, sparing muscle glycogen stores.

Calisthenics A system of exercise movements, without equipment, for the building of muscular strength and endurance, and flexibility. The Greeks formed the word from "kalos" (beautiful) and "sthenos" (strength).

Caloric cost The number of Calories burned to produce the energy for a task. Usually measured in Calories (kilocalories) per minute.

Calorie The Calorie used as a unit of metabolism (as in diet and energy expenditure) equals 1,000 small calories, and is often spelled with a capital C to make that distinction. It is the energy required to raise the temperature of one kilogram of water one degree Celsius. Also called a kilocalorie (kcal).

Cancer A large group of diseases characterized by uncontrolled growth and spread of abnormal cells.

Carbohydrate Chemical compound of carbon, oxygen and hydrogen, usually with the hydrogen and oxygen in the right proportions to form water. Common forms are starches, sugars, and dietary fibers.

Carbohydrate loading A dietary scheme emphasizing high amounts of carbohydrate to increase muscle glycogen stores before long endurance events.

Carbon dioxide A colorless, odorless gas that is formed in the tissues by the oxidation of carbon, and is eliminated by the lungs.

Carbon monoxide Produced mainly during combustion of fossil fuels such as coal and gasoline. Carbon monoxide is a tasteless, odorless, colorless gas.

Cardiac output The volume of blood pumped out by the heart in a given unit of time. It equals the stroke volume times the heart rate.

Cardiac rehabilitation A program to prepare cardiac patients to return to productive lives with a reduced risk of recurring health problems.

Cardiopulmonary resuscitation (CPR) A first-aid method to restore breathing and heart action through mouth-to-mouth breathing and rhythmic chest compressions. CPR instruction is offered by local American Heart Association and American Red Cross units, and is a minimum requirement for most fitness-instruction certifications.

Cardiorespiratory endurance The same as aerobic endurance. Can be defined as the ability to continue or persist in strenuous tasks involving large muscle groups for extended periods of time. It is the ability of the circulatory and respiratory systems to adjust to and recover from the effects of whole-body exercise or work.

Cardiovascular Pertaining to the heart and blood vessels.

Carotid artery The principal artery in both sides of the neck. A convenient place to detect a pulse.

Catecholamine Epinephrine and norepinephrine hormones.

Cellulite A commercially created name for lumpy fat deposits. Actually this fat behaves no differently from other fat; it is just straining against irregular bands of connective tissue.

Cerebral thrombosis Clot that forms inside the cerebral artery.

Cholesterol An alcohol steroid found in animal fats. This pearly, fatlike substance is implicated in the narrowing of the arteries in atherosclerosis. All Americans are being urged to decrease their serum cholesterol levels to less than 200 mg/dl.

Chronic Continuing over time.

Chronic diseases Lifestyle related diseases, such as heart disease, cancer, and stroke, and also accidents, which together account for 75 percent of all deaths in America.

Circuit training A series of exercises, performed one after the other, with little rest between.

Circuit weight training programs Involve 8-12 repetitions with various weight machines at 7 to 14 stations, while moving quickly from one station to the next.

Citric acid cycle See Krebs cycle.

Collateral circulation Blood circulation through small side branches that can supplement (or substitute for) the main vessel's delivery of blood to certain tissues.

Compliance Staying with a prescribed exercise program.

Concentric action Muscle action in which the muscle is shortening under its own power. This action is commonly called "positive" work, or, redundantly, "concentric contraction."

Contraindication Any condition which indicates that a particular course of action (or exercise) would be inadvisable.

Cool down A gradual reduction of the intensity of exercise to allow physiological processes to return to normal. Also called warm-down.

Continuous passive motion (CPM) Motorized machines that continuously move isolated muscle groups through their range of motion without requiring any effort by the user.

Coordination Relates to the ability to use the senses, such as sight and hearing, together with body parts in performing motor tasks smoothly and accurately.

Coronary arteries The arteries, circling the heart like a crown, that supply blood to the heart muscle. There are three major branches.

Coronary heart disease (CHD) Atherosclerosis of the coronary arteries.

Cortical bone Compact outer shaft bone.

Creatine phosphokinase (CPK) A muscle enzyme that can rise dramatically in the blood after unaccustomed exercise, indicating considerable muscle cell damage.

Cross-sectional study A study made at one point in time.

Cryokinetics A treatment that alternates cold and exercise for rehabilitation of traumatic musculoskeletal injuries in athletes.

Dehydration The condition resulting from the excessive loss of body water.

Delayed-onset muscle soreness (DOMS) Occurs from 1 to 5 days following unaccustomed or severe exercise, and involves actual damage to the muscle cell.

Detraining The process of losing the benefits of training by returning to a sedentary life.

Diastolic blood pressure The blood pressure when the heart is resting between beats.

DHEA This unapproved drug (dehydroepiandrosterone or dehydroandrosterone) is derived from human urine and other sources. Manufacturers tout DHEA as a "natural" weight-loss product, but this has not been substantiated.

Diabetes Mellitus A group of disorders that share glucose intolerance (high serum levels of glucose) in common. There are two common types: Type I, Insulin-Dependent Diabetes Mellitus (IDDM), and Type II, Non-Insulin-Dependent Diabetes Mellitus (IDDM). IDDM can occur at any age, but especially in the young, and is characterized by an abrupt onset of symptoms, and a need for insulin to sustain life. NIDDM is most common, usually occurring in people who are obese and over age 40.

Dietary fiber Complex plant cell wall materials that cannot be digested by the enzymes in the human small intestine. Examples from plants include cellulose, hemicellulose, pectin, mucilages, and lignin.

Diuretic Any agent which increases the flow of urine, ridding the body of water.

Drug dependence Criteria are: highly controlled or compulsive use, psychoactive effects, and drug-reinforced behavior.

Dry-bulb thermometer An ordinary instrument for indication temperature. Does not take into account humidity and other factors that combine to determine the heat stress experienced by the body.

Duration The time spent in a single exercise session. Duration, along with frequency and intensity, are factors called the F.I.T. which are related to improvement of cardiorespiratory endurance.

Dynamometer A device for measuring force. Common dynamometers include devices to test hand strength, and leg and back strength.

Dyspnea Difficult or labored breathing.

Eccentric action Muscle action in which the muscle resists while it is forced to lengthen. This action is commonly called "negative" work, or "eccentric contraction," but, since the muscle is lengthening, the word "contraction" is misapplied.

Economy Refers to ease of administration, the use of inexpensive equipment, the need for little time, and the simplicity of the test so that the person taking it can easily understand the purpose and results.

Ectomorphic A lean, thin, and linear body type.

Efficiency The ratio of energy consumed to the work accomplished.

EKG lead A pair of electrodes placed on the body and connected to an EKG recorder.

Elderly Individuals who reach of pass the age of 65. This group of Americans now represents the fastest growing minority in the United States.

Electrical muscle stimulators (EMS) EMS devices give a painless electrical stimulation to the muscle. Manufacturers claim that muscles are toned without exercise. Other benefits include face lifts without surgery, slimming and trimming, weight loss, bust development, spot reducing, and removal of cellulite. The Food and Drug Administration considers claims for EMS devices promoted for such purposes to be misbranded and fraudulent.

Electrolyte Scientists call minerals like sodium, chloride, and potassium "electrolytes" because in water they can conduct electrical currents. Sodium and potassium ions carry positive charges while chloride ions are negatively charged.

Electron transport system An additional metabolic pathway from which the products of Krebs cycle enter and yield ATP. This cycle requires oxygen.

Electrocardiogram (EKG, ECG) A graph of the electrical activity caused by the stimulation of the heart muscle. The millivolts of electricity are detected by electrodes on the body surface and recorded by an electrocardiograph.

Embolus A blood clot that breaks loose and travels to smaller arterial vessels where it may lodge and block the blood flow.

Endurance The capacity to continue a physical performance over a period of time.

Enzyme Complex proteins that induce and accelerate the speed of chemical reactions without being changed themselves. Enzymes are present in digestive juices, where they act on food substances, causing them to break down into simpler molecules.

Epidemiological studies Statistical study of the relationships between various factors that determine the frequency and distribution of disease in human populations.

Epinephrine A hormone primarily excreted from the adrenal medulla. This hormone is also called a catecholamine, and is involved in many important body functions, including the elevation of blood glucose levels during exercise or stress.

Ergogenic aids A physical, mechanical, nutritional, psychological, or pharmacological substance or treatment that either directly improves physiological variables associated with exercise performance or removes subjective restrains which may limit physiological capacity.

Ergometer A device that can measure work consistently and reliably. Stationary exercise cycles were the first widely available devices equipped with ergometers.

Estrogen replacement One of the major mainstays of prevention and management of osteoporosis is estrogen replacement. Women who are past menopause, and who are at high risk for osteoporosis, are often given estrogen replacements by physicians, and is highly effective.

Ethyl alcohol (ethanol) Grain alcohol. Ethyl alcohol is a social drug that is called a "sedative-hypnotic" because of its dramatic effects on the brain. Ethanol (CH_3CH_2OH) is a small water soluble molecule that is absorbed rapidly and completely from the stomach and small intestine.

Exercise Physical exertion of sufficient intensity, duration and frequency to achieve or maintain fitness, or other health or athletic, objectives.

Exercise-Induced Bronchospasm (EIB) EIB is defined as a diffuse bronchospastic response in both large and small airways following heavy exercise. Postexercise symptoms include difficulty in breathing, coughing, shortness of breath, and wheezing.

Exercise oxygen economy The oxygen cost of exercise, usually expressed as VO_2 at a certain running or exercise pace.

Exercise prescription A recommendation for a course of exercise to meet desirable individual objectives for fitness. Includes activity types; duration, intensity, and frequency of exercise.

Exercise program director Certification as exercise program director by the American College of Sports Medicine indicates the competency to design, implement and administer preventive and rehabilitative exercise programs, to educate staff in conducting tests and leading physical activity and to educate the community about such programs. Must have all the competencies of the certified fitness instructor, exercise test technologist and exercise specialist.

Exercise specialist A person certified by the American College of Sports Medicine as having the competency and skill to supervise preventive and rehabilitative exercise programs and prescribe activities for patients. Must also pass the ACSM standards for Exercise Test Technologist.

Exercise technologist A person certified by the American College of Sports Medicine as competent to administer graded exercise tests, calculate the data and implement any needed emergency procedures. Must have current CPR certification.

Expiratory reserve volume (ERV) The amount of air that can be pushed out of the lung following an expired resting tidal volume.

Extension A movement which moves the two ends of a jointed body part away from each other, as in straightening the arm.

Extensor A muscle that extends a jointed body part.

Extracellular Outside of the body cell.

Fartlek training Similar to interval training. Is a free form of training done out on trails or roads.

Fast-twitch fibers Muscle fiber type that contracts quickly and is used most in intensive, short-duration exercises, such as weightlifting or sprints. Also called Type II fibers.

Fats Fats serve as a source of energy. In food, the fat molecule is formed from one molecule of glycerol and is combined with three of fatty acids. Fats have a high caloric value yielding about 9 Calories per gram as compared with 4 Calories for carbohydrate and proteins. Saturated fats have no double bonds, are generally hard at room temperature, and have been associated with increased risk of heart disease. Monounsaturated fats and polyunsaturated fats have one and two double bonds respectively, are generally liquid at room temperature, and have been associated with decreased risk of heart disease.

Fat cell theory One of the many theories explaining obesity. Fat cell number can increase two to three times normal if an individual ingests too many Calories. And once formed, the extra fat cells cannot be removed by the body. This can happen anytime during the life-span of an individual, but appears to be particularly important during infancy when fat cells are still dividing.

Fat-free weight Lean body mass or bone, muscle, and water..

Fatigue A loss of power to continue a given level of physical performance.

Fitness See physical fitness.

Fitness instructor A person who directs classes or individuals in the performance of exercise. Certification by the American College of Sports Medicine indicates the competency to identify risk factors, conduct sub-maximal exercise tests, recommend exercise programs, lead classes and counsel with exercisers. Works with persons without known disease. CPR certification is required.

Flexibility The range of motion around a joint.

Flexion A movement which moves the two ends of a jointed body part closer to each other, as in bending the arm.

Food supplements Food supplements are substances or pills that are added to the diet. Most reputable nutritionists state that vitamin or mineral supplementation is unwarranted for people eating a balanced diet.

Forced vital capacity (FVC) The total amount of air that can be breathed into the lung on top of the residual volume.

Frame size Elbow breadth measurement for determination of small, medium, or large skeletal mass.

Frequency How often a person repeats a complete exercise session (eg. 3 times per week). Frequency, along with duration and intensity affect the cardiorespiratory response to exercise.

Functional capacity See maximal oxygen uptake.

Functional residual capacity (FRC) The combined expiratory reserve volume and residual volume.

Gastric stapling Surgery to radically reduce the volume of the stomach to less than 50 ml.

Genetic factors One of the several theories advanced to explain the high prevalence of obesity in Western countries. Some studies have demonstrated that certain people are more prone to obesity than others due to genetic factors. Such people have to be unusually careful in their dietary and exercise habits to counteract these inherited tendencies.

Gluconeogenesis The formation of glucose and glycogen from noncarbohydrate sources such as amino acids, glycerol, and lactate.

Glucose Blood sugar. The transportable form of carbohydrate, which reaches the cells.

Glucose polymers Four to six glucose units produced by partial breakdown of corn starch.

Glycogen The storage form of carbohydrate. Glycogen is used in the muscles for the production of energy.

Glucagon A hormone that is secreted by the pancreas, and helps to raise blood glucose levels by stimulating the breakdown of liver glycogen.

Glycolysis A metabolic pathway that converts glucose to lactic acid to produce energy in the form of ATP.

Glycosuria Glucose in the urine.

Golgi tendon organ Organs at the junction of muscle and tendon that send inhibitory impulses to the muscle when the muscle's contraction reaches certain levels. The purpose may be to protect against separating the tendon from bone when a contraction is too great.

Graded exercise test (GXT) A treadmill, or cycle-ergometer test with the workload gradually increased until exhaustion or a predetermined endpoint.

Grapefruit pills For several decades, grapefruit has been promoted by various people as having special fat burning properties. This myth has been spread far and wide. Grapefruit pills contain grapefruit extract, diuretics, and bulk-forming agents. Some contain phenylpropanolamine (PPA), along with herbs or other ingredients.

Growth hormone A hormone released from the pituitary that elevates blood glucose. As its name indicates, this hormone also helps in the regulation of growth.

Growth hormone releasers Various products such as Lipogene-GH, Nite Diet, Dream Away, Nite Time Diet, and HGH-3X are all sold with the claim that if they are taken before retiring, weight loss will occur overnight due to the increased release of growth hormone from the amino acids arginine and ornithine contained in the products. This is an erroneous concept.

Gynoid A form of obesity is characterized by excess body fat in the lower half of the body, especially the hips, buttocks, and thighs.

Haptoglobin A mucoprotein to which hemoglobin released into plasma is bound. It is increased in certain inflammatory conditions, and decreased during hemolysis.

HDL-C/TC The ratio of HDL-C to total cholesterol, which has been found to be highly predictive of heart disease.

Health The World Health Organization has defined health as a state of complete physical, mental, and social well-being, and not merely the absence of disease.

Health fraud Defined as the promotion, for financial gain, of fraudulent or unproven devices, treatments, services, plans or products (including, but not limited to, diets and nutritional supplements) that alter or claim to alter the human condition.

Health promotion The science and art of helping people change their lifestyle to move toward optimal health.

Health-related fitness Elements of fitness such as cardiorespiratory fitness, muscular strength and endurance, flexibility, and body composition that are related to improvement of health.

Heart attack Also called myocardial infarction. Often occurs when a clot blocks an atherosclerotic coronary blood vessel.

Heart rate Number of heart beats per minute.

Heart rate reserve The difference between the resting heart rate and the maximal heart rate.

Heat cramps Muscle twitching or painful cramping, usually following heavy exercise with profuse sweating. the legs, arms and abdominal muscles are the most often affected.

Heat exhaustion Caused by dehydration. Symptoms include a dry mouth, excessive thirst, loss of coordination, dizziness, headaches, paleness, shakiness and cool and clammy skin.

Heat stroke A life-threatening illness when the body's temperature-regulating mechanisms fail. Body temperature may rise to over 104 degrees F, skin appears red, dry and warm to the touch. The victim has chills, sometimes nausea and dizziness, and may be confused or irrational. Seizures and coma may follow unless temperature is brought down to 102 degrees within an hour.

Hegsted formula A formula to predict change in serum cholesterol from saturated fats (S) and polyunsaturated fats (P) and cholesterol in the diet. Change in serum cholesterol = (2.16 x change in S) - (1.65 x change in P) + (0.097 x change in dietary cholesterol).

Hematocrit Expressed as the percentage of total blood volume which consists of red blood cells and other solids.

Heme iron Forty percent of the iron in animal products is called heme iron. The remaining 60 percent of the iron in animal products and all the iron in vegetable products are called nonheme iron. Heme iron is more easily absorbed by the body.

Hemoconcentration Increase in the thickness of blood due to loss of plasma volume.

Hemorrhage Abnormal internal or external discharge of blood.

Hemoglobin The iron-containing pigment of the red blood cells. Its function is to carry oxygen from the lungs to the tissues. Low levels of hemoglobin is called anemia.

Hemolysis Breakdown of red blood cells, with liberation of hemoglobin, and loss through the kidneys.

Hepatic lipase (HL) An enzyme of the liver that removes HDL from circulation.

Herbalife Herbalife sells items described as "herbal-based" health, nutrition, weight-control, and skin-care products, marketing them through a multilevel program. Herbalife International has been sued for misrepresentation.

High blood pressure See hypertension.

High density lipoprotein cholesterol (HDL-C) Cholesterol is carried by the high density lipoprotein to the liver. The liver then uses the cholesterol to form bile acids which are finally excreted in the stool. Thus high levels of HDL-C have been associated with low cardiovascular disease risk.

Homeostasis State of equilibrium of the internal environment of the body.

Hormone A substance secreted from an organ or gland which is transported by the blood to another part of the body.

Human growth hormone Hormone which is liberated by the anterior pituitary and is important for regulating growth.

Hypercholesterolemia High blood cholesterol levels.

Hypertension A condition in which the blood pressure is chronically elevated above optimal levels. The diagnosis of hypertension in adults is confirmed when the average of two or more diastolic measurements on at least two separate visits is 90 mm Hg or higher. If the diastolic blood pressure is below 90 mm Hg, systolic hypertension is diagnosed when the average of multiple systolic blood pressure measurements on two or more separate visits is consistently greater than 140 mm Hg.

Hyperglycemia Excessive levels of glucose in the blood.

Hyperplastic obesity A high number of fat cells, two to three times normal.

Hyperthermia Body temperatures exceeding normal.

Hypertonic Describes a solution concentrated enough to draw water out of body cells.

Hypertriglyceridemia High blood triglyceride levels.

Hypertrophy An enlargement of a muscle by the increase in size of the cells.

Hypochromic Condition of the red blood cell in which they have a reduced hemoglobin content.

Hypoglycemia Blood sugar levels below 50 mg/dl accompanied by symptoms of dizziness, nausea, trembling, irritation, etc.

Hyponatremia Low sodium levels in the blood stream which can be caused by excessive sweating and inadequate electrolyte replacement during ultramarathons.

Hypothalamus A portion of the brain lying below the thalamus. Secretions from the hypothalamus are important in the control of important body functions, including the regulation of water balance, appetite, and body temperature.

Hypothermia Body temperature below normal. Usually due to exposure to cold temperatures, especially after exhausting ready energy supplies.

Hypotonic Describes a solution dilute enough to allow its water to be absorbed by body cells.

Hypoxia Insufficient oxygen flow to the tissues.

IDEA The International Dance-Exercise Association.

Iliac crest The upper, wide portion of the hip bone.

Impaired glucose tolerance Borderline hyperglycemia (between 115 and 140 mg/dl).

Indirect calorimetry Measurement of energy expenditure by analysis of expired air.

Infarction Death of a section of tissue from the obstruction of blood flow (ischemia) to the area.

Informed consent A procedure for obtaining a client's signed consent to a fitness center's testing and exercise program. Includes a description of the objectives and procedures, with associated benefits and risks, stated in plain language, with a consent statement and signature line in a single document.

Inspiration Breathing air into the lungs.

Inspiratory reserve volume (IRV) The amount of air that can be breathed into the lung on top of a resting inspired tidal volume.

Insulin A hormone secreted by special cells (beta cells) in the pancreas. Insulin is essential for the maintenance of blood glucose levels.

Insulin-dependent diabetes mellitus (IDDM) The form of diabetes mellitus in which the pancreas does not make or secrete insulin. The patient must use an external source of insulin to sustain life. This type of diabetes mellitus is also called Type I or juvenile-onset diabetes.

Intima The inner layer of arteries.

Intracellular Inside the cell.

Intensity The level of exertion during exercise. Intensity, along with duration and frequency, are important for improving the cardiorespiratory endurance.

Interval training An exercise session in which the intensity and duration of exercise are consciously alternated between harder and easier work. Often used to improve aerobic capacity and/or anaerobic endurance in exercisers who already have a base of endurance in training.

Iron deficiency Iron deficiency is the most common single nutritional deficiency in the world today and is characterized by low iron stores in the body. Severe iron deficiency or anemia is characterized by low blood hemoglobin.

Iron deficient erythropoiesis Stage 2 of iron deficiency, following the exhaustion of bone marrow iron stores, and characterized by a diminishing iron supply to the developing red cell. Iron-deficient erythropoiesis (formation of red blood cells) occurs and is measured by increased total iron binding capacity and reduced serum iron and percent saturation (<16 percent is abnormal).

Ischemia Inadequate blood flow to a body part, caused by constriction or obstruction of a blood vessel, leading to insufficient oxygen supply.

Isokinetic contraction A muscle contraction against a resistance that moves at a constant velocity, so that the maximum force of which the muscle is capable throughout the range of motion may be applied.

Isometric action Muscle action in which the muscle attempts to contract against an immovable object. This is sometimes called "isometric contraction," although there is not appreciable shortening of the muscle.

Isotonic contraction A muscle contraction against a constant resistance, as in lifting a weight.

Karvonen formula A method to calculate the training heart rate using a percentage of the "heart rate reserve" which is the difference between the maximum and resting heart rates.

Ketosis An elevated level of ketone bodies in the tissues. Seen in sufferers of starvation or diabetes, and a symptom brought about in dieters on very low carbohydrate diets.

Kilocalorie (kcal) A measure of the heat required to raise the temperature of one kilogram of water one degree Celsius. A large Calorie, used in diet and metabolism measures, that equals 1,000 small calories.

Kilogram (kg) A unit of weight equal to 2.204623 pounds; 1,000 grams (g).

Kilogram-meters (kgm) The amount of work required to lift one kilogram one meter.

Kilopond-meters (kpm) Equivalent to kilogram-meters, in normal gravity.

Korotkoff sounds Blood pressure sounds.

Krebs cycle Final common metabolic pathway for fats, proteins, and carbohydrates that yields additional ATP. Carbon dioxide and water are produced.

L-Carnintine An amine responsible for transporting fatty acids into the mitochondria for oxidation. Some have urged that L-carnitine supplements may increase the amount of fatty acid oxidation during exercise, sparing the glycogen. However, L-carnitine supplements have never been shown in reputable, double-blind, controlled studies to improve the athletic performance of a healthy individual.

Lactate Lactic acid.

Lactate dehydrogenase (LDH) A muscle enzyme that can leak out of ruptured muscle cells into the blood.

Lactic acid The end product of the metabolism of glucose (glycolysis) for the anaerobic production of energy.

Lactate system Exercise of 1 to 3 minutes duration depends on the lactate system or anaerobic glycolysis for ATP.

Late-onset (PEL) hypoglycemia Typically, PEL hypoglycemia happens during the night and occurs 6-15 hours after the completion of unusually strenuous exercise or play in diabetics.

Law of diminishing returns There appears to be a certain amount of training that most humans will respond quickly and fruitfully to. But every step beyond that level brings less return for the time and effort invested.

Lean body weight The weight of the body, less the weight of its fat.

Lecithin: cholesterol acyltransferase (LCAT) An enzyme from the liver that "matures" the incomplete HDL's by connecting fatty acids to the free cholesterol in the HDL particle. The incomplete HDL (HDL_3) swells into a mature sphere (HDL_3). The LCAT enzyme then grabs more cholesterol from the tissues and other circulating lipoproteins to form even bigger HDL particles (HDL_2).

Life expectancy The average number of years of life expected in a population at a specific age, usually at birth.

Life-span The maximal obtainable age by a particular member of the species, which is primarily related to one's genetic makeup.

Lipid A general term used for several different compounds which include both solid fats and liquid oils. There are three major classes of lipids: triglycerides, phospholipids, and sterols.

Lipid Research Center Program (LRCP) A study providing information on food and nutrient intake and blood lipid profiles of Americans. The LRCP is a program of the National Health, Lung, and Blood Institute (NHLBI) of the National Institutes of Health (NIH).

Lipoprotein A soluble aggregate of cholesterol, phospholipids, triglycerides, and protein. This package allows for easy transport through the blood. There are four types of lipoproteins: chylomicrons, low density lipoprotein (LDL), very low density lipoprotein (VLDL),and high density lipoprotein (HDL).

Lipoprotein lipase (LPL) An enzyme that breaks down VLDL, providing fatty acids for the muscle or adipose tissue.

Longitudinal study A study which observes the same subjects over a period of time.

Lordosis Forward pelvis tilt, often caused from weak abdominals and inflexible posterior thigh muscles allow the pelvis to tilt forward, causing curvature in the lower back.

Low Density Lipoprotein (LDL) Transports cholesterol from the liver to other body cells. LDL is often referred to as "bad" cholesterol because it may be taken up by muscle cells in arteries and it has been implicated in the development of atherosclerosis.

Low back pain (LBP) Pain in the lower back often caused from weak abdominal muscles and tight lower back and hamstring muscles.

Low-impact aerobics At least one foot is touching the floor throughout the aerobic portion.

Lumen Inside opening of artery.

Lung diffusion The rate at which gases diffuse from the lung air sacs to the blood in the pulmonary capillaries.

Mason-Likar The 12-lead exercise EKG system.

Maximal anaerobic power Anaerobic power is the ability to exercise for a short time period at high power levels, and is important for various sports where sprinting and power movements are common.

Maximal heart rate The highest heart rate of which an individual is capable. A broad rule of thumb for estimating maximal heart rate is 220 (beats per minute) minus the person's age (in years).

Maximal oxygen uptake The highest rate of oxygen consumption of which a person is capable. Usually expressed in milliliters of oxygen per kilogram of body weight per minute. Also called maximal aerobic power, maximal oxygen consumption, maximal oxygen intake.

Mean arterial pressure Equals 1/3 (systolic blood pressure - diastolic blood pressure) + diastolic blood pressure.

Mean corpuscular volume Stage 3 iron deficient anemia is characterized by a drop in hemoglobin. The bone marrow produces an increasing number of smaller and less brightly red colored red blood cells. This is measured when the mean corpuscular volume (MCV) falls below 80 fl.

Media Middle layer of muscle in artery wall.

Medical history A list of a person's previous illnesses, present conditions, symptoms, medications and health risk factors. Used to help classify an individual as apparently healthy, at risk for disease, or with known disease.

Mesomorphic An athletic, muscular body type.

Met A measure of energy output equal to the basal metabolic rate of a resting subject. Assumed to be equal to an oxygen uptake of 3.5 milliliters per kilogram of body weight per minute, or approximately 1 kilocalorie per kilogram of body weight per hour.

Microcytic A small red blood cell.

Mild obesity Defined as being 20 percent to 40 percent overweight.

Mineral Of the nearly 45 dietary nutrients known to be necessary for human life, 17 are minerals. Although mineral elements represent only a very small fraction of human body weight, they play very important roles throughout the body. They help form hard tissues such as bones and teeth, aid in normal muscle and nerve activity, act as catalysts in many enzyme systems, help control your body water levels, and are integral parts of organic compounds in the body like hemoglobin and the hormone thyroxine. Evidence is growing that certain minerals are related to prevention of disease and proper immune system function.

Minute ventilation The volume of air that is breathed into the body each minute.

Mitochondria The slender filament or rod inside of cells that are the source of energy. Enzymes important to producing energy from fat and carbohydrates are found inside the mitochondria.

Mode Type of exercise.

Moderate obesity Defined as being 40 percent to 100 percent overweight.

Monosaccharides The simplest carbohydrate containing only one molecule of sugar. Glucose, fructose, and galactose and the primary monosaccharides.

Monounsaturated fatty acids (See fats).

Motor neuron A nerve cell which conducts impulses from the central nervous system to a group of muscle fibers to produce movement.

Motor unit A motor neuron and the muscle fibers activated by it.

Muscle glycogen supercompensation The practice of exercising tapering combined with a high carbohydrate diet that stores very high levels of glycogen in the muscles before long endurance events.

Muscle spindle Organ in a muscle that senses changes in muscle length, especially stretches. Rapid stretching of the muscle results in messages being sent to the nervous system to contract the muscle, thereby limiting the stretch.

Musculoskeletal fitness Is comprised of three components: flexibility, muscular strength, and muscular endurance.

Muscular endurance Defined as the ability of the muscles to apply a submaximal force repeatedly or to sustain a muscular contraction for a certain period of time.

Myocardial infarction A common form of heart attack, in which the blockage of a coronary artery causes the death of a part of the heart muscle.

Myofilaments Within the muscle cell, actin and myosin protein fibers are called myofilaments.

Myoglobin A muscle protein molecule that contains iron. Myoglobin carries oxygen from the blood to the muscle cell.

National Health and Nutrition Examination Survey (NHANES) A periodic survey administered by the National Center for Health Statistics. These surveys provide a wealth of information about dietary patterns and practices of representative samples of the U.S. population.

Net energy expenditure Equals the Calories expended during the exercise session minus the Calories expended for the resting metabolic rate and other activities that would have occupied the individual had they not been formally exercising.

Non-insulin dependent diabetes mellitus (NIDDM) See diabetes mellitus.

Nonpharmacologic approaches Use of nondrug methods to treat hypertension, hypercholesterolemia, or other health problems.

Non-weight bearing activities Activities such as bicycling, swimming, and brisk walking, that do not overstress the musculoskeletal system.

Norms Represent the achievement level of a particular group to which the measured scores can be compared.

Nutritional assessment Involves the use of a wide variety of clinical and biochemical methods to assess the state of health as characterized by body composition, tissue function, and metabolic activity.

Obesity Excessive accumulation of body fat.

Oligomenorrhea Scanty or infrequent menstrual flow.

Omega-3-fatty acids A type of fat found in fish oils and associated with lower blood cholesterol levels, lower blood pressure, and reduced blood clotting.

One repetition maximum, 1 RM The maximum resistance with which a person can execute one repetition of an exercise movement.

Oral glucose tolerance test (OGTT) The OGTT is a 75 gram glucose solution given after an overnight fast of 10-16 hours.

Osmolarity The concentration of a solution participating in osmosis.

Osteoarthritis A noninflammatory joint disease of older person. The cartilage in the joint wears down, and there is bone growth at the edges of the joints. Results in pain and stiffness, especially after prolonged exercise.

Osteoclasts The cells that break down bone.

Osteoblasts Bone cells that build bone.

Osteoporosis Defined as an age-related disorder, characterized by decreased bone mineral content, and increased risk of fractures.

Overload Subjecting a part of the body to efforts greater than it is accustomed to, in order to elicit a training response. Increases may be in intensity or duration.

Overuse Excessive repeated exertion or shock which results in injuries such as stress fractures of bones or inflammation of muscles and tendons.

Oxygen debt The oxygen required to restore the capacity for anaerobic work after an effort has used those reserves. Measured by the extra oxygen that is consumed during the recovery from the work.

Oxygen deficit The energy supplied anaerobically while oxygen uptake has not yet reached the steady state which matches energy output. Becomes oxygen debt at end of exercise.

Oxygen uptake The amount of oxygen used up at the cellular level during exercise. Can be measured by determining the amount of oxygen exhaled as compared to the amount inhaled, or estimated by indirect means.

Ozone Produced by the photochemical reaction of sunlight on hydrocarbons and nitrogen dioxide from car exhaust.

Pangamic acid So called vitamin B-15 which is claimed to enhance performance. Reputable nutritionists do not support this claim or even the fact that a vitamin B-15 exists.

Parasympathetic The craniosacral division of the autonomic nervous system.

Parcourse An outdoor circuit system that combines calisthenics with running.

Passive smoking Breathing of air that has cigarette smoke in it.

Pellagra A disease of niacin deficiency.

Percentage of total Calories Nutritionists use this concept when representing the percentage of protein, carbohydrate, and fat Calories present in the diet. This is a useful skill to know, and is calculated from the fact that one gram carbohydrate, protein, and fat equals 4 Calories, 4 Calories, and 9 Calories respectively.

Percent saturation During iron-deficient erythropoiesis (stage 2 iron deficiency) percent saturation falls (<16 percent is abnormal).

Phenylpropanolamine (PPA) This is the active ingredient in most nonprescription weight-control products, such as Dexatrim, Appedrine, Control, Dietac, Prolamine and Adrinex. PPA is related to amphetamines and has similar side effects, such as nervousness, insomnia, headaches, nausea, tinnitus (ringing in the ears), and elevated blood pressure.

Phospholipids Substances found in all body cells. They are similar to lipids, but contain only two fatty acids and one phosphorus containing substance.

Physical activity Any form of muscular movement.

Physical activity readiness questionnaire (PAR-Q) A questionnaire for screening out high risk people prior to exercise testing that has been used very successfully in Canada.

Physical fitness A dynamic state of energy and vitality that enables one to carry out daily tasks, to engage in active leisure-time pursuits, and to meet unforeseen emergencies without undue fatigue. In addition, physically fit individuals have a decreased risk of hypokinetic diseases, and are more able to function at the peak of intellectual capacity while experiencing "joie de vivre."

Physical work capacity (PWC) An exercise test that measures the amount of work done at a given, submaximal heart rate. The work is measured in oxygen uptake, kilopond meters per minute, or other units, and can be used to estimate maximal heart rate and oxygen uptake.

Placebo An inactive substance given to satisfy a patient's demand for medicine.

Platelets The clotting material in the blood.

Polarized Charged heart cells in the resting state (negative ions inside the cell, positive outside), but when electrically stimulated, they depolarize (positive ions go inside the heart cell, negative ions go outside) and contract.

Polydipsia Excessive thirst.

Polyphagia Unsatisfied hunger.

Polyunsaturated fat Dietary fat whose molecules have more than one double bond open to receive more hydrogen. Found in safflower oil, corn oil, soybeans, sesame seeds, sunflower seeds.

Polyuria Excessive urination.

Power Work performed per unit of time. Measured by the formula: work equals force times distance divided by time. A combination of strength and speed.

Pre-event meal A meal 3 to 5 hours before an exercise event that emphasizes low fiber, high carbohydrate foods.

Premature ventricular contraction (PVC) One of the most common EKG abnormalities during the exercise test where a spot on the ventricle becomes the pacemaker, superseding the SA node.

Primary air pollutants Include carbon monoxide (CO), carbon dioxide (CO_2), sulfur dioxide (SO_2), nitrogen oxide (NO), and particulate material such as lead, graphite carbon, and fly ash.

Primary osteoporosis May occur in two types: Type I osteoporosis (post-menopausal) which is the accelerated decrease in bone mass that occurs when estrogen levels fall after menopause; and Type II osteoporosis (age-related) which is the inevitable loss of bone mass with age that occurs in both men and women.

Progressive resistance exercise Exercise in which the amount of resistance is increased to further stress the muscle after it has become accustomed to handling a lesser resistance.

Pronation Assuming a face-down position. Of the hand, turning the palm backward or downward. Of the foot, lowering the inner (medial) side of the foot so as to flatten the arch. The opposite of supination.

Proprioceptive neuromuscular facilitation (PNF) stretch Muscle stretches that use the proprioceptors (muscle spindles) to send inhibiting (relaxing) messages to the muscle that is to be stretched. Example: The contraction of an agonist muscle sends inhibiting signals that relax the antagonist muscle so that it is easier to stretch.

Protein A complex nitrogen carrying compound which occurs naturally in plants and animals and yield amino acids when broken down. The amino acids are essential for the growth and repair of living tissue. Proteins are also a source of heat and energy for the body. Protein is found widely in both animal and plant products.

Protoporphyrin A derivative of hemoglobin. Formed from heme by deletion of an atom of iron.

Prudent diet Defined in this book as the diet adhering to the 1988 *Surgeon General's Report on Nutrition and Health*

Puberty The period in life when one becomes functionally capable of reproduction.

P wave Transmission of electrical impulse through the atria.

QRS complex Impulse through the ventricles.

Quetelet index Body weight in kilograms divided by height in meters squared. This is the most widely accepted body mass index.

Racquet sports Sports like racquetball, squash, and tennis that use a racquet.

Radial pulse The pulse at the wrist.

Rating of perceived exertion (RPE) A means to quantify the subjective feeling of the intensity of an exercise. Borg scales, charts which describe a range of intensity from resting to maximal energy outputs, are used as a visual aid to exercisers in keeping their efforts in the effective training zone.

Reaction time Relates to the time elapsed between stimulation and the beginning of the reaction to it.

Recommended Dietary Allowances (RDA) The (RDA) established by the National Research Council of the National Academy of Sciences, have become the premier nutrient standard in both the U.S. and the world. The RDA are a technical standard used for nutrition policies and decision making. The RDA today are used for a wide variety of purposes ranging from development of new food products to being the standard for federal nutrition assistance programs.

Relative risk An expression of disease risk that usually compares death rates from groups varying in a certain practice.

Relative weight The body weight divided by the midpoint value of the weight range.

Relaxation therapy A treatment that involves teaching a patient to accomplish a state of both muscular and mental deactivation by the systematic use of relaxation or meditation exercises to reduce high blood pressure.

Reliability Deals with how consistently a certain element is measured by the particular test.

Residual volume The volume of air remaining in the lungs after a maximum expiration. Must be calculated in the formula for determining body composition through underwater weighing.

Respiratory exchange ratio (R) The ratio between the amount of carbon dioxide produced and the amount of oxygen consumed by the body during exercise.

Resting metabolic rate (RMR) This represents the energy expended by your body to maintain life and normal body functions, such as respiration and circulation.

R.I.C.E. Treatment of musculoskeletal pain and injury during the first 48 to 72 hours centers around rest, ice, compression, and elevation.

Risk factors Characteristics that are associated with higher risk of developing a specific health problem.

Sarcolemma The membrane of the muscle cell.

Sarcomere The smallest functional skeletal muscle subunit capable of contraction.

Satiety The feeling of fullness and satisfaction.

Saturated fat Dietary fat whose molecules are saturated with hydrogen. They are usually hard at room temperature and are readily converted into cholesterol in the body. Sources include animal products as well as hydrogenated vegetable oils.

Scurvy A disease of vitamin C deficiency.

Secondary air pollutants Formed by chemical action of the primary pollutants and the natural chemicals in the atmosphere. Examples include ozone (O_3), sulfuric acid (H_2SO_4), and nitric acid (HNO_3), peroxyacetyl nitrate, and a host of other inorganic and organic compounds.

Secondary osteoporosis May develop at any age as a consequence of hormonal, digestive, and metabolic disorders, as well as prolonged bedrest and weightlessness (space flight) that result in loss of bone mineral mass.

Senile dementia A form of organic brain syndrome, a mental disorder associated with impaired brain function in the elderly.

Serum erythropoietin A hormone that regulates red blood cell production.

Serum iron During iron-deficient erythropoiesis (stage 2 iron deficiency) serum iron levels fall.

Set A group of repetitions of an exercise movement done consecutively, without rest, until a given number, or momentary exhaustion, is reached.

Severe obesity Defined as more than 100 percent overweight.

Skeletal muscle Muscle which is connected with a bone.

Skill-related fitness Elements of fitness such as agility, balance, speed, coordination. While the elements of skill-related fitness are important for participation in various dual and team sports, they have little significance for the day-to-day tasks of Americans or their general health.

Skinfold measurements The most widely used method for determining obesity is based on the thickness of skinfolds. Calipers are used to measure the thickness of a double fold of skin at various sites.

Slow-twitch fibers Muscle fiber type that contracts slowly and is used most in moderate-intensity, endurance exercises, such as distance running. Also called Type I fibers.

Smokeless tobacco Use of smokeless tobacco takes two forms. Dipping involves placing a pinch of moist or dry powdered tobacco (snuff) between the cheek or lip and the lower gum. Chewing involves placing a golfball-sized amount of loose leaf tobacco between the cheek and lower gum where it is sucked and chewed.

Sodium This electrolyte is the major cation (positive ion) of fluids outside the body cells. Sodium and chloride ions tend to concentrate outside of body cell walls (extracellular), while potassium tends to concentrate inside of body cell walls (intracellular). This arrangement is essential in maintaining the balance of tissue fluids inside and outside of cells. Sodium, potassium, and chloride work with bicarbonate in regulating the acid-base balance of the body. Sodium has an important role in regulating normal muscle tone. The Food and Nutrition Board has established safe and adequate daily dietary intakes for sodium which is 1100-3300 mg.

Sodium bicarbonate A substance used by some athletes to enhance performance in events lasting 1-3 minutes. Sodium bicarbonate ingestion increases the pH of the body, allowing greater lactic acid to be produced and buffered.

Sodium to potassium ratio (Na:K) A ratio of the dietary sodium to potassium intake which may be important as an indicator of hypertension risk.

Specificity The principle that the body adapts very specifically to the training stimuli it is required to deal with. The body will perform best at the specific speed, type of contraction, muscle-group usage and energy-source usage it has been accustomed to in training.

Speed Relates to the ability to perform a movement within a short period of time.

Sphygmomanometer Consists of an inflatable, compression bag enclosed in an unyielding covering called the cuff, plus an inflating bulb, a manometer from which the pressure is read, and a controlled exhaust to deflate the system during measurement of blood pressure.

Spirulina This is a dark green powder or pill derived from algae that has been promoted as a weight-loss product.

Spot reducing An effort to reduce fat at one location on the body by concentrating exercise, manipulation, wraps, etc. on that location. Research indicates that any fat loss is generalized over the body, however.

Stadiometer A vertical ruler with a horizontal headboard that can be brought into contact with the most superior or highest point on the head.

Starch A polysaccharide made up of glucose monosaccharides.

Starch blockers: This enzyme inhibitor is supposed to block the digestion and absorption of ingested carbohydrate. Several studies have now shown these not only to be ineffective, but also a possible risk to health.

Step-care therapy An approach with lifestyle techniques and various drugs to treat hypertension.

Sterols are a type of lipid such as cholesterol, estrogen, testosterone, and vitamin D.

Stethoscope Made up of rubber tubing attached to a device that amplifies the sounds of blood passing through the blood vessels during measurement of blood pressure.

Strength The amount of muscular force that can be exerted.

Stress The general physical and psychological response of an individual to any real or perceived adverse stimulus, internal or external, that tends to disturb the individual's homeostasis.

Stretching Lengthening a muscle to its maximum extension; moving a joint to the limits of its extension.

Stroke A form of cardiovascular disease that affects the blood vessels that supply oxygen and nutrients to the brain.

Stroke volume The volume of blood pumped out of the heart (by the ventricles) in one contraction.

ST segment depression An indication of atherosclerotic blockage in the coronary arteries.

Sugars Defined as monosaccharides (glucose, fructose, galactose) and disaccharides (lactose, mannose, sucrose).

Supermarket diets A type of diet which includes such foods as chocolate chip cookies, salami, cheese, marshmallows, milk chocolate, peanut butter, and sweetened whole milk used to produce obesity in rats.

Supplementation Use of vitamin or mineral pills to supplement the regular diet.

Systolic blood pressure The pressure of the blood upon the walls of the blood vessels when the heart is contracting. A normal systolic blood pressure ranges between 90 and 139 mm Hg. When the systolic blood pressure is measured on more than one occasion to be more than 140 mm Hg, high blood pressure is diagnosed.

Submaximal Less than maximum. Submaximal exercise requires less than one's maximum oxygen uptake, heart rate or anaerobic power. Usually refers to intensity of the exercise, but may be used to refer to duration.

Supination Assuming a horizontal position facing upward. In the case of the hand, it also means turning the palm to face forward. The opposite of pronation.

Systolic blood pressure Blood pressure during the contraction of the heart muscle.

Tachycardia Excessively rapid heart rate. Usually describes a pulse of more than 100 beats per minute at rest.

Target heart rate (THR) The heart rate at which one aims to exercise. For example, the American College of Sports Medicine recommends that healthy adults exercise at a THR of 60 to 90 percent of maximum heart rate reserve. Also called training heart rate.

Testosterone An androgen hormone produced by the testicles and adrenal cortex. It accelerates growth in tissues.

Thermic effect of food (TEF) The increase in energy expenditure above the resting metabolic rate that can be measured for several hours after a meal.

Thrombosis Formation or existence of a blood clot within the blood vessel system.

Tidal volume The amount of air per breath.

Total iron binding capacity (TIBC) During iron-deficient erythropoiesis (inadequate formation of red blood cells), total iron binding capacity is increased.

Total lung capacity (TLC) Represents the total amount of air in the lung.

Total peripheral resistance The sum of all the forces that oppose blood flow in the body's blood vessel system. During exercise, total peripheral resistance decreases because the blood vessels in the active muscles increase in size.

Trabecular bone Spongy, internal end bone.

Triglyceride A type of fat made of glycerol with three fatty acids. Most animal and vegetable fats are triglycerides.

T wave Electrical recovery or repolarization of the ventricles.

Underwater weighing The most widely used laboratory procedure for measuring body density. In this procedure, whole body density is calculated from body volume according to Archimedes' principle of displacement which states that an object submerged in water is buoyed up by the weight of the water displaced.

US-RDA These are a set of standards developed by the Food and Drug Administration (FDA) for use in regulating nutrition labeling. Although these standards were taken from the RDA, they are based on very few categories, and only 19 vitamins and minerals were chosen.

Validity Refers to the degree to which the test measures what it was designed to measure.

Valsalva maneuver A strong exhaling effort against a closed glottis, which builds pressure in the chest cavity that interferes with the return of blood to the heart. May deprive the brain of blood and cause fainting.

Vasoconstriction The narrowing of a blood vessel to decrease blood flow to a body part.

Vasodilation The enlarging of a blood vessel to increase blood flow to a body part.

Very low calorie diets (VLCD) Also called the protein-sparing modified fast. The VLCD provides 400-700 Calories per day for people trying to lose weight. Protein is emphasized to help avoid loss of muscle tissue. Patients can use either special formula beverages or natural foods such as fish, fowl, or lean meat (along with mineral and vitamin supplements).

Very low density lipoproteins (VLDL) Transports triglycerides to body tissues.

Vital capacity The amount of air that can be expired after a maximum inspiration; the maximum total volume of the lungs, less the residual volume.

Vitamin Vitamins are nutrients which are essential for life itself. The body uses these organic substances to accomplish much of its work. Vitamins do not supply energy, but they do help release energy from carbohydrates, fats, and proteins. They also play a vital role in chemical reactions throughout the body. There are two types of vitamins—fat-soluble (A,D,E,K) and water-soluble (eight B-complex and vitamin C). Thirteen vitamins have been discovered, the most recent in 1948.

$\dot{V}O_{2max}$ Maximum volume of oxygen consumed per unit of time. In scientific notation, a dot appears over the V to indicate "per unit of time."

Waist to hip circumference (WHR) Ratio of waist and hip circumferences. A relatively high WHR predicts increased complications from obesity.

Warm-up A gradual increase in the intensity of exercise to allow physiological processes to prepare for greater energy outputs. Changes include: rise in body temperature, cardiorespiratory changes, increase in muscle elasticity and contractility, etc.

Watt A measure of power equal to 6.12 kilogram-meters per minute.

Weight reducing clothing Special weight-reducing clothing, including heated belts, rubberized suits, and oilskins rely chiefly on dehydration and localized pressure.

Wet-bulb thermometer A thermometer whose bulb is enclosed in a wet wick, so that evaporation from the wick will lower the temperature reading more in dry air than in humid air. The comparison of wet-and dry-bulb readings can be used to calculate relative humidity.

Wet-globe temperature A temperature reading that approximates the heat stress which the environment will impose on the human body. Takes into account not only temperature and humidity, but radiant heat from the sun and cooling breezes that would speed evaporation and convection of heat away from the body. Reading is provided by an instrument that encloses a thermometer in a wetted, black copper sphere. Cf. dry-bulb thermometer, wet-bulb thermometer.

White blood cells Special immune system cells that circulate in the blood. These include monocytes, neutrophils, basophils, eosinophils, and lymphocytes.

Index

A

Abdominal fat, 131–133, 320, 342
Abdominal muscle strength
  curl-up test for, 152
  exercises for, 528–531
  low back pain and, 142
  sit-up test for, 145, 151–152, 512t
Absenteeism
  cigarette smoking and, 279
  exercise and, 14–15
Acclimatization process, 235–236, 545
Acute effects of aerobic exercise, 157–166
  arterial-venous O_2 difference, increased, 159–160
  blood flow, increased to muscles, 163
  blood pressure, diastolic, unchanged, 161
  blood pressure, systolic, increased, 161
  cardiac output, increased, 159t, 165
  heart rate, increased, 158
  factors influencing, 157–158
  oxygen consumption, increased, 160–161
  stroke volume, increased, 158–159
  ventilation changes, 163, 164
Adenosine triphosphate (See ATP)
Administration
  of exercise programs, 212–214
  facility planning, 213
Aerobic, 545 (Also see Aerobic exercise)
  Ken Cooper and, 7, 32, 423
Aerobic capacity (See Aerobic power, maximal)
Aerobic capacity, tests of, 64, 70–96
  bicycle tests, 78–83, 85–87
  field tests, 70–71
  field test norms for children, 472t, 479t, 484t, 486t–489t, 483t, 495t–499t
  field test results for adults, 501t
  maximal laboratory tests, 83–87, 88–96
  step tests, 71–77
  submaximal laboratory tests, 71–83
  treadmill tests, 83–85, 503t
Aerobic dance, 197, 427–428, 545
  low impact aerobics, 197, 427–428
  musculoskeletal injuries and, 197, 427–428
Aerobic exercise
  appetite and, 338–340
  benefits of, 440t–441t
  cardiorespiratory endurance and, 32

duration of, 194–195
diabetic control and, 412–414
emphasis on, recently, 183, 184
F.I.T. frequency of, 188
fuel used as energy during, 230
goals for participation, 4,11
intensity of, 188, 194
mental stress and, 392–393
mode of, 195–199
mood and, 389–391, 393–394
precautions for obese
  progression of, 199
Resting Metabolic Rate and, 228
risks of, 440t–441t
self-concept and, 394
thermic effect of food and
  training methods, 199
weight loss and, 336–342
Aerobic power, maximal
  age, increasing and, effect of
    exercise on, 367–368
  aging and, 173, 363–368, 369
  anaerobic threshold and, 165–166
  average running speed and,
    predicted from, 71t
  Bruce treadmill equation for
    predicting, 84–85, 503t
  bicycle tests and, determination of,
    85, 87, 89–90
  definition of $\dot{V}O_{2max}$, 63–64, 160
  detraining and, 175
  duration of exercise session, 195
  effort expended and, 73
  estimation of, 71t–72t, 73, 76, 84–85,
    501t
  genetic component of, 173
  health benefits or, 183, 184, 195
  hemoglobin and, 242
  measurement of by tests, 65, 70–73,
    76, 84–85, 87, 89–90
  performance and, 176–Tn
  predicted, 73, 76, 84–85, 87
  training and, 166, 168–170, 340
  $\dot{V}O_2$, peak and, 190
  $\dot{V}O_2$ (steady state) and, estimated
    from, 85–87
  $\dot{V}O_2$ max norms, adult, 504t
  walking and, 197
  weight training and, 171
Agility, definition of, 30, 545
Aging, 359–375
  Alzheimer disease and, 361
  aerobic capacity and, 173, 363–368,
    369
  body composition and, 173, 319,
    362, 369
  cardiorespiratory fitness and, 173,
    368